BD Chaurasia's

Human Anatomy

Sixth Edition

Regional and Applied Dissection and Clinical

Volume 2

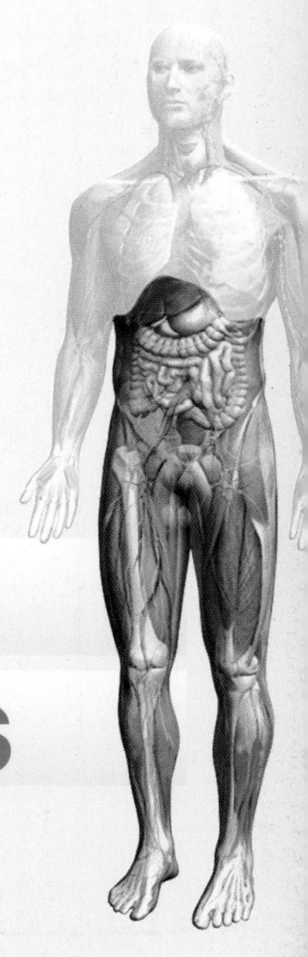

Lower Limb
Abdomen and Pelvis

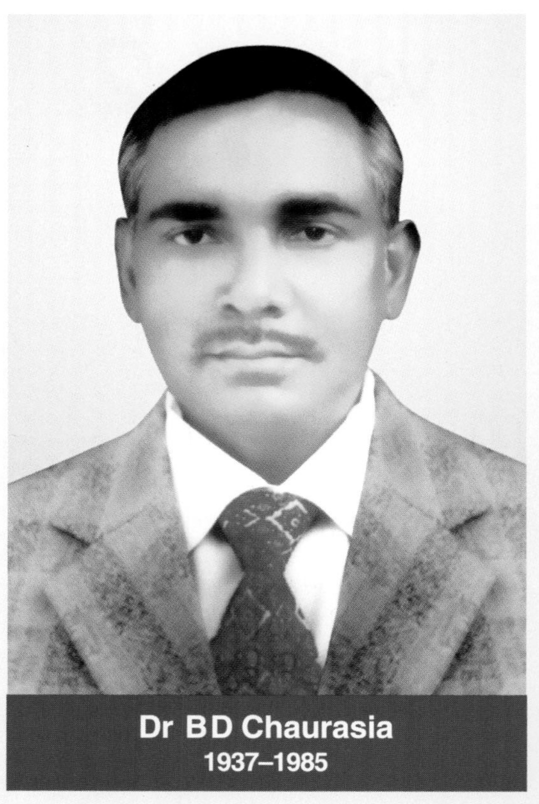

Dr BD Chaurasia (1937–1985)
was Reader in Anatomy at GR Medical College, Gwalior.
He received his MBBS in 1960, MS in 1965 and PhD in 1975.
He was elected fellow of National Academy of Medical Sciences (India) in 1982.
He was a member of the Advisory Board of the *Acta Anatomica* since 1981,
member of the editorial board of *Bionature*, and in addition
member of a number of scientific societies.
He had a large number of research papers to his credit.

BD Chaurasia's

Human Anatomy

Sixth Edition

Regional and Applied Dissection and Clinical

Volume 2

Lower Limb Abdomen and Pelvis

Chief Editor

Krishna Garg
MBBS, MS, PhD, FIMSA, FIAMS, FAMS, FASI
Ex-Professor and Head, Department of Anatomy
Lady Hardinge Medical College
New Delhi

Editors

PS Mittal MBBS, MS
Associate Professor, Department of Anatomy
Chattisgarh Institute of Medical Sciences
Bilaspur, CG

Mrudula Chandrupatla MBBS, MD
Associate Professor, Department of Anatomy
Apollo Institute of Medical Sciences
Hyderabad, AP

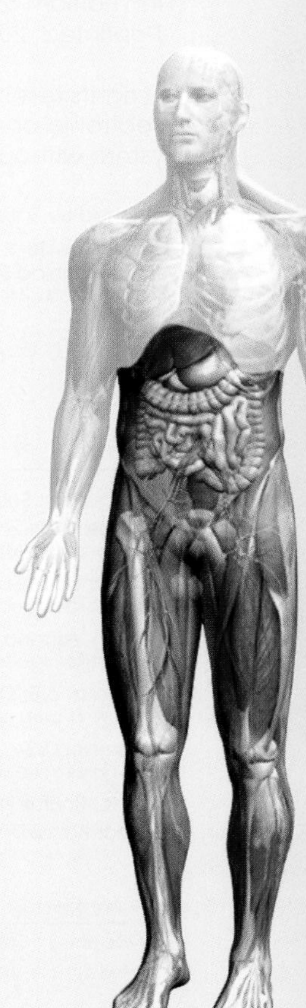

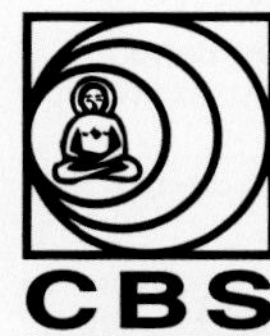

CBS Publishers & Distributors Pvt Ltd

New Delhi • Bengaluru • Chennai • Kochi • Kolkata • Mumbai • Pune
Hyderabad • Nagpur • Patna • Vijayawada

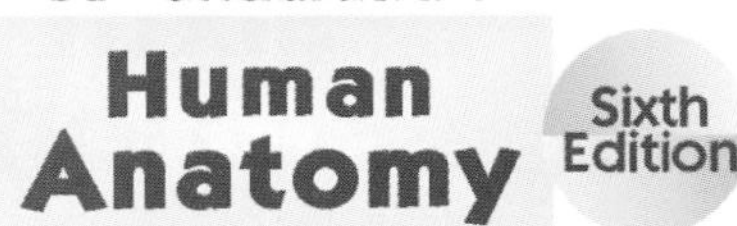

Regional and Applied
Dissection and Clinical

Volume 2

Disclaimer

Science and technology are constantly changing fields. New research and experi-ence broaden the scope of information and knowledge. The editors have tried their best in giving information available to them while preparing the material for this book. Although, all efforts have been made to ensure optimum accuracy of the material, yet it is quite possible some errors might have been left uncorrected. The publisher, the printer and the editors will not be held responsible for any inadvertent errors, omissions or inaccuracies.

Sixth Edition: 2013
Reprinted: 2014, 2015

ISBN: 978-81-239-2331-4

First Edition: 1979
Reprinted: 1980, 1981, 1982, 1983, 1984, 1985, 1986, 1987, 1988
Second Edition: 1989
Reprinted: 1990, 1991, 1992, 1993, 1994
Third Edition: 1995
Reprinted: 1996, 1997, 1998, 1999, 2000, 2001, 2002, 2003, 2004
Fourth Edition: 2004
Reprinted: 2005, 2006, 2007, 2008, 2009
Fifth Edition: 2010
Reprinted: 2011, 2012

Published by Satish Kumar Jain and produced by Varun Jain for
CBS Publishers & Distributors Pvt Ltd
4819/XI Prahlad Street, 24 Ansari Road, Daryaganj, New Delhi 110 002
Ph: 23289259, 23266861, 23266867 Fax: 011-23243014 Website: www.cbspd.com
e-mail: delhi@cbspd.com; cbspubs@airtelmail.in

Corporate Office: 204 FIE, Industrial Area, Patparganj, Delhi 110 092
Ph: 4934 4934 Fax: 4934 4935 e-mail: publishing@cbspd.com; publicity@cbspd.com

Branches

- **Bengaluru:** Seema House 2975, 17th Cross, K.R. Road, Banasankari 2nd Stage, Bengaluru 560 070, Karnataka
  Ph: +91-80-26771678/79 Fax: +91-80-26771680 e-mail: bangalore@cbspd.com
- **Chennai:** 7, Subbaraya Street, Shenoy Nagar, Chennai 600 030, Tamil Nadu
  Ph: +91-80-26771678/79 Fax: +91-80-26771680 e-mail: bangalore@cbspd.com
- **Kochi:** Ashana House, No. 39/1904, AM Thomas Road, Valanjambalam, Eranakulam 682 018, Kochi Kerala
  Ph: +91-484-4059061-65 Fax: +91-484-4059065 e-mail: kochi@cbspd.com
- **Kolkata:** 6/B, Ground Floor, Rameswar Shaw Road, Kolkata-700 014, West Bengal
  Ph: +91-33-22891126, +91-33-22891127, +91-33-22891128 e-mail: kolkata@cbspd.com
- **Mumbai:** 83-C, Dr E Moses Road, Worli, Mumbai-400018, Maharashtra
  Ph: +91-22-24902340/41 Fax: +91-22-24902342 e-mail: mumbai@cbspd.com
- **Pune:** Bhuruk Prestige, Sr. No. 52/12/2+1+3/2 Narhe, Haveli (Near Katraj-Dehu Road Bypass), Pune 411 041, Maharashtra
  Ph: +91-20-64704058, 59, 32392277 Fax: +91-20-24300160 e-mail: pune@cbspd.com

Representatives

- **Hyderabad** 0-9885175004
- **Nagpur** 0-9021734563
- **Patna** 0-9334159340
- **Vijayawada** 0-9000660880

Printed at Thomson Press (India) Ltd.

to

my teacher

Shri Uma Shankar Nagayach

— BD Chaurasia

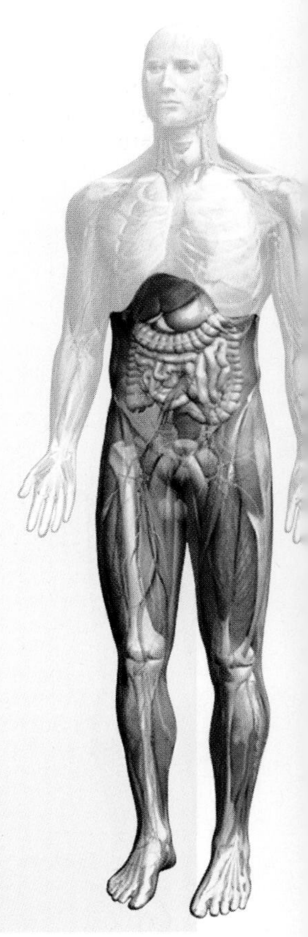

Volume **1**

UPPER LIMB and THORAX

Volume **2**

LOWER LIMB, ABDOMEN and PELVIS

Volume **3**

HEAD–NECK and BRAIN

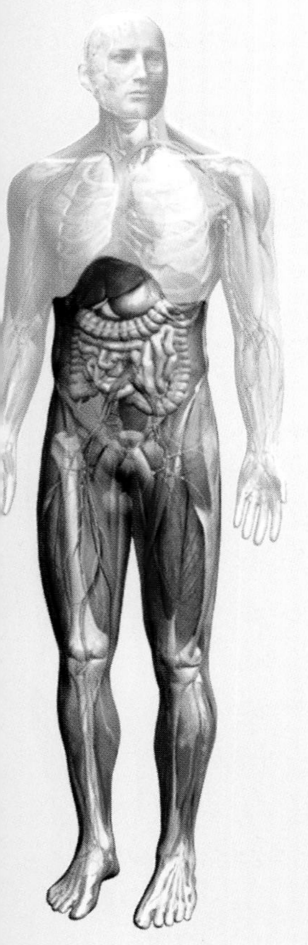

This human anatomy is not systemic but regional
Oh yes, it is theoretical as well as practical
Besides the gross features, it is chiefly clinical
Clinical too is very much diagrammatical.

Lots of tables for the muscles are provided
Even methods for testing are incorporated
Improved colour illustrations are added
So that right half of brain gets stimulated

Tables for muscles acting on joints are given
Tables for branches of nerves and arteries are given
Hope these volumes turn highly useful
Editor's hardwork under Almighty's guidance prove fruitful

Preface to the Sixth Edition

Volumes of the fifth edition of the book had illustrated clinical anatomy at the end of each chapter. An important suggestion came to subdivide this which prompted us to initiate the work on preparing the sixth edition under Almighty's guidance.

The text of each volume has been recast to match the level of international publications in the field of anatomy aimed at undergraduate medical students. To make the volumes still more student-friendly, the illustrated clinical anatomy has been put close to the relevant topic. In addition, the text has been revised and updated thoroughly. Each chapter starts with relevant words of wisdom — quotations from philosophers, leaders and diverse personalities.

All the graphics have been redrawn and prepared freshly to incorporate improvement and modification suggested by the huge following that the book commands. Illustrations have been colored systematically and thematically and many figures of embryology and histology introduced to render lucidity and understanding with ease.

Major attraction has been to take the sincere help and guidance of two young anatomists, Dr PS Mittal and Dr Mrudula Chandrupatla, now inducted in the editorial team.

The research work of well-known scientists has been recognized and elaborated. Many tables and flowcharts supplement the text for quick review. Mnemonics have been added at certain places.

To make each volume complete from practical point of view steps of dissection with line drawings are given. A few paper models based on "cut, paste and learn" pattern have been introduced as practical exercises. Relevant clinicoanatomical problems have been explained to induce clinical approach amongst the young readers. An attempt has been made to revise the topics of general anatomy through these problems.

An ultrashort summary of each chapter is provided as Facts to Remember. The knowledge acquired from the text can be tested by Multiple Choice Questions (MCQs) given at the end of each chapter. Further ten Spots of each section are given to improve the practical skills.

Layered anatomy of palm, sole and abdomen has been introduced to grasp the layered anatomy in depth.

Videos of bones and soft parts of human body, prepared at Kathmandu University School of Medical Sciences under my guidance and supervision, have been added in the CDs alongwith the Questions and Answers, and given free with each volume.

Hope and pray that we have achieved our benchmark in the field of textbooks in anatomy.

Please mail your valuable feedback to dr.krishnagarg@gmail.com.

Krishna Garg
Chief Editor

Preface to the First Edition

(Excerpts)

The necessity of having a simple, systematized and complete book on anatomy has long been felt. The urgency for such a book has become all the more acute due to the shorter time now available for teaching anatomy, and also to the falling standards of English language in the majority of our students in India. The national symposium on "Anatomy in Medical Education" held at Delhi in 1978 was a call to change the existing system of teaching the unnecessary minute details to the undergraduate students.

This attempt has been made with an object to meet the requirements of a common medical student. The text has been arranged in small classified parts to make it easier for the students to remember and recall it at will. It is adequately illustrated with simple line diagrams which can be reproduced without any difficulty, and which also help in understanding and memorizing the anatomical facts that appear to defy memory of a common student. The monotony of describing the individual muscles separately, one after the other, has been minimised by writing them out in tabular form, which makes the subject interesting for a lasting memory. The relevant radiological and surface anatomy have been treated in separate chapters. A sincere attempt has been made to deal, wherever required, the clinical applications of the subject. The entire approach is such as to attract and inspire the students for a deeper dive in the subject of anatomy.

The book has been intentionally split in three parts for convenience of handling. This also makes a provision for those who cannot afford to have the whole book at a time.

It is quite possible that there are errors of omission and commission in this mostly single-handed attempt. I would be grateful to the readers for their suggestions to improve the book from all angles.

I am very grateful to my teachers and the authors of numerous publications, whose knowledge has been freely utilised in the preparation of this book. I am equally grateful to my professor and colleagues for their encouragement and valuable help. My special thanks are due to my students who made me feel their difficulties, which was a great incentive for writing this book. I have derived maximum inspiration from Prof. Inderbir Singh (Rohtak), and learned the decency of work from Shri SC Gupta (Jiwaji University, Gwalior).

I am deeply indebted to Shri KM Singhal (National Book House, Gwalior) and Mr SK Jain (CBS Publishers & Distributors, Delhi), who have taken unusual pains to get the book printed in its present form. For giving it the desired get-up, Mr VK Jain and Raj Kamal Electric Press are gratefully acknowledged. The cover page was designed by Mr Vasant Paranjpe, the artist and photographer of our college; my sincere thanks are due to him. I acknowledge with affection the domestic assistance of Munne Miyan and the untiring company of my Rani, particularly during the odd hours of this work.

BD Chaurasia

Acknowledgements

Foremost acknowledgment is the gratefulness to God for the guidance and generosity in getting the sixth edition done. I am grateful to Dr PS Mittal and Dr Mrudula Chandrupatla for their expertise in improving the text and the diagrams. They have given their wholehearted support to this project.

Dr Hemant Juneja PhD (physiotherapy) of Amar Jyoti Institute of Physiotherapy (attached to University of Delhi) has been kind enough to add biomechanics, in addition to editing the chapters on joints of upper limb and lower limb. His skilled job is thankfully acknowledged.

Dr VG Sawant, Prof and Head, Department of Anatomy, Dr DY Patil Medical Collage, Navi Mumbai, has given enough inputs in editing these volumes. I am grateful to him.

The generosity shown by Dr R Koju, CEO of Dhulikhel Hospital and attached Kathmandu University Medical College, where the videos on osteology and soft parts were prepared, is highly recognised.

Dr DC Naik, Dr SD Joshi, Dr (Mrs) SS Joshi, Prof NA Faruqi, Prof SN Kazi, Dr Ved Prakash, Dr Mohini Kaul, Dr Indira Bahl, Dr SH Singh, Dr Rewa Choudhary, Dr Shipra Paul, Dr Anita Tuli, Dr Shashi Raheja, Dr Sneh Agarwal, Dr JM Kaul, Dr Smita Kakar, Dr Kumkum Rana, Dr Neelam Vasudeva, Dr Veena Bharihoke, Dr Jogesh Kaur, Dr Mahindra Nagar, Dr Vishram Singh, Dr Nisha Kaul, Dr Rani Kumar, Dr Shashi Wadhwa, Dr Pushpa Dhar, Dr TS Roy, Dr Satyam Khare, Dr AK Garg, Dr Archna Sharma, Dr Shilpi Jain, Dr Pooman Singh, Dr Gayatri Rath, Dr RK Suri, Dr Mangala Kohli, Dr Vandana Mehta, Dr Kamlesh Khatri, Dr Poonam Kharb, Dr Mahindra K Anand, Dr Usha Dhall, Dr Sudha Chhabra, Dr Madhur Gupta, Dr Daisy Sahni, Dr Kanchan, Dr Kiran Vasudeva, Dr Azmi Mohsin, Dr Rashmi Bhardwaj, Dr Medha Joshi and Dr Madhu Mohanty, Dr Farah Ghaus and Dr Neeraj Master had been providing necessary help.

The moral support of the family is also appreciated. Dr DP Garg and Dr Suvira Gupta have always been encouraging. Manoj, Rekha with her management skills, Surbhi (medical student), Shikhar, Meenakshi, Sanjay, Dr Manish and Dr Shilpa were very supportive.

Many students helped me, especially Ms Surbhi Ghai, Ms Resham Srivastava and Pooja Gole of Final year 2011–12 batch and Aishwarya Arya, Pooja Rani, Adhya Kumar, Diksha Tomer of 3rd year 2012–13 of Bachelor of Physiotherapy course at Pt Deen Dayal Upadhyaya Institute for Physically Handicapped, New Delhi.

The magnanimity shown by Mr SK Jain, Chairman, CBS Publishers & Distributors and Mr Varun Jain, Director, has been ideal and always forthcoming.

The unquestionable support from Mr YN Arjuna, Senior Vice President—Publishing, Editorial and Publicity, and his entire team comprising Mrs Ritu Chawla and support staff: It is only due to the untiring teamwork that the difficult task of bringing out the sixth edition has been achieved.

Any suggestions from the teachers and the readers for rectification and improvement are welcome.

Krishna Garg
Chief Editor

Thus spoke the cadaver

Handle me with little love and care
As I had missed it in my life affair
Was too poor for cremation or burial
That is why am lying in dissection hall

You dissect me, cut me, section me
But your learning anatomy should be precise
Worry not, you would not be taken to court
As I am happy to be with the bright lot

Couldn't dream of a fridge for cold water
Now my body parts are kept in refrigerator
Young students sit around me with friends
A few dissect, rest talk, about food, family and movies
How I enjoy the dissection periods
Don't you? Unless you are interrogated by a teacher

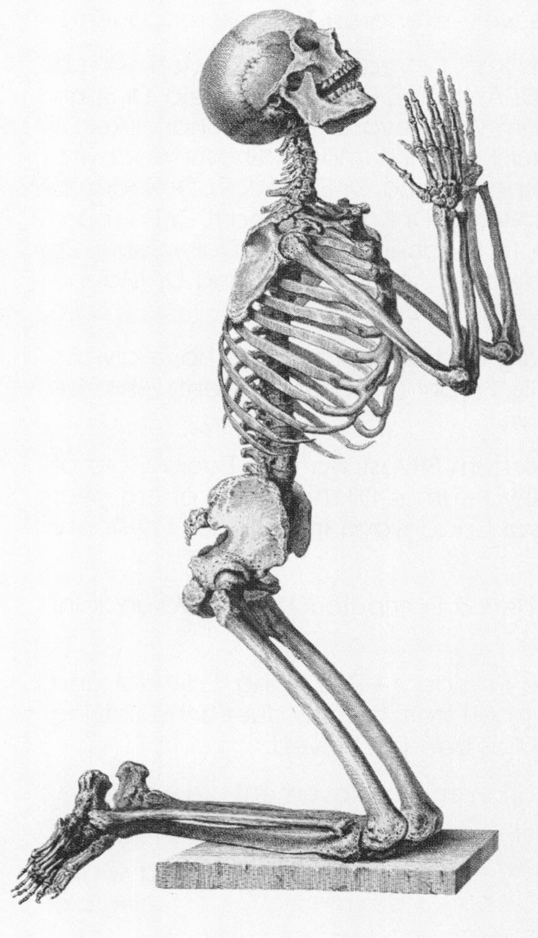

When my parts are buried post-dissection
Bones are taken out for the skeleton
Skeleton is the crown glory of the museum
Now I am being looked up by great enthusiasm

If not as skeletons as loose bones
I am in their bags and in their hostel rooms
At times, I am on their beds as well
Oh, what a promotion to heaven from hell

I won't leave you, even if you pass anatomy
Would follow you in forensic medicine and pathology
Would be with you even in clinical teaching
Medicine line is one where dead teach the living

One humble request I'd make
Be sympathetic to persons with disease
Don't panic, you'll have enough money
And I bet, you'd be singularly happy

Contents

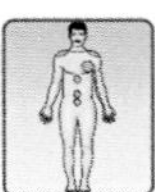

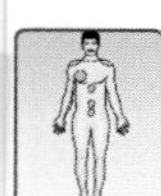

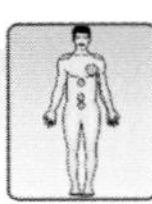

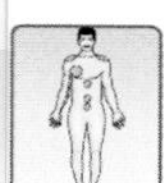

Section 2 ABDOMEN AND PELVIS

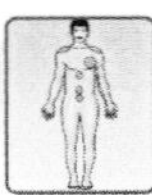

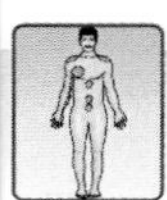

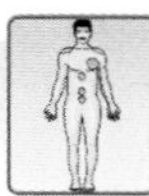

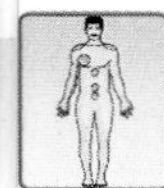

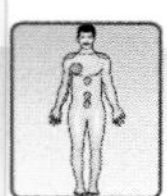

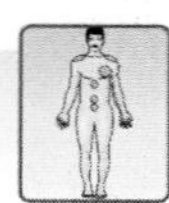

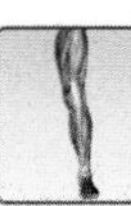

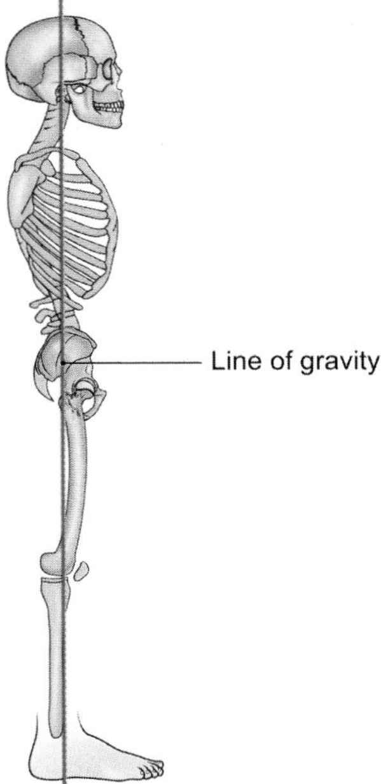

Fig. 1.3: The line of gravity

6 The foot or *pes* has an upper surface, called the *dorsal surface,* and a lower surface, called the *sole* or *plantar surface.* Sole is homologous with the palm of the hand.

The line of gravity passes through cervical and lumbar vertebrae. In the lower limbs, it passes behind the hip joint and in front of knee and ankle joints (Fig. 1.3).

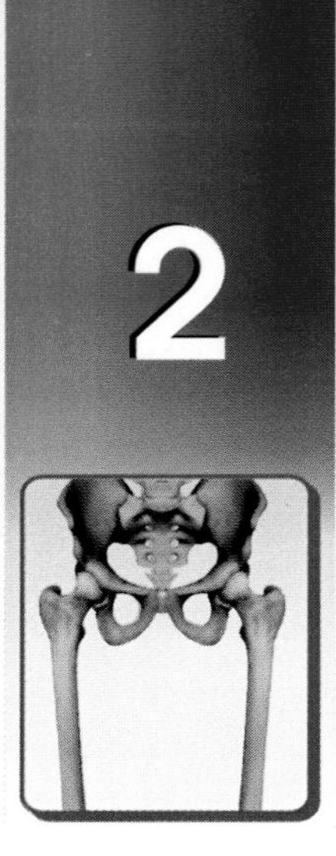

2 Bones of Lower Limb

Do instead of dream, move instead of meditate, work instead of wish
—Swami Vivekanand

INTRODUCTION

Various bones of the lower limb have been enumerated in the previous chapter. The bones are described one by one below. The description of each bone is given in two parts. The first part introduces the main features and the second part describes the muscular and ligamentous attachments.

HIP BONE

Hip/innominate bone is a large irregular bone. It is made up of three parts. These are the *ilium* (Latin *loin)* superiorly, the *pubis (*Latin *genital area)* anteroinferiorly, and the *ischium* (Greek *hip joint)* posteroinferiorly. The three parts are joined to each other at a cup-shaped hollow, called the *acetabulum (*Latin *vinegar cup)*. The pubis and ischium are separated by a large oval opening called the *obturator foramen.*

The acetabulum articulates with the head of the femur to form the *hip joint.* The pubic parts of the two hip bones meet anteriorly to form the *pubic symphysis.* The two hip bones form the *pelvic* or hip girdle. The bony pelvis is formed by the two hip bones along with the sacrum and coccyx.

Side Determination

1 The acetabulum is directed laterally.
2 The flat, expanded ilium forms the upper part of the bone, that lies above the acetabulum.
3 The obturator foramen lies below the acetabulum. It is bounded anteriorly by the thin pubis, and posteriorly by the thick and strong ischium.

Anatomical Position

1 The pubic symphysis and anterior superior iliac spine lie in the same coronal plane.
2 The pelvic surface of the body of the pubis is directed backwards and upwards.
3 The symphyseal surface of the body of the pubis lies in the median plane.

ILIUM

The ilium or *flank* forms the upper expanded plate like part of the hip bone. Its lower part forms the upper two-fifths of the acetabulum. The ilium has the following:

1 An upper end which is called the iliac crest.
2 A lower end which is smaller, and is fused with the pubis and the ischium at the acetabulum. The ilium forms the upper two-fifths of the acetabulum.
3 Three borders—anterior, posterior and medial.
4 Three surfaces—gluteal surface, iliac surface or iliac fossa, and a sacropelvic surface.

Iliac Crest

The iliac crest (Figs 2.1 to 2.3) is a broad convex ridge forming the upper end of the ilium. It can be felt in the living at the lower limit of the flank.

Curvatures: Vertically it is convex upwards, anteroposteriorly, it is concave inwards in front and concave outwards behind (Fig. 2.1).

The highest point of the iliac crest is situated a little behind the midpoint of the crest. It lies at the level of the interval between the spines of vertebrae L3 and L4.

Ends: The anterior end of the iliac crest is called the *anterior superior iliac spine* (ASIS). This is a prominent landmark that is easily felt in the living. The posterior end of the crest is called the *posterior superior iliac spine.* Its position on the surface of the body is marked by a *dimple* 5 cm lateral of the second sacral spine (S2) (*see* Fig. 5.1).

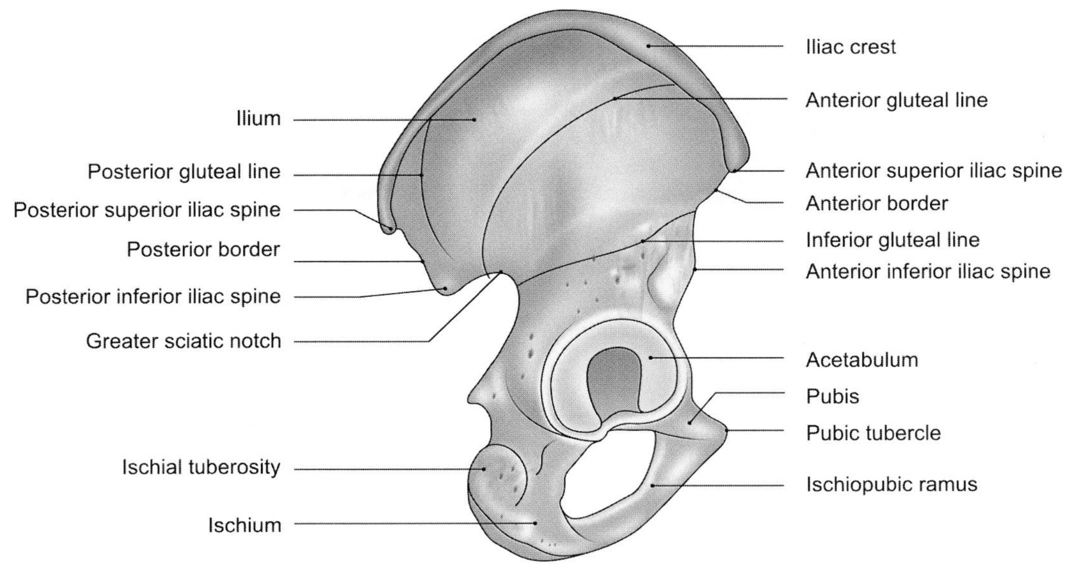

Fig. 2.1: Outer surface of right hip bone

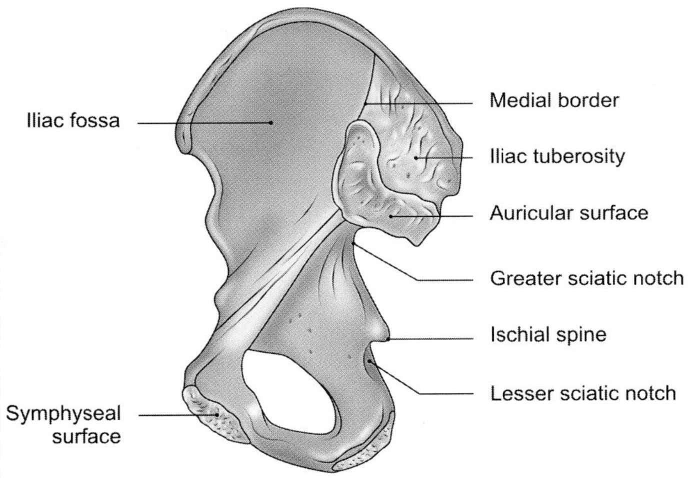

Fig. 2.2: Inner surface of right hip bone

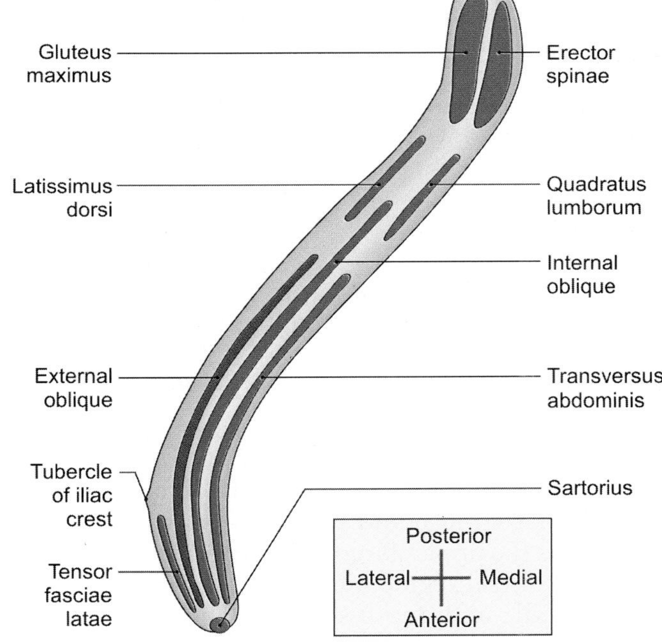

Fig. 2.3: Scheme to show the attachments on the right iliac crest (as seen from above)

Morphological divisions: Morphologically, the iliac crest is divided into a long *ventral segment* and a short *dorsal segment.*

The ventral segment forms more than the anterior two-thirds of the crest. It has an outer lip, an inner lip, and an intermediate area. The tubercle of the iliac crest is an elevation that lies on the outer lip about 5 cm behind the anterior superior iliac spine (Fig. 2.3).

The dorsal segment forms less than the posterior one-third of the crest. It has a lateral and a medial slope separated by a ridge.

Anterior Border of Ilium

Anterior border starts at the *anterior superior iliac* spine and runs downwards to the acetabulum. The upper part of the border presents a notch, while its lower part shows an elevated area called the *anterior inferior iliac spine.* The lower half of this spine is large, triangular and rough.

Posterior Border of Ilium

Posterior border extends from the *posterior superior iliac spine* to the upper end of the posterior border of

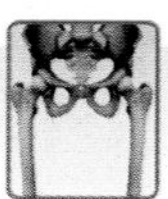

the ischium. A few centimetres below the posterior superior iliac spine it presents another prominence called the *posterior inferior iliac spine.* Still lower down the posterior border is marked by a large deep notch called the *greater sciatic notch.*

Medial Border

Medial border extends on the inner or pelvic surface of the ilium from the iliac crest to the iliopubic eminence. It separates the iliac fossa from the sacropelvic surface. Its lower rounded part forms the iliac parts of the *arcuate line* or inlet of pelvis.

Gluteal Surface

Gluteal surface is the outer surface of the ilium, which is convex in front and concave behind, like the iliac crest. It is divided into four areas by three gluteal lines (Fig. 2.1). The *posterior gluteal line,* the shortest, begins 5 cm in front of the posterior superior iliac spine, and runs downwards to end at upper part of greater sciatic notch. The *anterior gluteal line,* the longest, begins about 4 cm behind the anterior superior iliac spine, runs backwards and then downwards to end at the middle of the upper border of the greater sciatic notch. The *inferior gluteal line,* the most ill-defined, begins a little above and behind the anterior inferior spine, runs backwards and downwards to end near the apex of the greater sciatic notch.

Iliac Fossa

Iliac fossa is the large concave area on the inner surface of the ilium, situated in front of its medial border. It forms the lateral wall of the false pelvis (Fig. 2.2).

Sacropelvic Surface

Sacropelvic surface is the uneven area on the inner surface of the ilium, situated behind its medial border. It is subdivided into three parts; the iliac tuberosity, the auricular surface and the pelvic surface. The *iliac tuberosity* is the upper, large, roughened area, lying just below the dorsal segment of the iliac crest. It is raised in the middle and depressed both above and below. The *auricular surface* is articular but pitted. It lies anteroinferior to the iliac tuberosity. It articulates with the sacrum to form the sacroiliac joint. The *pelvic surface* is smooth and lies anteroinferior to the auricular surface. It forms a part of the lateral wall of the true pelvis. Along the upper border of the greater sciatic notch, this surface is marked by the *preauricular sulcus.* This sulcus is deeper in females than in males.

Attachments on the Ilium

1 The *anterior superior iliac spine* gives attachment to the lateral end of the inguinal ligament. It also gives origin to the *sartorius* muscle; the origin extends onto the upper half of the notch below the spine (Figs 2.3 and 2.4).

2 The *outer lip of the iliac crest* provides:
   a. Attachment to the *fascia lata* in its whole extent.
   b. Origin to the *tensor fasciae latae* in front of the tubercle.
   c. Insertion to the *external oblique muscle* in its anterior two-thirds.
   d. Origin to the *latissimus dorsi* just behind the highest point of the crest. The tubercle of the crest gives attachment to the *iliotibial tract* (Figs 2.3 and 3.8).

3 The *inner lip of the iliac crest* provides:
   a. Origin to the *transversus abdominis* in its anterior two-thirds (Fig. 2.3).
   b. Attachment to the *fascia transversalis* and to the *fascia iliaca* in its anterior two-thirds, deep to the attachment of the transversus abdominis.
   c. Origin to the *quadratus lumborum* in its posterior one-third (Fig. 2.3).
   d. Attachment to the *thoracolumbar fascia* around the attachment of the quadratus lumborum.

4 The *intermediate area of the iliac crest* gives origin to the *internal oblique* muscle in its anterior two-thirds (Figs 2.3 and 2.4).

5 The attachments on the *dorsal segment of the iliac crest* are as follows.
   a. The lateral slope gives origin to the *gluteus maximus* (Fig. 2.3).
   b. The medial slope gives origin to the *erector spinae.*
   c. The *interosseous* and *dorsal sacroiliac ligaments* are attached to the medial margin deep to the attachment of the *erector spinae* (Fig. 2.5).

6 The upper half of the *anterior inferior iliac spine* gives origin to the *straight head of the rectus femoris.* The rough lower part of this spine gives attachment to the *iliofemoral ligament* (Figs 2.4 and 2.14).

7 The *posterior border of the ilium* provides:
   a. Attachment to upper fibres of the *sacrotuberous ligament* above the greater sciatic notch.
   b. Origin to few fibres of the piriformis from upper margin of the greater sciatic notch.

8 The attachments on the *gluteal surface* are as follows.
   a. The area behind the posterior gluteal line gives origin to upper fibres of the *gluteus maximus* (Fig. 2.4).
   b. The *gluteus medius* arises from the area between the anterior and posterior gluteal lines (Fig. 2.4).
   c. The *gluteus minimus* arises from the area between the anterior and inferior gluteal lines (Fig. 2.4).

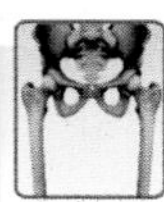

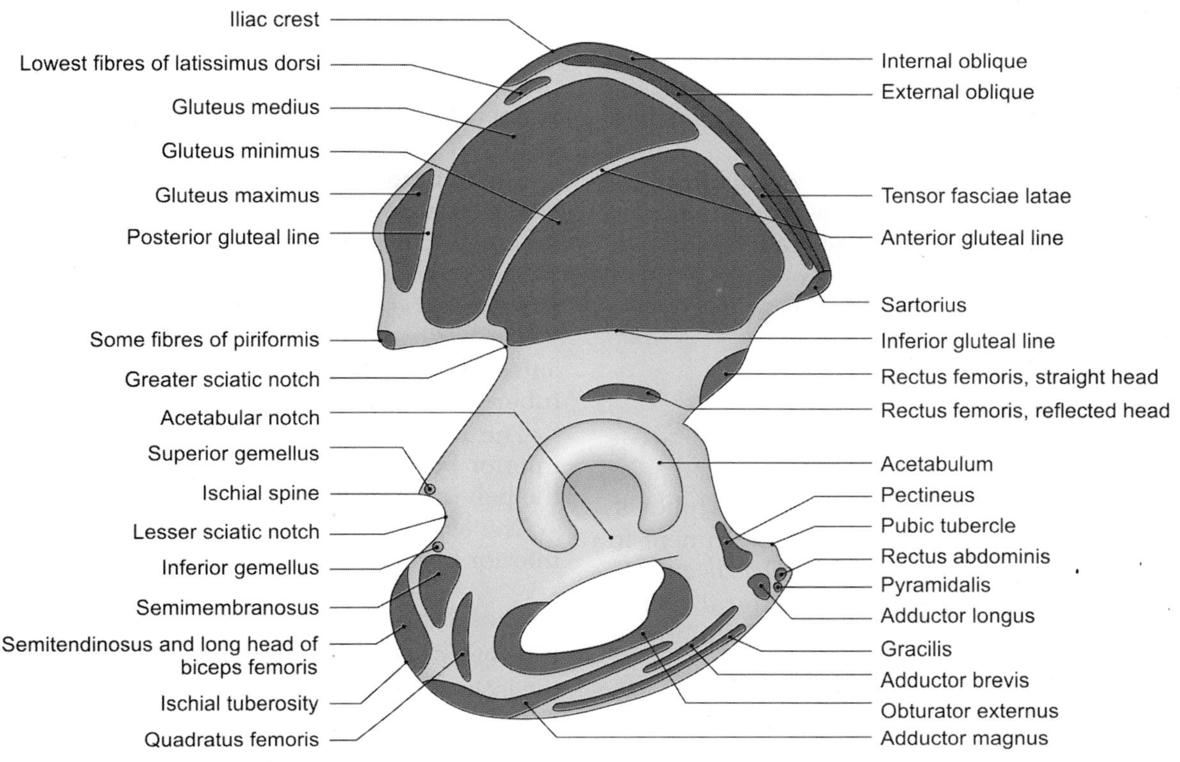

Fig. 2.4: Attachments on the outer surface of the right hip bone

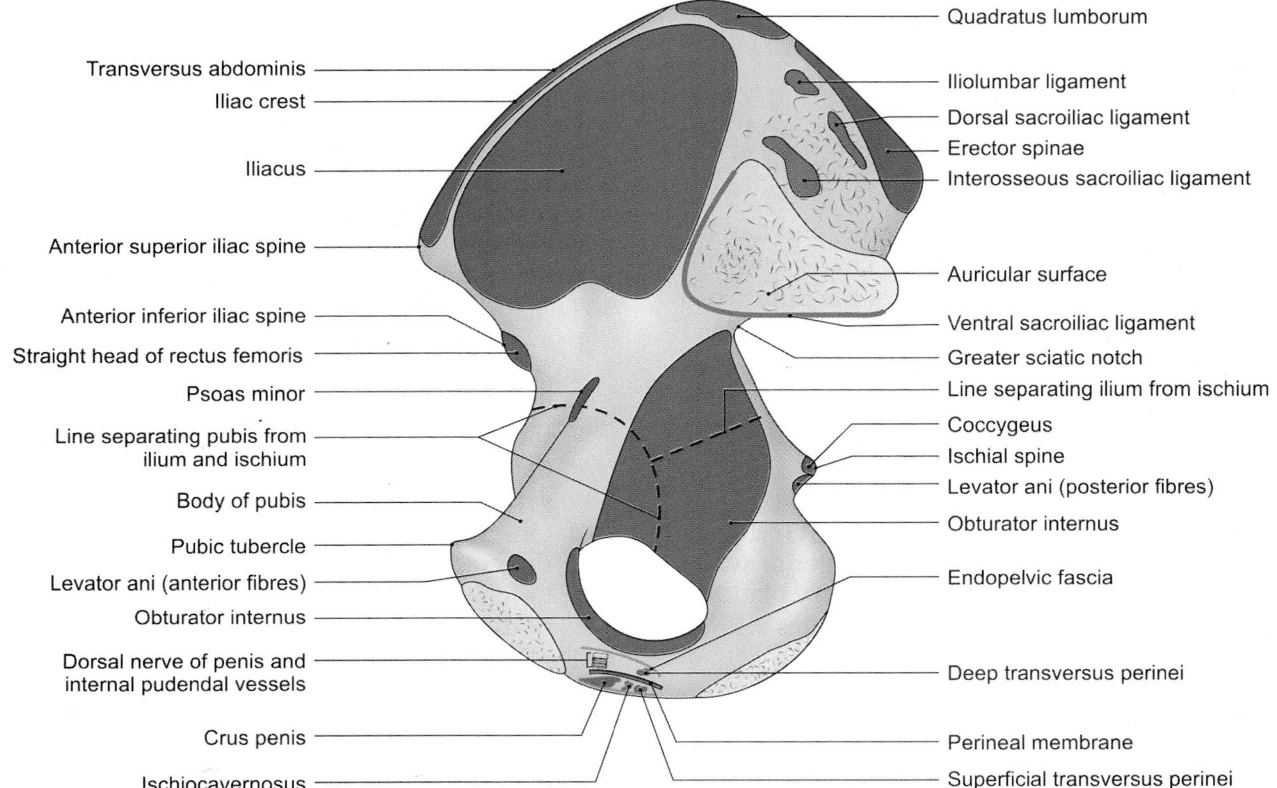

Fig. 2.5: Attachments of the inner surface of the right hip bone

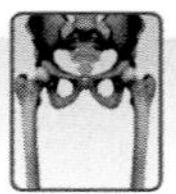

d. Below the inferior gluteal line, the *reflected head of the rectus femoris* arises from the groove above the acetabulum (Fig. 2.4).
e. The *capsular ligament of the hip joint* is attached along the margin of acetabulum.

9 The iliac fossa gives origin to the *iliacus* from its upper two-thirds (Fig. 2.5). The lower grooved part of the fossa is covered by the iliac bursa.

10 The *iliac tuberosity* provides attachment to:
a. The *interosseous sacroiliac ligament* in its greater part (Fig. 2.5).
b. The *dorsal sacroiliac ligament* posteriorly.
c. The *iliolumbar ligament* superiorly.

11 The convex margin of the *auricular surface* gives attachment to *ventral sacroiliac ligament*.

12 The attachments on the pelvic surface are as follows.
a. The preauricular sulcus provides attachment to the lower fibres of the *ventral sacroiliac ligament*.
b. The part of the pelvic surface lateral to the preauricular sulcus gives origin to a few fibres of the *piriformis*.
c. The rest of the pelvic surface gives origin to the upper half of the *obturator internus* (Fig. 2.5).

PUBIS

It forms the anteroinferior part of the hip bone and the anterior one-fifth of the acetabulum, forms the anterior boundary of the obturator foramen. It has:

a. A *body* anteriorly.
b. A *superior ramus* superolaterally.
c. An *inferior ramus* inferolaterally (Figs 2.1 and 2.2).

Body of Pubis

This is flattened from before backwards, and has:

1 A superior border called the *pubic crest*.
2 *A pubic tubercle* at the lateral end of the pubic crest.
3 Three surfaces, viz. anterior, posterior and medial.

The *pubic tubercle* is the lateral end of the pubic crest, forming an important landmark (Fig. 2.5).

The *anterior surface* is directed downwards, forwards and slightly laterally. It is rough superomedially and smooth elsewhere.

The *posterior* or *pelvic surface* is smooth. It is directed upwards and backwards. It forms the anterior wall of the true pelvis, and is related to the urinary bladder.

The *medial* or *symphyseal surface* articulates with the opposite pubis to form the pubic symphysis.

Superior Ramus

It extends from the body of the pubis to the acetabulum, above the obturator foramen. It has three borders and three surfaces.

The superior border is called the *pectineal line* or *pecten pubis*. It is a sharp crest extending from just behind the pubic tubercle to the posterior part of the iliopubic eminence. With the pubic crest it forms the pubic part of the arcuate line.

The anterior border is called the *obturator crest*. The border is a rounded ridge, extending from the pubic tubercle to the acetabular notch.

The *inferior border* is sharp and forms the upper margin of the obturator foramen.

The *pectineal surface* is a triangular area between the anterior and superior borders, extending from the pubic tubercle to the iliopubic eminence.

The *pelvic surface* lies between the superior and inferior borders. It is smooth and is continuous with the pelvic surface of the body of the pubis.

The *obturator surface* lies between the anterior and inferior borders. It presents the obturator groove.

Inferior Ramus

It extends from the body of the pubis to the ramus of the ischium, medial to the obturator foramen. It unites with the ramus of the ischium to form the conjoined ischiopubic rami. For convenience of description, the conjoined rami will be considered together at the end. (*refer to*).

Attachments and Relations of the Pubis

1 The *pubic tubercle* provides attachment to the *medial end of the inguinal ligament* and to *ascending loops of the cremaster muscle*. In males, the tubercle is crossed by the spermatic cord.

2 The medial part of the *pubic crest* is crossed by the medial head of the rectus abdominis. The lateral part of the crest gives origin to the lateral head of the rectus abdominis, and to the pyramidalis (Fig. 2.4).

3 The anterior surface of the body of the pubis provides:
a. Attachment to the *anterior pubic ligament* medially.
b. Origin to the *adductor longus* in the angle between the crest and the symphysis.
c. Origin to the *gracilis*, from the margin of symphysis, and from the inferior ramus.
d. Origin to the *adductor brevis* lateral to the origin of the gracilis (Fig. 2.4).
e. Origin to the obturator externus near the margin of the obturator foramen (*see* Fig. 4.1).

4 The *posterior surface* of the body of the pubis provides:
a. Origin to the *levator ani* from its middle part (Fig. 2.5).
b. Origin to the obturator internus laterally (Fig. 2.5).
c. Attachment to the *puboprostatic ligaments* medial to the attachment of the levator ani.

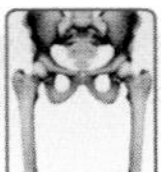

5 The *pectineal line* provides attachment to:
   a. The conjoint tendon at the medial end.
   b. The lacunar ligament at the medial end, in front of the attachment of the conjoint tendon.
   c. The pectineal ligament of Cooper along the whole length of the line lateral to the attachment of the lacunar ligament
   d. The pectineus muscle which arises from the whole length of the line (Figs 2.4 and 4.1).
   e. The fascia covering the pectineus.
   f. The psoas minor, which is inserted here when present.

6 The upper part of the *pectineal surface* gives origin to the pectineus (Fig. 2.4).

7 The pelvic surface is crossed by the ductus deferens in males, and the round ligament of the uterus in females (*see* Chapters 31 and 32).

8 The *obturator groove* transmits the obturator vessels and nerve (*see* Fig. 4.4).

9 See attachments on conjoined ischiopubic rami with ischium.

ISCHIUM

The ischium forms the posteroinferior part of the hip bone, and the adjoining two-fifths of the acetabulum. It forms the posterior boundary of the obturator foramen. The ischium has a body and a ramus (Figs 2.1, 2.2 and 2.4).

Body of the Ischium

This is a thick and massive mass of bone that lies below and behind the acetabulum. It has:

Two ends—upper and lower;
Three borders—anterior, posterior and lateral;
Three surfaces—femoral, dorsal and pelvic.

Two Ends

1 The *upper end* forms the posteroinferior two-fifths of the acetabulum. The ischium, ilium and pubis fuse with each other in the acetabulum.

2 The *lower end* forms the *ischial tuberosity.* It gives off the ramus of the ischium which forms an acute angle with the body.

Three Borders

1 The *anterior border* forms the posterior margin of the obturator foramen.

2 The *posterior border* is continuous above with the posterior border of the ilium. Below, it ends at the upper end of the ischial tuberosity. It also forms part of the lower border of the greater sciatic notch. Below the notch the posterior margin shows a projection called the *ischial spine.* Below the spine the posterior border shows a concavity called the *lesser sciatic notch.*

3 The *lateral border* forms the lateral margin of the ischial tuberosity, except at the upper end where it is rounded.

Three Surfaces

1 The *femoral surface* lies between the anterior and lateral borders.

2 The *dorsal surface* is continuous above with the gluteal surface of the ilium. From above downwards it presents a convex surface adjoining the acetabulum, a wide shallow groove, and the upper part of the ischial tuberosity.

The *ischial tuberosity* is divided by a transverse ridge into an upper and a lower area. The upper area is subdivided by an oblique ridge into a superolateral area and an inferomedial area. The lower area is subdivided by a longitudinal ridge into outer and inner area (Fig. 2.6).

3 The *pelvic surface* is smooth and forms part of the lateral wall of the true pelvis.

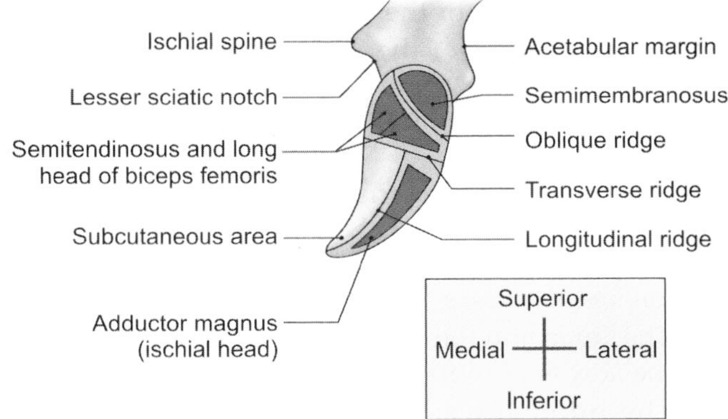

Fig. 2.6: Posterior view of the right ischial tuberosity and its attachments

Conjoined Ischiopubic Rami

The inferior ramus of the pubis unites with the ramus of the ischium on the medial side of the obturator foramen. The site of union may be marked by a localized thickening. The conjoined rami have:

Two Borders: Upper and lower

1 The *upper border* forms part of the margin of the obturator foramen.

2 The *lower border* forms the pubic arch along with the corresponding border of the bone of the opposite side.

Two Surfaces: Inner and outer

1 The *inner surface* is convex and smooth. It is divided into three areas, upper, middle and lower, by two ridges.

2 The outer surface is rough for the attachment of muscles.

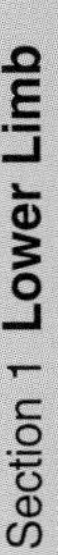

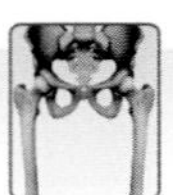

Attachments and Relations of the Ischium

1 The *ischial spine* provides:
   a. Attachment to the *sacrospinous ligament* along its margins.
   b. Origin for the posterior fibres of the *levator ani* from its pelvic surface. Its dorsal surface is crossed by pudendal nerve the internal pudendal vessels and by the nerve to the obturator internus (Figs 2.5 and 5.14).

2 The *lesser sciatic notch* is occupied by the tendon of the obturator internus. There is a bursa deep to the tendon. The notch is lined by hyaline cartilage. The upper and lower margins of the notch give origin to the *superior and inferior gemelli* respectively (Fig. 2.4). Gemellus is derived from gemini, which means 'twin'. Gemini is a sun sign.

3 The *femoral surface* of the ischium gives origin to:
   a. The *obturator externus* along the margin of the obturator foramen.
   b. The *quadratus femoris* along the lateral border of the upper part of the ischial tuberosity (Fig. 2.4).

4 The *dorsal surface* of the ischium has the following relationships. The upper convex area is related to the piriformis, the sciatic nerve, and the nerve to the quadratus femoris.

5 The attachments on the *ischial tuberosity* are as follows:
   - The superolateral area gives origin to the *semimembranosus*
   - The inferomedial area to the *semitendinosus* and the *long head* of the *biceps femoris*
   - The outer lower area to the *adductor magnus* (Figs 2.4 and 2.6).
   - The inner lower area is covered with fibrofatty tissue which supports body weight in the sitting position.
   - The sharp medial margin of the tuberosity gives attachment to the *sacrotuberous ligament*.
   - The lateral border of the ischial tuberosity provides attachment to the *ischiofemoral ligament*, just below the acetabulum.

6 The greater part of the pelvic surface of the ischium gives origin to the *obturator internus*. The lower end of this surface forms part of the lateral wall of the ischioanal fossa (Fig. 2.5).

7 The attachments on the *conjoined ischiopubic rami* are as follows:
   a. The upper border gives attachment to the *obturator membrane*.
   b. The lower border provides attachment to the *fascia lata*, and to the membranous layer of superficial fascia or *Colles' fascia* of the perineum.
   c. The muscles taking origin from the outer surface are:
      i. The *obturator externus*, near the obturator margin of both rami.
      ii. The *adductor brevis*, chiefly from the pubic ramus.
      iii. The *gracilis*, chiefly from the pubic ramus.
      iv. The *adductor magnus*, chiefly from the ischial ramus (Fig. 2.4).
   d. The attachments on the inner surface are as follows:
      i. The *perineal membrane* is attached to the lower ridge.
      ii. The upper area gives origin to the *obturator internus*.
      iii. The middle area gives origin to the *deep transversus perinei*, and is related to the dorsal nerve of the penis, and to the internal pudendal vessels.
      iv. The lower area provides attachment to crus penis, and gives origin to the *ischiocavernosus* and to *superficial transversus perinei* (Fig. 2.5).

ACETABULUM

1 It is a deep cup-shaped hemispherical cavity on the lateral aspect of the hip bone, about its centre (Fig. 2.1).

2 It is directed laterally, downwards and forwards.

3 The margin of the acetabulum is deficient inferiorly, this deficiency is called the *acetabular notch*. It is bridged by the transverse ligament.

4 The nonarticular roughened floor is called the *acetabular fossa*. It contains a mass of fat which is lined by synovial membrane.

5 A horseshoe-shaped articular surface or lunate surface is seen on the anterior, superior, and posterior parts of the acetabulum. It is lined with hyaline cartilage, and articulates with the head of the femur to form the *hip joint*. The fibrocartilaginous *acetabular labrum* is attached to the margins of the acetabulum; it deepens the acetabular cavity.

OBTURATOR FORAMEN

1 This is a large gap in the hip bone, situated anteroinferior to acetabulum, between the pubis and the ischium.

2 It is large and oval in males, and small and triangular in females (Fig. 2.2).

3 It is closed by the obturator membrane which is attached to its margins, except at the obturator groove where the obturator vessels and nerve pass out of the pelvis.

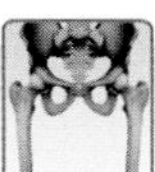

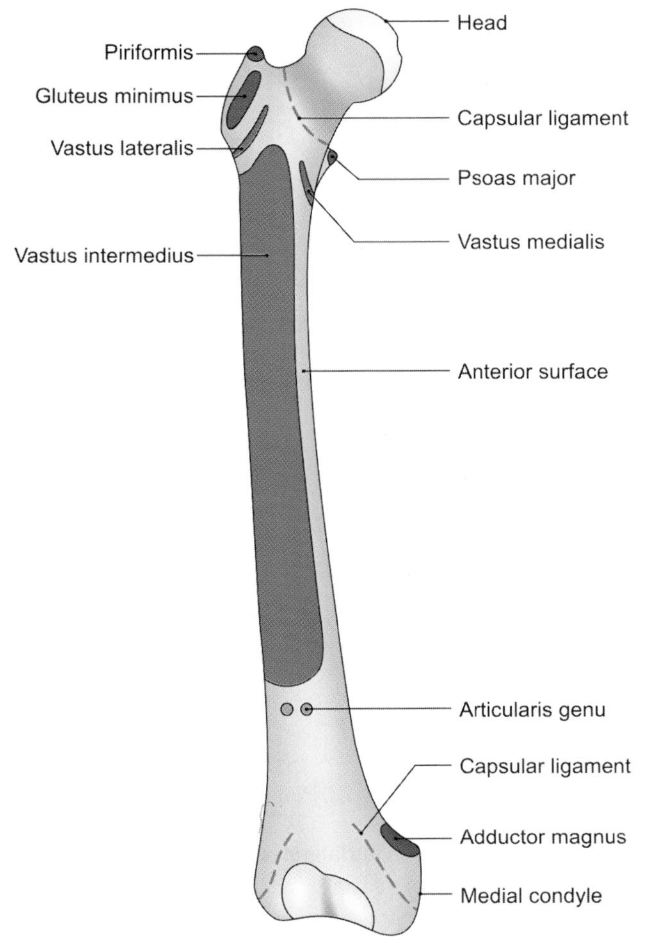

Fig. 2.11: Attachments on the anterior aspect of the right femur

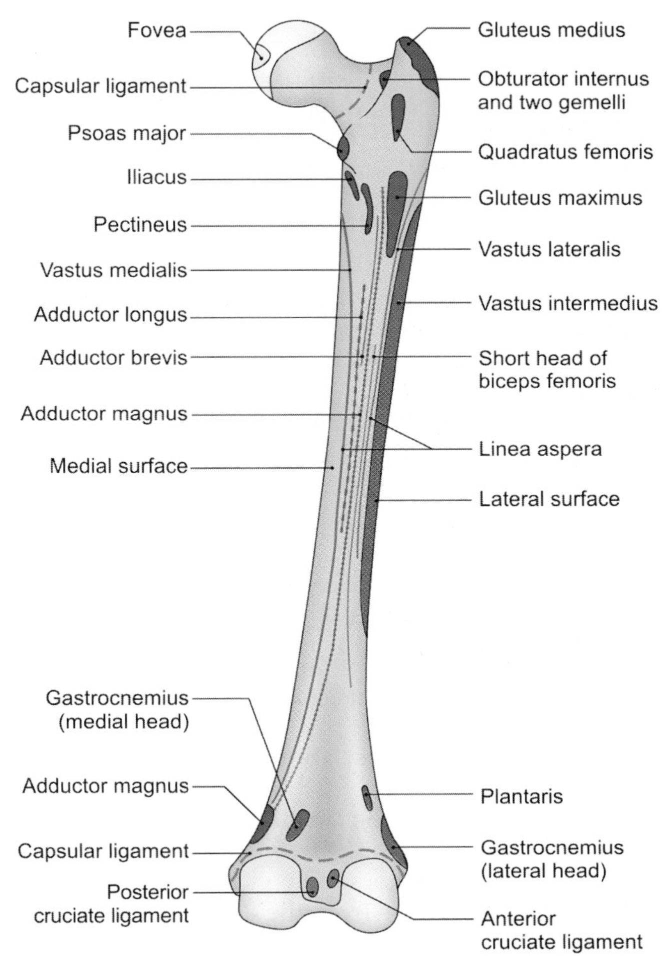

Fig. 2.12: Attachments on the posterior aspect of the right femur

e. The *vastus lateralis* arises from the upper part of the intertrochanteric line, anterior and inferior aspects of the greater trochanter, the lateral margin of the gluteal tuberosity, and the upper half of the lateral lip of the linea aspera (Figs 2.12 and 2.13).

f. The *vastus medialis* arises from the lower part of intertrochanteric line, the spiral line, medial lip of the linea aspera, and the medial supracondylar line (Fig. 2.13).

g. The deeper fibres of the lower half of the *gluteus maximus* are inserted into the gluteal tuberosity.

h. The *adductor longus* is inserted along the medial lip of the linea aspera between the vastus medialis and the adductors brevis and magnus.

i. The *adductor brevis* is inserted into a line extending from the lesser trochanter to the upper part of the linea aspera, behind the pectineus and the upper part of the adductor longus.

j. The *adductor magnus* is inserted into the medial margin of the gluteal tuberosity, the linea aspera, the medial supracondylar line, and the adductor tubercle, leaving a gap for the popliteal vessels (Fig. 2.13).

k. The *pectineus* is inserted on a line extending from the lesser trochanter to the linea aspera.

l. The *short head of the biceps femoris* arises from the lateral lip of the linea aspera between the vastus lateralis and the adductor magnus, and from the upper two-thirds of the lateral supracondylar line (Fig. 2.13).

m. The medial and lateral *intermuscular septa* are attached to the lips of the linea aspera and to the supracondylar lines. They separate the extensor muscles from the adductors medially, and from the flexors laterally (*see* Fig. 3.9).

n. The lower end of the lateral supracondylar line gives origin to the *plantaris* above and the upper part of the *lateral head of the gastrocnemius* below (Fig. 2.12).

o. The popliteal surface is covered with fat and forms the floor of the popliteal fossa. The origin of the *medial head of the gastrocnemius* extends to the

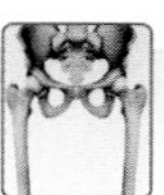

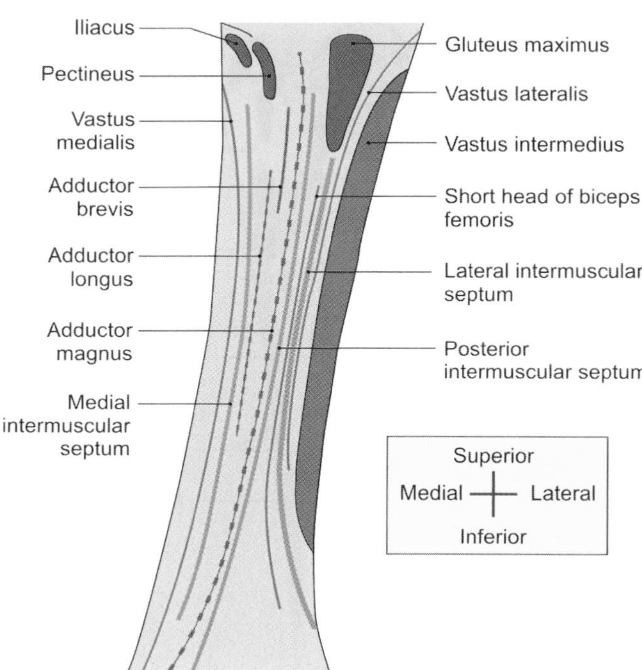

Fig. 2.13: Magnified view of structures attached to linea aspera

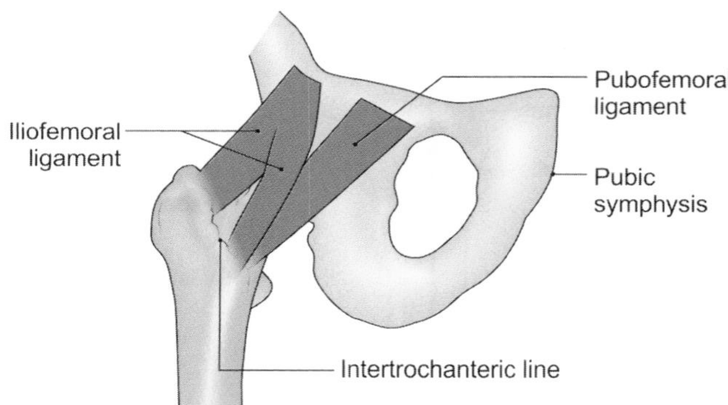

Fig. 2.14: Attachment of iliofemoral ligament

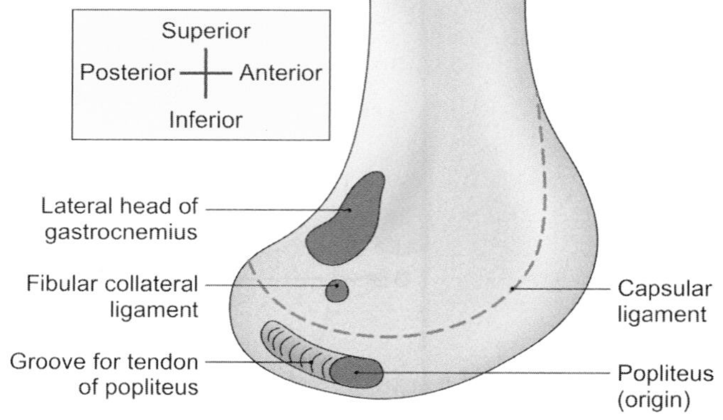

Fig. 2.15: Attachments on the lateral surface of the lateral condyle of the femur

popliteal surface just above the medial condyle (Fig. 2.12).

7 The attachments on the *lateral condyle* are:
   a. The *fibular collateral ligament* of the knee joint is attached to the lateral epicondyle (Fig. 2.15).
   b. The *popliteus* arises from the deep anterior part of the popliteal groove. When the knee is flexed the tendon of this muscle lies in the shallow posterior part of the groove.
   c. The muscular impression near the lateral epicondyle gives origin to the *lateral head of the gastrocnemius*.

8 The attachments on the *medial condyle* are as follows:
   a. The *tibial collateral ligament of the knee* joint is attached to the medial epicondyle (Fig. 12.11).
   b. The adductor tubercle receives the insertion of the hamstring part or the *ischial head of the adductor magnus* (Fig. 2.12).

9 The attachments on the *intercondylar notch* are as follows:
   a. The *anterior cruciate ligament* is attached to the posterior part of the medial surface of the lateral condyle, on a smooth impression.
   b. The *posterior cruciate ligament* is attached to the anterior part of the lateral surface of medial condyle, on a smooth impression (Fig. 2.12).
   c. The *intercondylar line* provides attachment to the capsular ligament and laterally to the oblique popliteal ligament.
   d. The *infrapatellar synovial fold* is attached to the anterior border of the intercondylar fossa (Fig. 2.12).

Nutrient Artery to the Femur

This is derived from the *second perforating artery,* branch of profunda femoris artery. The nutrient foramen is located on the medial side of the linea aspera, and is directed upwards.

Structure

The angles and curvatures of the femur are strengthened on their concave sides by bony buttresses. The concavity of the neck-shaft angle is strengthened by a thickened buttress of compact bone, known as the *calcar femorale.* Similarly, the linea aspera is also supported by another buttress. This mechanism helps in resisting stresses including that of body weight.

OSSIFICATION

The femur ossifies from one primary and four secondary centres. The primary centre for the shaft appears in the seventh week of intrauterine life. The secondary centres appear, one for the lower end at the end of the ninth month of intrauterine life, one for the head during the first six months of life, one for the greater trochanter during the fourth year, and one for the lesser trochanter during the twelfth year (Fig. 2.16).

There are three epiphyses at the upper end and one epiphysis at the lower end. The upper epiphyses; lesser trochanter, greater trochanter and head, in that order, fuse with the shaft at about eighteen years. The lower epiphysis fuses by the twentieth year.

The following points are noteworthy.

1. The neck represents the upper end of the shaft because it ossifies from the primary centre.
2. Ossification of the lower end of the femur is of medicolegal importance. Presence of its centre in a newly born child found dead indicates that the child was viable, i.e. it was capable of independent existence.
3. The lower end of the femur is the growing end.
4. The lower epiphyseal line passes through the adductor tubercle.
5. The epiphyseal line of the head coincides with the articular margins, except superiorly where a part of the monarticular area is included in the epiphysis for passage of blood vessels to the head. In addition, the plane of this epiphysis changes with age from an oblique to a more vertical one.

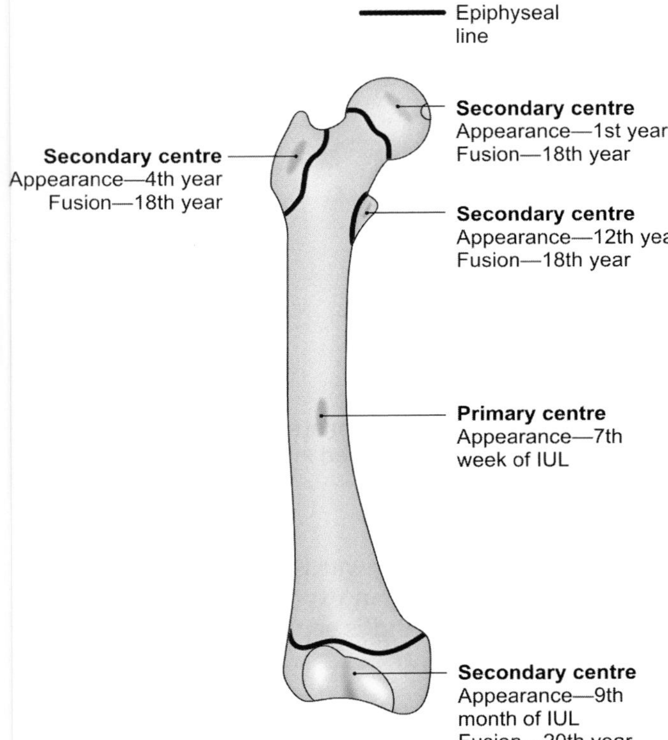

Fig. 2.16: Ossification of femur

CLINICAL ANATOMY

- Tripping over minor obstructions or other accidents causing forced medial rotation of the thigh and leg during the fall results in:
  a. The fracture of the shaft of femur in persons below the age of 16 years (Fig. 2.17).
  b. Bucket-handle tear of the medial meniscus between the ages of 14 and 40 years (Fig. 2.18).
  c. Pott's (British surgeon 1713–88) fracture of the leg between the ages of 40 and 60 years (Fig. 2.19).
  d. Fracture of neck of the femur over the age of 60 years (Fig. 2.17). This is common in females due to osteoporosis and degeneration of calcar femorale.
- The head of femur is partly supplied by a branch of obturator artery along the ligamentum teres. Main arterial supply is from retinacular arteries, branches of medial femoral circumflex artery. These arteries get injured in intracapsular fracture of neck of femur, leading to avascular necrosis of the head (Figs 2.20a and b). In such cases hip joint need to be replaced.
- The centre of ossification in lower end of femur and even in upper end of tibia seen by X-ray is used as a medicolegal evidence to prove that the newborn (found dead) was nearly full term and was viable.
- In fracture of upper third of shaft of femur, proximal segment is flexed by iliopsoas, laterally rotated by muscles attached to greater trochanter. Distal segment is pulled upwards by hamstrings and laterally rotated by adductor muscles.
- In normal knee, the obliquity of the line of quadriceps muscle and its insertion into the tibia, results in an angle called "Q angle". It is normally 15–20°. If the angle is increased, there may be lateral subluxation of the patella (*see* Fig. 3.27).

PATELLA

The patella (Latin *small plate*) is the largest sesamoid bone in the body, developed in the tendon of the quadriceps femoris. It is situated in front of the lower end of the femur about 1 cm above the knee joint (Fig. 2.21a).

Side Determination

1 The patella is triangular in shape with its apex directed downwards. The apex is nonarticular posteriorly.
2 The anterior surface is rough and nonarticular. The upper three-fourths of the posterior surface are smooth and articular.

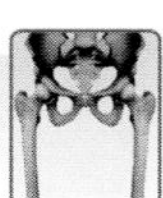

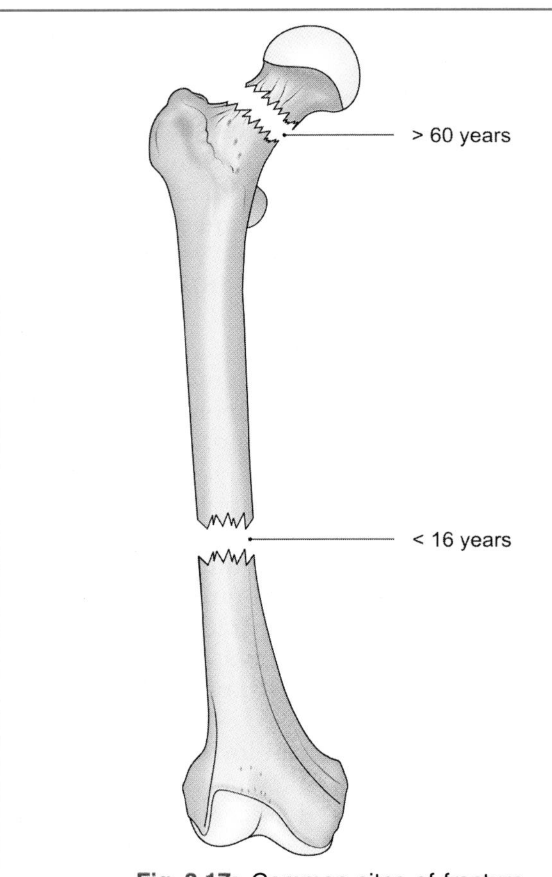

Fig. 2.17: Common sites of fracture

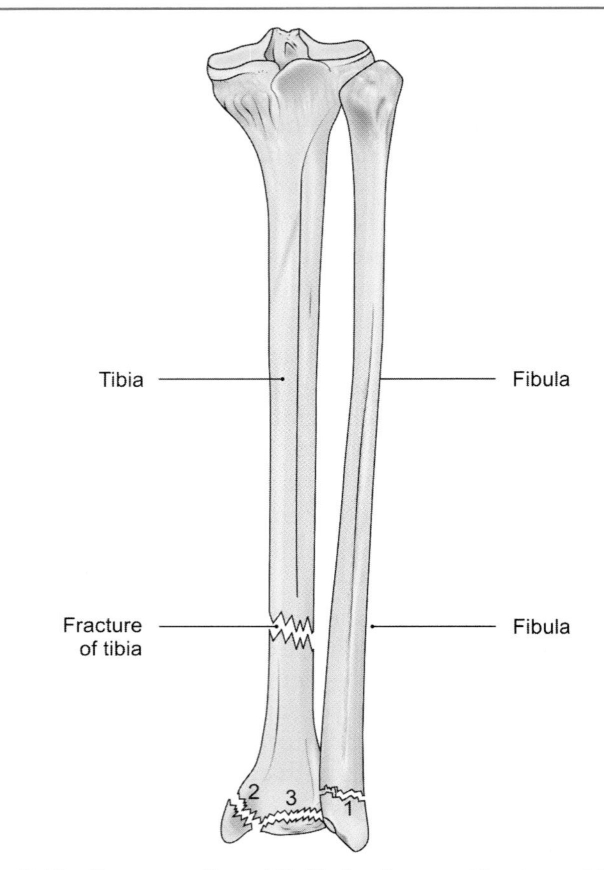

Fig. 2.19: Common sites of Pott's fracture and fracture of tibia

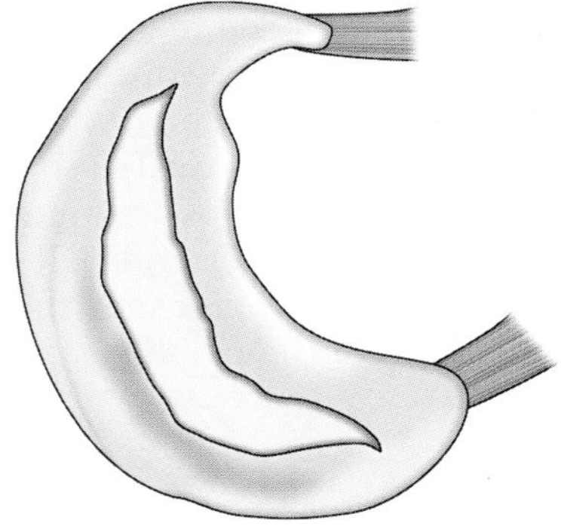

Fig. 2.18: Bucket-handle tear of medial meniscus

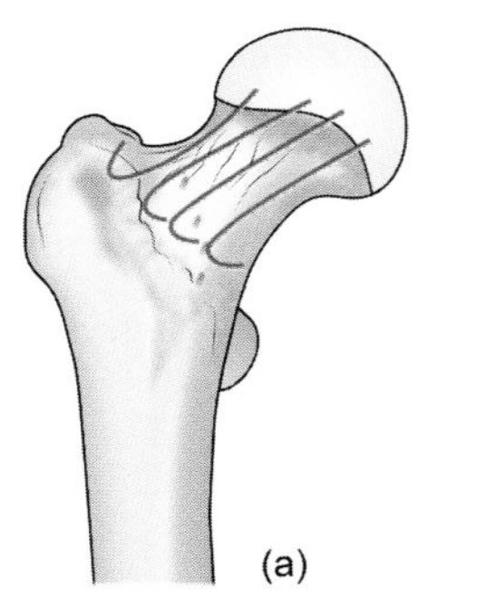

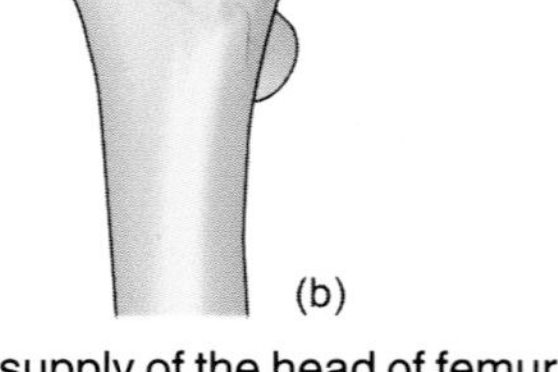

Figs 2.20a and b: (a) Normal arterial supply of the head of femur and (b) avascular necrosis of head in fracture neck femur

3 The posterior articular surface is divided by a vertical ridge into a larger lateral and a smaller medial areas.
4 The bone laid on a table rests on the broad lateral articular area and determines the side of the bone.

Features

The patella has an apex, three borders, superior, lateral and medial, and two surfaces, anterior and posterior.

The *apex* directed downwards, is rough and vertically ridged. It is covered by an expansion from the tendon of the rectus femoris, and is separated from the skin by the prepatellar bursa.

The *posterior surface* is articular in its upper three-fourths and monarticular in its lower one-fourth.

The articular area is divided by a vertical ridge into a larger lateral and smaller medial portion. Another

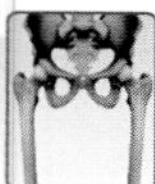

Attachment on the Tibial Tuberosity

The *ligamentum patellae* is attached to the upper smooth part of the *tibial tuberosity*. The lower rough area of the tuberosity is subcutaneous, but is separated from the skin by the subcutaneous infrapatellar bursa (Fig. 2.27).

Attachments on the Shaft

1 The *tibialis anterior* arises from the upper two-thirds of the lateral surface.
2 The upper part of the medial surface receives the insertions of the *sartorius*, the *gracilis* and the *semitendinosus*, from before backwards (Fig. 2.27). Still further posteriorly this surface gives attachment to the *tibial collateral ligament* along the medial border (Fig. 2.27).
3 The *soleus* arises from the soleal line (Fig. 2.28). The soleal line also gives attachment to the fascia covering the soleus, the fascia covering the popliteus, and the transverse fascial septum. The tendinous arch for origin of the soleus is attached to a tubercle at the upper end of the soleal line.
4 The *popliteus* is inserted on the posterior surface, into the triangular area above the soleal line.
5 The medial area of the posterior surface below the soleal line gives origin to the *flexor digitorum longus* while the lateral area gives origin to *the tibialis posterior*.
6 The anterior border of the tibia gives attachment to the *deep fascia of the leg* and, in its lower part, to the *superior extensor retinaculum*.
7 The rough upper part of the fibular notch gives attachment to the interosseous tibiofibular ligament.
8 The *capsular ligament of the ankle joint* is attached to the lower end along the margins of articular surface. The *deltoid ligament* of the ankle joint is attached to the lower border of the *medial malleolus* (Fig. 2.24).

Relations of the Tibia

Apart from the relations mentioned above, the following may be noted.

1 The lower part of the anterior surface of the shaft, and the anterior aspect of the lower end, are crossed from medial to lateral side by the tibialis anterior, the extensor hallucis longus, the anterior tibial artery, the deep peroneal nerve, the extensor digitorum longus, and the peroneus tertius (Fig. 2.27).
2 The lower most part of the posterior surface of the shaft and the posterior aspect of the lower end are related from medial to lateral side to the tibialis posterior, which lies in a groove, the flexor digitourm longus, the posterior tibial artery, the tibial nerve, and the flexor hallucis longus. The groove for the tendon of the tibialis posterior continues downwards on the posterior surface of the medial malleolus (Fig. 2.28).
3 The lower one-third of the medial surface of the shaft is crossed by the great saphenous vein (*see* Fig. 8.1).

Blood Supply

The nutrient artery to the tibia is the largest nutrient artery in the body. It is a branch of the posterior tibial artery which enters the bone on its posterior surface at the upper end of vertical ridge. It is directed downwards.

OSSIFICATION

The tibia ossifies from one primary and two secondary centres. The primary centre appears in the shaft during the seventh week of intrauterine life. A secondary centre for the upper end appears just *before birth*, and fuses with the shaft at 16–18 years. The upper epiphysis is prolonged downwards to form the tibial tuberosity. A secondary centre for the lower end appears during the first year, forms the medial malleolus by the seventh year, and fuses with the shaft by 15–17 years (Fig. 2.29).

CLINICAL ANATOMY

- The upper end of tibia is one of the commonest sites for acute osteomyelitis. The knee joint remains safe because the capsule is attached near the articular margins of the tibia, proximal to the epiphyseal line (Fig. 2.30).
- The tibia is commonly fractured at the junction of upper two-thirds and lower one-third of the shaft as the shaft is most slender here. Such fractures may unite slowly, or may not unite at all as the blood supply to this part of the bone is poor. This may also be caused by tearing of the nutrient artery.
- Forward dislocation of the tibia on the talus produces a characteristic prominence of the heel. This is the commonest type of injury of the ankle.

FIBULA

The fibula (Latin *clasp/pin*) is the lateral and smaller bone of the leg. It is very thin as compared to the tibia. It is homologous with the ulna of the upper limb (Figs 2.24 and 2.25). It forms a mortice of the ankle joint.

Side Determination

1 The upper end, or head, is slightly expanded in all directions. The lower end or lateral malleolus is expanded anteroposteriorly and is flattened from side to side.

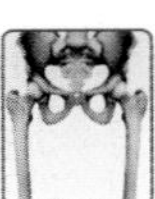

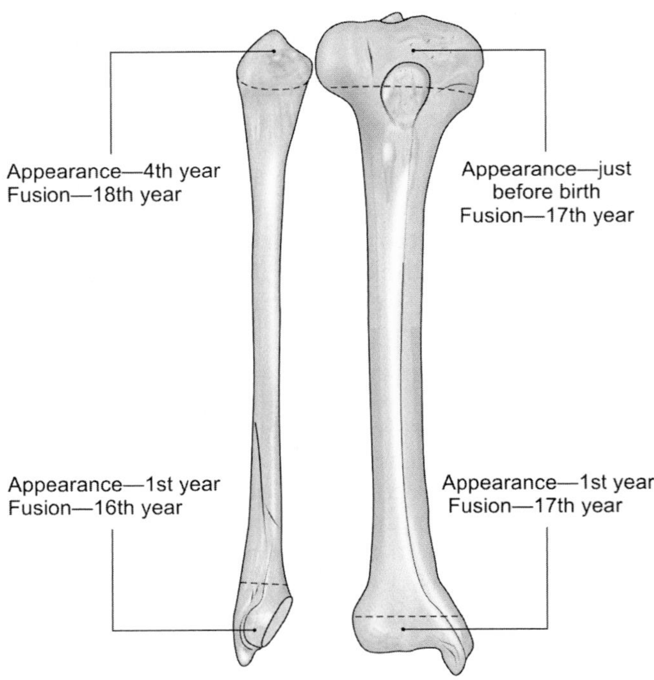

Fig. 2.29: Ossification of tibia and fibula

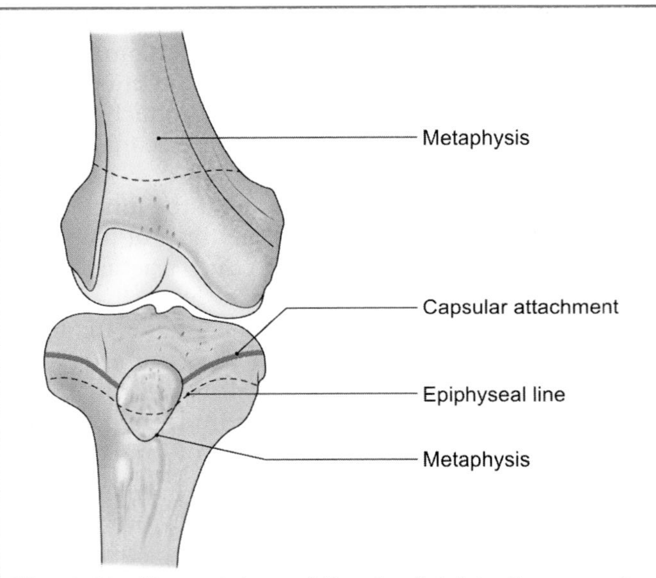

Fig. 2.30: The epiphyseal line is distal to the capsular attachment

2 The medial side of the lower end bears a triangular articular facet anteriorly, and a deep or *malleolar fossa* posteriorly (Fig. 2.31).

Features

The fibula has an upper end, a shaft (Fig. 2.32) and a lower end.

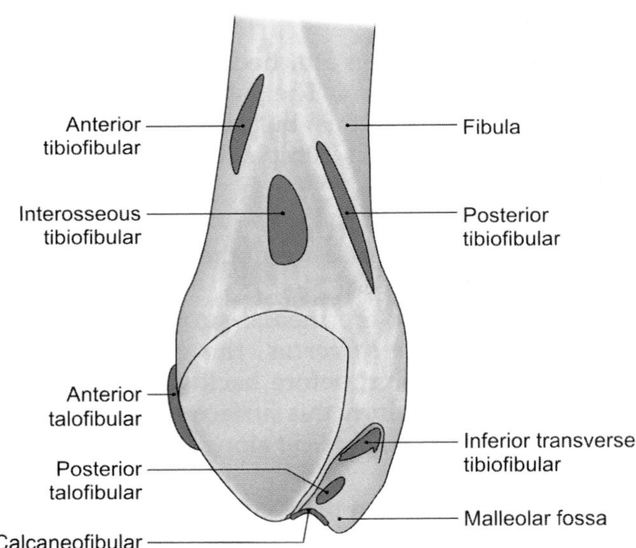

Fig. 2.31: Ligaments attached on the medial aspect of lower end of fibula

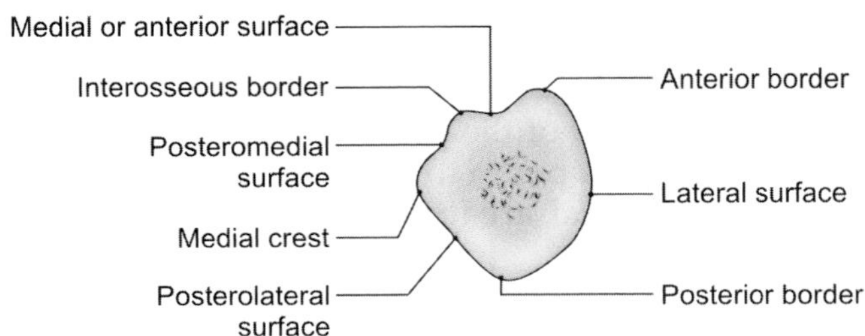

Fig. 2.32: Transverse section through shaft of middle two-fourths of fibula to show its borders and surfaces

Upper End or Head

It is slightly expanded in all directions. The superior surface bears a circular articular facet which articulates with the lateral condyle of the tibia. The *apex* of the head or the styloid process projects upwards from its posterolateral aspect.

The constriction immediately below the head is known as the *neck* of the fibula (Figs 2.25 and 2.33).

Shaft

The shaft shows considerable variation in its form because it is moulded by the muscles attached to it. It has three borders—anterior, posterior and interosseous; and three surfaces—medial, lateral and posterior (Fig. 2.32).

Borders

The *anterior border* begins just below the anterior aspect of the head. At its lower end it divides to enclose an elongated triangular area which is continuous with the lateral surface of the lateral malleolus (Fig. 2.33).

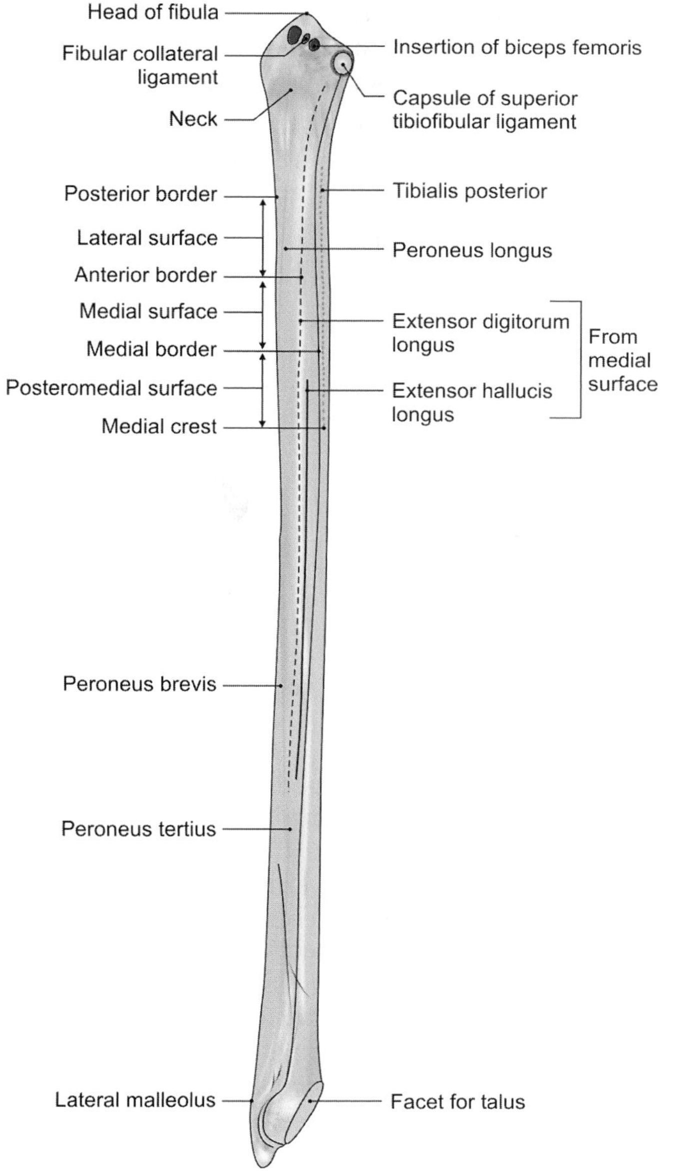

Fig. 2.33: Right fibula: Anterior aspect (schematic)

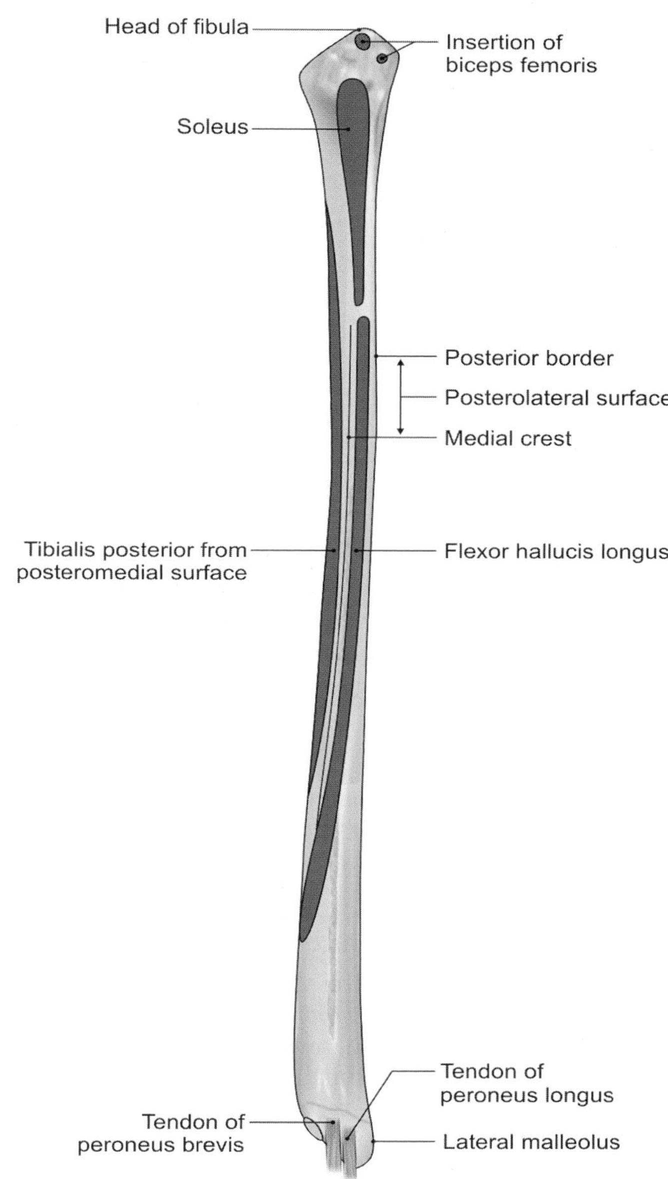

Fig. 2.34: Right fibula: Posterior aspect

The *posterior border* is rounded. Its upper end lies in line with the styloid process. Below, the border is continuous with the medial margin of the groove on the back of the lateral malleolus (Fig. 2.34).

The *interosseous* or *medial border* lies just medial to the anterior border, but on a more posterior plane. It terminates below at the upper end of a roughened area above the talar facet of the lateral malleolus. In its upper two-thirds, the interosseous border lies very close to the anterior border and may be indistinguishable from it.

Surfaces

The *medial surface* lies between the anterior and interosseous borders. In its upper two-thirds, it is very narrow, measuring 1 mm or less (Figs 2.33 and 2.35).

The *lateral surface* lies between the anterior and posterior borders. It is twisted backwards in its lower part.

The *posterior surface* is the largest of the three surfaces. It lies between the interosseous and posterior borders. In its upper two-thirds, it is divided into two parts by a vertical ridge called the *medial crest* (Fig. 2.34).

Lower End or Lateral Malleolus

The tip of the lateral malleolus is 0.5 cm lower than that of the medial malleolus, and its anterior surface is 1.5 cm posterior to that of the medial malleolus. It has the following four surfaces.

1 The anterior surface is rough and rounded.
2 The posterior surface is marked by a groove.

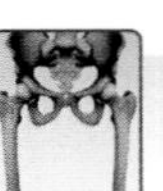

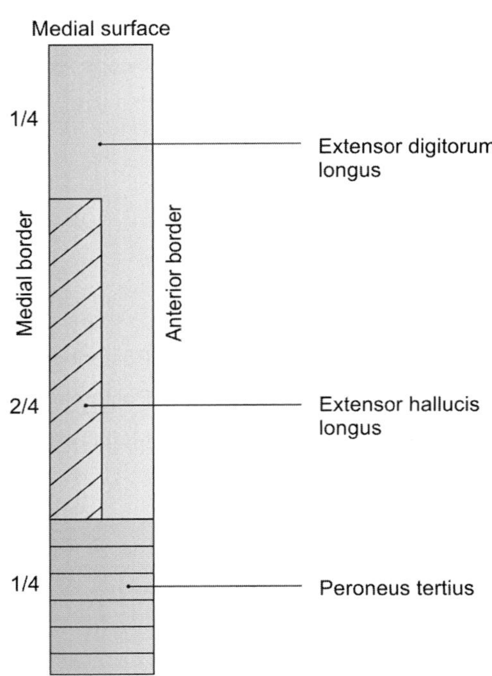

Fig. 2.35: Attachment on medial surface of fibula

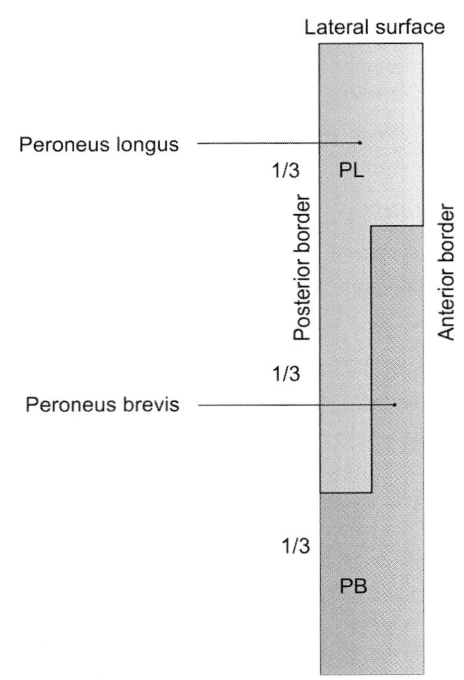

Fig. 2.36: Attachment on lateral surface of fibula

3 The lateral surface is subcutaneous.
4 The medial surface bears a triangular articular facet for the talus anteriorly and the malleolar fossa posteriorly.

Attachments and Relations of the Fibula

1 The medial surface of the shaft gives origin to:
   a. The *extensor digitorum longus*, from the whole of the upper one-fourth, and from the anterior half of the middle two-fourths.
   b. The *extensor hallucis longus*, from the posterior half of its middle two-fourths.
   c. The *peroneus tertius*, from its lower one-fourth (Fig. 2.35).
2 The part of the posterior surface between the medial crest and the interosseous border, the grooved part, gives origin to the *tibialis posterior*.
3 The part of the posterior surface between the medial crest and the posterior border gives origin to:
   a. *Soleus* from the upper one-fourth.
   b. *Flexor hallucis longus* from its lower three-fourths.
4 The lateral surface of the shaft gives origin to:
   a. *Peroneus longus (PL)* from its upper one-third, and posterior half of the middle one-third.
   b. The *peroneus brevis (PB)* from the anterior half of its middle one-third, and the whole of lower one-third (Fig. 2.36). The common peroneal nerve terminates in relation to the neck of fibula.
5 The head of the fibula receives the insertion of the *biceps femoris* on the anterolateral slope of the apex. This insertion is C-shaped. The *fibular collateral ligament* of the knee joint is attached within the C-shaped area (Fig. 2.33).

   The origins of the extensor digitorum, the peroneus longus, and the soleus, described above, extend on to the corresponding aspects of the head.
6 The *capsular ligament of the superior tibiofibular joint* is attached around the articular facet.
7 The anterior border of fibula gives attachment to:
   a. *Anterior intermuscular septum* of the leg (*see* Fig. 8.3).
   b. *Superior extensor retinaculum*, to lower part of the anterior margin of triangular area.
   c. *Superior peroneal retinaculum*, to the lower part of the posterior margin of triangular area.
8 The posterior border gives attachment to the *posterior intermuscular septum*.
9 The interosseous border gives attachment to the *interosseous membrane*. The attachment leaves a gap at the upper end for passage of the *anterior tibial vessels* (Fig. 2.24).
10 The triangular area above the medial surface of the lateral malleolus gives attachment to:
   a. The interosseous tibiofibular ligament, in the middle. The joint between lower ends of tibia and fibula is called *syndesmoses* (Greek *binding together*) (Fig. 2.24).
   b. The *anterior tibiofibular ligament*, anteriorly (Fig. 2.24).
   c. The *posterior tibiofibular*, posteriorly.

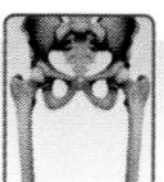

11 The attachments on the lateral malleolus are as follows:
   a. *Anterior talofibular ligament* to the anterior surface (Fig. 2.31).
   b. *Inferior transverse tibiofibular* (a part of posterior tibiofibular) ligament above and *posterior talofibular ligament* below to the *malleolar fossa* (Fig. 2.31).
   c. The *capsule of the ankle* joint along the edges of the malleolar articular surface.
   d. Slight notch on the lower border gives attachment to *calcaneofibular ligament* (Fig. 2.31).

12 The groove on the posterior surface of the malleolus lodges the tendon of the *peroneus brevis,* which is deep, and of the *peroneus longus,* which is superficial (Fig. 2.34).

Blood Supply

The peroneal artery gives off the nutrient artery for the fibula, which enters the bone on its posterior surface. The nutrient foramen is directed downwards.

OSSIFICATION

The fibula ossifies from one primary and two secondary centres. The primary centre for the shaft appears during the eighth week of intrauterine life. A secondary centre for the lower end appears during the first year, and fuses with the shaft by about sixteen years. A secondary centre for the upper end appears during the fourth year, and fuses with the shaft by about eighteen years (Fig. 2.29).

The fibula *violates* the law of ossification because the secondary centre which appears first in the lower end does not fuse last. The reasons for this violation are:

1. The secondary centre appears first in the lower end because it is a pressure epiphysis (law states that pressure epiphysis appears before the traction epiphysis).
2. The upper epiphysis fuses last because this is the growing end of the bone. It continues to grow afterwards along with the upper end of tibia which is a growing end.

CLINICAL ANATOMY

- Sometimes a surgeon takes a piece of bone from the part of the body and uses it to repair a defect in some other. This procedure is called a *bone graft*. For this purpose pieces of bone are easily obtained from the subcutaneous medial aspect of tibia and shaft of fibula.
- If the foot gets caught in a hole in the ground, there is forcible abduction and external rotation. In such an injury, first there occurs a spiral fracture of lateral malleolus, then fracture of the medial malleolus. Finally the posterior margin of the lower end of tibia shears off. These stages are termed 1st, 2nd and 3rd degrees of Pott's fracture (Fig. 2.19).
- The upper and lower ends of the fibula are subcutaneous and palpable (Fig. 2.37).
- The common peroneal nerve can be rolled against the neck of fibula. This nerve is commonly injured here resulting in *foot drop* (*see* Figs 6.8 and 7.11).
- Fibula is an ideal spare bone for a bone graft.
- Though fibula does not bear any weight, the lateral malleolus and the ligaments attached to it are very important in maintaining stability at the ankle joint.

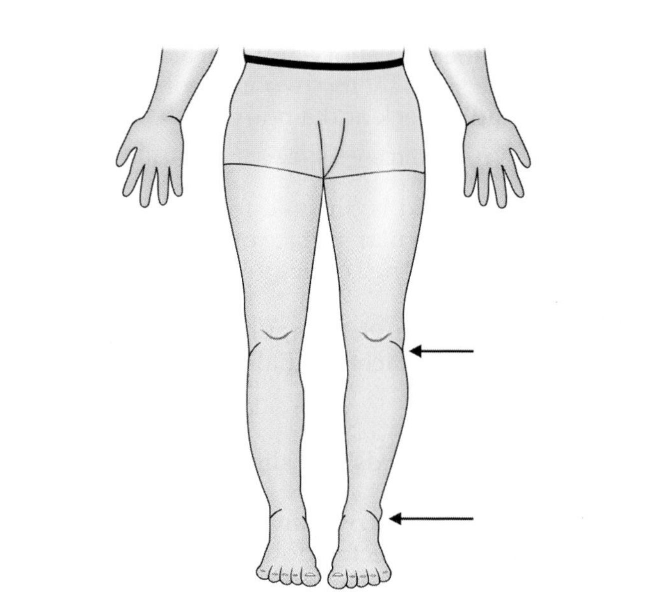

Fig. 2.37: Subcutaneous upper and lower ends of fibula

BONES OF THE FOOT

TARSUS/TARSALS

The tarsus is made up of seven tarsal bones, arranged in two rows. In the proximal row, there is the talus above, and the calcaneus below. In the distal row, there are four tarsal bones lying side by side. From medial to lateral side these are the medial cuneiform, the intermediate cuneiform, the lateral cuneiform and the cuboid. Another bone, the navicular, is interposed between the talus and the three cuneiform (Latin *wedge*) bones. In other words, it is interposed between the proximal and distal rows (Fig. 2.38).

The tarsal bones are much larger and stronger than the carpal bones because they have to support and

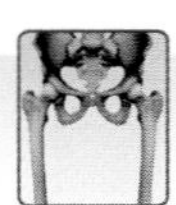

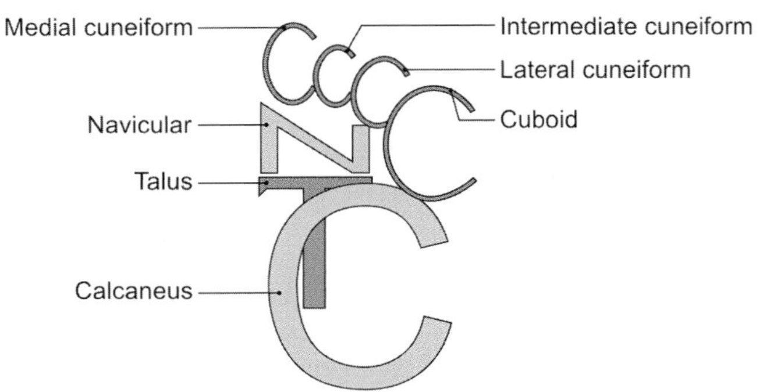

Fig. 2.38: Tarsus

distribute the body weight. Each tarsal bone is roughly cuboidal in shape, having six surfaces.

TALUS

The talus (Latin *ankle*) is the second largest tarsal bone. It lies between the tibia above and the calcaneum below, gripped on the sides by the two malleoli.

It has a head, a neck and a body.

Side Determination

1 The rounded head is directed forwards.
2 The trochlear articular surface of the body is directed upwards, and the concave articular surface downwards.
3 The body bears a large triangular, facet laterally, and a comma-shaped facet medially.

Head

1 It is directed forwards and slightly downwards and medially.
2 Its anterior surface is oval and convex. The long axis of this surface is directed downwards and medially. It articulates with the posterior surface of the navicular bone.
3 The inferior surface is marked by three articular areas separated by indistinct ridges. The posterior facet is largest, oval and gently convex; it articulates with the middle facet on sustentaculum tali of the calcaneum. The anterolateral facet articulates with the anterior facet of the calcaneum, and the medial facet with the spring ligament (Fig. 2.39b) (*refer* to).

Neck

1 This is the constricted part of the bone between the head and the body.
2 It is set obliquely on the body, so that inferiorly it extends further backwards on the medial side than on the lateral side. However, when viewed from dorsal side, the long axis of the neck is directed downwards, forwards and medially. The *neck–body angle* is 130 to 140 degrees in infants and 150 degrees in adults. The smaller angle in young children accounts for the inverted position of their feet.
3 The medial part of its plantar surface is marked by a deep groove termed the *sulcus tali.* The sulcus tali lies opposite the sulcus calcanei on the calcaneum, the two together enclosing a space called the *sinus tarsi.*
4 In habitual squatters, a squatting facet is commonly found on the upper and lateral part of the neck. The facet articulates with the anterior margin of the lower end of the tibia during extreme dorsiflexion of the ankle.

Body

The body is cuboidal in shape and has five surfaces.

The *superior surface* bears an articular surface, which articulates with the lower end of the tibia to form the ankle joint (Fig. 2.39a). This surface is also called the *trochlear surface.* It is convex from before backwards and concave from side to side. It is wider anteriorly than posteriorly. The medial border of the surface is straight, but the lateral border is directed forwards and laterally. The trochlear surface articulates with the inferior surface of lower end of tibia.

The *inferior surface* bears an oval, concave articular surface which articulates with the posterior facet of the calcaneum to form the subtalar joint (Fig. 12.22a).

The *medial surface* is articular above and nonarticular below. The articular surface is comma-shaped and articulates with the medial malleolus of tibia (Fig. 2.39c).

The *lateral surface* bears a triangular articular surface for the lateral malleolus. The surface is concave from above downwards, and its apex forms the lateral tubercle of the talus. The posterior part of the lateral surface is separated from the trochlea by an ill-defined, small triangular area which articulates with the inferior transverse tibiofibular ligament (Fig. 2.39d).

The *posterior process* is small and is marked by an oblique groove. The groove is bounded by medial and lateral tubercles. The lateral tubercle is occasionally separate (5%) and is then called the *os trigonum* (Fig. 2.39a).

Attachments on the Talus

The talus is devoid of muscular attachments, but numerous ligaments are attached to it because it takes part in three joints, e.g. ankle, talocalcanean and talonavicular:

1 The following ligaments are attached to the neck
   a. The distal part of the dorsal surface provides attachment to the *capsular ligament of the ankle joint* and to the *dorsal talonavicular ligament*. The proximal part of the dorsal surface lies within the ankle joint.
   b. The inferior surface provides attachment to the *interosseous talocalcanean and cervical ligaments*.

Section 1 Lower Limb

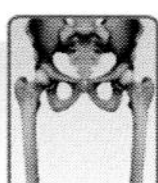

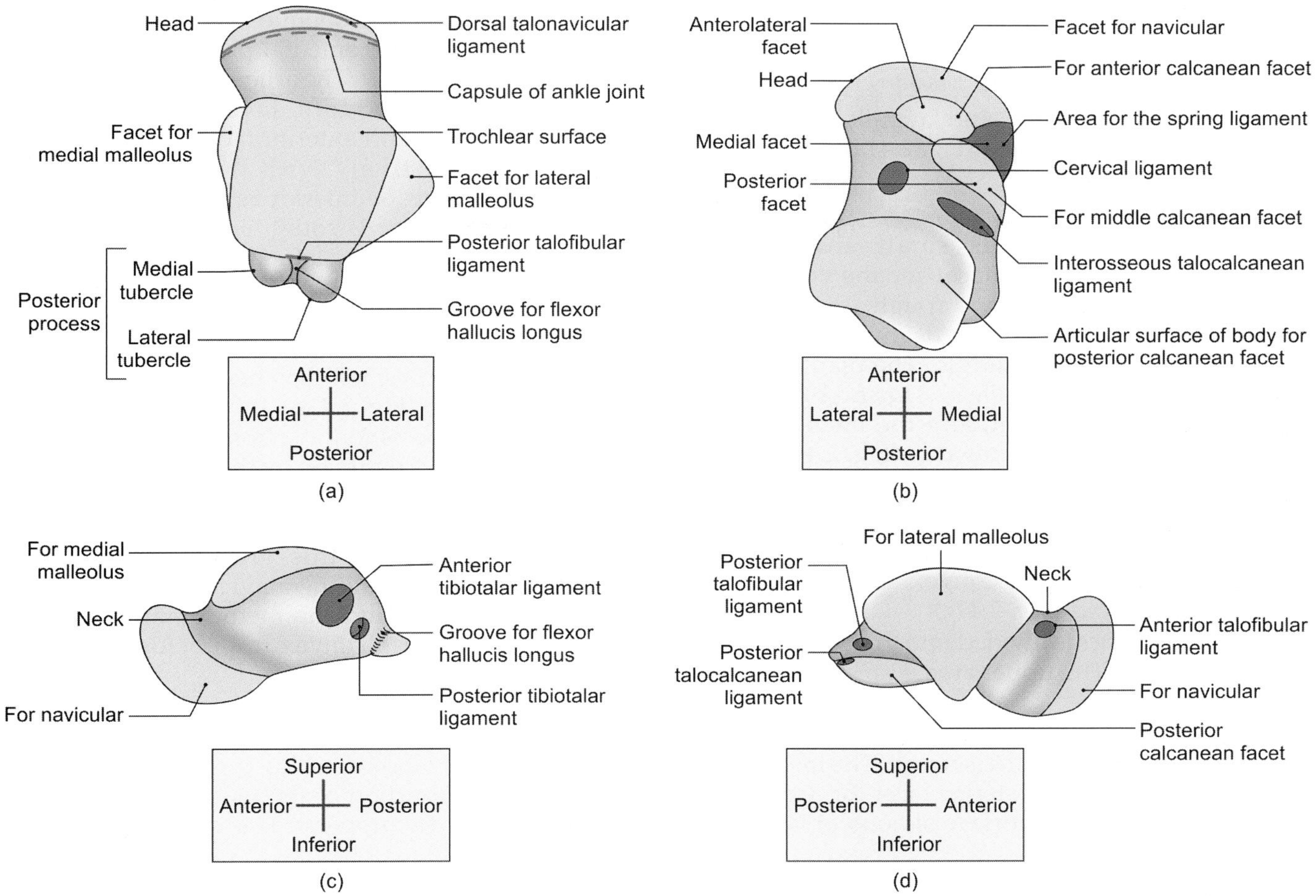

Figs 2.39a to d: Right talus: (a) Superior view, (b) inferior view, (c) medial view, and (d) lateral view

c. The lateral part of the neck provides attachment to the anterior talofibular ligament (Figs 2.31 and 2.39d).

2 The lower, nonarticular part of the medial surface of the body gives attachment to the *deep fibres of the deltoid* or *anterior tibiotalar ligament* (Fig. 2.39c).

3 The groove on the posterior process lodges the tendon of the flexor hallucis longus (Fig. 2.39a).

The medial tubercle provides attachment to the *superficial fibres of the deltoid ligament (posterior tibiotalar)* above and the *medial talocalcanean ligament* below.

Posterior talofibular ligament is attached to upper part of posterior process while *posterior talocalcanean ligament* is attached to its plantar border (Figs 2.39a and d).

OSSIFICATION

The talus ossifies from one centre which appears during the 6th month of intrauterine life.

CLINICAL ANATOMY

- Forced dorsiflexion may cause fracture of the neck of the talus.
- If arteries to body of talus go through the neck only as occurs in some cases, the body would get avascular necrosis in fracture of its neck (Fig. 2.40).

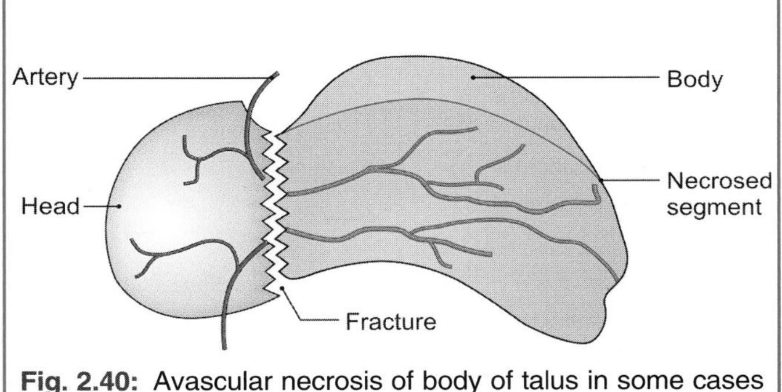

Fig. 2.40: Avascular necrosis of body of talus in some cases

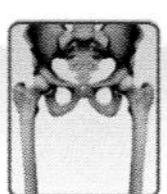

CALCANEUS OR CALCANEUM

The calcaneus (Latin *heel*) is the largest tarsal bone. It forms the prominence of the heel. Its long axis is directed forwards, upwards and laterally. It is roughly cuboidal and has six surfaces (Fig. 2.41a).

Side Determination

1 The anterior surface is small and bears a concavoconvex articular facet for the cuboid. The posterior surface is large and rough.
2 The dorsal or upper surface bears a large convex articular surface in the middle. The plantar surface is rough and triangular (Figs 2.41a and b).
3 The lateral surface is flat, and the medial surface concave from above downwards (Fig. 2.41c).

Features

The *anterior surface* is the smallest surface of the bone. It is covered by a concavoconvex, sloping articular surface for the cuboid (Fig. 2.41c).

The *posterior surface* is divided into three areas, upper, middle and lower. The upper area is smooth while the others are rough.

The *dorsal* or *superior surface* can be divided into three areas. The posterior one-third is rough. The middle one-third is covered by the posterior facet for articulation with the facet on inferior surface of body of talus. This facet is oval, convex and oblique. The anterior one-third is articular in the anteromedial part, and nonarticular in its posterolateral part. The articular part is in the form of an elongated middle facet present on the sustentaculum tali and anterior facet. These two facets articulate respectively with posterior facet and anteromedial facets on inferior aspect of head of talus.

The *plantar surface* is rough and marked by three tubercles. The medial and lateral tubercles are situated posteriorly, whereas the anterior tubercle lies in the anterior part.

The *lateral surface* is rough and almost flat. It presents in its anterior part, a small elevation termed the *peroneal trochlea* or *tubercle* (Fig. 2.41d).

The *medial surface* is concave from above downwards. The concavity is accentuated by the presence of a shelf-like projection of bone, called the *sustentaculum tali,* which projects medially from its anterosuperior border. The upper surface of this process assists in the formation of the talocalcaneonavicular joint. Its lower surface is grooved; and the medial margin is in the form of a rough strip convex from before backwards (Fig. 2.41c).

Attachments and Relations of the Calcaneus

1 The middle rough area on the posterior surface receives the insertion of the tendocalcaneus and of the plantaris. The upper area is covered by a bursa.

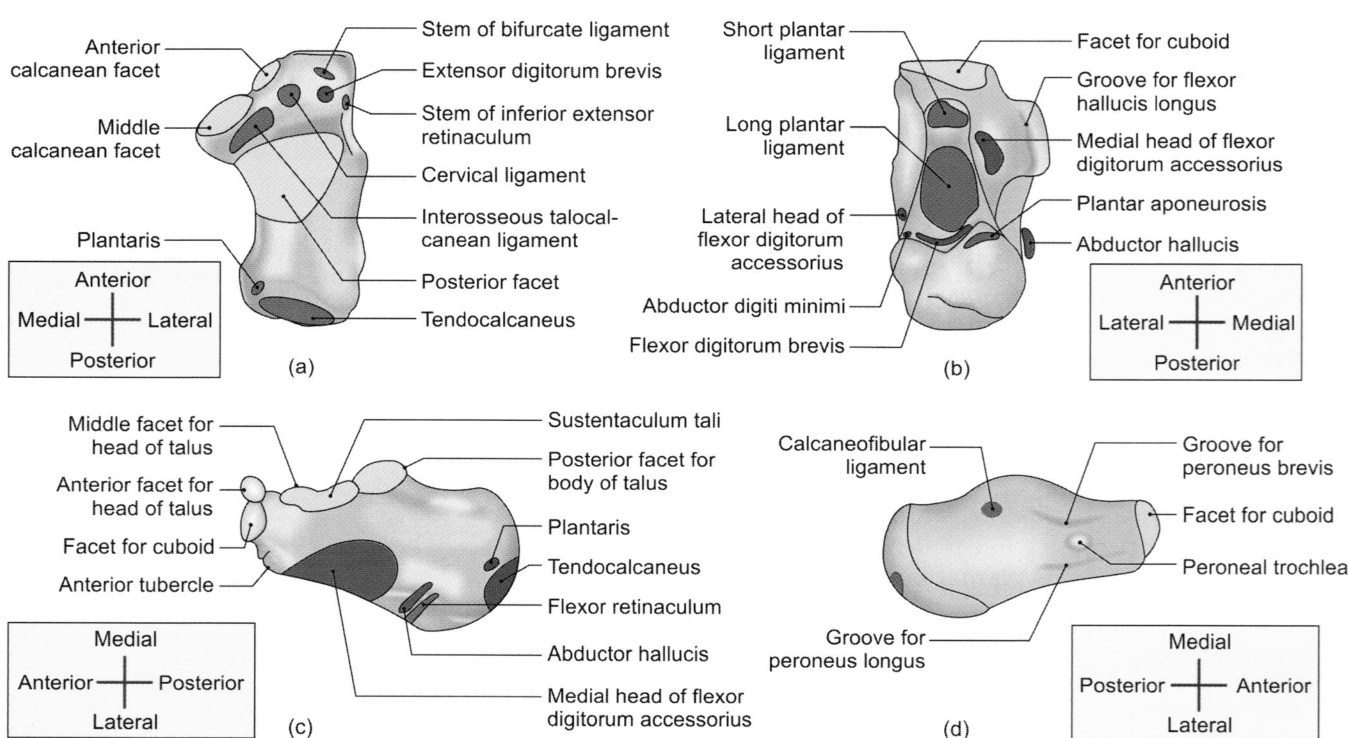

Figs 2.41a to d: Right calcaneus: (a) Superior view, (b) inferior view, (c) medial view, and (d) lateral view

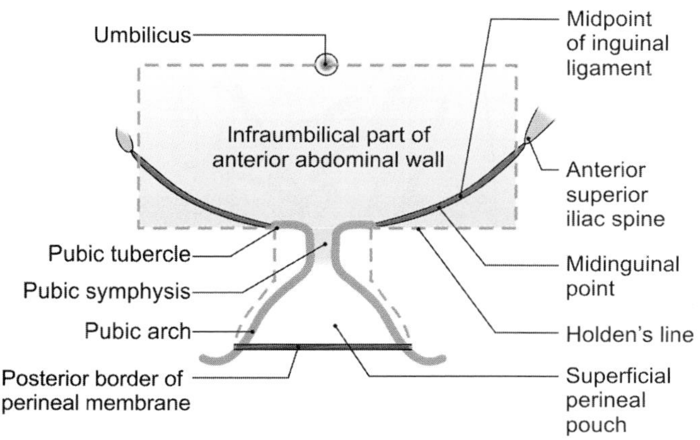

Fig. 3.2: The superficial area into which urine may pass when urethra is injured. The areas within the interrupted lines have a well-defined membranous layer of superficial fascia

It is easily seen and felt in front of the knee. It can be moved freely in a fully extended knee.

Tibial tuberosity is a blunt prominence in front of the upper end of tibia, marking the upper end of the shin.

Ligamentum patellae extends from the apex of patella to the tibial tuberosity. It represents the tendon (5 × 2.5 cm) of the quadriceps femoris which can be felt best in a half flexed knee.

The medial and lateral *condyles of the femur* and *of the tibia* form large bony masses at the sides of the knee. The most prominent points on the sides of the femoral condyles are called the medial and lateral epicondyles. Vastus medialis forms a fleshy prominence above the medial condyle of femur, particularly in an extended knee.

Adductor tubercle is a bony projection from the uppermost part of the medial condyle of femur to which the tendon of adductor magnus is attached. To palpate the tubercle, flex the knee partly and note the wide, shallow groove that appears posterior to the mass of vastus medialis. The tendon of adductor magnus can be felt in this groove. The tendon can be traced down to the adductor tubercle.

SKIN AND SUPERFICIAL FASCIA

DISSECTION

Make a curved incision from anterior superior iliac spine to the pubic tubercle.

Give a curved incision around the scrotum/pudendal cleft towards upper medial side of thigh. Extend it vertically down below the medial condyle of tibia till the level of tibial tuberosity.

Now make a horizontal incision below the tibial tuberosity till the lateral side of leg (Fig. 3.1).

Reflect the skin laterally, exposing the superficial fatty and deeper membranous layers of superficial fascia. Remove the fatty layer.

Identify the great saphenous vein in the medial part of anterior surface of thigh. Draining into its upper part are its three superficial tributaries, namely superficial circumflex iliac, superficial epigastric and superficial external pudendal. The vertical group of superficial inguinal lymph nodes lie along the upper part of great saphenous vein.

Dissect the superficial inguinal ring 1 cm above and lateral to the pubic tubercle. The spermatic cord and ilioinguinal nerve leave the abdomen through this ring.

Trace the great saphenous vein backwards till it pierces the specialised deep fascia known as cribriform fascia to drain into the femoral vein enclosed in the femoral sheath.

SKIN

The skin of thigh in the region around pubic symphysis, is studded with hair. The presence of few stitches indicates that embalming for preservation of the body has been done from this site.

Procedure for embalming: A 6 cm long vertical incision is given in the upper medial side of thigh. After reflecting skin and fasciae, femoral sheath is incised to visualise the femoral artery. About 10 litres of embalming fluid prepared by mixing appropriate amounts of formalin, glycerine, water, red lead, common salt, etc. is put in the embalming machine connected to a cannula.

A small nick is given in the femoral artery and cannula introduced so that its tip points towards the head end and 8.5 litres of fluid is pumped under 20 lb pressure. Then the direction of cannula is reversed and rest of fluid is pumped in. Lastly, the skin and fasciae are sutured.

SUPERFICIAL FASCIA

The superficial fascia has *two layers*, a superficial fatty layer and a deep membranous layer, which are continuous with the corresponding layers of the anterior abdominal wall. The two layers are most distinct in the uppermost part of the thigh, near the groin, where the cutaneous nerves, vessels and lymph nodes lie between the two layers.

The membranous layer is loosely attached to the deep fascia of the thigh except near the inguinal ligament, where it is firmly attached along a horizontal line. The line of firm attachment is called *Holden's line.* It begins a little lateral to the pubic tubercle and extends laterally for about 8 cm (Fig. 3.2).

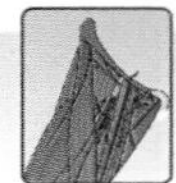

The importance of this Holden's line is as follows.

When the urethra is injured in the perineum, urine may flow out or extravasate into the interval deep to the membranous layer of superficial fascia. This urine can pass up into the anterior abdominal wall from where it can enter the upper part of the thigh. However, the firm attachment of the membranous layer of superficial fascia to the deep fascia along Holden's line prevents urine from descending into the thigh beyond the line.

The superficial fascia contains cutaneous nerves, cutaneous arteries, the great saphenous vein and its tributaries, and the superficial inguinal lymph nodes. The nerves and vessels are described below. The inguinal lymph nodes are described later.

Cutaneous Nerves

The skin of the front of the thigh is supplied by following cutaneous nerves derived directly, or indirectly, from the lumbar plexus (Fig. 3.3).

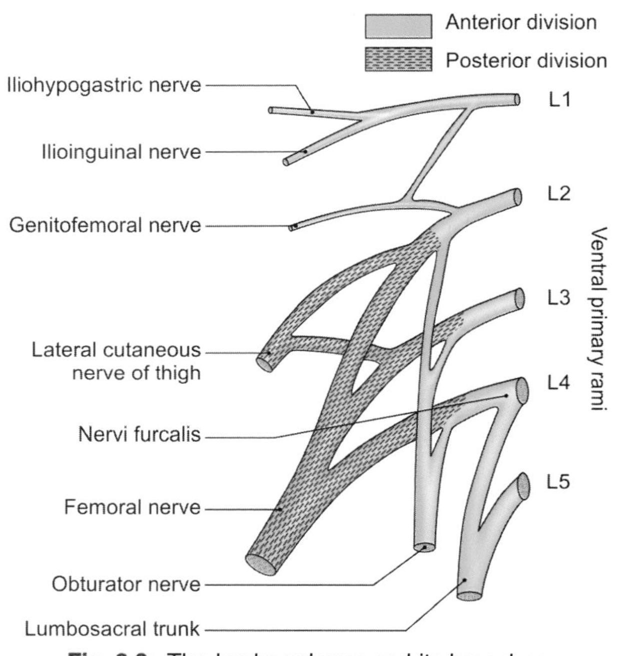

Fig. 3.3: The lumbar plexus and its branches

The *ilioinguinal nerve* (L1) emerges at the superficial inguinal ring, and supplies the skin at the root of the penis or over the mons pubis in the female, the anterior one-third of the scrotum or labium majus, and the superomedial part of the thigh (Fig. 3.4).

The *femoral branch of genitofemoral nerve* (L1, L2) pierces the femoral sheath and the overlying deep fascia 2 cm below the midinguinal point, and supplies most of the skin over the femoral triangle (Fig. 3.4).

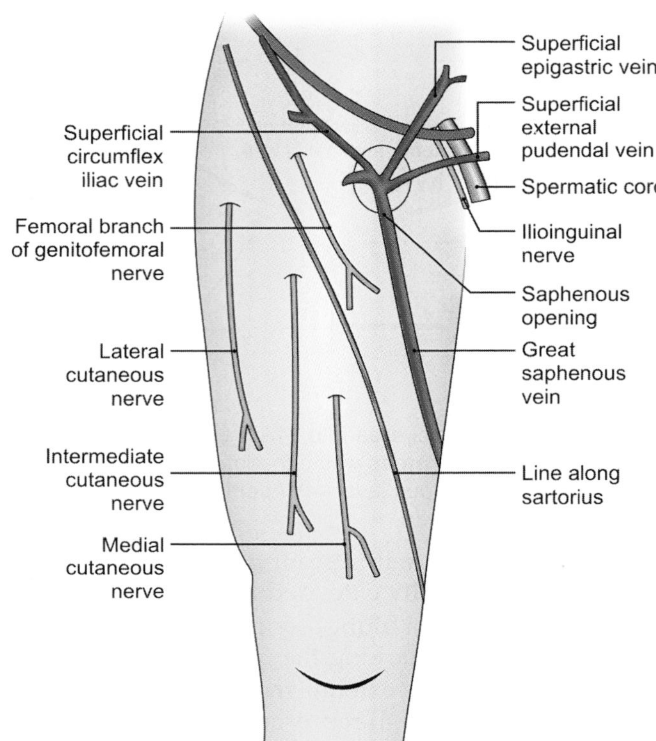

Fig. 3.4: Superficial veins and nerves seen on the front of the thigh

The *lateral cutaneous nerve of thigh* (L2, L3) is a branch of the lumbar plexus. It emerges behind the lateral end of the inguinal ligament, divides into anterior and posterior branches, and supplies the skin on the anterolateral side of the thigh and on the anterior part of the gluteal region.

The *intermediate cutaneous nerve of thigh* (L2, L3) is a branch of the anterior division of the femoral nerve. It pierces the deep fascia at the junction of the upper one-third and middle one-third of the thigh. It divides into two or more branches and supplies a strip of skin on the front of the thigh extending from the sartorius to the knee.

The *medial cutaneous nerve of the thigh* (L2, L3) is a branch of the anterior division of the femoral nerve. It divides into anterior and posterior divisions. The nerve supplies the skin on the medial side of the lower two-thirds of the thigh.

The *saphenous nerve* (L3, L4) is a branch of the posterior division of the femoral nerve. It pierces the deep fascia on the medial side of the knee, runs down in front of the great saphenous vein, and supplies the skin on the medial side of the leg and foot up to the ball of the big toe (*see* Fig. 8.2).

Before piercing the deep fascia the saphenous nerve gives off the *infrapatellar branch* which runs downwards

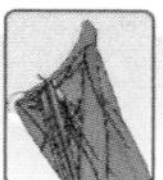

and laterally, and supplies the skin over the ligamentum patellae.

Patellar Plexus

It is a plexus of fine nerves situated in front of the patella, the ligamentum patellae and the upper end of the tibia. It is formed by contributions from:

1 The anterior division of the lateral cutaneous nerve
2 The intermediate cutaneous nerve
3 The anterior division of the medial cutaneous nerve
4 The infrapatellar branch of the saphenous nerve.

Cutaneous Arteries

Three small arteries arising from the femoral artery can be seen a little below the inguinal ligament (Fig. 3.11).

1 *Superficial external pudendal artery* pierces the cribriform fascia, runs medially in front of the spermatic cord, and supplies the external genitalia.
2 *Superficial epigastric artery* pierces the cribriform fascia, runs towards the umbilicus, and supplies the lower part of anterior abdominal wall.
3 *Superficial circumflex iliac artery* pierces the fascia lata lateral to saphenous opening, runs upwards below the inguinal ligament, and anastomoses at the anterior superior iliac spine with deep circumflex iliac, superior gluteal and lateral circumflex femoral arteries.

Great or Long Saphenous Vein

This is the largest and longest superficial vein of the lower limb (*Saphes* = easily seen).

It begins on the dorsum of the foot from the medial end of the dorsal venous arch, and runs upwards in front of the medial malleolus, along the medial side of the leg, and behind the knee. In the thigh, it inclines forwards to reach the saphenous opening where it pierces the cribriform fascia and opens into the femoral vein. Before piercing the cribriform fascia, it receives three named tributaries corresponding to the three cutaneous arteries, and also many unnamed tributaries (*see* Figs 3.4 and 11.1).

Superficial Inguinal Lymph Nodes

The superficial inguinal lymph nodes are variable in their number and size. Their arrangement is T-shaped, there being a lower vertical group and an upper horizontal group. The upper nodes can be subdivided into the upper lateral and upper medial groups (Fig. 3.5).

1 Lower vertical group drains lymph from most of the lower limb.
2 Upper lateral group drains lymph from infra-umbilical part of anterior abdominal wall and gluteal region.

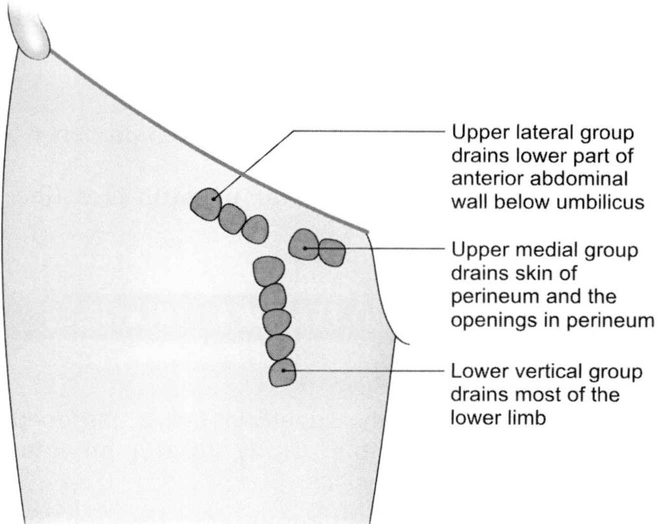

Fig. 3.5: Superficial inguinal lymph nodes

3 Upper medial group drains lymph from external genital organs including the terminal ends of the *urethra, anal canal* and *vagina*.

Subcutaneous Bursae

Bursae are lubricating mechanisms which are provided at sites of friction to smoothen movement. Undue pressure on them may cause their pathological enlargement. Bursae present in relation to the patella are described here (Fig. 3.6).

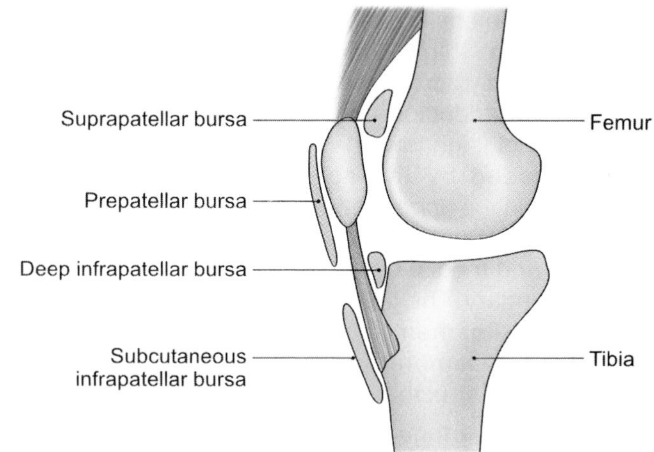

Fig. 3.6: The patellar bursae

Prepatellar Bursa

It lies in front of the lower part of the patella and of the upper part of the ligamentum patellae.

Subcutaneous Infrapatellar Bursa

It lies in front of lower part of the tibial tuberosity and of the lower part of the ligamentum patellae.

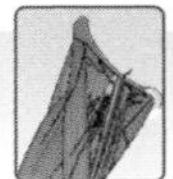

Two deep bursae are also present. These are suprapatellar bursa and deep infrapatellar bursa.

CLINICAL ANATOMY

- Prepatellar bursitis is called "housemaids knee" or miner's knee.
- Subcutaneous infrapatellar bursitis is called "clergyman's knee."

DEEP FASCIA AND FEMORAL TRIANGLE

DISSECTION

After the reflection of the superficial fascia, the deep fascia of thigh is visible. Study its attachments, modifications and extensions.

Follow the great saphenous vein through the cribriform fascia and the anterior wall of femoral sheath into the femoral vein. The femoral vein occupies the intermediate compartment of the femoral sheath. Medial compartment of femoral sheath is the femoral canal occupied by a lymph node while the lateral compartment is occupied by the femoral artery.

Give a vertical incision in the deep fascia of thigh from tubercle of iliac crest till the lateral condyle of femur and remove the deep fascia or fascia lata in lateral part of thigh. This will expose the tensor fasciae latae muscle and gluteus maximus muscle getting attached to iliotibial tract. Identify the four heads of quadriceps femoris muscle.

Remove the entire deep fascia from upper one-third of the front of thigh. Identify the sartorius muscle stretching gently across the thigh from lateral to medial side and the adductor longus muscle extending from medial side of thigh towards lateral side into the femur, being crossed by the sartorius. This triangular depression in the upper one-third of thigh is the femoral triangle. The medial border of sartorius forms lateral boundary and medial border of adductor longus forms medial boundary. The base of this triangle is formed by the inguinal ligament. Dissect its boundaries, and contents, e.g. femoral nerve, artery and vein, and accompanying structures.

Expose the sartorius muscle till its insertion into the upper medial surface of shaft of tibia.

DEEP FASCIA/FASCIA LATA

The fascia lata is a tough fibrous sheath that envelops the whole of the thigh like a sleeve. Its attachments, shown in Fig. 3.7, are as follows:

Superiorly it is attached to the boundary line between the lower limb and the pelvis. Thus anteriorly it is attached to the inguinal ligament; laterally to the iliac

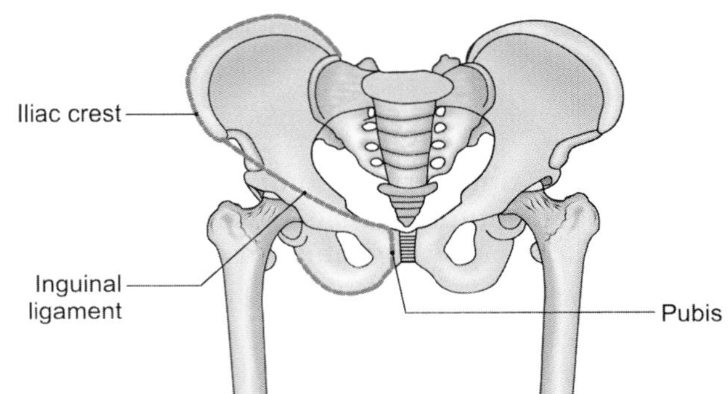

Fig. 3.7: The upper attachments of the fascia lata

crest; posteriorly, through the gluteal fascia to the sacrum, coccyx and sacrotuberous ligament; and medially to the pubis, the pubic arch and the ischial tuberosity.

Inferiorly, on the front and sides of the knee, the fascia lata is attached to subcutaneous bony prominences and the capsule of the knee joint. Posteriorly, it forms the strong popliteal fascia which is continuous below with the fascia of the back of the leg.

Modifications of Fascia Lata

Iliotibial Tract

The fascia lata is thickened laterally where it forms a 5 cm wide band called the iliotibial tract (Fig. 3.8). Superiorly the tract splits into two layers. The superficial lamina is attached to tubercle of iliac crest, and deep lamina to the capsule of hip joint. Inferiorly, the tract is attached to a smooth area on anterior surface of the lateral condyle of tibia. The importance of the iliotibial tract is as follows.

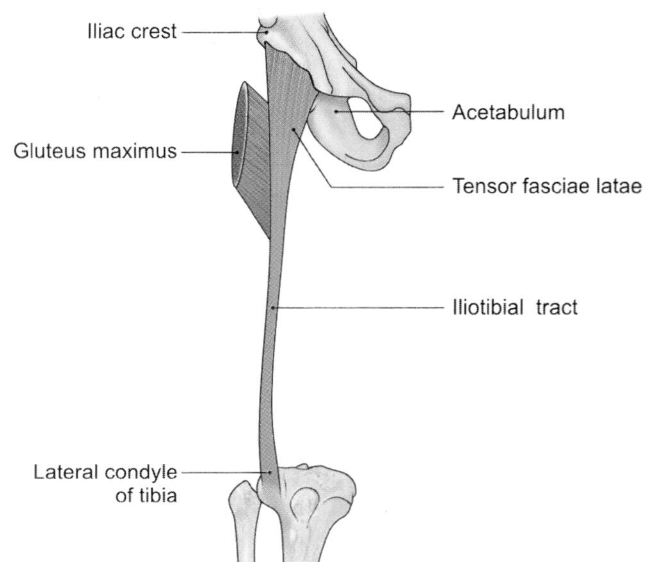

Fig. 3.8: The iliotibial tract with insertion of two muscles

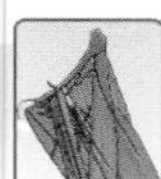

a. Two important muscles are inserted into its upper part, between the superficial and deep laminae. These are the three-fourths part of the *gluteus maximus*; and the *tensor fasciae latae*.

b. The iliotibial tract stabilizes the knee both in extension and in partial flexion; and is, therefore, used constantly during walking and running. In leaning forwards with slightly flexed knees, the tract is the main support of the knee against gravity.

Saphenous Opening

This is an oval opening in the fascia lata. The centre of the opening is 4 cm below and 4 cm lateral to the pubic tubercle. It is about 2.5 cm long and 2 cm broad with its long axis directed downwards and laterally. The opening has a sharp crescentic lateral margin or falciform margin which lies in front of the femoral sheath. The medial well defined margin of the opening lies at a deeper level. It is formed by the fascia overlying the pectineus. The fascia passes behind the femoral sheath (Fig. 3.4).

The saphenous opening is closed by the *cribriform fascia* formed by modification of superficial fascia which covers the opening.

Intermuscular Septa

Three intermuscular septa divide the thigh into three compartments (Fig. 3.9).

The *lateral intermuscular septum* is the thickest of these septa. It extends from the iliotibial tract to the lateral lip of the linea aspera. It separates the anterior compartment of the thigh from the posterior compartment.

The *medial intermuscular septum* is attached to the medial lip of the linea aspera, and separates the anterior compartment of the thigh from the medial compartment.

The *posterior intermuscular septum* is poorly defined. It separates the medial compartment of the thigh from the posterior compartment.

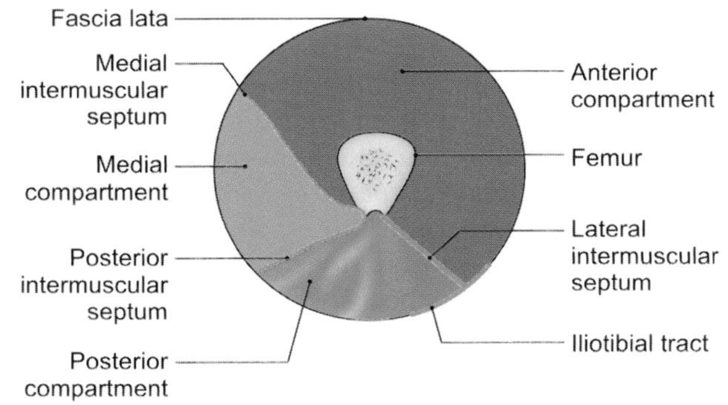

Fig. 3.9: Intermuscular septa and compartments of thigh

CLINICAL ANATOMY

The fascia lata is attached to the inguinal ligament. Extension of the thighs pulls the abdominal wall downwards and makes it tense. To relax the abdomen fully for palpation by an examining physician, the patient is asked to draw the legs up. This overcomes the pull of the fascia lata on the abdominal wall.

FEMORAL TRIANGLE

It is a triangular depression on the front of the upper one-third of the thigh immediately below the inguinal ligament.

Boundaries

The femoral triangle is bounded *laterally* by the medial border of *sartorius*; and *medially* by the medial border of the *adductor longus* (Figs 3.10 to 3.12). Its *base* is formed by the *inguinal ligament*. The *apex*, which is directed downwards, is formed by the point where the medial and lateral boundaries cross.

The apex is continuous, below, with the adductor canal.

The *roof* of the femoral triangle is formed by:

a. Skin.
b. Superficial fascia containing the superficial inguinal lymph nodes, the femoral branch of the genitofemoral nerve, branches of the ilioinguinal nerve, superficial branches of the femoral artery with accompanying veins, and the upper part of the great saphenous vein.
c. *Deep fascia*, with the saphenous opening and the cribriform fascia (Fig. 3.10b).

The *floor* of the triangle is formed medially by the *adductor longus* and *pectineus*, and laterally by the *psoas major* and *iliacus* (Figs 3.10 a and b).

Contents

The contents of the femoral triangle (Fig. 3.11) are as follows:

1 *Femoral artery and its branches:* The femoral artery traverses the triangle from its base at the midinguinal point to the apex. In the triangle, it gives off six branches, three superficial and three deep.

2 *Femoral vein and its tributaries:* The femoral vein accompanies the femoral artery. The vein is medial to the artery at base of triangle, but posteromedial to artery at the apex.

The femoral vein receives the great saphenous vein, circumflex veins and veins corresponding to the branches of femoral artery.

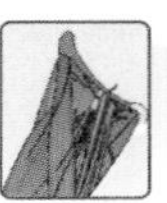

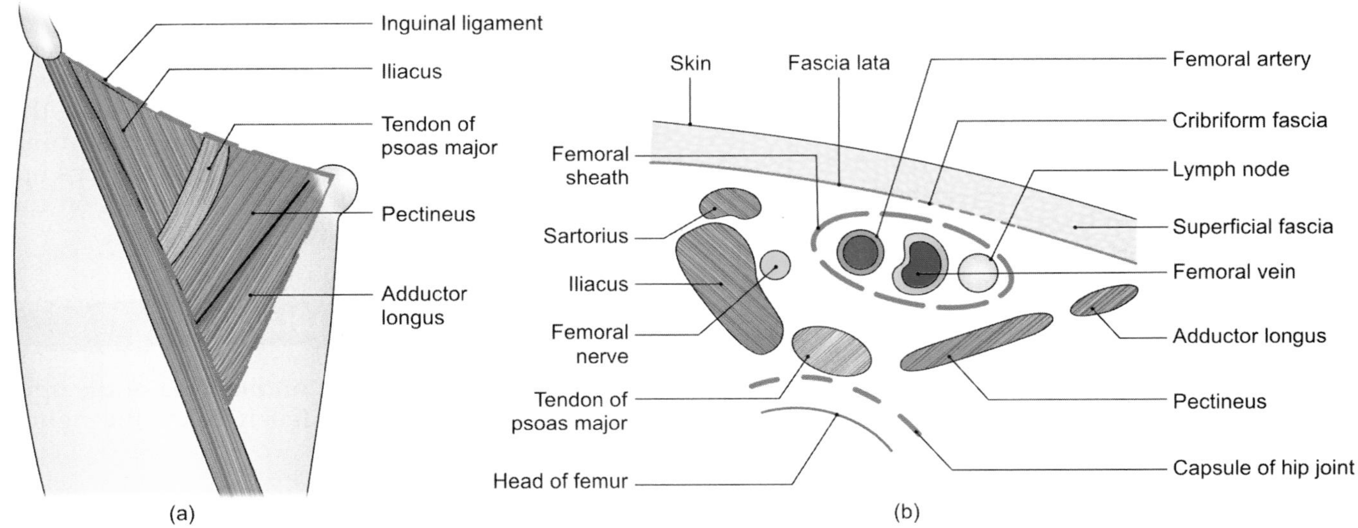

Figs 3.10a and b: Floor of the femoral triangle: (a) Surface view, and (b) sectional view

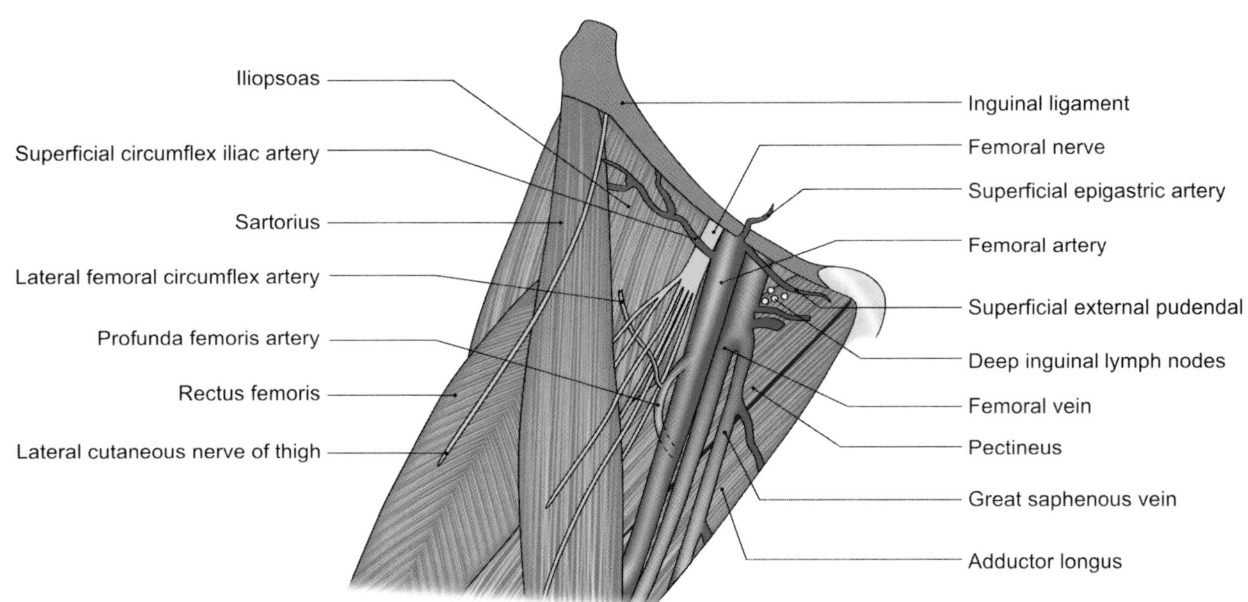

Fig. 3.11: Contents of the right femoral triangle

3 The *femoral sheath* encloses the upper 4 cm of the femoral vessels (Fig. 3.12).

4 *Nerves:*

a. The *femoral nerve* lies lateral to the femoral artery, *outside the femoral sheath,* in the groove between the iliacus and the psoas major muscles. It is described later.

b. The *nerve to the pectineus* arises from the femoral nerve just above the inguinal ligament. It passes behind femoral sheath to reach the anterior surface of pectineus.

c. The *femoral branch of the genitofemoral nerve* occupies the lateral compartment of the femoral sheath along with the femoral artery. It supplies most of the skin over the femoral triangle.

d. The *lateral cutaneous nerve of the thigh* crosses the lateral angle of the triangle. Runs on the lateral side of thigh and ends by dividing into anterior and posterior branches. These supply anterolateral aspect of front of thigh and lateral aspect of gluteal region respectively.

5 The *deep inguinal lymph nodes* lie deep to the deep fascia. These lie medial to upper part of femoral vein

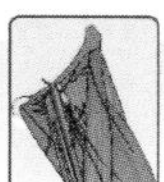

3 Both are supplied by spinal segments L2 and L3. The psoas is supplied by the branches from the nerve roots, whereas the iliacus is supplied by the femoral nerve.

CLINICAL ANATOMY

- *Testing for Quadriceps Femoris:* A person lies supine with one bare lower limb and hip and knee joints partially flexed. The right hand of physician presses the person's right leg downwards. He is requested to straighten the knee against resistance of the physician's right hand, while his left hand feels the contracting quadriceps muscle above the knee (Fig. 3.29).
- Patellar tendon reflex or knee jerk (L3, L4). The knee joint gets extended on tapping the ligamentum patellae (Fig. 3.30).
- Psoas abscess formed due to tubercular infection of lumbar vertebrae can track down between psoas major muscles and its fascia to reach behind the inguinal ligament into the femoral triangle. It may be mistaken for enlarged lymph nodes (Fig. 3.31).
- Intramuscular injection can be given in anterolateral region of thigh in the vastus lateralis muscle (Fig. 3.32).

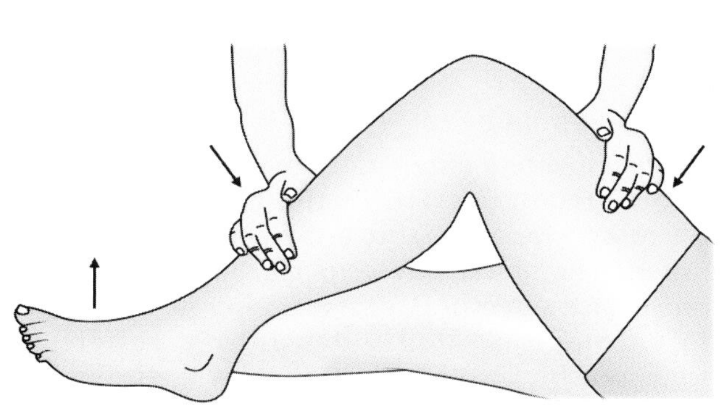

Fig. 3.29: Shows how to test the quadriceps femoris muscle

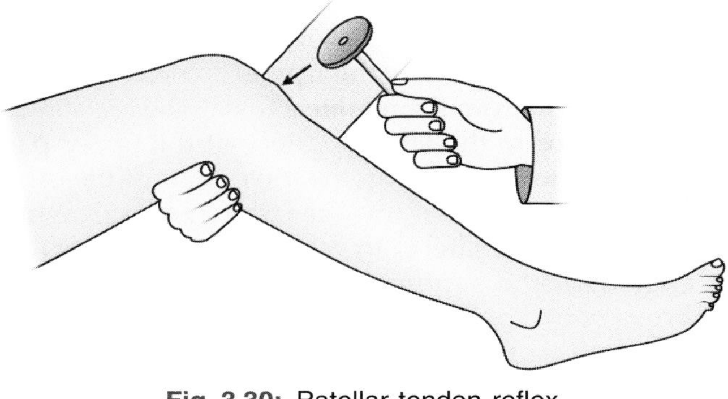

Fig. 3.30: Patellar tendon reflex

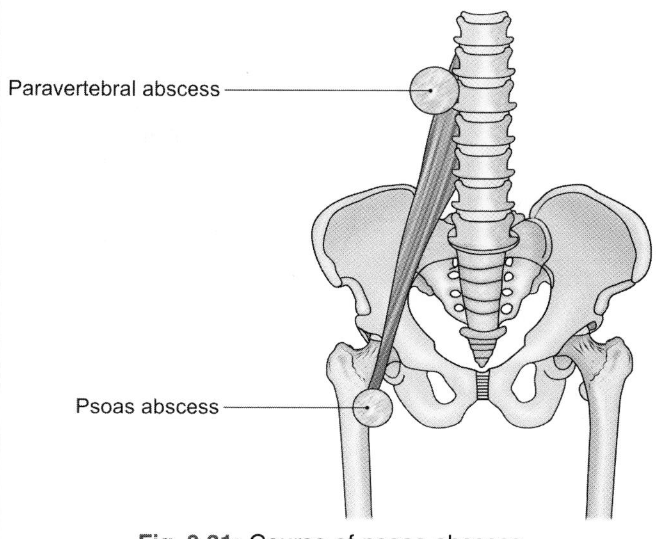

Fig. 3.31: Course of psoas abscess

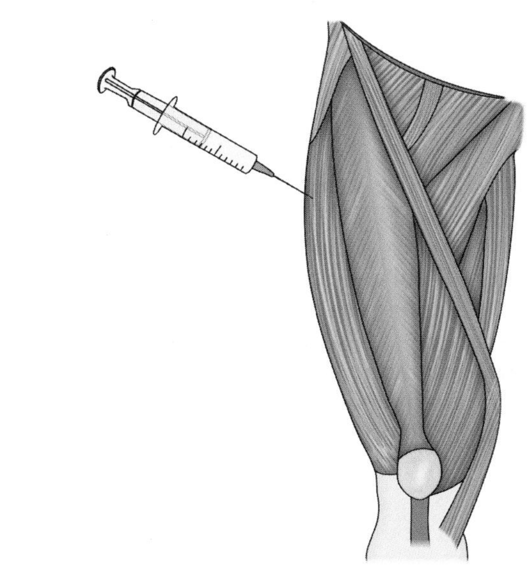

Fig. 3.32: Anterolateral region of thigh

ADDUCTOR/HUNTER'S/SUBSARTORIAL CANAL

DISSECTION

Upper one-third of sartorius forms the lateral boundary of the femoral triangle.

On lifting the middle one-third of sartorius, a part of deep fascia stretching between vastus medialis and adductor muscles is exposed. On longitudinal division of this strong fascia, the adductor canal subsartorial canal/Hunter's canal is visualised (Fig. 3.33).

Dissect its contents, e.g. femoral vessels, saphenous nerve and nerve to vastus medialis, and distal parts of both divisions of obturator nerve.

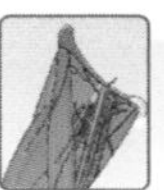

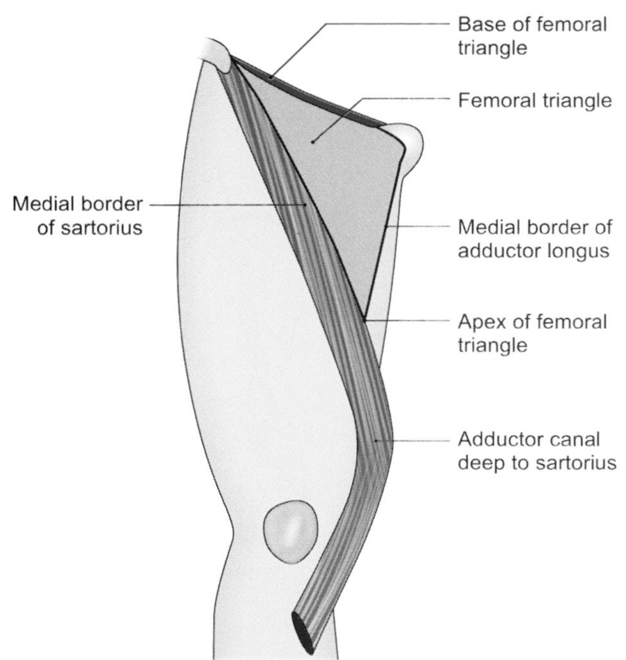

Fig. 3.33: Location of the adductor canal

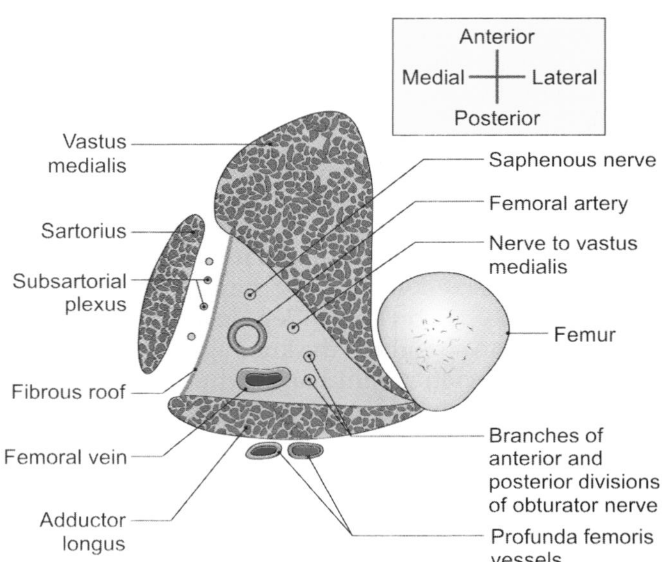

Fig. 3.34: Transverse section through the middle of the right adductor canal, seen from above. Note the boundaries and contents of the canal

Features

This is also called the subsartorial canal or Hunter's canal. John Hunter (1729–93) was an anatomist and surgeon at London. Hunter's operation for the treatment of popliteal aneurysm by ligating the femoral artery in the adductor canal is a landmark in the history of vascular surgery.

The adductor canal is an intermuscular space situated on the medial side of the middle one-third of the thigh (Figs 3.33 and 3.34).

Extent

The canal extends from the apex of the femoral triangle, above, to the tendinous opening in the adductor magnus, below.

Shape

The canal is triangular on cross-section.

Boundaries

- It has anterolateral, posteromedial and medial walls.
- The anterolateral wall is formed by the vastus medialis.
- The posteromedial wall or floor is formed by the adductor longus, above, and the adductor magnus, below.
- The medial wall or roof is formed by a strong fibrous membrane joining the anterolateral and posteromedial walls. The roof is overlapped by the sartorius.

The *subsartorial plexus* of nerves lies on the fibrous roof of the canal under cover of the sartorius. The plexus is formed by branches from the medial cutaneous nerve of the thigh, the saphenous nerve, and the anterior division of the obturator nerve. It supplies the overlying fascia lata and the neighbouring skin.

Contents

These are as follows (Fig. 3.35).

1. The *femoral artery* enters the canal at the apex of the femoral triangle. Within the canal it gives off muscular branches and a descending genicular branch. The *descending genicular artery* is the last branch of the femoral artery arising just above the hiatus magnus. It divides into a superficial saphenous branch that accompanies the saphenous nerve, and a deep muscular branch that enters the vastus medialis and reaches the knee. Femoral artery leaves the adductor canal through the opening in adductor magnus muscle to continue as popliteal artery in the popliteal fossa.
2. Femoral vein begins as the upward continuation of popliteal vein from the popliteal fossa. The *femoral vein* lies posterior to the femoral artery in the upper part, and lateral to the artery in the lower part of the canal.
3. The *saphenous nerve* crosses the femoral artery anteriorly from lateral to medial side. It leaves the canal with the saphenous artery by piercing the fibrous roof.
4. The *nerve* to the *vastus medialis* lies lateral to the femoral artery, and enters the vastus medialis in the upper part of the canal.

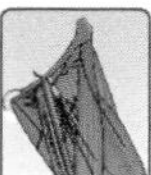

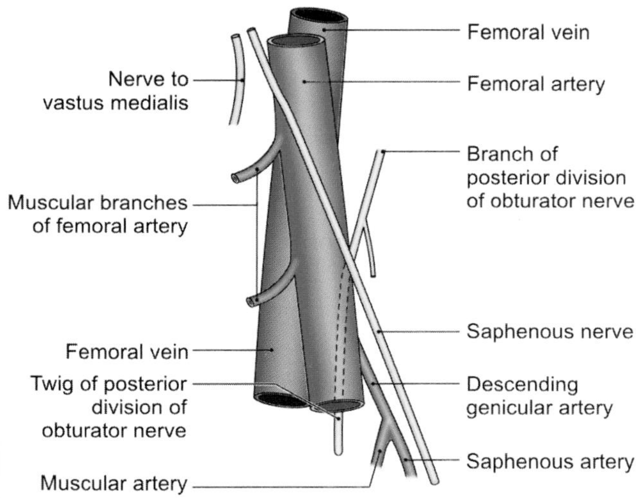

Fig. 3.35: Contents of the adductor canal

5 *Branches of two divisions of obturator nerve:* The anterior division emerges at the lower border of the adductor longus, gives branches to the subsartorial plexus, and ends by supplying the femoral artery. The posterior division of the obturator nerve runs on the anterior surface of the adductor magnus, accompanies the femoral and popliteal arteries, and ends by supplying the knee joint (Fig. 3.34).

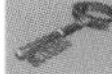

FACTS TO REMEMBER

- Sartorius is the longest muscle of the body.
- Saphenous is the longest cutaneous nerve.
- Femoral hernia is common in female, while inguinal hernia is common in male
- Embalming for preservation of the dead body is also done through femoral artery
- Insertion of vastus medialis extends to lower level on patella than that of vastus lateralis to stabilise the patella.

CLINICOANATOMICAL PROBLEM

A 50-year-old woman complained of a swelling in upper medial side of her right thigh, when she coughs.
- Where is the swelling and why does it appear when she coughs?
- What is the position of the swelling in relation to pubic tubercle?

Ans: The swelling is the femoral hernia which appears at saphenous opening when she coughs due to raised intra-abdominal pressure. The swelling is inferolateral to the pubic tubercle. The femoral hernia is more common in females due to larger pelvis, larger femoral canal and smaller femoral vessels.

MULTIPLE CHOICE QUESTIONS

1. Which is longest superficial vein of lower limb?
   a. Long saphenous
   b. Femoral
   c. Popliteal
   d. None of the above
2. Which of these pair of muscle are inserted into upper part of iliotibial tract?
   a. Gluteus maximus and tensor fasciae latae
   b. Gluteus maximus and pectineus
   c. Pectineus and tensor fasciae latae
   d. Adductor longus and pectineus
3. Iliotibial tract stabilizes knee in:
   a. Extension b. Partial flexion
   c. Both a and b d. None of above
4. Which one of the following make lateral boundary of femoral triangle?
   a. Inguinal ligament
   b. Adductor longus
   c. Medial border of sartorius muscle
   d. Pectineus
5. Femoral artery is the continuation of which artery?
   a. Popliteal
   b. External iliac
   c. Profunda femoris
   d. Obturator
6. Medial boundary of femoral ring is formed by:
   a. Inguinal ligament
   b. Pectineus
   c. Lacunar ligament
   d. Femoral vein
7. Which is the largest branch of femoral artery?
   a. Superficial external pudendal
   b. Superficial epigastric
   c. Deep external pudendal
   d. Profunda femoris artery
8. Which is not a part of quadriceps femoris?
   a. Rectus femoris
   b. Vastus medialis
   c. Sartorius
   d. Vastus lateralis

9. Which muscles have common insertion on lesser trochanter of femur?
   a. Iliacus and psoas major
   b. Pectineus and adductor longus
   c. Psoas major and Pectineus
   d. None of these
10. A femoral hernia is more common in female due to:
   a. Wider pelvis
   b. Smaller size of femoral vessel
   c. Femoral canal is wider
   d. All of above
11. Which region of thigh is preferred to give intramuscular injection in children?
   a. Anterolateral
   b. Anteromedial
   c. Posterolateral
   d. Posteromedial
12. Which vein is commonly used for intravenous infusions in children?
   a. Femoral
   b. Long saphenous
   c. Popliteal
   d. Short saphenous

ANSWERS

1. a	2. a	3. c	4. c	5. b	6. c	7. d	8. c	9. a	10. d	11. a	12. a

4

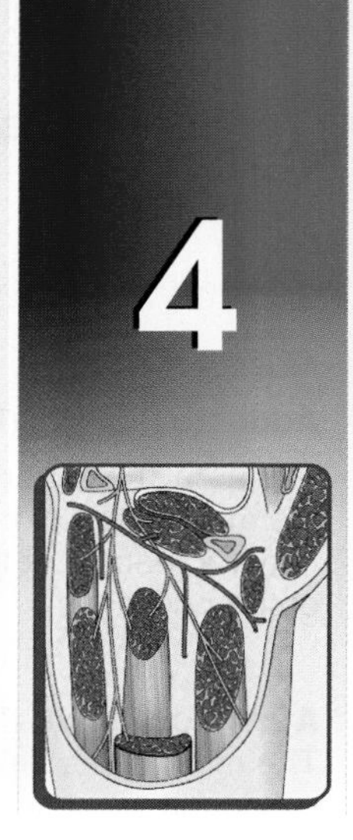

Medial Side of Thigh

We make a living by what we get, but we make a life by what we give.

INTRODUCTION

The adductor or medial compartment of thigh is very well developed and is derived, as indicated by its nerve supply from both the flexors and extensors between which it lies. Its counterpart in the arm is represented only by coracobrachialis muscle, as the arm can be adducted by pectoralis major and latissimus dorsi muscles.

ADDUCTOR COMPARTMENT

DISSECTION

The triangular adductor longus was seen to form the medial boundary of femoral triangle (*see* Fig. 3.11). Cut this muscle 3 cm below its origin and reflect the distal part laterally. On its deep surface, identify the anterior division of obturator nerve which supplies both adductor longus and gracilis muscles.

Lateral to adductor longus on the same plane is the pectineus muscle. Cut it close to its origin and reflect laterally, tracing the branch of anterior division of obturator nerve to this muscle. Obturator nerve is accompanied by the branches of obturator artery and medial circumflex femoral arteries.

Deeper to adductor longus and pectineus is the adductor brevis. Look for its nerve supply either from anterior/posterior division.

Divide adductor brevis close to its origin. Deepest plane of muscles comprises adductor magnus (Fig. 4.2) and obturator externus, both supplied by posterior division of obturator nerve.

Lying vertically along the medial side of thigh is the graceful gracilis. Study these muscles and the course of obturator nerve.

Look for accessory obturator nerve. If present, it supplies pectineus.

Lastly, remove the obturator externus from its origin to expose the obturator artery and its branches.

BOUNDARIES

The adductor or medial compartment of the thigh is bounded anteriorly by the medial intermuscular septum which separates it from the extensor (anterior) compartment; and posteriorly by an ill-defined posterior intermuscular septum which separates it from the flexor (posterior) compartment (*see* Fig. 3.9).

The structures to be studied in this region are muscles, nerves and arteries. These are as follows.

Muscles

Intrinsic

1 Adductor longus
2 Adductor brevis
3 Adductor magnus
4 Gracilis
5 Pectineus.

Extrinsic

The obturator externus lies deep in this region. It is functionally related to the gluteal region.

Nerves

1 Obturator nerve.
2 Accessory obturator nerve.

Arteries

1 Obturator artery.
2 Medial circumflex femoral artery.

MUSCLES OF ADDUCTOR COMPARTMENT OF THIGH

The attachments of the muscles are given in Table 4.1. Their nerve supply and actions are given in Table 4.2.

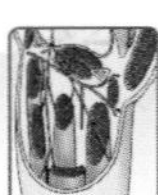

Table 4.1: Muscles of the medial compartment of thigh

Muscle	*Origin from*	*Insertion into*
Adductor longus (Fig. 4.1) This is a triangular muscle, forming the medial part of the floor of the femoral triangle. It lies in the plane of the pectineus	It arises by a narrow, flat tendon from the front of the body of the pubis in the angle between the pubic crest and the pubic symphysis. Sometimes sesamoid bone is seen near its origin (rider's bone)	The linea aspera in middle one-third of the shaft of the femur between the vastus medialis and the adductor brevis and magnus (Fig. 4.2a)
Adductor brevis (Fig. 4.1) The muscle lies behind the pectineus and adductor longus	a. Anterior surface of body of the pubis b. Outer surface of inferior ramus of the pubis between the gracilis and obturator externus c. Outer surface of ramus of the ischium between gracilis and the adductor magnus	Line extending from the lesser trochanter to upper part of linea aspera, behind the upper part of adductor longus (Fig. 4.2a)
Adductor magnus (Fig. 4.1) This is the largest muscle of this compartment. Because of its double nerve supply, it is called a hybrid muscle	a. Inferolateral part of the ischial tuberosity b. Ramus of the ischium c. Lower part of inferior ramus of the pubis	a. Medial margin of gluteal tuberosity b. Linea aspera c. Medial supracondylar line d. Adductor tubercle
Gracilis (Fig. 4.1) (Greek *slender*)	a. Medial margin of the lower half of the body of the pubis b. Inferior ramus of the pubis c. Adjoining part of the ramus of the ischium	Upper part of the medial surface of tibia behind the sartorius and in front of the semitendinosus (Fig. 4.2b)
Pectineus (*see* Figs 3.11 and 4.1) This is flat, quadrilateral muscle It forms a part of the floor of the femoral triangle	a. Pecten pubis b. Upper half of the pectineal surface of superior ramus of the pubis c. Fascia covering the pectineus	Line extending from lesser trochanter to the linea aspera

Table 4.2: Nerve supply and actions of muscles

Muscle	*Nerve supply*	*Actions*
Adductor longus	Anterior division of obturator nerve	Powerful adductor of thigh at hip joint These act as posture controllers
Adductor brevis	Anterior or posterior division of obturator nerve	Adductor longus, adductor brevis help in adduction and flexion of thigh
Adductor magnus (hybrid muscle)	Double nerve supply: Adductor part by posterior division of obturator nerve Hamstring part by tibial part of sciatic nerve	Adductor part causes adduction of thigh and hamstring part helps in extension of hip and flexion of knee
Gracilis	Anterior division of obturator nerve	Flexor and medial rotator of thigh. It is a weak adductor of thigh. It is used for transplantation of any damaged muscles
Pectineus (hybrid or composite muscle)	Double nerve supply: Anterior fibres by femoral nerve Posterior fibres by anterior division of obturator nerve	Flexor of thigh Adductor of thigh

The obturator externus is described in Chapter 5 (*see* also Tables 5.1 and 5.2).

RELATIONS OF ADDUCTOR LONGUS

The relations of the adductor longus are important. They are as follows.

Anterior Surface

1 Spermatic cord
2 Great saphenous vein with fascia lata
3 Femoral vessels
4 Sartorius (Fig. 4.3).

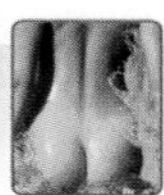

Table 5.2: Nerve supply and actions of muscles

Muscle	*Nerve supply*	*Actions*
Gluteus maximus	Inferior gluteal nerve (L5, S1, S2)	Chief extensor of the thigh at the hip joint. This action is very important in rising from a sitting position. It is essential for maintaining the erect posture. Other actions are: a. Lateral rotation of the thigh b. Abduction of the thigh (by upper fibres) c. Along with the tensor fasciae latae the muscle stabilises the knee through the iliotibial tract. It supports both the hip and the knee when these joints are slightly flexed. It is an antigravity muscle as well.
Gluteus medius **Gluteus minimus**	Superior gluteal nerve (L4, L5, S1) Superior gluteal nerve (L4, L5, S1)	The *gluteus medius* and *gluteus minimus* are: Powerful abductors of the thigh. Their anterior fibres are also medial rotators. However, their most important action is to maintain the balance of the body when the opposite foot is off the ground, as in walking and running. They do this by preventing the opposite side of the pelvis from tilting downwards under the influence of gravity.
Piriformis	Ventral rami of S1, S2	Lateral rotators of thigh at the hip joint
Gemellus superior	Nerve to obturator internus (L5, S1, S2)	
Gemellus inferior	Nerve to quadratus femoris (L4, L5, S1)	
Obturator internus	Nerve to obturator internus (L5, S1, S2)	
Quadratus femoris	Nerve to quadratus femoris (L4, L5, S1)	
Obturator externus	Posterior division of obturator nerve (L2, L3, L4)	
Tensor fasciae latae	Superior gluteal nerve (L4, L5, S1)	Abductor and medial rotator of thigh and an extensor of knee joint

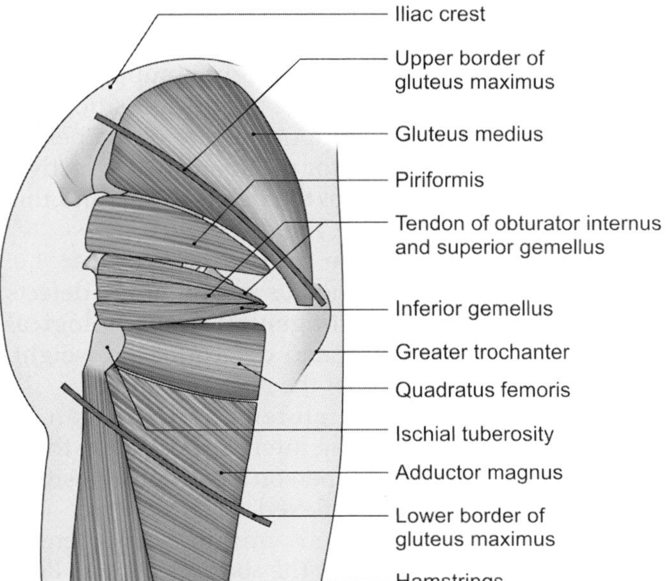

Fig. 5.5: Muscles under cover of the gluteus maximus. The upper and lower borders of this muscle are indicated in thick lines

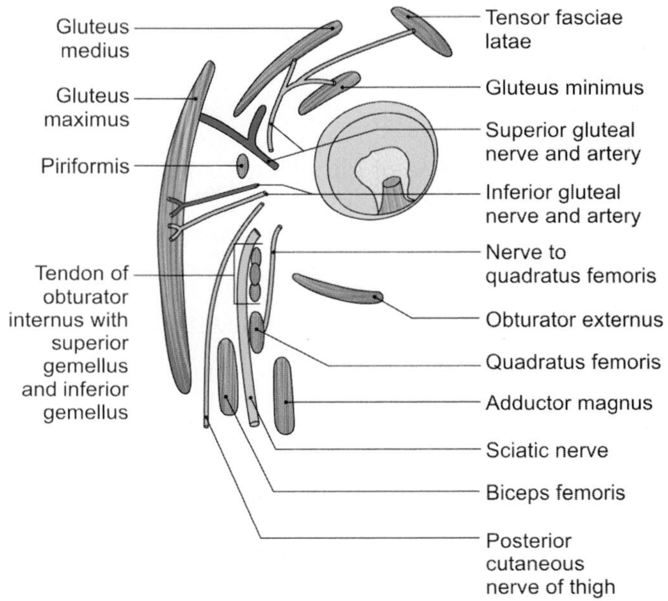

Fig. 5.6: Scheme of an oblique vertical section showing muscles of the gluteal region. Structures under cover of the gluteus maximus

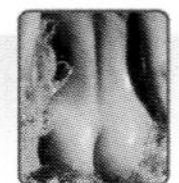

Vessels

1 Superior gluteal vessels (Fig. 5.6).
2 Inferior gluteal vessels.
3 Internal pudendal vessels.
4 Ascending branch of the medial circumflex femoral artery.
5 Trochanteric anastomoses (described with arteries of gluteal region).
6 Cruciate anastomoses (described with arteries of gluteal region).
7 The first perforating artery.

Nerves

1 Superior gluteal (L4, L5, S1) as in Fig. 5.6.
2 Inferior gluteal (L5, S1, S2).
3 Sciatic (L4, S5, S1, S2, S3).
4 Posterior cutaneous nerve of thigh (S1, S2, S3).
5 Nerve to the quadratus femoris (L4, L5, S1).
6 Pudendal nerve (S2, S3, S4).
7 Nerve to the obturator internus (L5, S1, S2).
8 Perforating cutaneous nerves (S2, S3).

Bones and Joints

1 Ilium.
2 Ischium with ischial tuberosity.
3 Upper end of femur with the greater trochanter.
4 Sacrum and coccyx.
5 Hip joint.
6 Sacroiliac joint.

Ligaments

1 Sacrotuberous.
2 Sacrospinous.
3 Ischiofemoral.

Bursae

1 Trochanteric bursa of gluteus maximus.
2 Bursa over the ischial tuberosity.
3 Bursa between the gluteus maximus and vastus lateralis.

STRUCTURES DEEP TO THE GLUTEUS MEDIUS

The gluteus medius covers:

- The superior gluteal nerve,
- The deep branch of the superior gluteal artery,
- The gluteus minimus,
- The trochanteric bursa of the gluteus medius.

STRUCTURES DEEP TO THE GLUTEUS MINIMUS

Structures lying deep to the gluteus minimus include the reflected head of the rectus femoris, and the capsule of the hip joint.

CLINICAL ANATOMY

- Testing gluteus maximus the patient lies prone. The right hand of physician presses the patient's right leg downwards. Patient is requested to extend his hip against resistance provided by the physician's right hand; while his left hand feels the contracting gluteus maximus muscle (Fig. 5.7).
- *When the gluteus maximus is paralysed* as in muscular dystrophy, the patient cannot stand up from a sitting posture without support. Such patients, while trying to stand up, rise gradually, supporting their hands first on legs and then on the thighs; they climb on themselves (Fig. 5.8).
- *Intramuscular injections* are given in the anterosuperior quadrant of the gluteal region, i.e. in the glutei medius and minimus, to avoid injury to large vessels and nerves which pass through the lower part of this region (Fig. 5.9). Gluteal region is not the prominence of the buttock only. It is a very big area over the iliac bone.
- *When the glutei medius and minimus (of right side) are paralysed,* the patient cannot walk normally. He bends or waddles on the right side or paralysed side to clear the opposite foot, i.e. left, off the ground. This is known as *lurching gait;* when bilateral, it is called *waddling gait* (Fig. 5.10).
- The normal gait depends on the proper abductor mechanism at both hips (Fig. 5.11). This mechanism comprises:
  a. The adequate power, provided by the glutei medius and minimus (Figs 5.12a to c).
  b. The fulcrum, formed by a normal relationship of the head of the femur with the acetabulum.
  c. The weight transmitted by the head and neck of the femur.
- Normally when the body weight is supported on one limb, the glutei of the supported side raise the opposite and unsupported side of the pelvis. However, if the abductor mechanism is defective, the unsupported side of the pelvis drops, and this is known as a positive *Trendelenburg's sign.*

  The sign is positive in defects of power, i.e. paralysis of the glutei medius and minimus; defects of the fulcrum, i.e. congenital or pathological dislocation of the hip; and defects of the weight, i.e. ununited fracture of the neck of femur.
- Gluteus medius and gluteus minimus can be tested together by doing internal rotation of thigh against resistance. The person is in supine position with the hip and knee flexed.
- Gluteus medius, gluteus minimus and tensor fasciae latae are tested by the abducting lower limb against resistance. The person in the supine position and the knee is extended (Fig. 5.13).

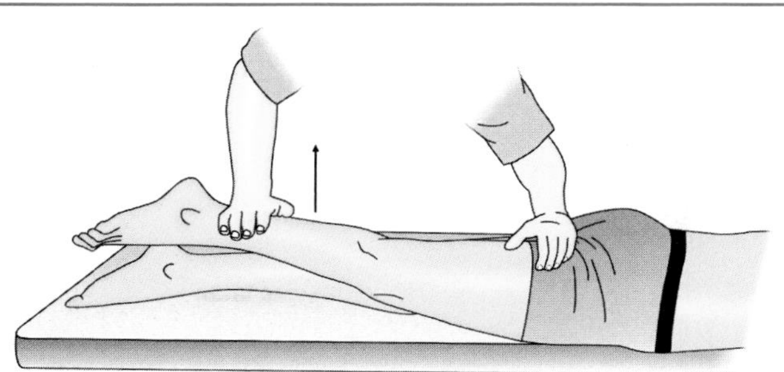
Fig. 5.7: How to test the gluteus maximus

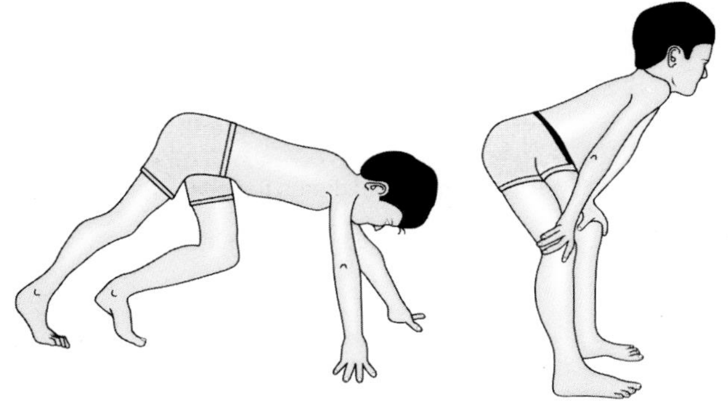
Fig. 5.8: Trying to stand up in paralysis of gluteus maximus muscle

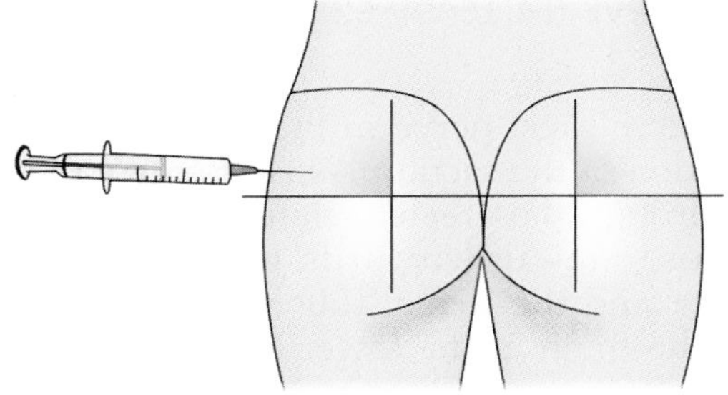
Fig. 5.9: Site of intramuscular injection

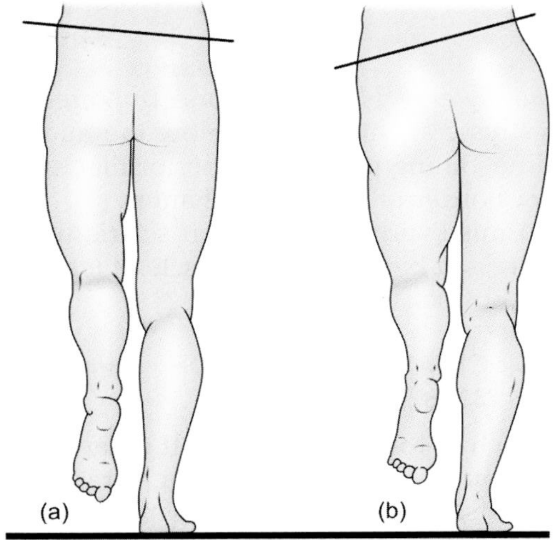

Figs 5.10a and b: (a) Normal gait, and (b) lurching gait

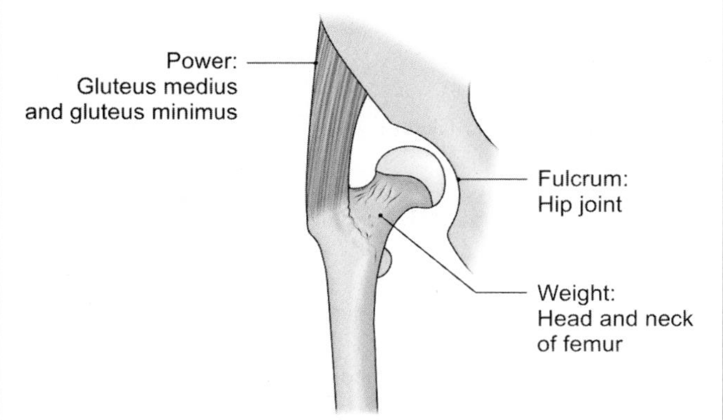

Fig. 5.11: Abductor mechanism at the hip joint

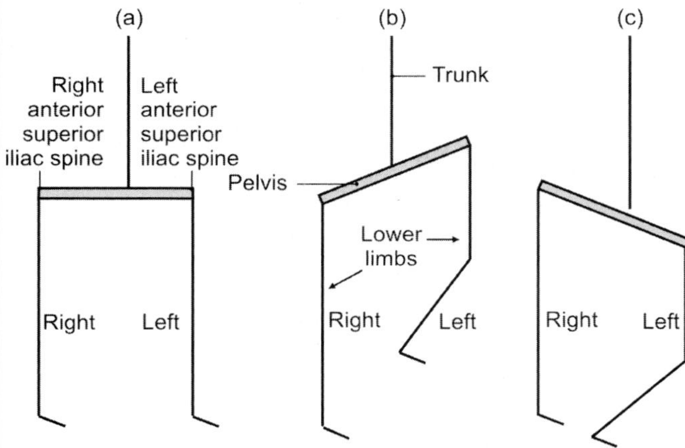

Figs 5.12a to c: Trendelenburg's sign. (a) When both feet are supporting the body weight, the pelvis (anterior superior iliac spine) on the two sides lies in the same horizontal plane, (b) when only the right foot is supporting the body weight, the unsupported side of the pelvis is normally raised by the opposite gluteal medius and minimus, and (c) if the right glutei medius and minimus are paralysed, the unsupported left side of the pelvis drops. This is a positive Trendelenburg's sign

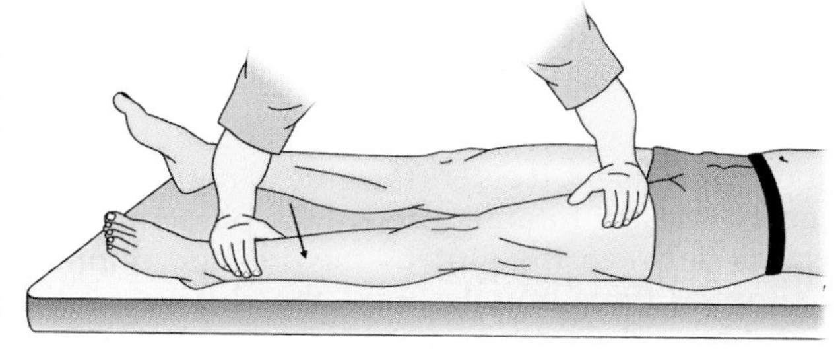
Fig. 5.13: How to test the gluteus medius

SACROTUBEROUS AND SACROSPINOUS LIGAMENTS

These two ligaments convert the greater and lesser sciatic notches of the hip bone into foramina of the same name.

The *sacrotuberous ligament* is a long and strong ligament extending between the medial margin of

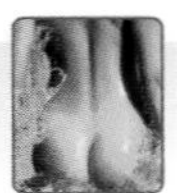

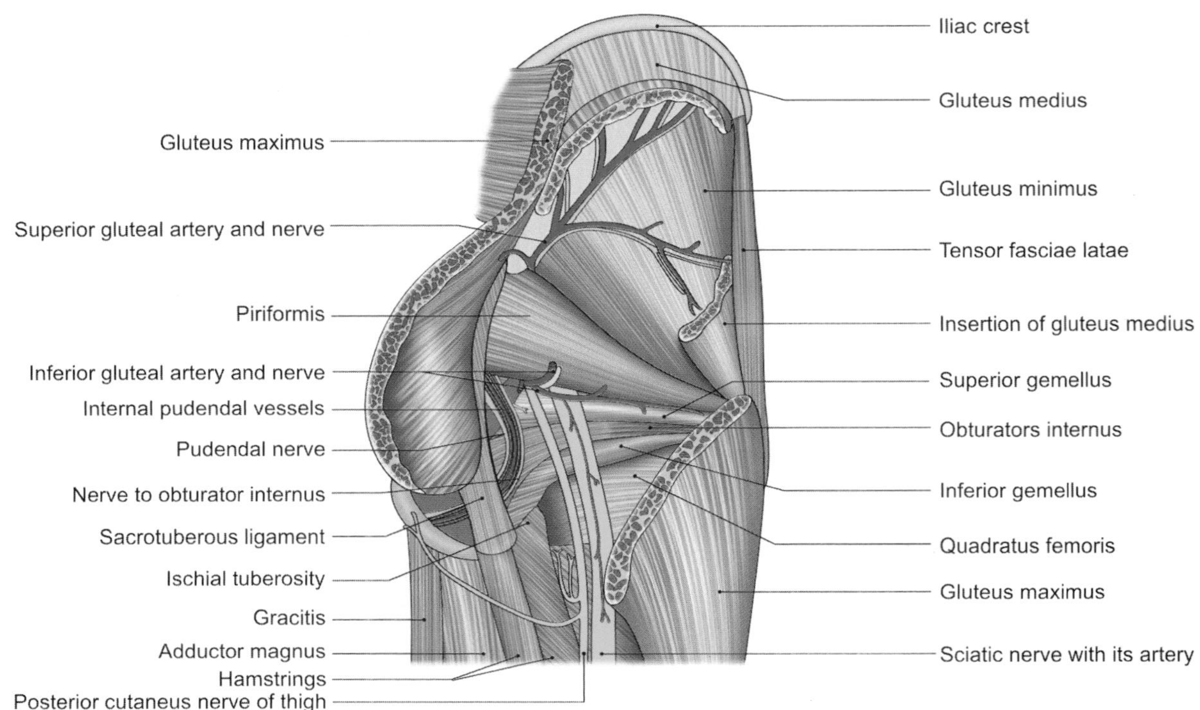

Fig. 5.14: Structures in the gluteal region

ischial tuberosity and the posterior iliac spines. It forms the posterolateral boundary of the outlet of the pelvis (Fig. 5.14).

The *sacrospinous ligament* is a short, thick, triangular band situated deep to the sacrotuberous ligament. It is attached:

a. Laterally to the ischial spine
b. Medially to the sacrococcygeal junction.

NERVES OF THE GLUTEAL REGION

SUPERIOR GLUTEAL NERVE (L4, L5, S1)

The superior gluteal nerve is a branch of the lumbosacral plexus. It enters the gluteal region through the greater sciatic foramen, above the piriformis, runs forwards between the gluteus medius and minimus, and supplies three muscles, viz., the gluteus medius, the gluteus minimus and the tensor fasciae latae (Fig. 5.14).

INFERIOR GLUTEAL NERVE (L5, S1, S2)

This is also a branch of the sacral plexus given off in the pelvis. It enters the gluteal region through the greater sciatic foramen below the piriformis, and ends by supplying the gluteus maximus only, to which it is fully committed (Fig. 5.14).

SCIATIC NERVE (L4, L5; S1, S2, S3)

Course

This is the thickest nerve in the body. It is the main continuation of the sacral plexus. It enters the gluteal region through the greater sciatic foramen below the piriformis, runs downwards between the greater trochanter and the ischial tuberosity, and enters the back of the thigh at the lower border of the gluteus maximus. It does not give any branches in the gluteal region (Fig. 5.14).

It is described in detail in Chapter 7.

CLINICAL ANATOMY

- *"Sciatic nerve block"* is done by injecting an anaesthetic agent few cm below the midpoint of the line joining posterior superior iliac spine and upper border of greater trochanter.
- Piriformis syndrome occurs if sciatic nerve gets compressed by piriformis muscle. It leads to pain in the buttock.

POSTERIOR CUTANEOUS NERVE OF THE THIGH (S1, S2, S3)

It is a branch of the sacral plexus. It enters the gluteal region through the greater sciatic foramen, below the piriformis, and runs downwards medial or posterior to the sciatic nerve. It continues in the back of the thigh immediately deep to the deep fascia (Figs 5.6 and 5.14).

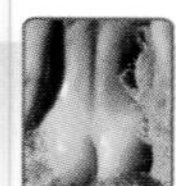

The nerve gives:

a. A perineal branch which crosses the ischial tuberosity, enters the urogenital triangle of the perineum, and supplies the skin of the posterior two-thirds of the scrotum, or labium majus.
b. Gluteal branches which wind upwards round the lower border of the gluteus maximus, and supply the skin of the posteroinferior quadrant of the gluteal region.

NERVE TO QUADRATUS FEMORIS (L4, L5, S1)

This nerve arises from the sacral plexus, enters the gluteal region through the greater sciatic foramen below the piriformis, and runs downwards deep to the sciatic nerve, the obturator internus and the gemelli. It supplies the quadratus femoris, the gemellus inferior and the hip joint (Fig. 5.9).

PUDENDAL NERVE (S2, S3, S4)

This is a branch of the sacral plexus. Only a small part of this nerve is seen in the gluteal region. It enters this region through the greater sciatic foramen. It then crosses the apex or lateral end of the sacrospinous ligament, medial to the internal pudendal vessels. It leaves the gluteal region by passing into the lesser sciatic foramen through which it enters the ischioanal fossa (Fig. 5.14).

NERVE TO THE OBTURATOR INTERNUS (L5, S1, S2)

This is a branch of the sacral plexus. It enters the gluteal region through the greater sciatic foramen and crosses the ischial spine, lateral to the internal pudendal vessels, to re-enter the pelvis. It supplies both the obturator internus and the gemellus superior muscles.

PERFORATING CUTANEOUS NERVE (S2, S3)

This is a branch of the sacral plexus. It pierces the lower part of the sacrotuberous ligament, winds round the lower border of the gluteus maximus, and supplies the skin of the posteroinferior quadrant of the gluteal region.

ARTERIES OF GLUTEAL REGION

SUPERIOR GLUTEAL ARTERY

It is a branch of the posterior division of the internal iliac artery.

Course and Distribution

It enters the gluteal region through the greater sciatic foramen passing above the piriformis along with the superior gluteal nerve. In the foramen, it divides into superficial and deep branches. The *superficial branch* supplies the gluteus maximus (Figs 5.6 and 5.14).

The *deep branch* subdivides into superior and inferior branches, which run along the anterior and inferior gluteal lines respectively, between the gluteus medius and the gluteus minimus. The superior division ends at the anterior superior iliac spine by anastomosing with the ascending branch of the lateral circumflex femoral artery. The inferior division takes part in the trochanteric anastomoses.

INFERIOR GLUTEAL ARTERY

It is a branch of the anterior division of the internal iliac artery.

Course and Distribution

It enters the gluteal region by passing through the greater sciatic foramen, below the piriformis, along with the inferior gluteal nerve. It supplies:

1 *Muscular branches* to gluteus maximus and to all the muscles deep to it below the piriformis.
2 *Cutaneous branches* to the buttock and the back of the thigh (Figs 5.6 and 5.14).
3 An *articular branch* to the hip joint.
4 A *cruciate anastomotic branch.*
5 An *artery to the sciatic nerve,* which represents the axis artery in this region, and may at times be quite large.
6 A *coccygeal branch* which supplies the area over the coccyx.

INTERNAL PUDENDAL ARTERY

This is a branch of the anterior division of the internal iliac artery.

It enters the gluteal region through the greater sciatic foramen (Fig. 5.14). It has a very short course in the gluteal region.

It crosses the ischial spine and leaves the gluteal region by passing into the lesser sciatic foramen through which it reaches the ischioanal fossa.

TROCHANTERIC ANASTOMOSES

This is situated near the trochanteric fossa, and supplies branches to the head of the femur. It is shown in Flow chart 5.1.

CRUCIATE ANASTOMOSES

This anastomosis is situated over the upper part of the back of the femur at the level of the middle of the lesser trochanter. It is shown in Flow chart 5.2.

STRUCTURES PASSING THROUGH THE GREATER SCIATIC FORAMEN (GATEWAY OF GLUTEAL REGION)

1 The piriformis, emerging from the pelvis fills the foramen almost completely. It is the key muscle of the region.

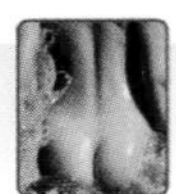

Flow chart 5.1: Trochanteric anastomoses

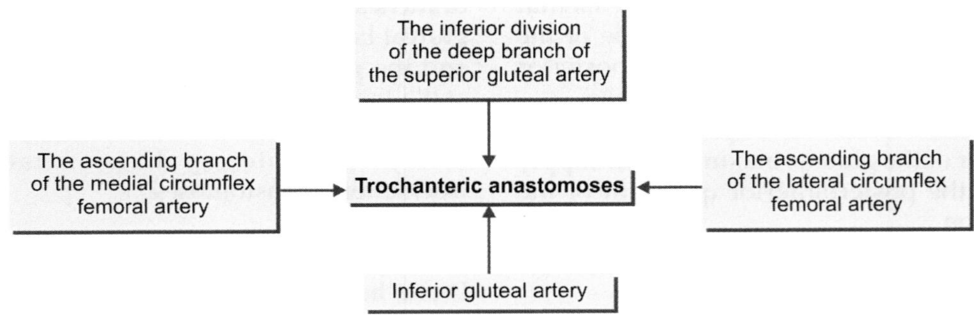

Flow chart 5.2: Cruciate anastomoses

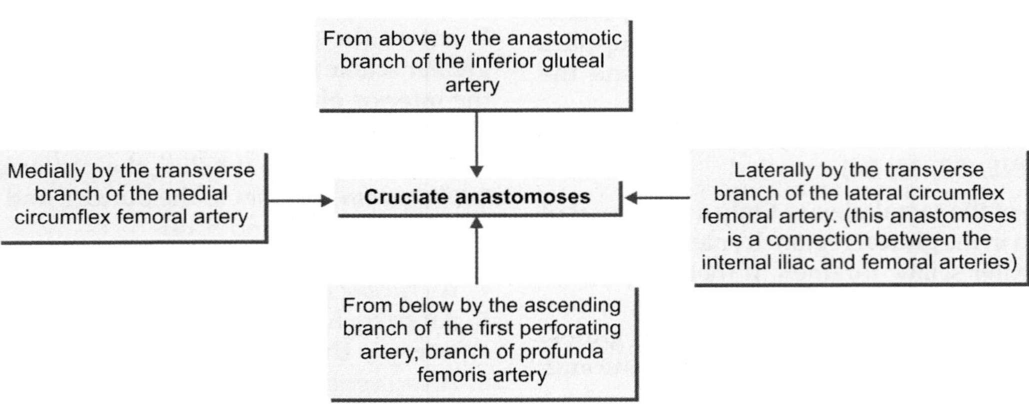

2 Structures passing above the piriformis are:
 a. Superior gluteal nerve.
 b. Superior gluteal vessels (Fig. 5.14).

3 Structures passing below the piriformis are:
 a. Inferior gluteal nerve.
 b. Inferior gluteal vessels.
 c. Sciatic nerve (Fig. 5.14).
 d. Posterior cutaneous nerve of thigh.
 e. Nerve to quadratus femoris.
 f. Pudendal nerve.
 g. Internal pudendal vessels.
 h. Nerve to obturator internus.

The last three structures, after a short course in the gluteal region, enter the lesser sciatic foramen, where the pudendal nerve and internal pudendal vessels run in the pudendal canal.

STRUCTURES PASSING THROUGH THE LESSER SCIATIC FORAMEN

1 Tendon of obturator internus.
2 Pudendal nerve (Fig. 5.14).
3 Internal pudendal vessels.
4 Nerve to obturator internus.

The upper and lower parts of the foramen are filled up by the origins of the two gemelli muscles.

FACTS TO REMEMBER

- Gluteus maximus is the antigravity, postural thickest muscle of the body. It contains red fibres.
- Sciatic nerve is the thickest nerve of the body.
- Intramuscular injections are given in the upper and lateral quadrant of the gluteal region.
- Greater sciatic notch is the gateway of the gluteal region
- Sciatic nerve and pudendal nerve do not supply any structure in the gluteal region.
- Piriformis is the key muscle of the gluteal region.
- Sciatic nerve and its branches supply the hamstring muscles, muscles of all the three compartments of the leg and the muscles of the sole.
- Sciatic nerve is accompanied by a thin artery, the sciatic artery, which is part of the axial artery of the lower limb.
- Lesser sciatic foramen is the gateway of the perineal region.
- Sciatic nerve lies on the femur for a very short distance between lower border of quadratus femoris and upper border of adductor magnus muscles. At this site it may get compressed when one sits on a stool or a bench; leading to harmless condition, the sleeping foot.

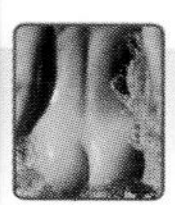

CLINICOANATOMICAL PROBLEM

A woman of 30 years complained of pain in her elbow joints. She also has pain in her calf muscles, and was advised "Neurobion injections".

Where should the injection be given and why?

Ans: The "neurobion injections" are to be given by intramuscular route. The site of the injection is upper lateral quadrant of the gluteal region. Gluteal region is a big region extending along the iliac crest till the midline posteriorly. It extends below on the ischial tuberosity and laterally till the greater trochanter of femur. The upper lateral quadrant is safe as there are no important nerve or blood vessel here. The lower and medial quadrant contains sciatic nerve and must be avoided. The injection is given in big gluteus medius muscle and is well absorbed in the circulating system.

MULTIPLE CHOICE QUESTIONS

1. Intramuscular injections in upper and lateral quadrant of gluteal region are given in:
   a. Glutei maximus and minimus
   b. Gluteus medius
   c. Glutei maximus and erector spinae
   d. Gluteus maximus

2. Lurching gait is due to paralysis of which two muscles?
   a. Glutei medius and minimus
   b. Glutei maximus and minimus
   c. Glutei maximus and medius
   d. Gluteus maximus

3. Which muscle is not under cover of gluteus maximus?
   a. Piriformis
   b. Quadratus femoris
   c. Sartorius
   d. Obturator internus with two gemelli

4. What is origin of piriformis?
   a. From upper three sacral vertebrae
   b. Lower margin of lesser sciatic notch
   c. Upper margin of lesser sciatic notch
   d. Lower margin of greater sciatic notch

5. Which of the following is not supplied by superior gluteal nerve?
   a. Gluteus medius
   b. Gluteus minimus
   c. Gluteus maximus
   d. Tensor fasciae latae

6. Which muscle is one of the most powerful and bulkiest muscle in human?
   a. Gluteus maximus
   b. Obturator internus
   c. Quadriceps femoris
   d. Soleus

ANSWERS

1. b **2.** a **3.** c **4.** a **5.** c **6.** a

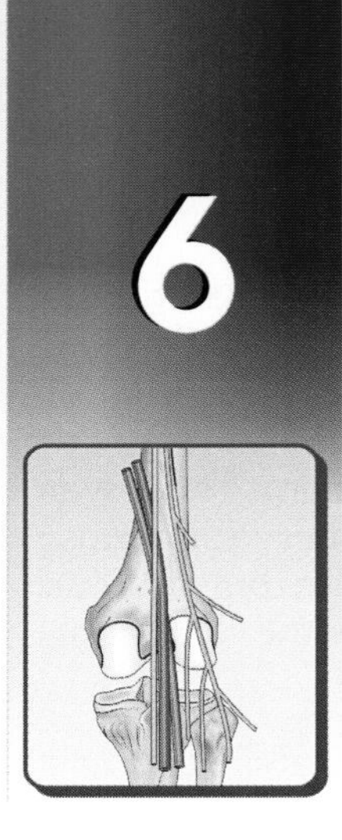

6 Popliteal Fossa

The popliteal artery is auscultated for measuring the blood pressure in the lower limb.

INTRODUCTION

Popliteal (Latin *hamstring of knee*) fossa is a shallow diamond shaped depression felt best at the back of knee joint, when the joint is semi-flexed. It corresponds to the cubital fossa of the forearm.

SURFACE LANDMARKS

1 *Lateral* and *medial condyles* of femur and tibia can be identified easily on the sides and front of the knee.

2 *Head of the fibula* is a bony prominence situated just below the posterolateral aspect of the lateral condyle of tibia.

3 *Common peroneal nerve* can be palpated against the posterolateral aspect of the neck of fibula, medial to the tendon of biceps femoris, by moving the finger from below upwards.

4 *Fibular collateral ligament* of the knee joint is felt like a rounded cord just above the head of the fibula in a flexed knee.

5 When the knee is flexed against resistance, the *hamstrings* can be seen and palpated easily right up to their insertion. Medially, the rounded tendon of the *semitendinosus* lies superficial to the flat tendon of *semimembranosus.* In front of these tendons there is a groove bounded anteriorly by the tendon of *adductor magnus.* Laterally, there is the tendon of *biceps femoris.* In front of this tendon there is a shallow groove bounded anteriorly by the *iliotibial tract.*

6 Pulsations of the *popliteal artery* can be felt in the middle of the popliteal fossa by applying deep pressure.

7 In the lower part of popliteal fossa, two heads of the *gastrocnemius* form rounded cushions that merge inferiorly into the calf.

POPLITEAL FOSSA

DISSECTION

Make a horizontal incision across the back of thigh at its junction of upper two-thirds with lower one-third and another horizontal incision at the back of leg at its junction of upper one-third and lower two-thirds (v), (vi) (*see* Fig. 5.2).

Draw a vertical incision joining the midpoints of the two horizontal incisions made (vii) (*see* Fig. 5.2). Reflect the skin and fascia on either side.

Find the cutaneous nerves, e.g. posterior cutaneous nerve of thigh, posterior division of medial cutaneous nerve, sural communicating nerve and short saphenous vein. Cut and clean the deep fascia.

Identify the boundaries and contents of the fossa.

Trace the tibial nerve as it courses through the centre of the popliteal fossa. Its three delicate articular branches are given off in the upper part of the fossa, cutaneous branch in the middle part and muscular branches in lower part of the fossa.

Common peroneal nerve is lying just medial to the tendon of biceps femoris muscle. Trace its branches.

Popliteal vein is deep to the tibial nerve and popliteal artery is the deepest as seen from the back. Trace all the muscular, cutaneous, genicular and terminal branches of the popliteal artery (*refer* to).

LOCATION

The popliteal fossa is a diamond-shaped depression lying behind the knee joint, the lower part of the femur, and the upper part of the tibia.

Boundaries

Superolaterally: The biceps femoris (Fig. 6.1).

Superomedially: The semitendinosus and the semimembranosus, supplemented by the gracilis, the sartorius and the adductor magnus.

7

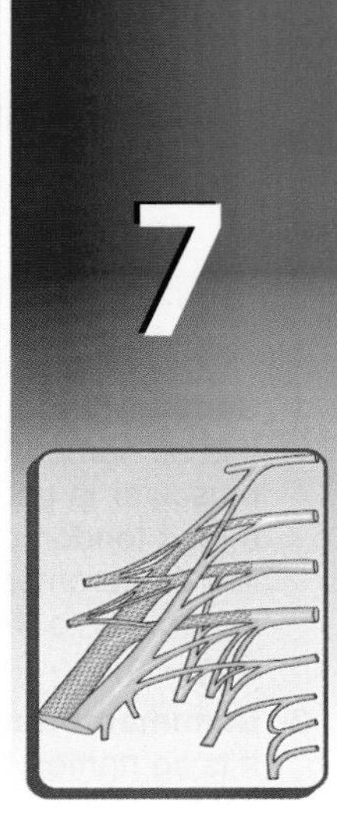

Back of Thigh

Pressure on the sciatic nerve between the edge of a chair and the hard femur results in sleeping foot, even if one is wide awake.
—Krishna Garg

INTRODUCTION

The posterior compartment of the thigh is also called the flexor compartment. It is incompletely separated from the medial compartment by the poorly defined posterior intermuscular septum. The adductor magnus is a component of both these compartments.

MUSCLES AND NERVES

DISSECTION

Give a vertical incision on the back of intact skin left after the dissections of gluteal region and the popliteal fossa (viii) (*see* Fig. 5.2). Reflect the skin and fasciae on either side. Clean the hamstring muscles and study their features from the Tables 7.1 and 7.2.

Sciatic nerve was seen in the gluteal region. Identify its branches in back of thigh to each of the hamstring muscles including occasionally for the short head of biceps femoris muscle. Trace the two terminal divisions of this nerve.

Separate the hamstring muscles to expose the ischial part of the composite or hybrid adductor magnus muscle.

Look for insertion of adductor longus, into the linea aspera of femur.

Trace the profunda femoris vessels behind adductor longus including its perforating branches (*refer to*).

Cutaneous Innervation

The skin over the back of the thigh is supplied by branches from the posterior cutaneous nerve of the thigh (*see* Fig. 6.2).

MUSCLES OF THE BACK OF THIGH

The muscles of the back of the thigh are called the *hamstring muscles*. They are the semitendinosus, the semimembranosus, the long head of the biceps femoris, and the ischial head of the adductor magnus (Figs 7.1 to 7.4).

The hamstrings share the following characters.

a. Origin from the ischial tuberosity (*see* Fig. 2.6).
b. Insertion into one of the bones of the leg.
   The adductor magnus reaches only up to the adductor tubercle of the femur, but is included amongst the hamstrings because the tibial collateral ligament of the knee joint is, morphologically, the degenerated tendon of this muscle. The ligament is attached to medial epicondyle, two millimeters from the adductor tubercle.
c. Nerve supply from the tibial part of the sciatic nerve.
d. The muscles act as flexors of the knee and extensors of the hip.

The attachments hamstrings are given in Tables 7.1 and 7.2.

CLINICAL ANATOMY

- Hamstring muscles lying at the back of the knee can be accidently or deliberately slashed or cut. If cut, the person cannot run, as these muscles are required for extension of the hip and flexion of the knee, movements essential in walking/ running.
- Hamstrings have variable length. Some persons cannot touch their toes with fingers while standing straight as their hamstring muscles are rather short.
- The inflammation of semimembranous bursa is called *semimembranosus bursitis*. The bursa becomes more prominent during extension of knee, and disappears during flexion of knee (Fig. 7.5).

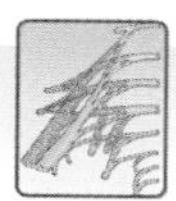

Table 7.1: Muscles of the back of thigh

Muscle	*Origin from*	*Insertion into*
1. **Semitendinosus** It is so named because it is muscular in upper part and has a long tendon of insertion. It lies posteromedially in the thigh, superficial to the semimembranosus (Fig. 7.1)	From the inferomedial impression on the upper part of the ischial tuberosity, in common with the long head of the biceps femoris (Fig. 7.1)	Into the upper part of the medial surface of the tibia behind the sartorius and the gracilis (*see* Fig. 4.2b)
2. **Semimembranosus** It is so named because it has a flat tendon of origin. It lies posteromedially in the thigh, deep to the semitendinosus (Fig. 7.2)	From the superolateral impression on the upper part of the ischial tuberosity.	Into the groove on the posterior surface of the medial condyle of the tibia. Expansions from the tendon form the oblique popliteal ligament, and the fascia covering the popliteus (*see* Fig. 6.3a)
3. **Biceps femoris** It has two heads of origin long and short. It lies posterolaterally in the thigh (Fig. 7.1)	a. *Long head:* From the inferomedial impression on the upper part of the ischial tuberosity; in common with the semitendinosus, and also from the lower part of the sacrotuberous ligament b. *Short head:* From the lateral lip of the linea aspera between the adductor magnus and the vastus lateralis, from the upper two-thirds of the lateral supracondylar line, and from the lateral intermuscular septum	The tendon is either folded around, by the fibular collateral ligament. It is inserted into the head of the fibula in front of its apex or styloid process (*see* Fig. 2.24)
4. **Adductor magnus** (*see* Fig. 4.1) This is the largest muscle of this compartment. Because of its double nerve supply, it is called a hybrid muscle (Figs 7.3 and 7.4)	a. Lower lateral part of the ischial tuberosity b. Ramus of the ischium c. Lower part of the inferior ramus of the pubis	a. Medial margin of gluteal tuberosity b. Linea aspera c. Medial supracondylar line d. Adductor tubercle

Table 7.2: Nerve supply and actions of muscles

Muscle	*Nerve supply*	*Actions*
1. **Semitendinosus**	Tibial part of sciatic nerve (L5, S1, S2)	Chief flexor of the knee and medial rotator of the leg in semiflexed knee. Weak extensor of the hip
2. **Semimembranosus**	Tibial part of sciatic nerve (L5, S1, S2)	Chief flexor of the knee and medial rotator of the leg in semiflexed knee. Weak extensor of the hip
3. **Biceps femoris**	a. Long head, by tibial part of sciatic nerve b. Short head, by common peroneal part of sciatic nerve (L5, S1, S2)	Chief flexor of the knee and lateral rotator of leg in semiflexed knee. Weak extensor of the hip
4. **Adductor magnus** (hybrid muscle)	Double nerve supply: Adductor part by posterior division of obturator nerve Hamstring part by tibial part of sciatic nerve	Adductor part causes adduction of thigh; Ischial part helps in extension of hip and flexion of knee

SCIATIC NERVE

The sciatic nerve is the thickest nerve in the body. In its upper part, it forms a band about 2 cm wide. It begins in the pelvis and terminates at the superior angle of the popliteal fossa by dividing into the tibial and common peroneal nerves.

Origin and Root Value

This is the largest branch of the sacral plexus. Its root value is L4, L5, S1, S2, S3. It is made up of two parts, the tibial part and the common peroneal part. The tibial part is formed by the ventral divisions of the anterior primary rami of L4, L5, S1, S2, S3. The common peroneal

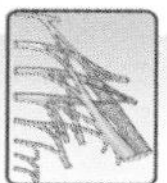

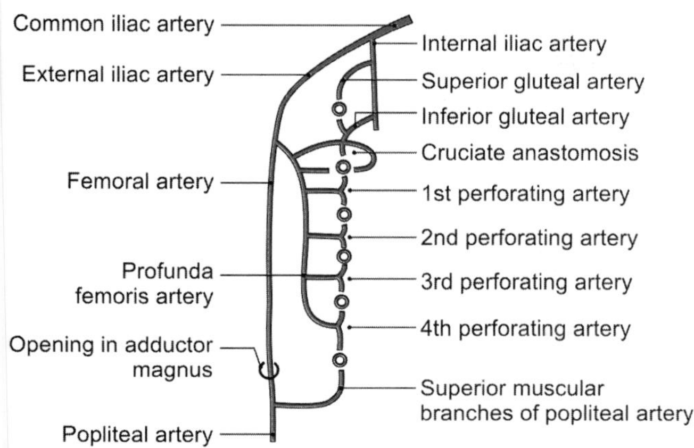

Fig. 7.14: Anastomoses on the back of thigh

2 The circumflex femorals anastomose with the first perforating artery (cruciate anastomoses) (Fig. 7.14 and *see* Flow chart 5.2).
3 The perforating arteries anastomose with one another.
4 The fourth perforating artery anastomoses with the upper muscular branches of the popliteal artery.

Another anastomosis is found on the sciatic nerve. This is formed by the companion artery of the sciatic nerve and the perforating arteries.

These longitudinal anastomoses provide an alternative route of blood supply to the lower limb, bypassing the external iliac and femoral arteries.

FACTS TO REMEMBER

- Sciatic nerve is the thickest nerve of the body.
- Sleeping foot is a temporary condition.
- Hamstrings are flexors knee and weak extensors of hip.
- Adductor magnus is a hybrid muscle.
- Thin artery accompanying sciatic nerve is part of the axial artery of lower limb.

CLINICOANATOMICAL PROBLEM

A 26-year-old woman complained of severe pain in the back of her right thigh and leg.

- Which nerve is involved and what is its root value?
- What is straight leg raising test? If done on this patient, why does it cause pain?

Ans: The nerve involved is sciatic nerve. Its root value is ventral rami of L4, L5, S1, S2, S3 segments of spinal cord. The pain on the back of thigh indicates compression of the roots of sciatic and radiating pain along cutaneous branches of tibial and common peroneal nerves.

Straight leg raising test:

The patient lies supine on the bed. The affected leg is extended at both hip and knee joints. Then it is raised up from the bed by holding the foot. As the nerve is stretched, it causes severe pain.

MULTIPLE CHOICE QUESTIONS

1. The posterior compartment is also known as:
a. Flexor compartment
b. Extensor compartment
c. Abductor compartment
d. Adductor compartment

2. Biceps femoris is inserted into:
a. Head of fibula
b. Adductor tubercle of femur
c. On styloid process of fibula
d. Medial condyle of tibia

3. Compression of which nerve leads to numbness of lower limb
a. Sciatic nerve b. Tibial nerve
c. Femoral nerve d. Deep peroneal nerve

4. Which is not a character of hamstring muscle?
a. Origin from ischial tuberosity
b. Nerve supply by deep peroneal muscle
c. The muscle act as flexor of knee and extensor of hip
d. Insertion into one of bones of leg

5. Semimembranosus is supplied by:
a. Tibial part of sciatic nerve
b. Common peroneal part of sciatic nerve
c. Obturator nerve
d. Femoral nerve

6. Sciatic nerve is largest branch of:
a. Sacral plexus b. Lumbar plexus
c. Cervical plexus d. Brachial plexus

7. Tibial collateral ligament of knee is the morphological continuation of:
a. Adductor magnus muscle
b. Adductor brevis muscle
c. Adductor longus muscle
d. None of above

ANSWERS

1. a **2.** a **3.** a **4.** b **5.** a **6.** a **7.** a

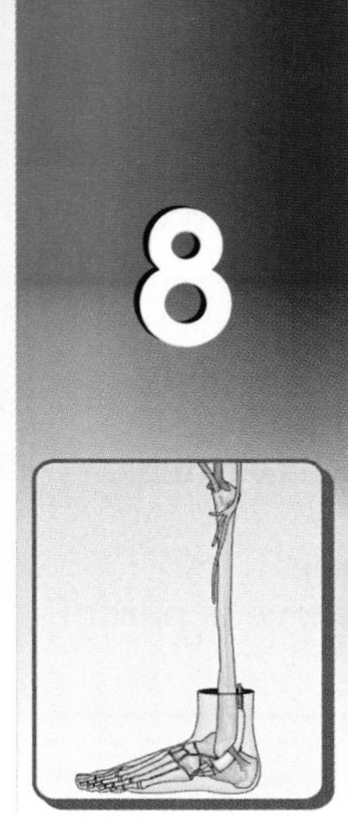

8

Front, Lateral and Medial Sides of Leg and Dorsum of Foot

Human life is but a series of footnotes to a vast obscure unfinished masterpiece.
—V Nabokov

INTRODUCTION

The great saphenous vein starts on the medial side of the dorsum of the foot and runs up just anterior to the medial malleolus, where it can be "slit open" for transfusion purposes. Dorsalis pedis artery, the distal continuation of the anterior tibial artery, is used for palpation in some clinical conditions. The dorsiflexors of foot supplied by deep peroneal nerve lie in the anterior compartment of leg. Tibialis anterior is an invertor of the foot as well. The two big evertors of the foot with superficial peroneal nerve are placed in the lateral compartment of the leg. The tendons of all these muscles are retained in position by two extensor and two peroneal retinacula. The three muscles inserted on the upper medial surface of tibia stabilise the pelvis on the thigh and leg (*see* Fig. 4.2b).

SURFACE LANDMARKS

1 *Medial and lateral condyles of tibia* are felt better in a flexed knee with the thigh flexed and laterally rotated (Fig. 8.1).
2 *Tibial tuberosity* is a bony prominence on the front of the upper part of tibia, 2.5 cm distal to the knee joint line passing through the upper margins of the tibial condyles. The tuberosity provides attachment to ligamentum patellae above, and is continuous with the shin below.
3 *Head of the fibula* lies posterolaterally at the level of tibial tuberosity. It serves as a guide to common peroneal nerve which winds around the posterolateral aspect of the neck of fibula.
4 *Shin* is the subcutaneous anterior border of tibia. It is sinuously curved and extends from the tibial tuberosity to the anterior margin of the medial malleolus. It is better defined in the upper part than in the lower part.

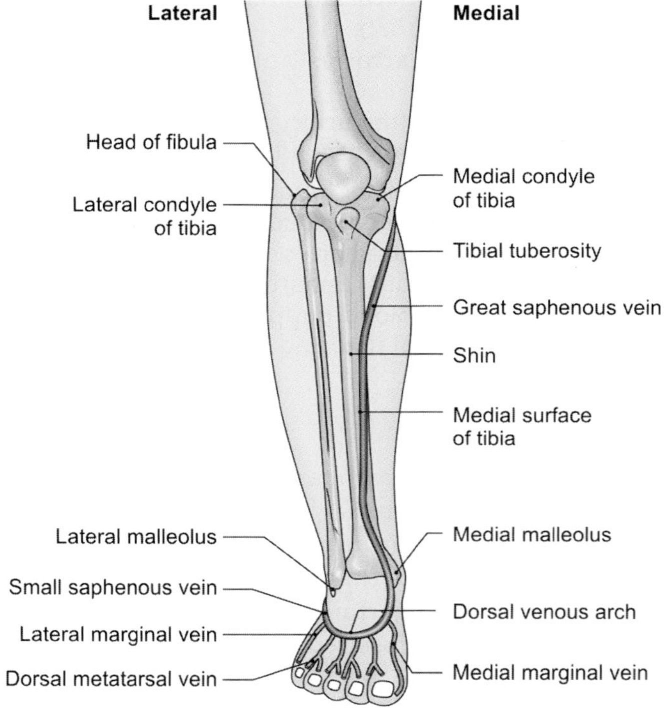

Fig. 8.1: Landmarks on leg and foot with superficial veins on the front

5 *Medial surface of tibia* is subcutaneous, except in the uppermost part where it is crossed by the tendons of sartorius, gracilis and semitendinosus. Great saphenous vein crosses lower one-third of the surface, running obliquely upwards and backwards from the anterior border of medial malleolus.
6 *Medial border of tibia* is palpable throughout its whole extent. The saphenous nerve and great saphenous vein run partly along it.
7 *Gastrocnemius* and the underlying *soleus* form the fleshy prominence of the *calf*. These muscles become

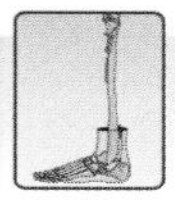

prominent when heel is raised as standing on toes. *Tendocalcaneus* is the strong, thick tendon of these muscles; it is attached below to the posterior surface of calcaneum.

8 *Medial malleolus* is the bony prominence on the medial side of ankle. It is formed by a downwards projection from the medial surface of the lower end of tibia.

9 *Lateral malleolus* is the bony prominence on the lateral side of ankle. It is formed by the lower end of fibula. It is larger but narrower than the medial malleolus, and its tip is 0.5 cm below that of the medial malleolus. The posterior borders of two malleoli are in the same coronal plane, but the anterior border of lateral malleolus is about 1.5 cm behind that of the medial malleolus.

10 *Peroneal trochlea,* when present, is felt as a little prominence about a finger-breadth below the lateral malleolus. Peroneus brevis passes above and the peroneus longus below the trochlea.

11 *Sustentaculum tali* can be felt about a thumb-breadth below the medial malleolus.

12 *Tuberosity of navicular bone* is a low bony prominence felt 2.5 to 3.75 cm anteroinferior to the medial malleolus, about midway between the back of the heel and root of the big toe.

13 *Head of the talus* lies above the line joining the sustentaculum tali and tuberosity of navicular bone.

14 *Tuberosity of the base of fifth metatarsal bone* is the most prominent landmark on the lateral border of the foot. It lies midway between the point of the heel and the root of the little toe.

15 *Posterior tibial artery* pulsations can be felt against calcaneum about 2 cm below and behind the medial malleolus (*see* Fig. 9.9).

16 *Dorsalis pedis artery* pulsations can be felt best on the dorsum of foot about 5 cm distal to the malleoli, lateral to the tendon of extensor hallucis longus, over the intermediate cuneiform bone (Fig. 8.11).

17 *Tendon of tibialis anterior* becomes prominent on active inversion of the foot, passing downwards and medially across the medial part of the anterior surface of ankle.

18 *Tendon of extensor hallucis longus* becomes prominent when the foot is dorsiflexed.

19 *Extensor digitorum brevis* produces an elevation on the lateral part of the dorsum of foot when the toes are dorsiflexed or extended (Fig. 8.7).

20 *First metatarsophalangeal joint* lies a little in front of the centre of the ball of big toe. The *other metatarsophalangeal joints* are placed about 2.5 cm behind the webs of the toes.

SUPERFICIAL FASCIA

DISSECTION

1. Make a horizontal incision across the leg at its junction with foot (*see* Fig. 3.1).
2. Provide a vertical incision up from the centre of incision (1) to the middle of incision drawn just below the level of tibial tuberosity.
3. Carry this vertical incision on to the dorsum of foot till the middle of the second toe.

   Reflect the skin on both the sides. Look for various veins and cutaneous nerves in the leg and foot according to the description given in the text (*refer* to).

CONTENTS

The superficial fascia of the front of the leg and the dorsum of the foot contains: The superficial veins, cutaneous nerves, lymphatics, and small unnamed arteries.

Superficial Veins

1 The *dorsal venous arch* lies on the dorsum of the foot over the proximal parts of the metatarsal bones. It receives four dorsal metatarsal veins each of which is formed by the union of two dorsal digital veins (Fig. 8.1).

2 The *great* or *long saphenous vein* is formed by the union of the medial end of the dorsal venous arch with the medial marginal vein which drains the medial side of the great toe. It passes upwards in front of the medial malleolus, crosses the lower one-third of the medial surface of tibia obliquely, and runs along its medial border to reach the back of the knee. The saphenous nerve runs in front of the great saphenous vein.

3 The *small* or *short saphenous vein* is formed by the union of the lateral end of the dorsal venous arch with the lateral marginal vein, draining the lateral side of the little toe. It passes upwards behind the lateral malleolus to reach the back of the leg. The sural nerve accompanies the small saphenous vein.

Both saphenous veins are connected to the deep veins through the perforating veins.

Cutaneous Nerves

1 The *infrapatellar branch of the saphenous nerve* pierces the sartorius and the deep fascia on the medial side of the knee, curves downwards and forwards, and supplies the skin over the ligamentum patellae (Fig. 8.2).

2 The *saphenous nerve* is a branch of the posterior division of the femoral nerve. It pierces the deep fascia on the medial side of the knee between the

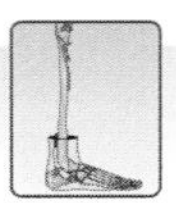

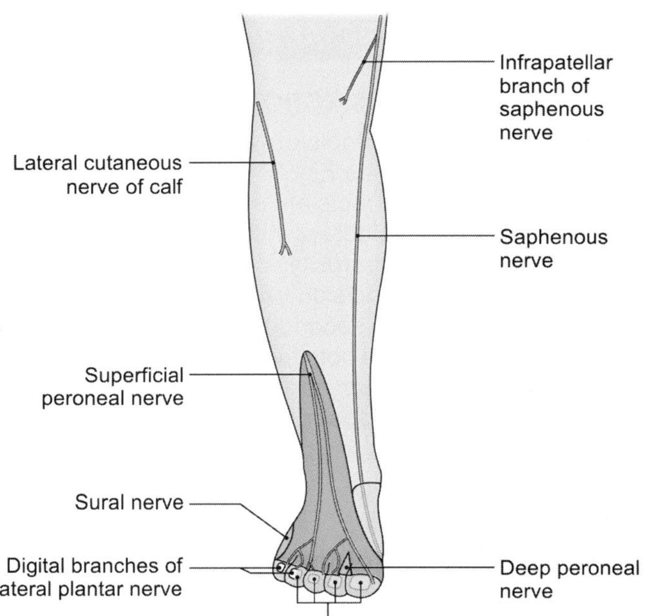

Fig. 8.2: Cutaneous nerves on the front of the leg and dorsum of foot

sartorius and the gracilis, and runs downwards in front of the great saphenous vein. It supplies the skin of the medial side of the leg and the medial border of the foot up to the ball of the great toe.

3 The *lateral cutaneous nerve of the calf* is a branch of the common peroneal nerve. It pierces the deep fascia over the lateral head of the gastrocnemius, and descends to supply the skin of the upper two-thirds of the lateral side of the leg (Fig. 8.2).

4 The *superficial peroneal nerve* is a branch of the common peroneal nerve. It arises on the lateral side of the neck of the fibula deep to the fibres of the peroneus longus. It descends between the peroneal muscles, pierces the deep fascia at the junction of the upper two-thirds and lower one-third of the lateral side of the leg, and divides into medial and lateral branches. These branches supply the following area:
   a. The skin over the lower one-third of the lateral side of the leg (Fig. 8.2).
   b. The skin over the entire dorsum of the foot with the exception of the following areas.
      i. Lateral border, supplied by sural nerve.
      ii. Medial border up to the base of the great toe, supplied by the saphenous nerve.
      iii. Cleft between the first and second toes, supplied by the deep peroneal nerve.

5 The *sural nerve* is a branch of the tibial nerve. It arises in the middle of the popliteal fossa. It runs vertically downwards, pierces the deep fascia in the middle of the back of leg, accompanies the small saphenous vein, and supplies the skin of the lower half of the back of leg and of the whole of the lateral border of the foot up to the tip of the little toe (*see* Fig. 9.1).

6 The *deep peroneal nerve* terminates by supplying the skin adjoining the cleft between the first and second toes.

7 The *digital branches of the medial and lateral plantar nerves* curve upwards and supply the distal parts of the dorsum of the toes. Medial plantar nerve supplies medial 3½ toes; lateral plantar nerve supplies lateral 1½ toes.

CLINICAL ANATOMY

Saphenous nerve may be subjected to entrapment neuropathy as it leaves the adductor canal, leading to pain in the area of its supply.

DEEP FASCIA

DISSECTION

Underlying the superficial fascia is the dense deep fascia of leg. Divide this fascia longitudinally as it stretches between tibia and fibula.

Expose the superior extensor retinaculum 5 cm above the ankle joint and the inferior extensor retinaculum in front of the ankle joint.

Features

The following points about the fascia are noteworthy.

1 In the leg, tibia and fibula are partly subcutaneous, the most notable being the medial surface of the tibia, and the malleoli. Over these subcutaneous areas, the deep fascia is replaced by periosteum.

2 Extensions of deep fascia form intermuscular septa that divide the leg into compartments (Fig. 8.3).

   The *anterior* and *posterior* intermuscular septa are attached to the anterior and posterior borders of the fibula. They divide the leg into three compartments: *anterior, lateral,* and *posterior.* The posterior compartment is subdivided into superficial, intermediate and deep parts by *superficial* and *deep transverse fascial septa.*

3 Around the ankle, the deep fascia is thickened to form bands called *retinacula.* These are so called because they retain tendons in place. On the front of the ankle there are the *superior and inferior extensor retinacula.* Laterally, there are the *superior and inferior peroneal retinacula.* Posteromedially, there is the *flexor retinaculum.* The extensor retinacula are described below. The peroneal retinacula are considered with the lateral compartment of the leg and the flexor retinaculum with the posterior compartment.

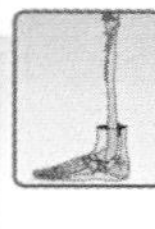

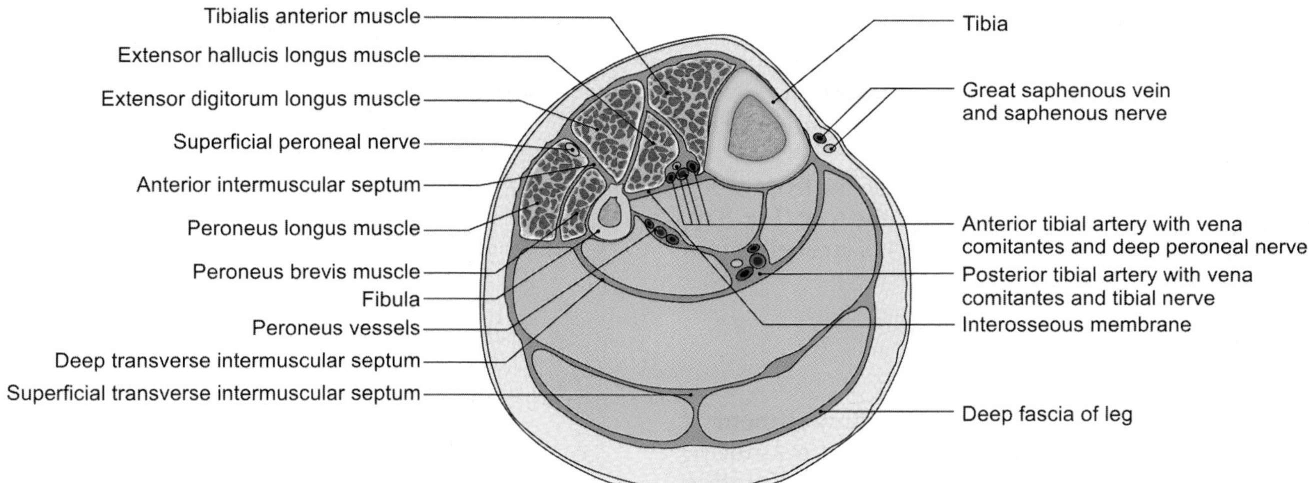

Fig. 8.3: Transverse section through the middle of the leg showing the intermuscular septa and the arrangement of structures in the anterior and lateral compartments

Superior Extensor Retinaculum

Attachments

Medially, it is attached to the lower part of the anterior border of the tibia, and *laterally* to the lower part of the anterior border of the fibula forming the anterior boundary of the elongated triangular area just above the lateral malleolus (Fig. 8.4).

Inferior Extensor Retinaculum

This is a Y-shaped band of deep fascia, situated in front of the ankle joint and over the posterior part of the dorsum of the foot. The stem of the Y lies laterally, and the upper and lower bands, medially (Fig. 8.4).

Attachments

1 The *stem* is attached to the anterior non-articular part of the superior surface of the calcaneum, in front of the sulcus calcanei.

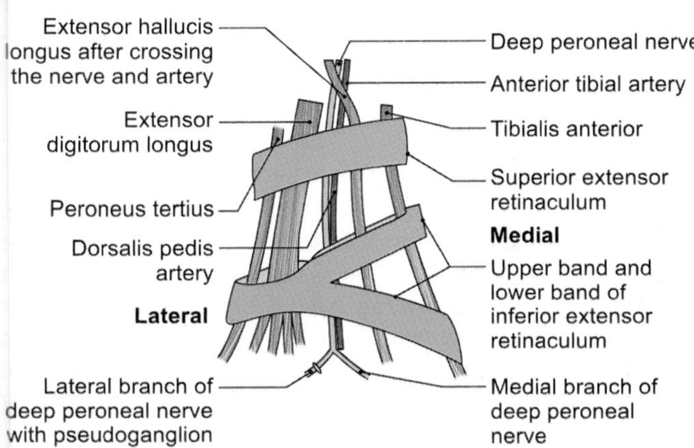

Fig. 8.4: Tendons, vessels and nerves related to the extensor retinacula

2 The *upper band* passes upwards and medially, and is attached to the anterior border of the medial malleolus.

3 The *lower band* passes downwards and medially and is attached to the plantar aponeurosis.

Structures Passing under

1 Tibialis anterior.
2 Extensor hallucis longus.
3 Anterior tibial vessels.
4 Deep peroneal nerve
5 Extensor digitorum longus.
6 The peroneus tertius.

CLINICAL ANATOMY

Anterior tibial compartment syndrome/fresher's syndrome: The muscles of anterior compartment of leg get pain because of too much sudden exercise. The muscles are tender to touch.

MUSCLES OF FRONT OF LEG

DISSECTION

Identify the muscles of anterior compartment of leg as these are lying close together on the lateral surface of tibia, adjoining interosseous membrane and medial surface of fibula.

Trace their tendons deep to the two retinacula on the dorsum of foot till their insertion. Learn about these muscles given in Tables 8.1 and 8.2.

Look for anterior tibial artery and accompanying deep peroneal nerve as these lie on the upper part of interosseous membrane of leg. Study their course, relations and branches.

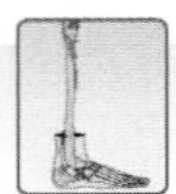

MUSCLES OF ANTERIOR COMPARTMENT OF THE LEG

The muscles of the anterior compartment of the leg are the tibialis anterior, the extensor hallucis longus, the extensor digitorum longus and the peroneus tertius (Fig. 8.5).

These muscles are tested *by palpation* on the front of leg and requesting the patient to dorsiflex the foot (Fig. 8.6).

The attachments of these muscles are given in Tables 8.1 and 8.2.

ANTERIOR TIBIAL ARTERY

Introduction

This is the main artery of the anterior compartment of the leg (Fig. 8.8). The blood supply to the anterior compartment of the leg is reinforced by the perforating branch of the peroneal artery, the size of which is inversely proportional to that of the anterior tibial artery.

Beginning, Course and Termination

The anterior tibial artery is the smaller terminal branch of the popliteal artery.

It begins on the back of the leg at the lower border of the popliteus, opposite the tibial tuberosity.

It enters the anterior compartment of the leg by passing forwards close to the fibula, through an opening in the upper part of the interosseous membrane.

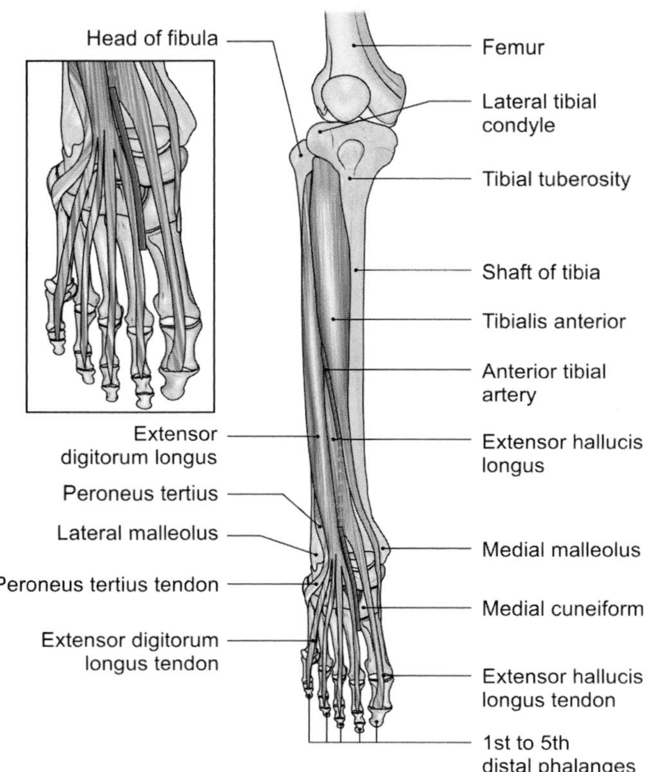

Fig. 8.5: Muscles of front of leg and dorsum of foot (inset)

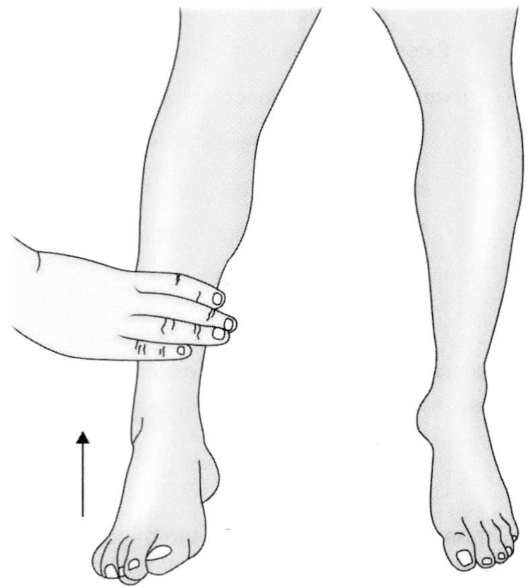

Fig. 8.6: How to test the dorsiflexors of the ankle joint

In the anterior compartment, it runs vertically downwards to a point midway between the two malleoli where it changes its name to become the dorsalis pedis artery.

Relations

In the upper one-third of the leg, the artery lies between the *tibialis anterior* and the *extensor digitorum longus* (Fig. 8.5).

In the middle one-third it lies between the *tibialis anterior* and the *extensor hallucis longus* (Fig. 8.3).

In the lower one-third it lies between the *extensor hallucis longus* and the *extensor digitorum longus*. In understanding these relations note that the artery is crossed from lateral to medial side by the tendon of the *extensor hallucis longus* (Fig. 8.4).

The artery is accompanied by the venae comitantes.

The deep peroneal nerve is lateral to it in its upper and lower thirds, and anterior to it in its middle one-third (Fig. 8.4).

Branches

1 *Muscular* branches supply adjacent muscles.
2 *Anastomotic* branches are given to the knee and ankle. The *anterior* and *posterior tibial recurrent branches* take part in the anastomoses round the knee joint (*see* Fig. 6.10). The *anterior medial malleolar* and *anterior lateral malleolar branches* take part in the anastomoses round the ankle joint or malleolar networks (Fig. 8.8).

The *lateral malleolar network* lies just below the lateral malleolus.

The *medial malleolar network* lies just below the medial malleolus.

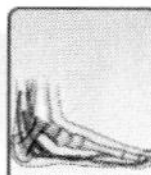

Table 9.2: Nerve supply and actions of superficial muscles

Muscle	Nerve supply	Actions
1. **Gastrocnemius**	Tibial nerve (S1, S2)	The gastrocnemius and soleus are strong plantar flexors of the foot, at the ankle joint. The gastrocnemius is also a flexor of the knee. Plantar
2. **Soleus**	Tibial nerve (S1, S2)	flexion, produced by the gastrocnemius and the soleus, is very important in walking and running The soleus is more powerful than the gastrocnemius, but the latter is faster acting. In walking, the soleus overcomes the inertia of the body weight, like the bottom gear of a car. When movement is under way, the quicker acting gastrocnemius increases the speed like the top gear of a car. Soleus is chiefly a postural muscle, to steady the leg on the foot
3. **Plantaris**	Tibial nerve (S1, S2)	The plantaris is a rudimentary muscle, and is accessory to the gastrocnemius. Its functional importance is of transplantation

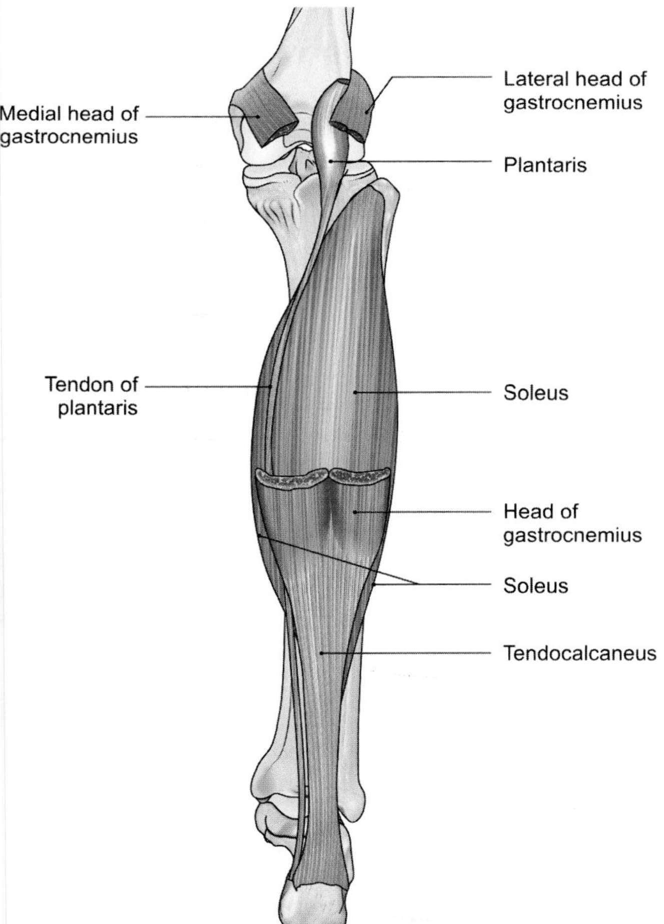

Fig. 9.3: Superficial muscles of the back of the leg

the only unprotected part of his body. His mother had held him by one heel, and the water over this heel had not flowed.

DEEP MUSCLES, ARTERIES AND NERVE

DISSECTION

Once the soleus has been studied, separate it from its attachment on tibia and reflect it laterally. Look for a number of deep veins which emerge from this muscle.

Identify popliteus, situated above the soleus muscle. Deep to soleus is the first intermuscular septum. Incise this septum vertically to reach the long flexors of the toes, e.g. flexor hallucis longus laterally and flexor digitorum longus medially. Trace these tendons till the flexor retinaculum. Turn the flexor hallucis longus laterally and expose the second intermuscular septum.

Divide this septum to reveal the deepest muscle of the posterior compartment of leg, e.g. tibialis posterior. Trace its tendon also till flexor retinaculum. Study these deep muscles.

Clean the lowest part of popliteal vessels and trace its two terminal branches, anterior tibial into anterior compartment and posterior tibial into the posterior compartment of leg. Identify posterior tibial vessels and tibial nerve in fibrofatty tissue between the two long flexors of the leg deep to the first intermuscular septum.

Peroneal vessels are identified in the connective tissue of the second intermuscular septum. Study their origin, course and branches from the following text.

The nerve to popliteus deserves special mention. Being a branch of tibial nerve it descends over the popliteus to reach its distal border. There it supplies the muscle after winding around its distal border. It also supplies a branch to tibialis posterior muscle, both tibiofibular joints and interosseous membrane.

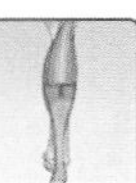

Table 9.3: Deep muscles of the posterior compartment of the leg		
Name	*Origin*	*Insertion*
Popliteus (Fig. 9.4)	Lateral surface of lateral condyle of femur; origin is intracapsular Outer margin of lateral meniscus of the knee joint	Posterior surface of shaft of tibia above soleal line
Flexor digitorum longus (Fig. 9.4)	Upper two-thirds of medial part of posterior surface of tibia below the soleal line	Bases of distal phalanges of shaft of lateral four toes. Muscle ends in a tendon which divides into four slips, one for each of the lateral four toes. Each slip is attached to the plantar surface of the distal phalanx of the digit concerned
Flexor hallucis longus (Fig. 9.4)	Lower three-fourths of the posterior surface of the fibula (except the lowest 2.5 cm) and interosseous membrane (*see* Fig. 2.34)	Plantar surface of base of distal phalanx of big toe
Tibialis posterior (Fig. 9.4)	Upper two-thirds of lateral part of posterior surface of tibia below the soleal line (*see* Fig. 2.28). Posterior surface of fibula in front of the medial crest and posterior surface of interosseous membrane	Tuberosity of navicular bone and other tarsal bones except talus. Insertion is extended into 2nd, 3rd and 4th metatarsal bones at their bases

Table 9.4: Nerve supply and actions of deep muscles of the posterior compartment of the leg		
Name	*Nerve supply*	*Actions*
Popliteus	Tibial nerve	Unlocks knee joint by lateral rotation of femur on tibia prior to flexion
Flexor digitorum longus	Tibial nerve	Flexes distal phalanges, plantar flexor of ankle joint; supports medial and lateral longitudinal arches of foot
Flexor hallucis longus	Tibial nerve	Flexes distal phalanx of big toe; plantar flexor of ankle joint; supports medial longitudinal arch of foot
Tibialis posterior	Tibial nerve	Plantar flexor of ankle joint; inverts foot at subtalar joint, supports medial longitudinal arch of foot (Fig. 9.4)

DEEP MUSCLES

The deep muscles of the back of the leg are the popliteus, the flexor digitorum longus, the flexor hallucis longus, and the tibialis posterior. They are described in Tables 9.3 and 9.4.

Important Relations of Flexor Digitorum Longus

1 The tendon crosses the tibialis posterior in lower part of the leg. It passes deep to the flexor retinaculum to enter the sole of foot. Here it crosses the tendon of flexor hallucis longus (Fig. 9.4).
2 The tendon receives the insertion of the flexor digitorum accessorius.
3 The slips for the digits give origin to the four lumbrical muscles.

Important Relations of Flexor Hallucis Longus

The tendon runs across the lower part of the posterior surface of the tibia. Reaching the calcaneus it turns forwards below the sustentaculum tali which serves as a pulley for it. As the tendon lies on the medial side of calcaneum, it runs deep to the flexor retinaculum and is surrounded by a synovial sheath. The tendon then runs forwards in the sole when it is crossed by the tendon of flexor digitorum longus.

Important Relations of Tibialis Posterior

The tendon passes behind the medial malleolus, grooving it. The tendon then passes deep to the flexor retinaculum. The terminal part of the tendon supports the spring ligament.

CLINICAL ANATOMY

- The deep muscles are tested by palpating the calf while the foot is being plantarflexed (Fig. 9.5).
- Tendo-Achilles reflex or ankle jerk (S1, S2): The foot gets plantar flexed on tapping the tendocalcaneus (Fig. 9.6).
- For thromboangiitis obliterans or occlusive disease of lower limb arteries, sympathetic fibres to the arteries are removed, so as to denervate the arteries. Lumbar 2 and 3 ganglia with intervening sympathetic trunk is removed, as these supply the arteries of lower limb.

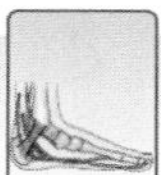

- In long distance air travel, sitting immobile can lead to thrombosis of soleal venous sinuses. The thrombus may get dislodged to block any other artery. One must stretch the legs frequently.
- Dislocation or subluxation of ankle is common during plantarflexion. Lower end of the leg bones, i.e. medial malleolus, tibia, thin fibula and lateral malleolus form tibiofibular mortice. This is wider anteriorly and narrow posteriorly.
  The trochlear surface of talus forming ankle joint is also wider anteriorly and narrow posteriorly.
  During dorsiflexion, wider trochlear surface fits into narrow posterior part of the mortice. The joint is stable and close packed.
  During plantarflexion the narrow posterior trochlear surface lies loosely in wider anterior part of the mortice. The joint is unstable and can easily get subluxated or dislocated. This occurs while walking in high heels (Fig. 9.10).

POSTERIOR TIBIAL ARTERY

Beginning, Course and Termination

It begins at the lower border of the popliteus, between the tibia and the fibula, deep to the gastrocnemius (Fig. 9.7).

It enters the back of leg by passing deep to the tendinous arch of the soleus.

In the leg, it runs downwards and slightly medially, to reach the posteromedial side of the ankle, midway between the medial malleolus and the medial tubercle of the calcaneum.

It terminates deep to flexor retinaculum (and the origin of the abductor hallucis) by dividing, into the lateral and medial plantar arteries (Fig. 9.2).

Relations

Superficial

1. In the upper two-thirds of the leg, it lies deep to the gastrocnemius, the soleus and the superficial transverse fascial septum (Fig. 9.8).
2. In the lower one-third of the leg, it runs parallel to, and 2.5 cm in front of, the medial border of the tendocalcaneus. It is covered by skin and fasciae.
3. At the ankle, it lies deep to the flexor retinaculum and the abductor hallucis (Fig. 9.2).

Deep

1. In the upper two-thirds of the leg, it lies on the tibialis posterior (Fig. 9.8).
2. In the lower one-third of the leg, it lies on the flexor digitorum longus and on the tibia.
3. At the ankle, it lies directly on the capsule of the ankle joint between the flexor digitorum longus and the flexor hallucis longus (Fig. 9.2).

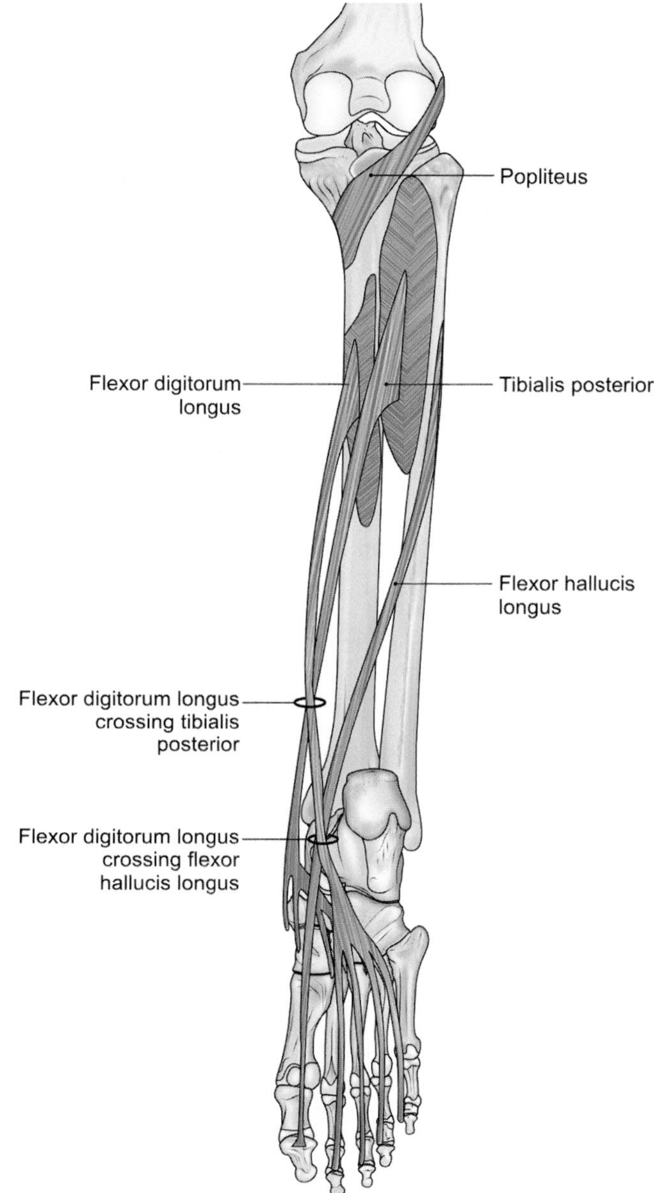

Fig. 9.4: Deep muscles of the back of the leg

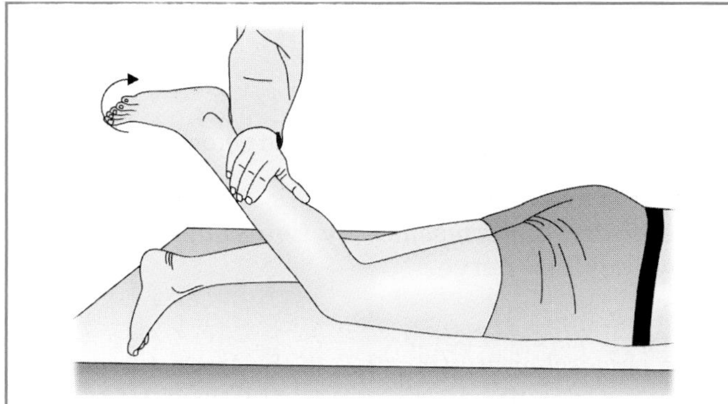

Fig. 9.5: Testing the deep muscles of the calf by plantar flexing the foot

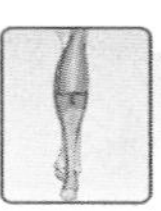

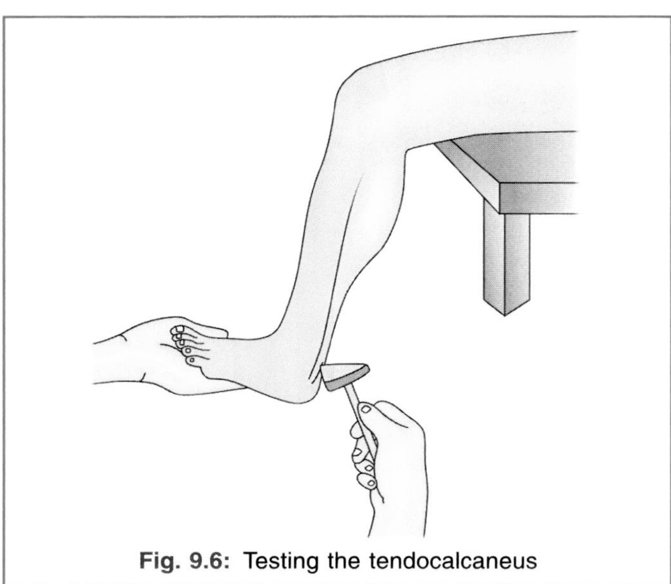

Fig. 9.6: Testing the tendocalcaneus

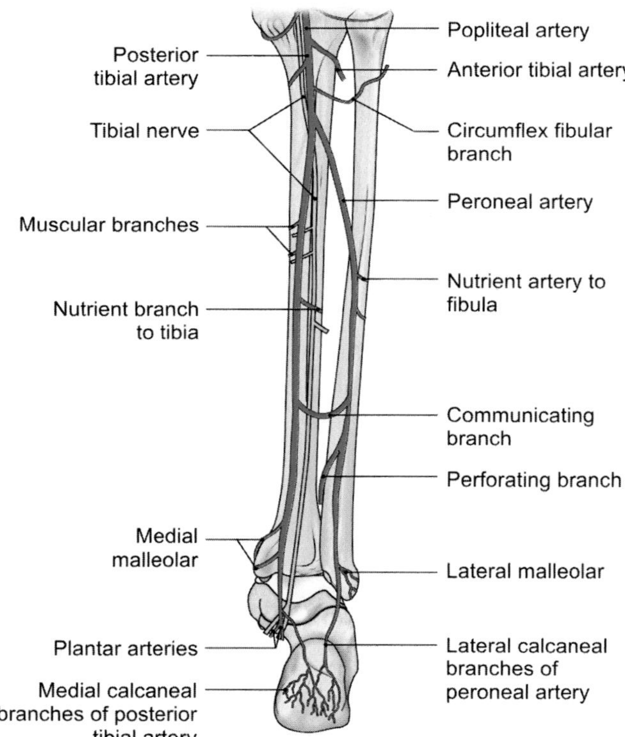

Fig. 9.7: Course of the posterior tibial and peroneal arteries and the tibial nerve

The artery is *accompanied* by two venae comitantes and by the tibial nerve.

Branches

1 The *peroneal artery* (Fig. 9.7) is the largest branch of the posterior tibial artery. It is described later.
2 Several *muscular branches* are given off to muscles of the back of the leg.
3 A *nutrient artery* is given off to the tibia.
4 The *anastomotic branches* of the posterior tibial artery are as follows.
   a. The circumflex fibular branch winds round the lateral side of the neck of the fibula to reach the front of the knee where it takes part in the anastomoses around the knee joint.
   b. A communicating branch forms an arch with a similar branch from the peroneal artery about 5 cm above the ankle.
   c. A malleolar branch anastomoses with other arteries over the medial malleolus.
   d. Calcaneal branches anastomose with other arteries in the region.
5 *Terminal branches:* These are the medial and lateral plantar arteries. They will be studied in the sole (Fig. 9.7).

PERONEAL ARTERY

Beginning, Course and Termination

This is the largest branch of the posterior tibial artery. It supplies the posterior and lateral compartments of the leg (Fig. 9.7).

It begins 2.5 cm below the lower border of the popliteus.

It runs obliquely towards the fibula, and descends along the medial crest of the fibula, accompanied by the nerve to the flexor hallucis longus. It passes behind the inferior tibiofibular and ankle joints, medial to peroneal tendons. It terminates by dividing into a number of lateral calcanean branches (Fig. 9.7).

Branches

1 *Muscular branches,* to the posterior and lateral compartments.
2 *Nutrient artery,* to the fibula.
3 *Anastomotic branches:*
   a. The large perforating branch pierces the interosseous membrane 5 cm above the ankle, and joins the lateral malleolar network.
   b. The communicating branch anastomoses with a similar branch from the posterior tibial artery, about 5 cm above the lower end of the tibia.
   c. The calcanean branches join the lateral malleolar network.

The perforating branch of the peroneal artery may reinforce, or even replace the dorsalis pedis artery.

TIBIAL NERVE

Course

The course and relations of the tibial nerve in the leg are similar to those of the posterior tibial artery. Like the artery, the tibial nerve also terminates by dividing into the medial plantar and lateral plantar nerves (Fig. 9.2).

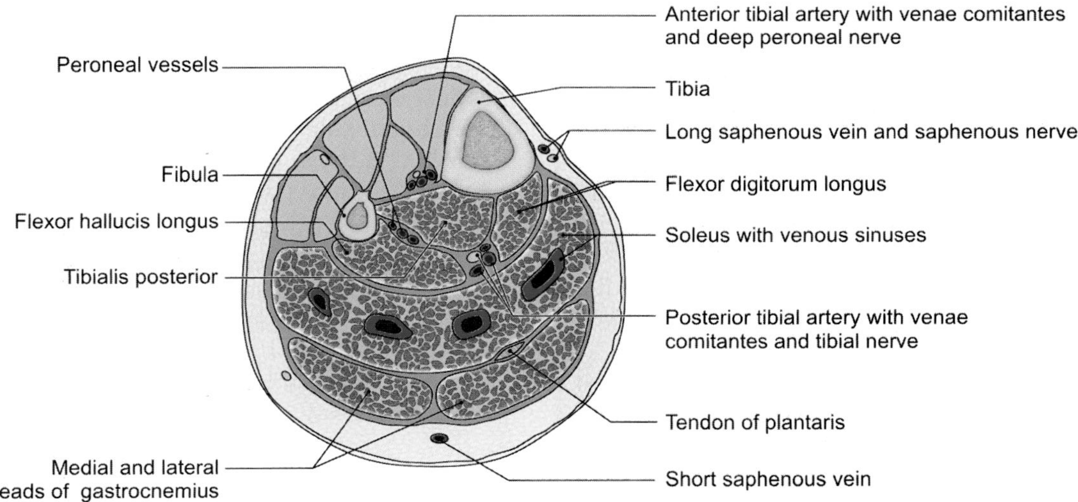

Fig. 9.8: Transverse section through the middle of the leg, showing the arrangement of structures in the posterior compartment

Branches

Muscular

To the tibialis posterior, the flexor digitorum longus; the flexor hallucis longus, and the deep part of the soleus (Figs 9.7 and 9.8).

Cutaneous

Medial calcanean branches pierce the flexor retinaculum, and supply the skin on the back and lower surface of the heel.

Articular

To the ankle joint.

Terminal

Medial plantar and lateral plantar nerves (Fig. 9.2).

CLINICAL ANATOMY

- The posterior tibial pulse is palpated in doubtful cases of intermittent claudication where a person gets cramps and severe pain in calf muscles due to lack of blood supply.
- The posterior tibial pulse can be felt against the calcaneum about 2 cm below and behind the medial malleolus (Fig. 9.9).
- The long tendon of plantaris is used for tendon transplantation in the body.
- Tendocalcaneus can rupture in tennis players 5 cm above its insertion. Plantar flexion is not possible. The two ends must be stitched.
- High heels for long periods causes change in posture. Knees are excessively bent, with lumbar vertebrae pushed forwards. There is a lot of stress on the muscles of back and those of the calf. So many fashionable ladies wear high heels for short time and change to flat ones soon (Fig. 9.10).

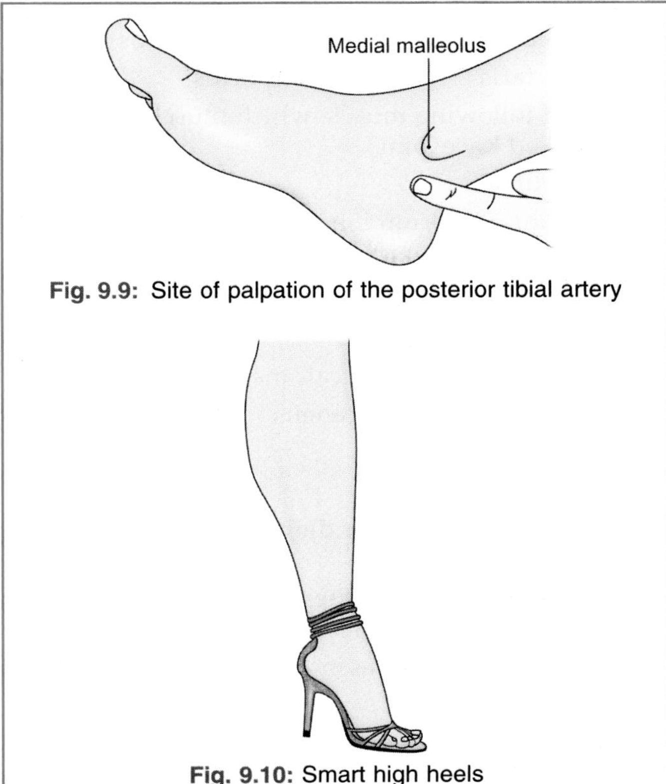

Fig. 9.9: Site of palpation of the posterior tibial artery

Fig. 9.10: Smart high heels

Mnemonics

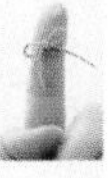

Structures under flexor retinaculum

Talented **d**octors **ar**e **n**ever **h**ungry
Tibialis posterior
Flexor **d**igitorum longus
Posterior tibial **ar**tery
Tibial **n**erve
Flexor **h**allucis longus

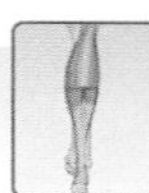

FACTS TO REMEMBER

- Soleus acts as the peripheral heart, as it pushes the venous blood upwards.
- Soleus acts like first gear while gastrocnemius act like second and third gears during walking.
- Tendocalcaneus is the strongest tendon in the body
- All the muscles of back of leg/calf are supplied by the tibial nerve
- Posterior tibial artery is palpated between medial malleolus and calcaneus under the flexor retinaculum.
- Posterior tibial artery ends by dividing into medial and lateral plantar arteries.

CLINICOANATOMICAL PROBLEM

An elderly man complained of pain on the inner aspect of right ankle joint. The pain was also felt in the area of sole.

- What is the syndrome called?
- Why is there pain in the sole?

Ans: The syndrome is called *tarsal tunnel syndrome* if tibial nerve gets entrapped under the flexor retinaculum of the ankle. Since the tibial nerve gets constricted, there is pain in the sole as the medial and lateral plantar nerves are affected. There may be paralysis of intrinsic muscles of the sole due to compression of medial and lateral plantar nerves.

MULTIPLE CHOICE QUESTIONS

1. Which muscle is called peripheral heart?
   a. Soleus
   b. Gastrocnemius
   c. Plantaris
   d. Sartorius

2. Out of following muscle which muscle acts as key of locked knee joint?
   a. Popliteus
   b. Flexor digitorum longus
   c. Tibialis posterior
   d. Flexor hallucis longus

3. Plantaris is inserted in:
   a. Posterior surface of calcaneum
   b. Medial to tendocalcaneus
   c. Both a and b
   d. None of above

4. What relation of flexor digitorum longus is wrong (not correct)?
   a. The tendon crosses the tibialis posterior in lower part of leg
   b. The tendon receives insertion of flexor digitorum accessorius
   c. The 4 slips of the tendon give origin to 3 lumbrical muscles
   d. The tendon crosses the tendon of flexor hallucis longus

5. If tibial nerve is injured under flexor retinaculum, the condition is called:
   a. Tarsal tunnel syndrome
   b. Foot drop
   c. Morton's neuroma
   d. Pes calcaneus

6. Tibialis posterior is chiefly inserted into:
   a. Base of distal phalanges of shaft of lateral 4 toes
   b. Base of distal phalanges of big toe
   c. Posterior surface of shaft of tibia
   d. Tuberosity of navicular bone

7. Deep muscles of posterior compartment of leg are supplied by which nerve?
   a. Tibial
   b. Deep peroneal
   c. Obturator
   d. Femoral

ANSWERS

1. a **2.** a **3.** c **4.** c **5.** a **6.** d **7.** a

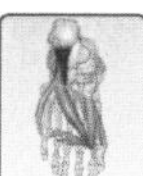

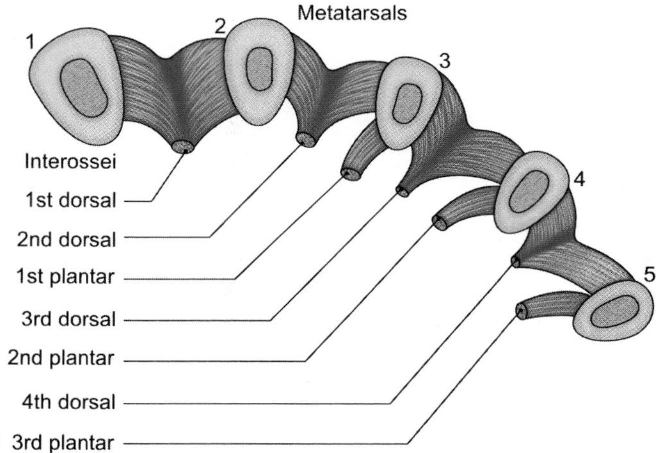

Fig. 10.15: Schematic transverse section through the metatarsal bones (1–5) to show the origins of the interossei

FACTS TO REMEMBER

- Muscles of the sole are disposed in four layers.
- Medial plantar nerve supplies 4 intrinsic muscles.
- Lateral plantar nerve supplies 14 intrinsic muscles.
- Extrinsic muscles are supplied by the nerve of the respective compartments of the leg.
- Only one arterial arch, the plantar arch is present.
- The muscles of the sole maintain the arches of the foot.
- Between 1st and 2nd layers of muscles are the trunks of medial plantar and lateral plantar nerves and vessels.
- Between the 3rd and 4th layers are the plantar arch and deep branch of lateral plantar nerve.

CLINICOANATOMICAL PROBLEM

A young female complains of severe pain along the middle of her right sole.

- What is the condition called?
- Name the branches of medial plantar nerve?

Ans: This may due to a "neuroma" in the common digital nerve between third and fourth metatarsal bones. This is a benign proliferation of the nerve fibres.

The condition is painful. The treatment is surgery.

Medial plantar nerve gives:

a. Muscular branches to abductor hallucis, flexor digitorum brevis, both of 1st layer of sole; first lumbrical of 2nd layer of sole and flexor hallucis brevis of 3rd layer of sole
b. The nerve gives 7 digital branches to adjacent sides of medial 3½ toes, including their nail beds and distal phalanges on the dorsum of foot
c. It also gives articular branches to the joints in its territory of distribution.

MULTIPLE CHOICE QUESTIONS

1. Muscles of first layer of sole are all *except*:
a. Abductor hallucis
b. Flexor digitorum brevis
c. Abductor digiti minimi
d. Extensor digitorum brevis

2. Which is not inserted into plantar aspect of foot?
a. Flexor hallucis longus
b. Peroneus longus
c. Peroneus tertius
d. Flexor digitorum longus

3. In the movement of eversion of foot, all of the following muscles are involved *except*:
a. Peroneus longus b. Peroneus brevis
c. Tibialis anterior d. Peroneus tertius

4. The bone devoid of muscular attachment:
a. Cuboid b. Talus
c. Navicular d. Medial cuneiform

5. All muscles form second layer of sole *except*:
a. Flexor digitorum accessorius
b. Lumbricals
c. Flexor hallucis longus
d. Flexor digitorum brevis

6. All of following structures pass behind medial malleolus beneath flexor retinaculum of ankle region *except*:
a. Tibialis posterior
b. Flexor digitorum longus
c. Deep peroneal nerve
d. Tibial nerve

7. How many plantar interossei are present in the sole?
a. Four b. Three
c. Two d. Five

8. Medial plantar nerve supplies all muscles *except*:
a. Abductor hallucis
b. Adductor hallucis
c. Flexor digitorum brevis
d. Flexor hallucis brevis

ANSWERS

1. d **2.** c **3.** c **4.** b **5.** d **6.** c **7.** b **8.** b

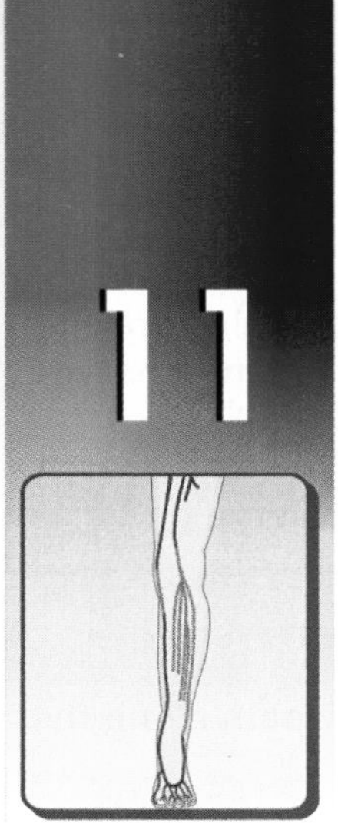

11 Venous and Lymphatic Drainage, Segmental Innervation, and Comparison of Lower and Upper Limbs

Doctors are lucky. The sun sees their success—the earth covers their mistake
—Bushnell

INTRODUCTION

Venous drainage acquires importance as blood has to flow up against the gravity.

The saphenous veins can be "easily seen" in the leg. The varicose veins, if occur, look quite ugly under the skin. Effort should be made not to develop the varicose veins. The lymph travels mostly to the inguinal group of lymph nodes.

The sensory nerves are derived only from ventral rami of L1 to L5 and S1 to S3 segments of spinal cord.

Lower limb bud rotates medially, so that extensor compartment lies on front, while flexor compartment is present on the back of thigh. Tibia and big toe lie along the pre-axial border while fibula and little toe are along the post-axial border of the limb.

VENOUS DRAINAGE

Consideration of the venous drainage is of great importance because in the lower limb venous blood has to ascend against gravity. This is aided by a number of local factors, the failure of which gives rise to varicose veins.

Factors Helping Venous Return

General Factors

1 Negative intrathoracic pressure, which is made more negative during inspiration;
2 Arterial pressure and overflow from the capillary bed;
3 Compression of veins accompanying arteries by arterial pulsation; and
4 The presence of valves, which support and divide the long column of blood into shorter columns. These also maintain a unidirectional flow.

Local Factors

These are venous, muscular and fascial.

1 *Venous:* The veins of the lower limb are more muscular than the veins of any other part of the body. They have greater number of valves. Superficial veins are connected to deep veins by perforators.
2 *Muscular:* When the limb is active, muscular contraction compresses the deep veins and drives the blood in them upwards.
   It is helped by the suction action of the diaphragm
3 *Fascial:* The tight sleeve of deep fascia makes muscular compression of the veins much more effective by limiting outward bulging of the muscles.

VEINS OF LOWER LIMB

The veins may be classified into three groups: superficial, deep and perforating.

Superficial Veins

They include the great and small saphenous veins, and their tributaries. They lie in the superficial fascia, on the surface of deep fascia (*see* Figs 3.4 and 8.1). They are thick-walled because of the presence of smooth muscle and some fibrous and elastic tissues in their walls. Valves are more numerous in the distal parts of these veins than in their proximal parts. A large proportion of their blood is drained into the deep veins through the perforating veins.

Deep Veins

These are the medial plantar, lateral plantar, dorsalis pedis, anterior and posterior tibial, peroneal, popliteal, and femoral veins, and their tributaries. They accompany the arteries, and are supported by powerful surrounding muscles. The valves are more numerous in deep veins than in superficial veins. They are more efficient channels than the superficial veins because of the driving force of muscular contraction.

Perforating Veins

They connect the superficial with the deep veins. Their valves permit only one way flow of blood, from the superficial to the deep veins. There are about five perforators along the great saphenous vein, and one perforator along the small saphenous vein.

The relevant details of these veins are given below.

LONG SAPHENOUS VEINS

1 The dorsal venous arch lies on the dorsum of the foot over the proximal parts of the metatarsal bones. It receives four dorsal metatarsal veins each of which is formed by the union of two dorsal digital veins (*see* Fig. 8.1).

2 The great or long saphenous vein is formed by the union of the medial end of dorsal venous arch with the medial marginal vein which drains the medial side of great toe. It passes upwards in front of the medial malleolus, crosses the lower one-third of the medial surface of tibia obliquely, and runs along its medial border to reach the back of the knee. The saphenous nerve runs in front of the great saphenous vein.

3 In the thigh, it inclines forwards to reach the saphenous opening where it pierces the cribriform fascia and opens into the femoral vein. Before piercing the cribriform fascia, it receives three named tributaries corresponding to the three cutaneous arteries, and also many unnamed tributaries (Fig. 11.1).

It contains about 10 to 15 valves which prevent back flow of the venous blood, which tends to occur because of gravity. One valve is always present at the saphenofemoral junction. Incompetence of these valves makes the vein dilated and tortuous leading to varicose veins.

The vein is also connected to the deep veins of the limb by perforating veins. There are three medial perforators just above the ankle, one perforator just below the knee, and another one in the region of the adductor canal (Fig. 11.2). The perforating veins are also provided with valves which permit flow of blood only from the superficial to the deep veins. Failure of the valves also gives rise to varicose veins.

Tributaries

At the commencement: Medial marginal vein from the sole.

In the leg: It communicates freely with the small saphenous vein and with deep veins.

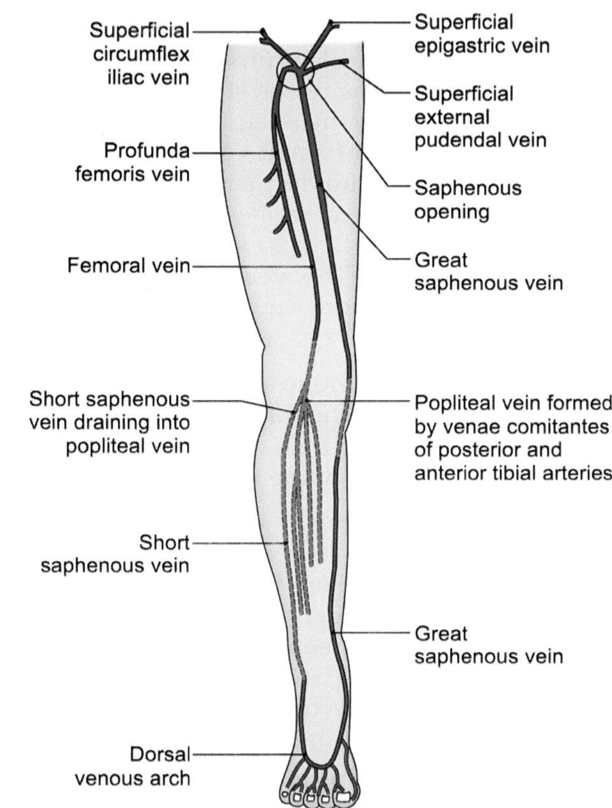

Fig. 11.1: Scheme to show the arrangement of the veins of lower limb. Popliteal, short saphenous and venae comitantes of posterior tibial artery are on posterior aspect

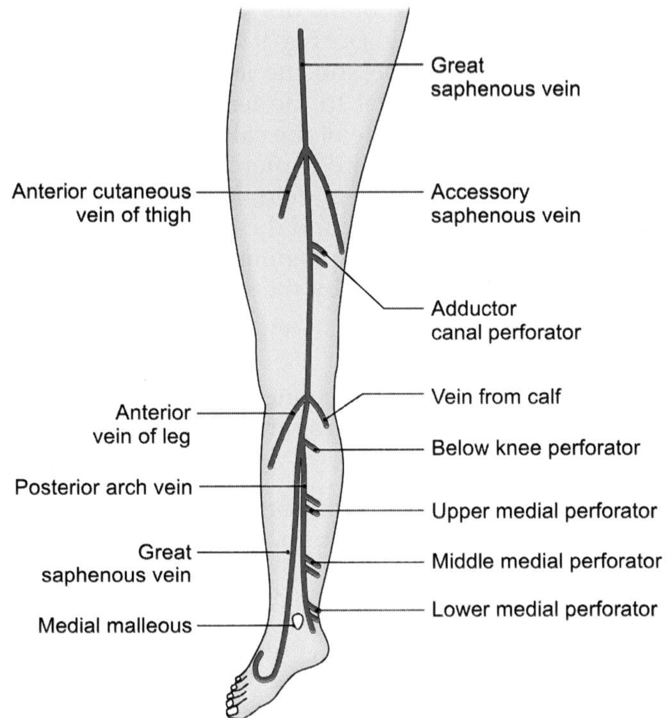

Fig. 11.2: Tributaries and perforating veins of the great saphenous vein

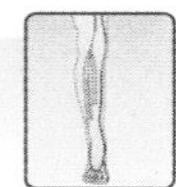

Just below the knee:

1 The anterior vein of the leg runs upwards, forwards and medially, from the lateral side of the ankle.
2 The posterior arch vein is large and constant. It begins from a series of small venous arches which connect the medial ankle perforators, and runs upwards to join the great saphenous vein just below the knee.
3 A vein from the calf: This vein also communicates with the small saphenous vein.

In the thigh:

1 The accessory saphenous vein drains the posteromedial side of the thigh.
2 The anterior cutaneous vein of the thigh drains the lower part of the front of the thigh.

Just before piercing the cribriform fascia:

1 Superficial epigastric,
2 Superficial circumflex iliac, and
3 Superficial external pudendal.

Just before termination: Deep external pudendal vein.

The *thoracoepigastric vein* runs along the anterolateral wall of the trunk. It connects the superficial epigastric vein with the lateral thoracic vein. Thus it is an important connection between the veins of the upper and lower limbs.

SMALL OR SHORT SAPHENOUS VEIN

The vein is formed on the dorsum of the foot by the union of the lateral end of the dorsal venous arch with the lateral marginal vein (*see* Fig. 9.1). It enters the back of the leg by passing behind the lateral malleolus. In the leg, it ascends lateral to the tendocalcaneus, and then along the middle line of the calf, to the lower part of the popliteal fossa. Here it pierces the deep fascia and opens into the popliteal vein. It drains the lateral border of the foot, the heel, and the back of the leg. It is connected with the great saphenous and with the deep veins, and is accompanied by the sural nerve.

PERFORATING VEINS

As already mentioned, they connect the superficial with the deep veins (Fig. 11.2). These are classified as follows.

Indirect perforating veins

Indirect perforating veins connect the superficial veins with the deep veins through the muscular veins (Fig. 11.3).

Direct perforating veins

Direct perforating veins (Fig. 11.4) connect the superficial veins directly with the deep veins. The great and small saphenous veins are the large direct perforators. The small direct perforating veins (Fig. 11.5) are follows:

1 *In the thigh:* The *adductor canal perforator* connects the great saphenous vein with the femoral vein in the lower part of the adductor canal.

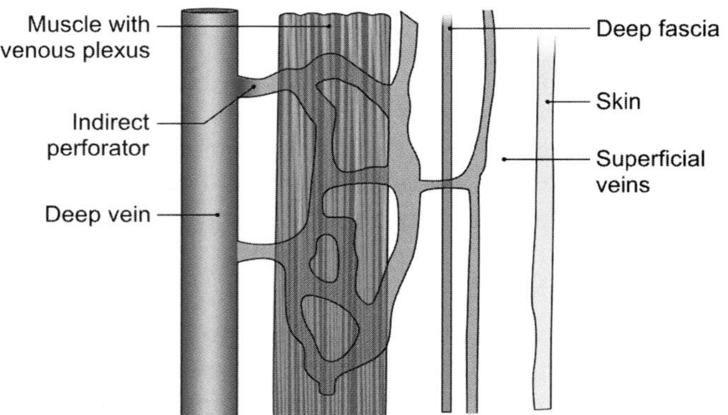

Fig. 11.3: Indirect perforating vein

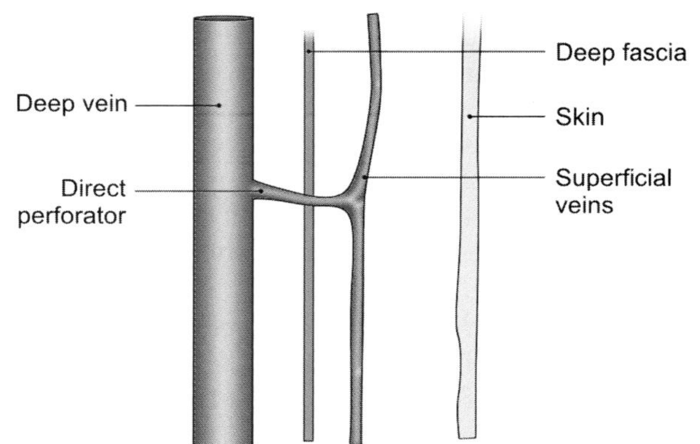

Fig. 11.4: Direct perforating vein

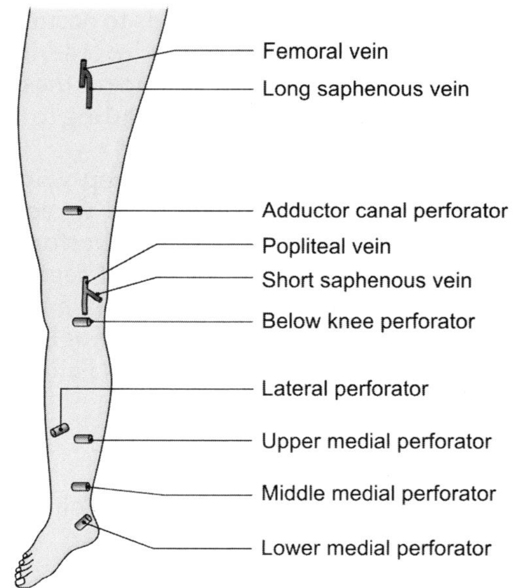

Fig. 11.5: Perforating veins of the lower limb

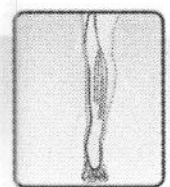

2 *Below the knee:*
One perforator connects the great saphenous vein or the posterior arch vein with the posterior tibial vein.

3 *In the leg:*
A *lateral perforator* is present at the junction of the middle and lower thirds of the leg. It connects the small saphenous vein, or one of its tributaries with the peroneal vein.

Medially there are three perforators which connect the posterior arch vein with the posterior tibial vein.

- The *upper medial perforator* lies at the junction of the middle and lower thirds of the leg.
- The *middle medial perforator* lies above the medial malleolus.
- The *lower medial perforator* lies posteroinferior to the medial malleolus.

CLINICAL ANATOMY

- *Calf pump* and *peripheral heart.* In the upright position of the body, the venous return from the lower limb depends largely on the contraction of calf muscles. These muscles are, therefore, known as the "calf pump".

  For the same reason the soleus is called the *peripheral heart* (*see* Fig. 9.3). When this muscle contracts, blood contained in large sinuses within it is pumped into the deep veins; and when the muscle relaxes, blood flows into the sinuses from the superficial veins. Unidirectional blood flow is maintained by the valves in the perforating veins (Fig. 11.6).
- "Cut open procedure"/venesection is done on the great saphenous vein as it lies in front of medial malleolus. This vein is used for transfusion of blood/fluids in case of non-availability or collapse of other veins. Saphenous nerve is identified and not injured as it lies anterior to the great saphenous vein (Fig. 11.7).
- Great saphenous vein is used for bypassing the blocked coronary arteries. The vein is reversed so that valves do not block the passage of blood.
- *Varicose veins and ulcers:* If the valves in perforating veins or at the termination of superficial veins become incompetent, the defective veins become "high pressure leaks" through which the high pressure of the deep veins produced by muscular contraction is transmitted to the superficial veins. This results in dilatation of the superficial veins and to gradual degeneration of their walls producing varicose veins and varicose ulcers (Fig. 11.8).
- Varicose veins often occur during third trimester of pregnancy, as the iliac vein get pressed due to enlarged uterus. These mostly subside after delivery.
- *Trendelenburg's test*: This is done to find out the site of leak or defect in a patient with varicose veins. Only the superficial veins and the perforating veins can be tested, not the deep veins.
- The patient is made to lie down, and the veins are emptied by raising the limb and stroking the varicose veins in a proximal direction. Now pressure is applied with the thumb at the saphenofemoral junction and the patient is asked to stand up quickly. To test the superficial veins, the pressure is released. Quick filling of the varicose veins from above indicates incompetency of the superficial veins.

  To test the perforating veins, the pressure at the saphenofemoral junction is not released, but maintained for about a minute. Gradual filling of the varices indicates incompetency of the perforating veins, allowing the blood to pass from deep to superficial veins.
- After a deep vein thrombosis affecting the perforators, they recanalise without valves. So the muscle pump will force blood from deep to superficial veins, causing varicosity of the veins.
- Varicose veins are treated with sclerosing injections or laser treatment.

Comparison between long saphenous and short saphenous veins is as follows.

Features	*Long saphenous vein*	*Short saphenous vein*
Beginning	Medial end of dorsal venous plexus	Lateral end of dorsal venous plexus
Position	Anterior to medial malleolus	Posterior to lateral malleolus
Number of valves	15–20 valves	8–10 valves
Relation of a sensory nerve	Saphenous nerve	Sural nerve
Termination	Femoral vein	Popliteal vein

LYMPHATIC DRAINAGE

Most of the lymph from the lower limb drains into the inguinal lymph nodes, either mostly directly or partly indirectly through the popliteal and anterior tibial nodes. The deep structures of the gluteal region and the upper part of the back of the thigh drain into the internal iliac nodes along the gluteal vessels.

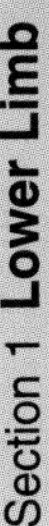

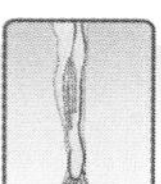

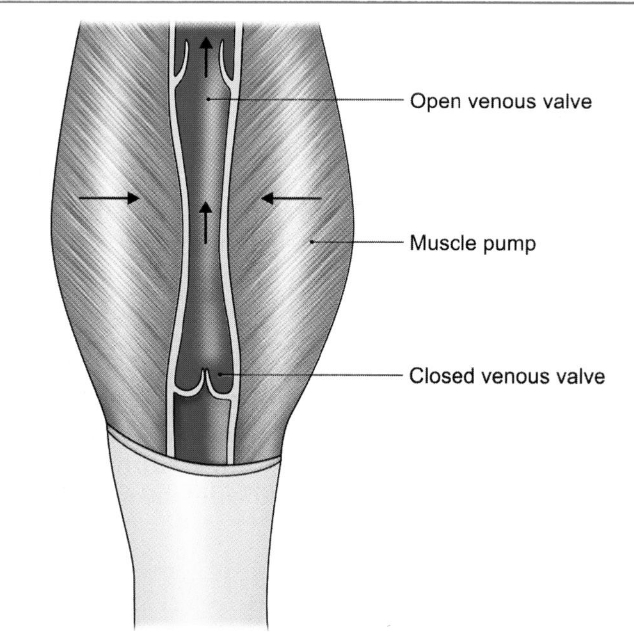

Fig. 11.6: Venous valves for unidirectional flow of blood

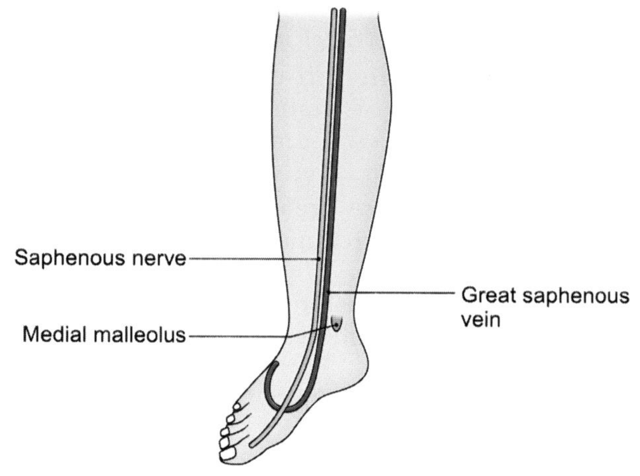

Fig. 11.7: Cut open vene section procedure on great saphenous vein

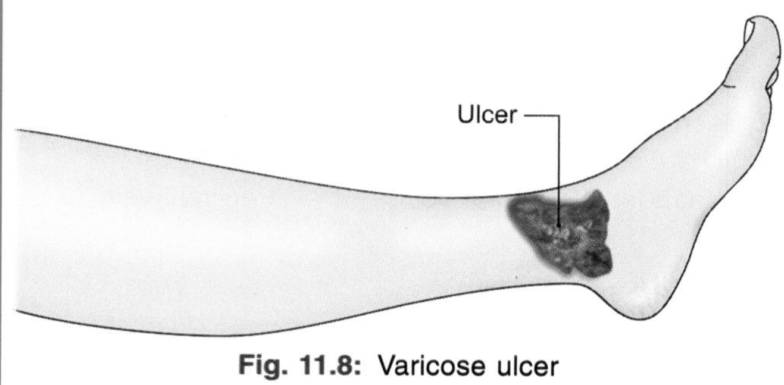

Fig. 11.8: Varicose ulcer

Classification

I. Lymph nodes
   a. Superficial inguinal lymph nodes.
   b. Deep:
      - Deep inguinal lymph nodes
      - Popliteal lymph nodes
      - Anterior tibial lymph nodes.

II. Lymphatics:
   a. Superficial, and
   b. Deep.

Superficial Inguinal Lymph Nodes

These are very important because they drain the skin and fasciae of the lower limb; the perineum and the trunk below the umbilical plane (*see* Fig. 3.5). They are divided into three sets.

1 The *lower vertical group* is placed along both sides of the terminal part of the great saphenous vein, and contains about four or five nodes. They drain the skin and fasciae of the lower limb (great saphenous territory), except the buttock and the short saphenous territory. A few lymphatics, accompanying the short saphenous vein, cross the leg, accompany the great saphenous vein, and drain into this group of nodes.

2 The *upper lateral group* is placed below the lateral part of the inguinal ligament, and contains about two or three nodes. They drain the skin and fasciae of the upper part of the lateral side of the thigh, the buttock, the flank and the back below the umbilical plane.

3 The *upper medial group* is placed below the medial end of the inguinal ligament. One or two nodes may lie above the inguinal ligament along the course of the superficial epigastric vessels. The group contains two to three nodes. They drain:
   a. The anterior abdominal wall below the level of the umbilicus.
   b. The perineum, including external genitalia, except the glans, the anal canal below the pectinate line, the vagina below hymen and the penile part of the male urethra.
   c. The superolateral angle of the uterus, via the round ligament.

Efferents from all superficial inguinal nodes pierce the cribriform fascia, and terminate in the deep inguinal nodes. A few may pass directly to the external iliac nodes.

Deep Inguinal Lymph Nodes

These are about four to five in number, and lie medial to the upper part of the femoral vein. The most proximal node of this group; gland of Cloquet or of Rosenmüller, lies in the femoral canal. These nodes receive afferents from:

1 The superficial inguinal nodes.
2 The popliteal nodes.
3 Glans penis or clitoris.
4 The deep lymphatics of the lower limb accompanying the femoral vessels.

Their efferents pass to the external iliac nodes.

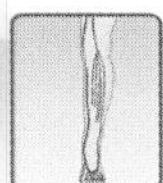

Popliteal Lymph Nodes

These nodes lie near the termination of the small saphenous vein, deep to the deep fascia. One node lies between the popliteal artery and the oblique popliteal ligament. They receive afferents from:

1 The territory of the small saphenous vein.
2 The deep parts of the leg (through vessels running along the anterior and posterior tibial vessels).
3 The knee joint.

Their efferents run along the popliteal and femoral vessels, and terminate in the deep inguinal nodes.

Anterior Tibial Lymph Node

One inconstant node may lie along the upper part of the anterior tibial artery. When present, it collects lymph from the anterior compartment of the leg, and passes it on to the popliteal nodes.

Superficial Lymphatics

These lymph vessels are larger and are more numerous than the deep lymphatics. They run in the superficial fascia and ultimately form two streams. The main stream follows the great saphenous vein, and ends in the lower vertical group of superficial inguinal lymph nodes shown in (Fig. 11.9a). The accessory stream follows the small saphenous vein and ends in the popliteal lymph nodes (Fig. 11.9b).

Deep Lymphatics

These are smaller and fewer than the superficial lymphatics, although they drain all structures lying deep to the deep fascia. They run along the principal blood vessels, and terminate mostly into the deep inguinal nodes, either directly or indirectly through the popliteal nodes. The deep lymphatics from the gluteal region and from the upper part of the back of the thigh accompany the gluteal vessels and end in the internal iliac nodes.

CLINICAL ANATOMY

- *Elephantiasis:* Lymphatic obstruction caused by the parasite filaria is very common in the lower limb. This results in great hypertrophy of the skin and of subcutaneous tissue (elephantiasis) (Fig. 11.10).
- The commonest cause of a swelling in the inguinal area is enlargement of the inguinal lymph nodes. This can be caused by infection, or carcinoma, anywhere in the area drained by these nodes (Fig. 11.11).

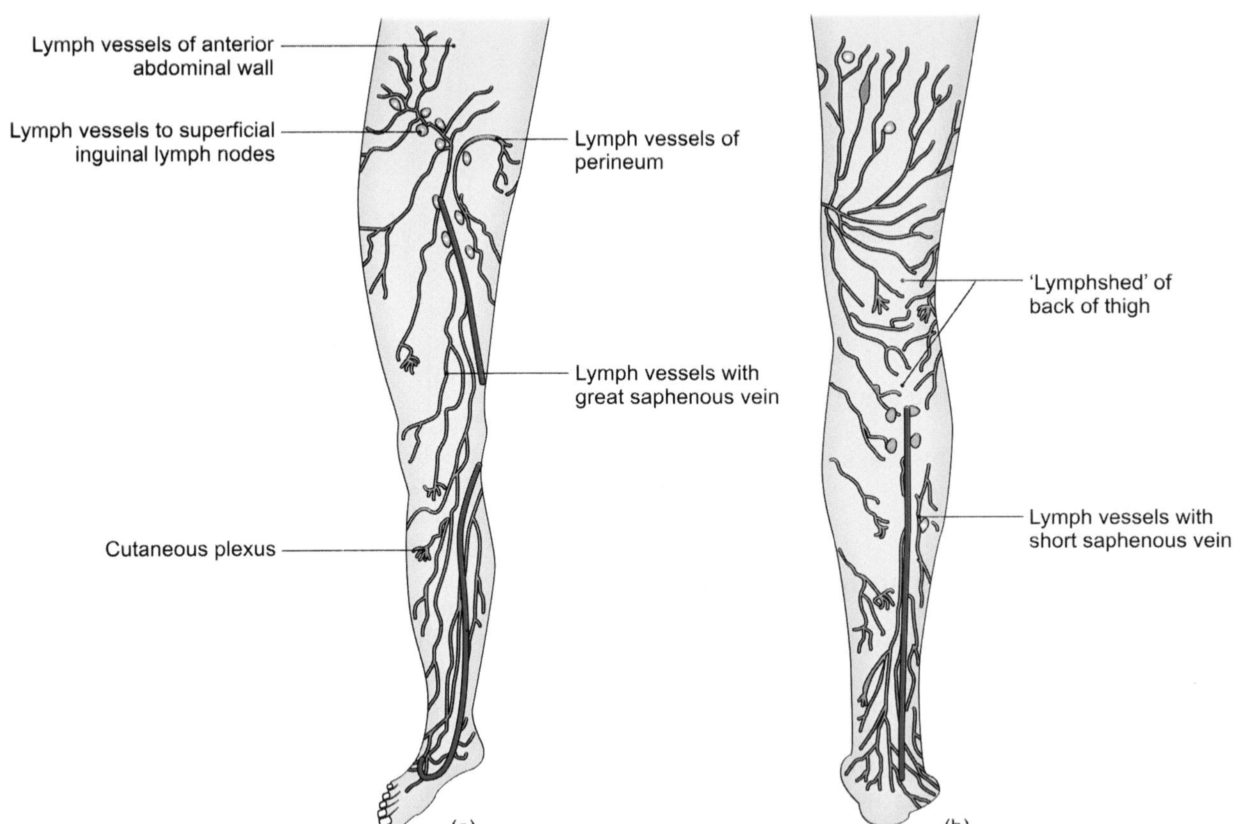

Figs 11.9a and b: Superficial lymphatics of the lower limb: (a) Anterior aspect, and (b) posterior aspect

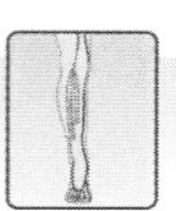

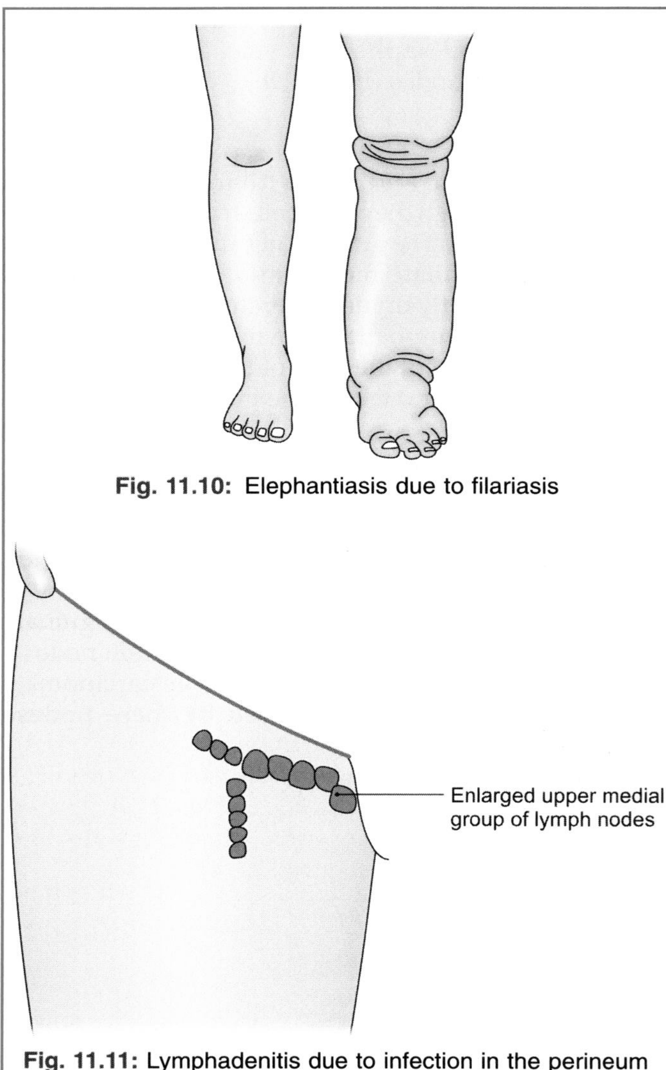

Fig. 11.10: Elephantiasis due to filariasis

Fig. 11.11: Lymphadenitis due to infection in the perineum

SEGMENTAL INNERVATION

Dermatomes

The principles involved are the same as described in the upper limb.

The area of skin supplied by one spinal segment is called a dermatome.

Important Features

1 The cutaneous innervation of the lower limb is derived:
   a. Mainly from segments L1 to L5 and S1 to S3 of the spinal cord; and
   b. Partly from segments T12 and S4.

2 As a rule, the limb is supplied only by anterior primary rami. The exception to this rule is that the skin of the superomedial quadrant of the gluteal region is supplied by the posterior primary rami of nerves L1 to L3 and S1 to S3.

3 There is varying degree of overlap of adjoining dermatomes, so that the area of sensory loss following damage to the spinal cord or nerve roots is always less than the actual area of the dermatome.

4 Initially, each limb bud has a cephalic border, and a caudal border. These are known as the *preaxial* and the *postaxial* borders, respectively. In the embryo, the great toe and tibia lie along the preaxial border, and the little toe and fibula along the postaxial border. Later, the limb bud rotates medially through 90°, so that the great toe and tibia are carried medially, and the little toe and fibula laterally. Thus, the tibial border is the original preaxial border, and the fibular border, the postaxial border, of the lower limb.

5 The dermatomes of the lower limb are distributed in an orderly numerical sequence (Figs 11.12a and b).

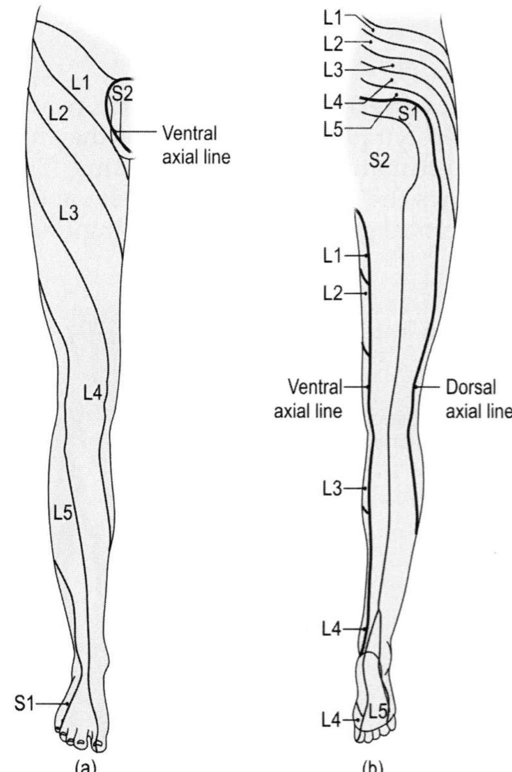

Figs 11.12a and b: Dermatomes of the lower limb: (a) Anterior view, and (b) posterior view

Along the preaxial border from above downwards, there are dermatomes T12, L1 to L4.

The middle three toes, the adjoining area of the dorsum of the foot and the lateral side of the leg are supplied by segment L5.

Along the postaxial border from below upwards, there are dermatomes S1, S2, S3.

6 As the limb elongates, the central dermatomes (L4, L5, S1) get pulled in such a way that these are

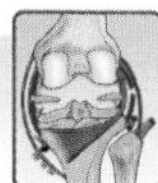

Ligaments

The ligaments include:

- The fibrous capsule,
- The iliofemoral ligament,
- The pubofemoral ligament,
- The ischiofemoral ligament,
- The ligament of the head of the femur,
- The acetabular labrum, and
- The transverse acetabular ligament.

1 The *fibrous capsule* is attached *on the hip bone* to the acetabular labrum including the transverse acetabular ligament, and to bone above and behind the acetabulum; and *on the femur* to the intertrochanteric line in front, and 1 cm medial to the intertrochanteric crest behind (Fig. 12.2).

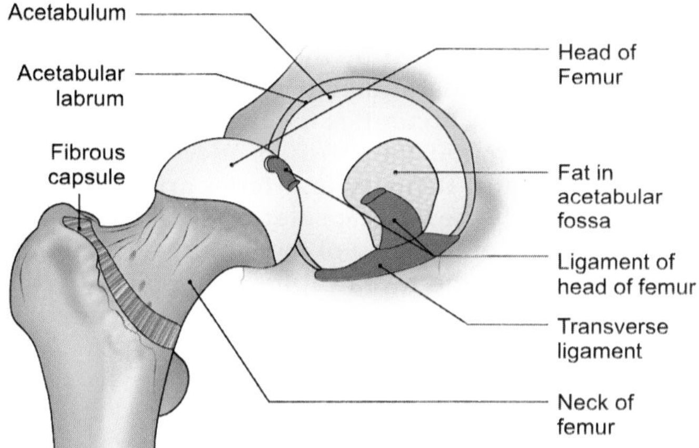

Fig. 12.2: Fibrous capsule of the hip joint

Anterosuperiorly, the capsule is thick and firmly attached. This part is subjected to maximum tension in the standing posture. Posteroinferiorly, the capsule is thin and loosely attached to bone.

The capsule is made up of two types of fibres. The outer fibres are longitudinal and the inner circular ones are called as *zona orbicularis*. The longitudinal fibres are best developed anterosuperiorly, where many of them are reflected along the neck of the femur to form the *retinacula*. Blood vessels supplying the head and neck of the femur, travel along these retinacula. The synovial membrane lines the fibrous capsule, the intracapsular portion of the neck of the femur, both surfaces of the acetabular labrum, the transverse ligament, and fat in the acetabular fossa. It also invests the round ligament of the head of the femur (Fig. 12.2).

The joint cavity communicates with a bursa lying deep to the tendon of psoas major, through a circular opening in the capsule located between the pubofemoral ligament and vertical band of the iliofemoral ligament (Fig.12.3).

2 The *iliofemoral ligament*, or inverted Y-shaped ligament of *Bigelow*, lies anteriorly. It is one of the strongest ligaments in the body. It prevents the trunk from falling backwards in the standing posture. The ligament is triangular in shape. Its apex is attached to the lower half of the anterior inferior iliac spine; and the base to the intertrochanteric line. The upper oblique and lower vertical fibres form thick and strong bands, while the middle fibres are thin and weak (Fig. 12.3).

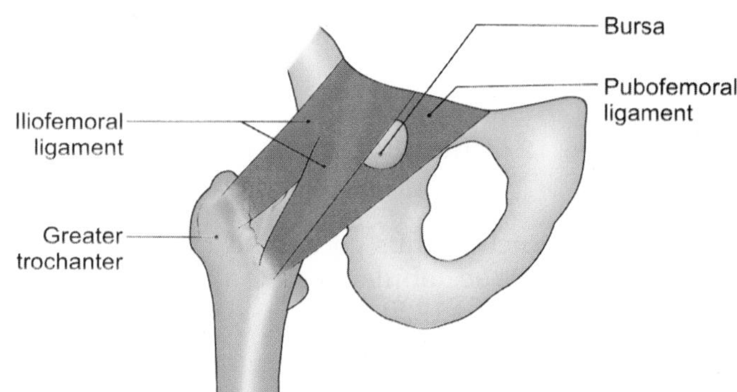

Fig. 12.3: The iliofemoral and pubofemoral ligaments

3 The *pubofemoral ligament* supports the joint inferomedially. It is also triangular in shape. Superiorly, it is attached to the iliopubic eminence, the obturator crest and the obturator membrane. Inferiorly, it merges with the anteroinferior part of the capsule and with the lower band of the iliofemoral ligament.

4 The *ischiofemoral ligament* is comparatively weak. It covers the joint posteriorly. Its fibres are twisted and extend from the ischium to the acetabulum. The fibres of the ligament form the zona orbicularis. Some of them are attached to the greater trochanter (Fig. 12.4).

5 The *ligament of the head of the femur,* round ligament or ligamentum teres is a flat and triangular ligament. The apex is attached to the fovea capitis, and the base to the transverse ligament and the margins of the acetabular notch. It may be very thin, or even absent. It transmits arteries to the head of the femur, from the acetabular branches of the obturator and medial circumflex femoral arteries (*see* Fig. 4.7).

6 The *acetabular labrum* is a fibrocartilaginous rim attached to the margins of the acetabulum. It narrows the mouth of the acetabulum. This helps in holding the head of the femur in position (Fig. 12.5).

7 The *transverse ligament of the acetabulum* is a part of the acetabular labrum which bridges the acetabular

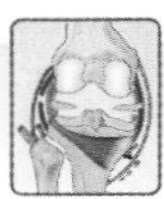

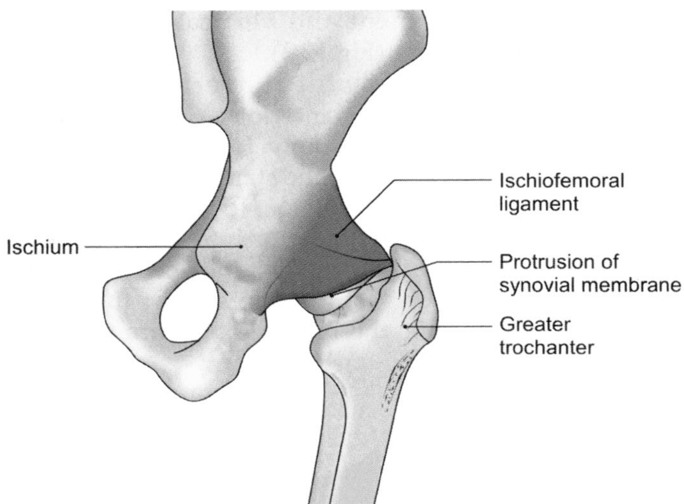

Fig. 12.4: The ischiofemoral ligament

notch. The notch is thus converted into a foramen which transmits acetabular vessels and nerves to the joint (Figs 12.1 and 12.5).

Relations of the Hip Joint

Anterior Relations

Tendon of the iliopsoas separated from the joint by a bursa and femoral vein, femoral artery and femoral nerve (Fig. 12.5).

Posterior Relations

The joint, from below upwards, is related to the following muscles: Tendon of obturator externus covered by the quadratus femoris, obturator internus and gemelli, piriformis, sciatic nerve and the gluteus maximus muscle.

Superior Relations

Reflected head of the rectus femoris covered by the gluteus minimus, gluteus medius and partly by gluteus maximus.

Inferior Relations

Lateral fibres of the pectineus and the obturator externus. In addition there are gracilis, adductors longus, brevis, magnus and hamstring muscles.

Blood Supply

The hip joint is supplied by the obturator artery, two circumflex femorals and two gluteal arteries. The medial and lateral circumflex femoral arteries form an arterial circle around the capsular attachment on the neck of the femur. Retinacular arteries arise from this circle and supply the intracapsular part of the neck and the greater part of the head of the femur. A small part of the head, near the fovea capitis is supplied by the acetabular branches of the obturator and medial circumflex femoral arteries (*see* Fig. 4.7).

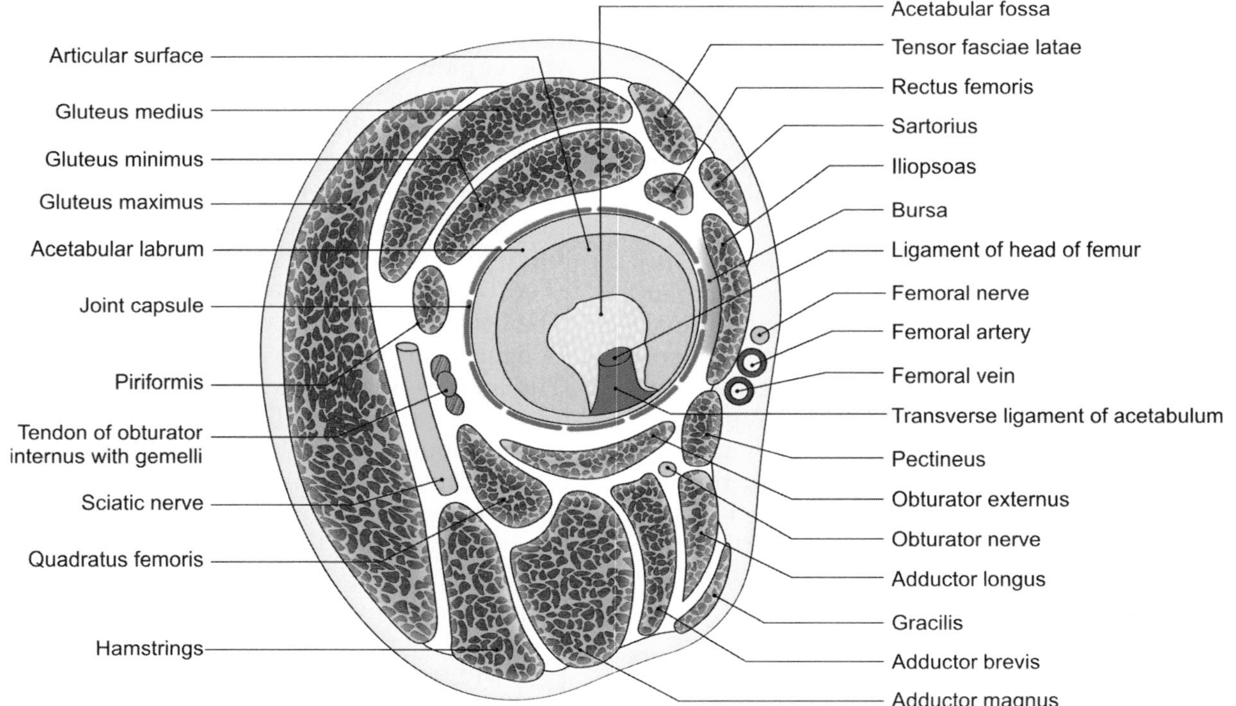

Fig. 12.5: Relations of the hip joint

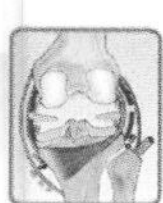

Nerve Supply

The hip joint is supplied by the femoral nerve, through the nerve to the rectus femoris; the anterior division of the obturator nerve; the nerve to the quadratus femoris; and the superior gluteal nerve.

Movements

1 Flexion and extension occur around a transverse axis.
2 Adduction and abduction occur around an anteroposterior axis.
3 Medial and lateral rotation occur around a vertical axis.
4 Circumduction is a combination of the foregoing movements.

Hip joint extension and slight abduction and medial rotation is the close packed position for the hip joint which means the ligaments and the capsules are most taut in this position. But the surfaces are most congruent in slightly flexed, abducted and laterally rotated position of the hip.

In general, all axes pass through the centre of the head of the femur, but none of them is fixed because the head is not quite spherical.

Flexion is limited by contact of the thigh with the anterior abdominal wall. Similarly, adduction is limited by contact with the opposite limb. The range of the other movements is different from one another: Extension 15°, abduction 50°, medial rotation 25°, and lateral rotation 60°.

The movement of the hip is closely related to the position of the knee because of the presence of two muscles which act on both hip and knee. In the extended position of the knee, the stretch on the hamstring muscles does not allow the hip to move into its complete flexion range. Similarly with knee completely flexed, the hip joint may not attain complete extension due to tension in the rectus femoris which gets stretched at the hip and the knee.

When the hip joints are bearing weight, the femur is fixed. But like any other joint, here also the proximal bone, i.e. pelvis is capable of moving on the fixed distal femur. The pelvis can either move into anterior tilting (equivalent to flexion of hip) or posterior tilting (equivalent to extension of the hip).

The muscles producing these movements are given in Table 12.1.

CLINICAL ANATOMY

- *Congenital dislocation* is more common in the hip than in any other joint of the body. The head of the femur slips upwards on to the gluteal surface of the ilium because the upper margin of the acetabulum is developmentally deficient (Fig. 12.6). This causes lurching gait, and Trendelenburg's test is positive (*see* Fig. 5.12).
- *Perthes' disease* or pseudocoxalgia is characterized by destruction and flattening of the head of the femur, with an increased joint space in X-ray pictures.
  Coxa vara is a condition in which the neck-shaft angle is reduced from the normal angle of about 150° in a child, and 127° in an adult (Fig. 12.7).
- *Dislocation of the hip* may be posterior (more common), anterior (less common), or central (rare). The sciatic nerve may be injured in posterior dislocations.
- Injuries in the region of hip joint may produce shortening of the lower limb. The length of lower limb is measured from the anterior superior iliac spine to the medial malleolus.
- Disease of the hip like tuberculosis, may cause *referred pain* in the knee because of the common nerve supply of the two joints.
- *Aspiration of the hip joint* can be done by passing a needle from a point 5 cm below the anterior superior iliac spine, upwards, backwards and medially. It can also be done from the side by passing the needle from the posterior edge of the greater trochanter, upwards and medially, parallel with the neck of the femur.

Table 12.1: Muscles producing movements at the hip joint

Movement	*Chief muscles*	*Accessory muscles*
1. Flexion	Psoas major and iliacus	Pectineus, rectus femoris, and sartorius; adductors (mainly adductor longus) participate in early stages
2. Extension	Gluteus maximus and hamstrings	—
3. Adduction	Adductors longus, brevis and magnus	Pectineus and gracilis
4. Abduction	Glutei medius and minimus	Tensor fasciae latae and sartorius
5. Medial rotation	Tensor fasciae latae and the anterior fibres of the glutei medius and minimus	—
6. Lateral rotation	Two obturators, two gemelli and the quadratus femoris	Piriformis, gluteus maximus and sartorius

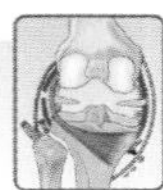

- Hip diseases show an interesting age pattern:
  a. Below 5 years : Congenital dislocation and tuberculosis (Fig. 12.6)
  b. 5 to 10 years : Perthes' disease
  c. 10 to 20 years : Coxa vara (Fig. 12.7)
  d. Above 40 years: Osteoarthritis
- In arthritis of hip joint, the position of joint is partially flexed, abducted and laterally rotated.
- Fracture of the neck of the femur may be subcapital, near the head (Fig. 12.8), cervical in the middle, or basal near the trochanters. Damage to retinacular arteries causes avascular necrosis of the head. Such a damage is maximal in subcapital fractures and least in basal fractures. These fractures are common in old age, between the age of 40 and 60 years. Femur neck fracture is usually produced by trivial injuries.

  Trochanteric fracture may be intertrochanteric, i.e. between the trochanters or subtrochanteric, i.e. below the trochanters. These fractures occur in strong, adult subjects, and are produced by severe, violent injuries (Fig. 12.8).
- Shenton's line, in an X-ray picture, is a continuous curve formed by the upper border of the obturator foramen and the lower border of the neck of the femur. In fracture neck femur, line becomes abnormal (Fig. 12.9).

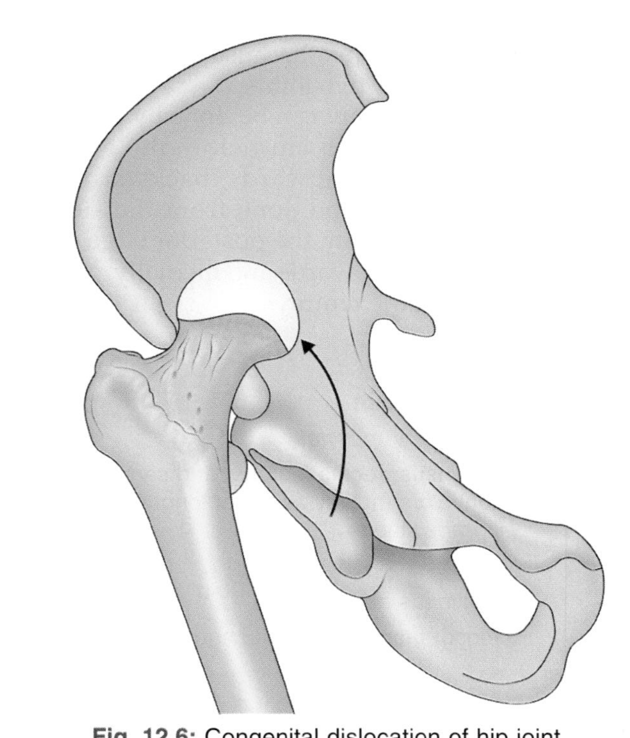

Fig. 12.6: Congenital dislocation of hip joint

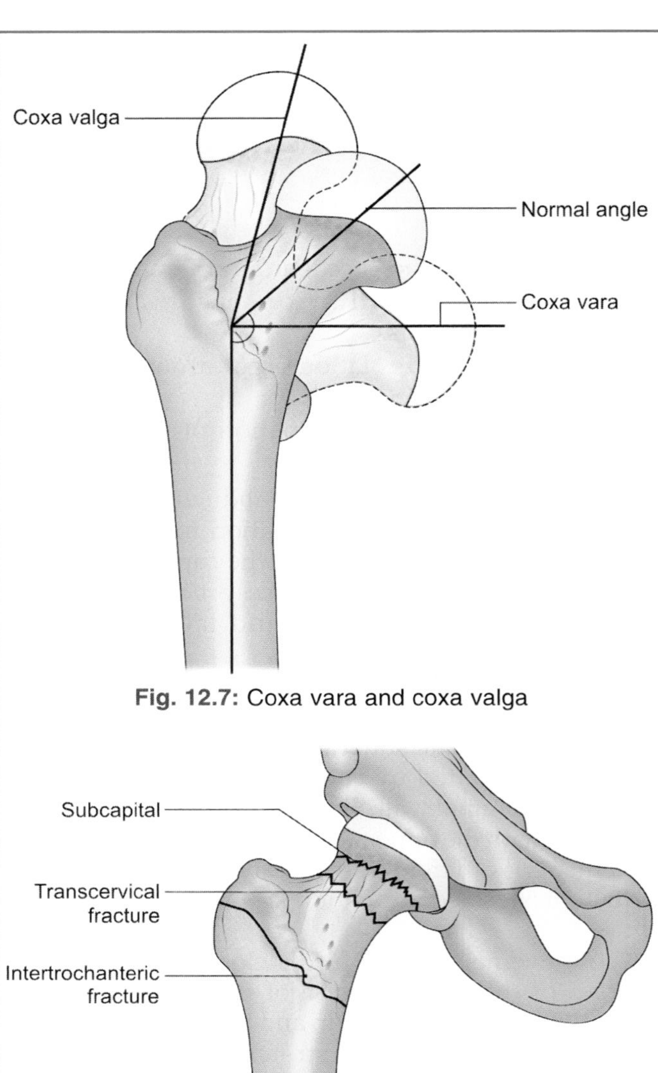

Fig. 12.7: Coxa vara and coxa valga

Fig. 12.8: Fracture of neck and trochanteric fracture

KNEE JOINT

DISSECTION

Strip the extra structures around the knee joint, leaving behind the fibrous capsule, ligaments and parts of muscles/tendons attached to the bones/ligaments.

Study the articular surfaces, articular capsule, medial and lateral collateral ligaments, oblique popliteal ligament and arcuate popliteal ligament.

Features

The knee is the largest and most complex joint of the body. The complexity is the result of fusion of three joints in one. It is formed by fusion of the lateral

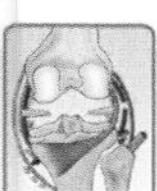

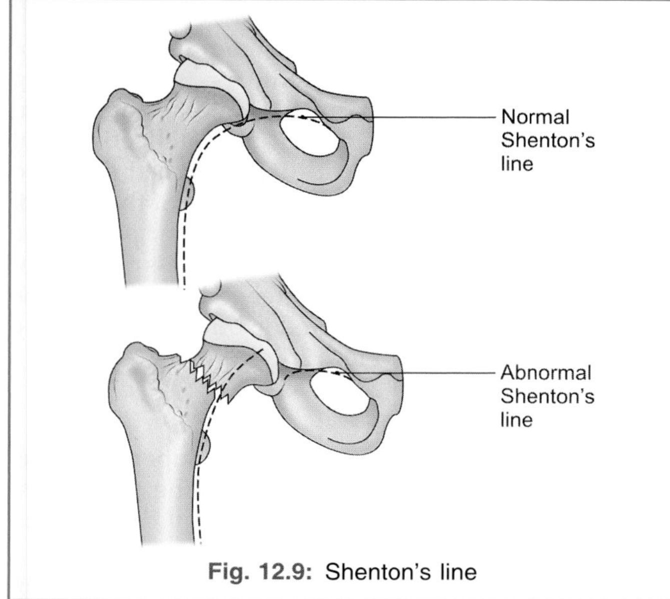

Fig. 12.9: Shenton's line

femorotibial, medial femorotibial, and femoropatellar joints.

Type

It is condylar synovial joint, incorporating two condylar joints between the condyles of the femur and tibia, and one saddle joint between the femur and the patella. It is also a complex joint as the cavity is divided by the menisci.

Articular Surfaces

The knee joint is formed by:

1 The condyles of the femur.
2 The patella (Figs 12.10 to 12.12).
3 The condyles of the tibia. The femoral condyles articulate with the tibial condyles below and behind, and with the patella in front.

Ligaments

The knee joint is supported by the following ligaments.

1 Fibrous capsule (Fig. 12.11).
2 Ligamentum patellae (Fig. 12.12).
3 Tibial collateral or medial ligament (Fig. 12.11).
4 Fibular collateral or lateral ligament (Fig. 12.11).

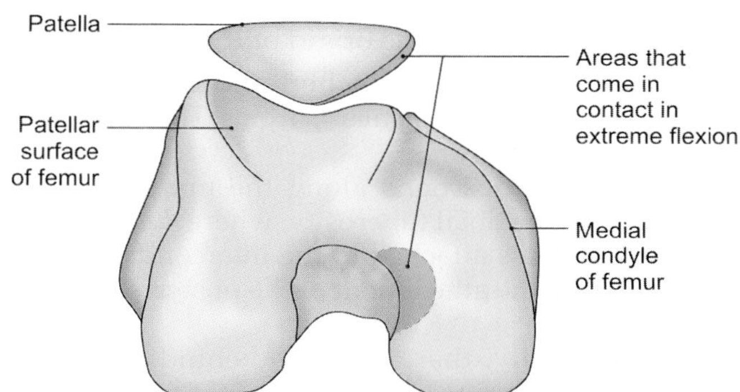

Fig. 12.10: Lower end of the femur and patella

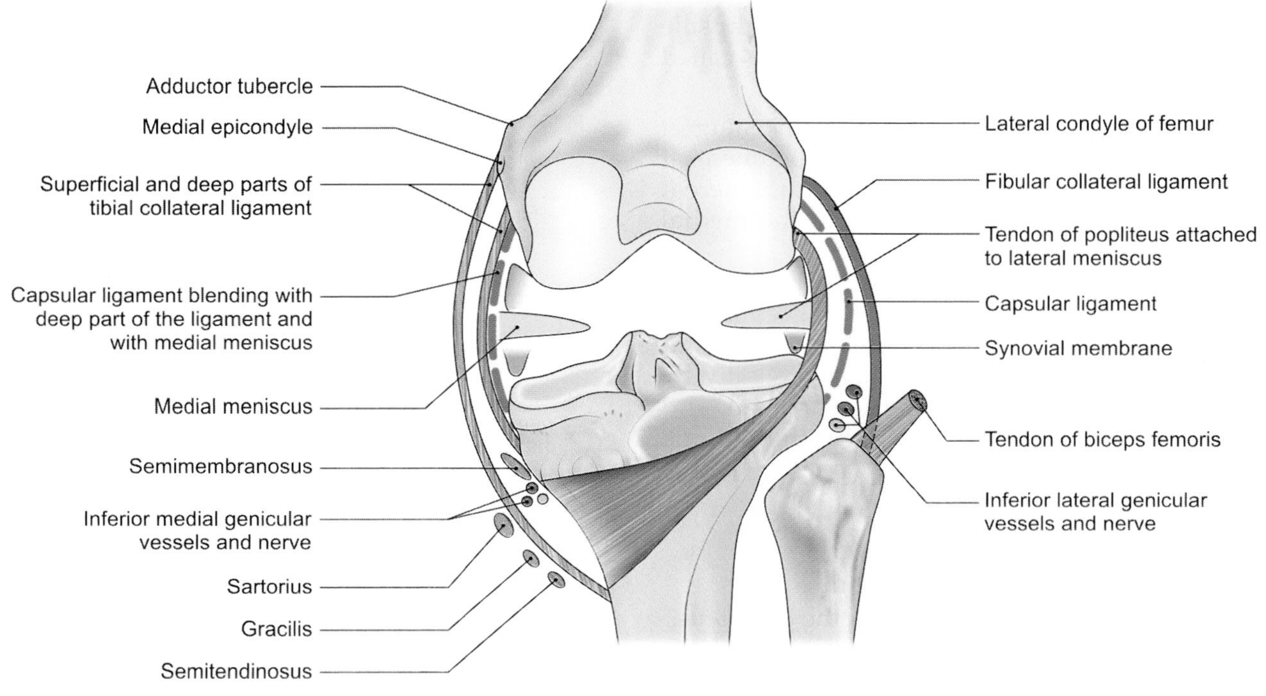

Fig. 12.11: Tibial and fibular collateral ligaments

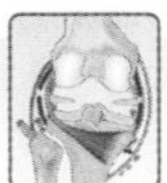

5 Oblique popliteal ligament (Fig. 12.11).
6 Arcuate popliteal ligament.
7 Anterior cruciate ligament (Fig. 12.12).
8 Posterior cruciate ligament (Fig. 12.12).
9 Medial meniscus (Fig. 12.11).
10 Lateral meniscus (Fig. 12.11).
11 Transverse ligament.

Fibrous (Articular) Capsule

The fibrous capsule is very thin, and is deficient anteriorly, where it is replaced by the quadriceps femoris, the patella and the ligamentum patellae.

Femoral attachment: It is attached about half to one centimeter beyond the articular margins. The attachment has three special features.

1 Anteriorly, it is deficient.
2 Posteriorly, it is attached to the intercondylar line.
3 Laterally, it encloses the origin of the popliteus.

Tibial attachment: It is attached about half to one centimeter beyond the articular margins. The attachment has three special features.

1 Anteriorly, it descends along the margins of the condyles to the tibial tuberosity, where it is deficient.
2 Posteriorly, it is attached to the intercondylar ridge which limits the attachment of the posterior cruciate ligament.
3 Posterolaterally, there is a gap behind the lateral condyle for passage of the tendon of the popliteus.

Some terms applied to parts of the capsule are as follows.

Coronary ligament: The fibrous capsule is attached to the periphery of the menisci. The part of the capsule between the menisci and the tibia is sometimes called the coronary ligament.

Short lateral ligament: This is a cord-like thickening of the capsule deep to the fibular collateral ligament. It extends from the lateral epicondyle of femur, where it blends with the tendon of popliteus, to the medial border of the apex of the fibula.

The capsular ligament is weak. It is strengthened anteriorly by the medial and lateral patellar retinacula, which are extensions from the vastus medialis and lateralis; laterally by the iliotibial tract; medially by expansions from the tendons of the sartorius and semimembranosus; and posteriorly, by the oblique popliteal ligament.

Openings

The capsule has two constant gaps.

1 One leading into the suprapatellar bursa.
2 Another for the exit of the tendon of the popliteus.

Sometimes there are gaps that communicate with the bursae deep to the medial head of the gastrocnemius, and deep to the semimembranosus.

Ligamentum Patellae

This is the central portion of the common tendon of insertion of the quadriceps femoris; the remaining portions of the tendon form the medial and lateral patellar retinacula. The ligamentum patellae is about 7.5 cm long and 2.5 cm broad. It is attached above to the margins and rough posterior surface of the apex of the patella, and below to the *smooth, upper part* of the tibial tuberosity. The superficial fibres pass in front of the patella. The ligamentum patellae is related to the superficial and deep infrapatellar bursae, and to the infrapatellar pad of fat (Fig. 12.12).

Tibial Collateral or Medial Ligament

This is a long band of great strength. Superiorly, it is attached to the medial epicondyle of the femur just below the adductor tubercle. Inferiorly, it divides into anterior and posterior parts.

The *anterior* or *superficial part* is about 10 cm long and 1.25 cm broad, and is separated from the capsule by one or two bursae. It is attached below to the medial border and posterior part of the medial surface of the shaft of the tibia. It covers the inferior medial genicular vessels and nerve, and the anterior part of the tendon of the semimembranosus, and is crossed below by the tendons of the sartorius, gracilis and the semitendinosus (Fig. 12.11).

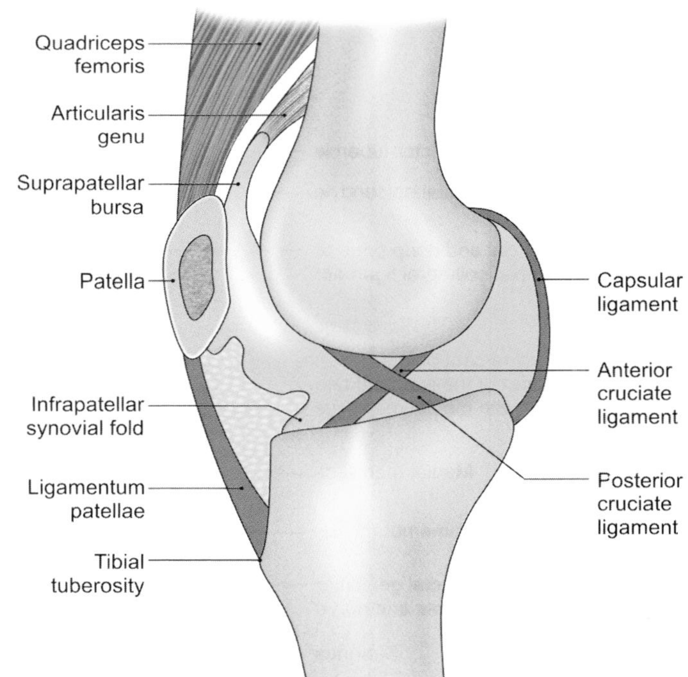

Fig. 12.12: Sagittal section through the knee joint of right side seen from the medial aspect to show the reflection of the synovial membrane (note the cruciate ligaments)

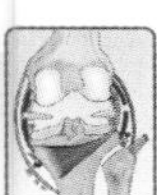

The *posterior (deep) part* of the ligament is short and blends with the capsule and with the medial meniscus. It is attached to the medial condyle of the tibia above the groove for the semimembranosus.

Morphologically, the tibial collateral ligament represents the degenerated tendon of the adductor magnus muscle.

Fibular Collateral or Lateral Ligament

This ligament is strong and cord-like. It is about 5 cm long. Superiorly, it is attached to the lateral epicondyle of the femur just above the popliteal groove. Inferiorly, it is embraced by the tendon of the biceps femoris, and is attached to the head of the fibula in front of its apex. It is separated from the lateral meniscus by the tendon of the popliteus. It is free from the capsule. The inferior lateral genicular vessels and nerve separate it from the capsule (Fig. 12.11).

Morphologically, it represents the femoral attachment of the peroneus longus.

Oblique Popliteal Ligament

This is an expansion from the tendon of the semimembranosus. It runs upwards and laterally, blends with the posterior surface of the capsule, and is attached to the intercondylar line and lateral condyle of the femur. It is closely related to the popliteal artery, and is pierced by the middle genicular vessels and nerve, and the terminal part of the posterior division of the obturator nerve (Fig 12.13).

Arcuate Popliteal Ligament

This is a posterior expansion from the short lateral ligament. It extends backwards from the head of the fibula, arches over the tendon of the popliteus, and is attached to the posterior border of the intercondylar area of the tibia.

Cruciate Ligaments

These are very thick and strong fibrous bands, which act as direct bonds of union between tibia and femur, to maintain anteroposterior stability of knee joint. They are named according to the attachment on tibia.

Anterior cruciate ligament begins from anterior part of intercondylar area of tibia, runs upwards, backwards and laterally and is attached to the posterior part of medial surface of lateral condyle of femur. It is taut during extension of knee (*see* Fig. 2.12).

Posterior cruciate ligament begins from the posterior part of intercondylar area of tibia, runs upwards, forwards and medially and is attached to the anterior part of the lateral surface of medial condyle of femur. It is taut during flexion of the knee.

These are supplied by middle genicular vessels and nerves (*see* Figs 2.26 and 12.13).

Menisci or Semilunar Cartilages

The menisci are two fibrocartilaginous discs. They are shaped like crescents. They deepen the articular surfaces of the condyles of the tibia, and partially divide the joint cavity into upper and lower compartments. Flexion and extension of the knee take place in the *upper* compartment, whereas rotation takes place in the *lower* compartment (Fig. 12.11).

Each meniscus has the following.

a. *Two ends:* The anterior and posterior ends of menisci are attached to the tibia and are referred to as anterior and posterior horns.
b. *Two borders:* The 'outer' border is thick, convex and close to the fibrous capsule; while the 'inner' border is thin, concave and free.
c. *Two surfaces:* The upper surface is concave for articulation with the femur. The lower surface is flat and rests on the peripheral two-thirds of the tibial condyle. The peripheral thick part is vascular. The inner part is avascular and is nourished by synovial fluid.

The *medial meniscus* is nearly semicircular, being wider behind than in front. The posterior fibres of the anterior end are continuous with the transverse ligament. Its peripheral margin is adherent to the deep part of the tibial collateral ligament (Fig. 12.11).

The *lateral meniscus* is nearly circular (*see* Fig. 2.26). The posterior end of the meniscus is attached to the medial condyle of femur through two meniscofemoral ligaments. The tendon of the popliteus and the capsule separate this meniscus from the fibular collateral ligament. The more medial part of the tendon of the popliteus is attached to the lateral meniscus. The mobility of the posterior end of this meniscus is controlled by the popliteus and by the two meniscofemoral ligaments.

Because of the attachments of the menisci to multiple structures, the motion of the menisci is limited to a great extent. Out of the two menisci the medial meniscus has more firm attachments to the tibia.

In a young person the peripheral 25–33% of the meniscus is vascularised and is innervated. The remaining part of the meniscus receives its nutrition from the synovial fluid. Therefore, movement is important for cartilage nutrition since movement causes diffusion of nutrients from synovial fluid to the cartilage.

Functions of menisci

1 They help in making the articular surfaces more congruent. Because of their flexibility they can adapt

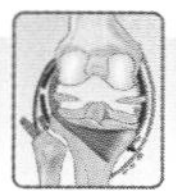

their contour to the varying curvature of the different parts of the femoral condyles, as the latter glide over the tibia.
2 The menisci serve as shock absorbers.
3 They help in lubricating the joint cavity.
4 Because of their nerve supply, they also have a sensory function. They give rise to proprioceptive impulses.

Transverse Ligament

It connects the anterior ends of the medial and lateral menisci (Fig. 12.13).

SYNOVIAL MEMBRANE

DISSECTION

Cut through the tendon of quadriceps femoris muscle just above the knee joint. Extend this incision on either side of patella and ligamentum patellae anchored to the tibial tuberosity. Reflect patella downwards to peep into the cavity of knee joint.

Note the huge infrapatellar synovial fold and pad of fat in it. Remove the fat and posterior part of fibrous capsule so that the cruciate ligaments and menisci are visualised.

Features

The synovial membrane of the knee joint lines the capsule, except posteriorly where it is reflected forwards by the cruciate ligaments, forming a common covering for both the ligaments (Figs 12.11 and 12.12).

In front, it is absent from the patella. Above the patella, it is prolonged upwards for 5 cm or more as the suprapatellar bursa. Below the patella, it covers the deep surface of the infrapatellar pad of fat, which separates it from the ligamentum patellae. A median fold, the *infrapatellar synovial fold,* extends backwards from the pad of fat to the intercondylar fossa of the femur. An alar fold diverges on each side from the median fold to reach the lateral edges of the patella (Fig. 12.12).

Bursae around the Knee

As many as 12 bursae have been described around the knee—four anterior, four lateral, and four medial. These bursae are as follows.

Anterior

1 Subcutaneous prepatellar bursa (*see* Fig. 3.6).
2 Subcutaneous infrapatellar bursa.
3 Deep infrapatellar bursa.
4 Suprapatellar bursa.

Lateral

1 A bursa deep to the lateral head of the gastrocnemius.
2 A bursa between the fibular collateral ligament and the biceps femoris.
3 A bursa between the fibular collateral ligament and the tendon of the popliteus.
4 A bursa between the tendon of the popliteus and the lateral condyle of the tibia.

Medial

1 A bursa deep to the medial head of the gastrocnemius.
2 The *anserine bursa* is a complicated bursa which separates the tendons of the sartorius, the gracilis and the semitendinosus from one another, from the tibia, and from the tibial collateral ligament (*see* Fig. 8.14).
3 A bursa deep to the tibial collateral ligament.
4 A bursa deep to the semimembranosus.

Relations of Knee Joint

Anteriorly

Anterior bursae (*see* Fig. 3.6), ligamentum patellae (Fig. 12.12), and patellar plexus of nerves.

Posteriorly

1 *At the middle:* Popliteal vessels, tibial nerve.
2 *Posterolaterally:* Lateral head of gastrocnemius, plantaris, and common peroneal nerve.
3 *Posteromedially:* Medial head of gastrocnemius, semitendinosus, semimembranosus, gracilis, and popliteus at its insertion (Fig. 12.13).

Medially

1 Sartorius, gracilis and semitendinosus (*see* Fig. 8.14).
2 Great saphenous vein with saphenous nerve.
3 Semimembranosus (Fig. 12.13).

Laterally

Biceps femoris, and tendon of origin of popliteus.

Blood Supply

The knee joint is supplied by the anastomoses around it. The chief sources of blood supply are:

1 Five genicular branches of the popliteal artery.
2 The descending genicular branch of the femoral artery.
3 The descending branch of the lateral circumflex femoral artery.
4 Two recurrent branches of the anterior tibial artery.
5 The circumflex fibular branch of the posterior tibial artery (*see* Fig. 6.10).

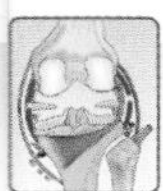

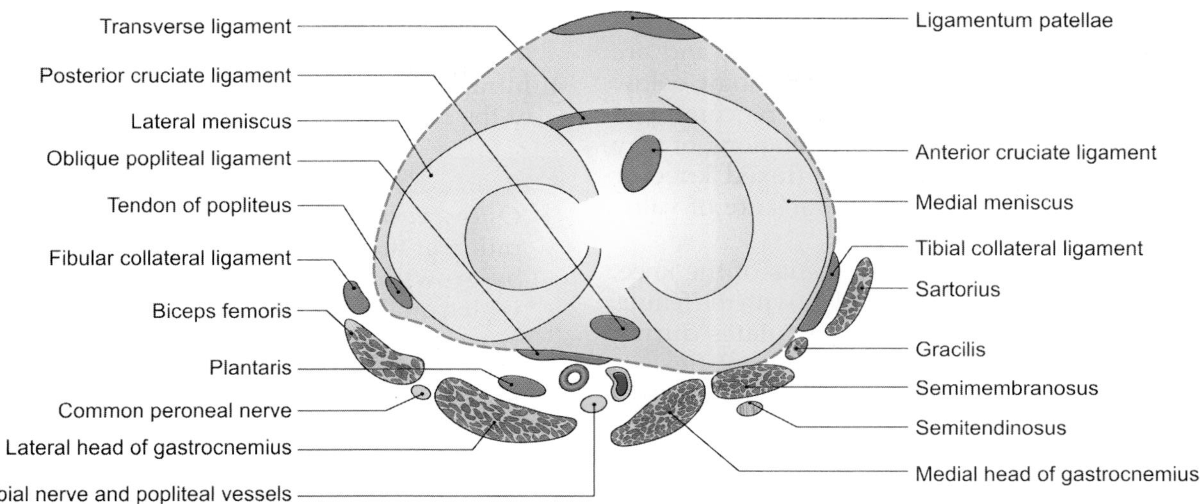

Fig. 12.13: Transverse section through the left knee joint showing the synovial relations

Nerve Supply

1. Femoral nerve, through its branches to the vasti, especially the vastus medialis.
2. Sciatic nerve, through the genicular branches of the tibial and common peroneal nerves.
3. Obturator nerve, through its posterior division.

MOVEMENTS AT THE KNEE JOINT

DISSECTION

Clean the articular surfaces of femur, tibia and patella on the soft specimen and on dried bones. Analyse the movements on them. Try all these movements on yourself and on your friends as well.

Features

Active movements at the knee are flexion, extension, medial rotation and lateral rotation (Table 12.2).

Flexion and *extension* are the chief movements. These take place in the upper compartment of the joint, above the menisci. They differ from the ordinary hinge movements in two ways.

1. The transverse axis around which these movements take place is not fixed. During extension, the axis moves forwards and upwards, and in the reverse direction during flexion.
2. These movements are invariably accompanied by rotations or conjunct rotation. When the foot is on the ground, while standing erect, medial rotation of femur occurs during last 30 degrees of extension as in position of "attention" by the vastus medialis. It is called conjunct rotation. During the position of "stand at ease", there is lateral rotation of femur, during initial stages of flexion, by popliteus muscle.

   Medial rotation of the femur occurs during the last 30 degrees of extension, and lateral rotation of the femur occurs during the initial stages of flexion.

   When the foot is off the ground as while sitting on a chair the tibia rotates instead of the femur, in the opposite direction.

Table 12.2: Muscles producing movements at the knee joint

Movement	*Principal muscles*
A. Extension (from sitting on a chair to standing)	Quadriceps femoris (four heads)
B. Locking (standing in "attention")	Vastus medialis
C. Unlocking (standing "at ease")	Popliteus
D. Flexion	1. Biceps femoris 2. Semitendinosus 3. Semimembranosus
E. Medial rotation of flexed leg	1. Popliteus 2. Semimembranosus 3. Semitendinosus
F. Lateral rotation of flexed leg	Biceps femoris

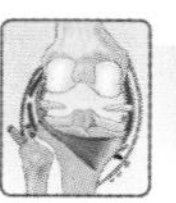

Rotatory movements at the knee are of a small range. Rotations take place around a vertical axis, and are permitted in the lower compartment of the joint, below the menisci. Rotatory movements may be combined with flexion and extension or conjunct rotations, or may occur independently in a partially flexed knee or adjunct rotations. The conjunct rotations are of value in locking and unlocking of the knee.

During different phases of movements of the knee, different portions of the patella articulate with the femur. The lower pair of articular facets articulates during extension; middle pair during beginning of flexion; upper pair during midflexion; and the medial strip during full flexion of the knee (*see* Figs 2.21 and 12.10).

Locking and Unlocking of the Knee Joint

Locking is a mechanism that allows the knee to remain in the position of full extension as in standing without much muscular effort.

Locking occurs as a result of medial rotation of the femur during the last stage of extension. The anteroposterior diameter of the lateral femoral condyle is less than that of the medial condyle. As a result, when the lateral condylar articular surface is fully 'used up' by extension, part of the medial condylar surface remains unused. At this stage the lateral condyle serves as an axis around which the medial condyle rotates backwards, i.e. medial rotation of the femur occurs, so that the remaining part of the medial condylar surface is also 'taken up'. This movement locks the knee joint. Locking is aided by the oblique pull of ligaments during the last stages of extension. When the knee is locked, it is completely rigid and all ligaments of the joint are taut. Locking is produced by continued action of the same muscles that produce extension, i.e. the quadriceps femoris, especially the vastus medialis part.

The locked knee joint can be flexed only after it is unlocked by a reversal of the medial rotation, i.e. by lateral rotation of the femur. Unlocking is brought about by the action of the popliteus muscle.

Accessory or *passive movements* can be performed in a partially flexed knee. These movements include:

a. A wider range of rotation.
b. Anteroposterior gliding of the tibia on the femur.
c. Some adduction and abduction.
d. Some separation of the tibia from the femur.

Morphology of Knee Joint

1 The tibial collateral ligament is the degenerated tendon of the adductor magnus.
2 The fibular collateral ligament is the degenerated tendon of the peroneus longus.
3 Cruciate ligaments represent the collateral ligaments of the originally separate femorotibial joints.
4 Infrapatellar synovial fold indicates the lower limit of the femoropatellar joint.

CLINICAL ANATOMY

- *Osteoarthritis* is an age related cartilage degeneration of the articular surfaces. It is characterized by growth of osteophytes at the articular ends, which make movements limited and painful. However, osteoarthritis may set in at an early age also due to underlying congenital deformities or fractures around the knee joint.
- Structurally, the knee is a weak joint because the articular surfaces are not congruent. The tibial condyles are too small and shallow to hold the large, convex, femoral condyles in place. The femoropatellar articulation is also quite insecure because of the shallow articular surfaces, and because of the outward angulation between the long axis of the thigh and of the leg.
  The stability of the joint is maintained by a number of factors.
  a. The cruciate ligaments maintain anteroposterior stability.
  b. The collateral ligaments maintain side to side stability.
  c. The factors strengthening the capsule have been enumerated earlier (*see* page 142, col. 1).
  d. The iliotibial tract plays an important role in stabilizing the knee (*see* Fig. 3.8).
- *Deformities of the knee:* The angle between the long axis of the thigh and that of the leg may be abnormal and the leg may be abnormally abducted (genu valgum or knock knee) or abnormally adducted (genu varum or bow knee). This may occur due to rickets, and posture, or as a congenital abnormality (Fig. 12.14).
- *Diseases of the knee:* The knee joint may be affected by various diseases. These include osteoarthritis and various infections. Infections may be associated with collections of the fluid in the joint cavity. This gives rise to swelling above, and at the sides of the patella. The patella appears to float in the fluid. Aspiration of fluid can be done by passing a needle into the joint on either side of the patella. Bursae around the joint may get filled with fluid resulting in swellings.
- *Injuries to the knee:*
  a. *Injuries to menisci*: Strains in a slightly flexed knee, as in kicking a football, the meniscus may get separated from the capsule, or may be torn longitudinally (bucket-handle tear) or transversely (*see* Fig. 2.18).

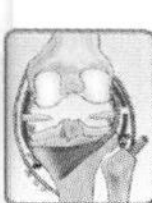

The medial meniscus is more vulnerable to injury than the lateral because of its fixity to the tibial collateral ligament, and because of greater excursion during rotatory movements. The lateral meniscus is protected by the popliteus which pulls it backwards so that it is not crushed between the articular surfaces.

b. *Injuries to cruciate ligaments* are also common. The anterior cruciate ligament is more commonly damaged than the posterior. It may be injured in violent hyperextension of the knee or in anterior dislocation of the tibia. The posterior ligament is injured in posterior dislocation of the tibia. The injury may vary from simple sprain to complete tear. Tear of the ligaments leads to abnormal anteroposterior mobility (Figs 12.15a and b).
c. *Injuries to collateral ligaments* are less common, and may be produced by severe abduction and adduction strains (Figs 12.16a and b).

- *Mal-alignment of patella:* Ideally the patella is resting in the centre of the width of the femur in a relaxed standing position. However, the patellar position may be altered congenitally or due to tightness of surrounding structures which may lead to painful conditions of the patello-femoral joint.
- Semimembranosus bursitis is quite common. It causes a swelling in the popliteal fossa region on the posteromedial aspect (*see* Fig. 7.5).
- Baker's cyst is a central swelling, occurs due to osteoarthritis of knee joint. The synovial membrane protrudes through a hole in the posterior part of capsule of knee joint.
- Hip joint and knee joint may need to be replaced if beyond repair.
- In knee joint disease vastus medialis is first to atrophy and last to recover (*see* Fig. 3.27).

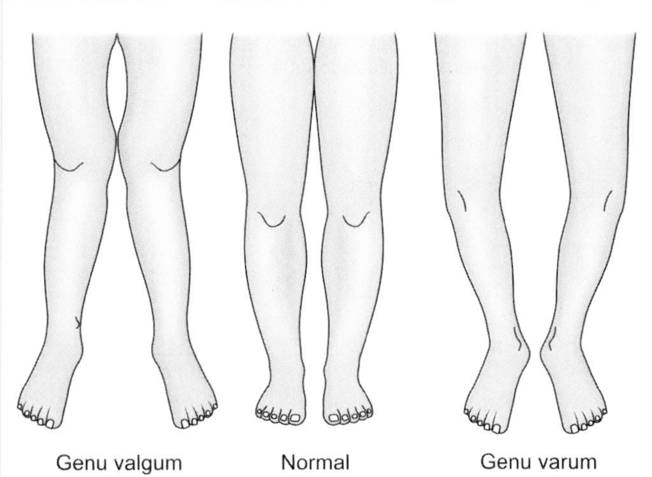

Fig. 12.14: Deformities of the knee

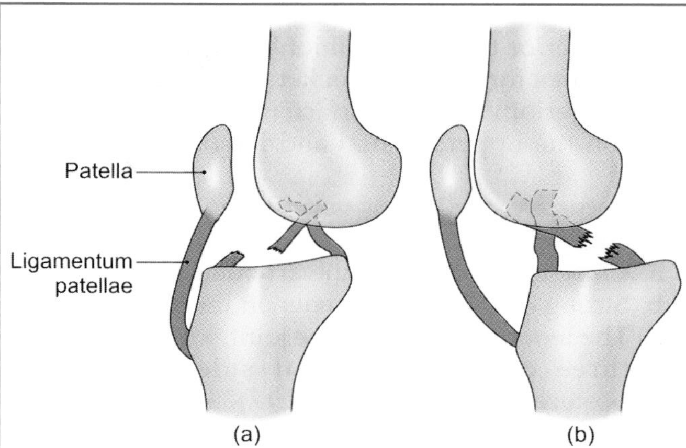

Figs 12.15a and b: Rupture of: (a) Anterior, and (b) posterior cruciate ligaments

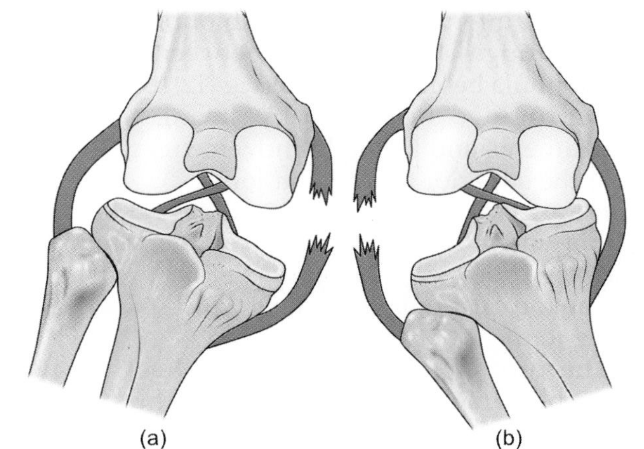

Figs 12.16a and b: Injury of: (a) Medial, and (b) lateral collateral ligaments

ANKLE JOINT

DISSECTION

Define the margins of both extensor retinacula, one flexor retinaculum and both peroneal retinacula. Identify the tendons enclosed in synovial sheaths, nerves and blood vessels passing under them. Displace these structures without removing them.

Clean and define the strong medial and lateral ligaments of ankle joint. Also demarcate the thin anterior and posterior parts of the capsule of the joint.

Type

This is a synovial joint of the hinge variety.

Articular Surfaces

The upper articular surface is formed by:

1 The lower end of the tibia including the medial malleolus.

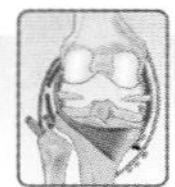

2 The lateral malleolus of the fibula, and
3 The inferior transverse tibiofibular ligament. These structures form a deep socket (Fig. 12.18).

The inferior articular surface is formed by articular areas on the upper, medial and lateral aspects of the talus.

Structurally, the joint is very strong. The stability of the joint is ensured by:

a. Close interlocking of the articular surfaces.
b. Strong collateral ligaments on the sides.
c. The tendons that cross the joint, four in front, and three on posteromedial side and two on posterolateral side (Fig. 12.17).

The depth of the superior articular socket is contributed by:

a. The downward projection of medial and lateral malleoli, on the corresponding sides of talus.
b. By the inferior transverse tibiofibular ligament that bridges across the gap between the tibia and the fibula behind the talus (Fig. 12.18). The socket is provided flexibility by strong tibiofibular ligaments and by slight movements of the fibula at the superior tibiofibular joint.

There are two factors, however, that tend to displace the tibia and fibula forwards over the talus. These factors are:

a. The forward pull of tendons which pass from the leg to the foot.
b. The pull of gravity when the heel is raised. Displacement is prevented by the following factors.
   i. The talus is wedge-shaped, being wider anteriorly. The malleoli are oriented to fit this wedge.
   ii. The posterior border of the lower end of the tibia is prolonged downwards.
   iii. The presence of the inferior transverse tibiofibular ligament.
   iv. The tibiocalcanean, posterior tibiotalar, calcaneofibular and posterior talofibular ligaments pass backwards and resist forward movement of the tibia and fibula.

Ligaments

The joint is supported by:

a. Fibrous capsule.
b. The deltoid or medial ligament.
c. A lateral ligament.

Fibrous Capsule

It surrounds the joint but is weak anteriorly and posteriorly. It is attached all around the articular margins with two exceptions.

1 Posterosuperiorly, it is attached to the inferior transverse tibiofibular ligament.
2 Anteroinferiorly, it is attached to the dorsum of the neck of the talus at some distance from the trochlear surface.

The anterior and posterior parts of the capsule are loose and thin to allow hinge movements. On each side, however, it is supported by strong collateral ligaments.

The synovial membrane lines the capsule. The joint cavity ascends for some distance between the tibia and the fibula.

Deltoid or Medial Ligament

This is a very strong triangular ligament present on the medial side of the ankle. The ligament is divided

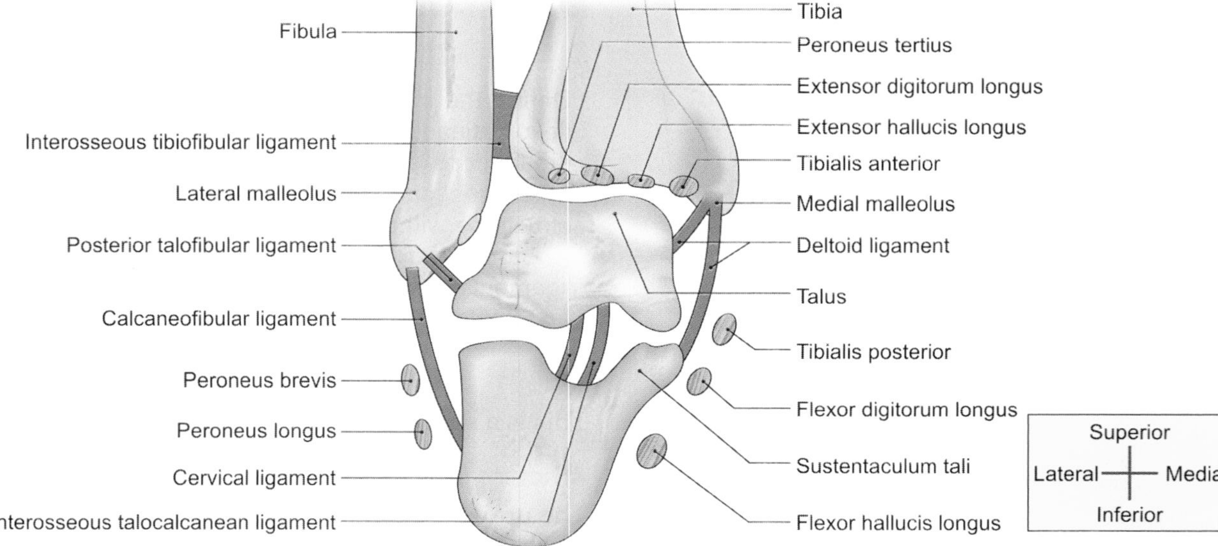

Fig. 12.17: Anterior view of coronal section through the right ankle joint to show its relations

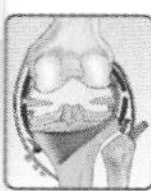

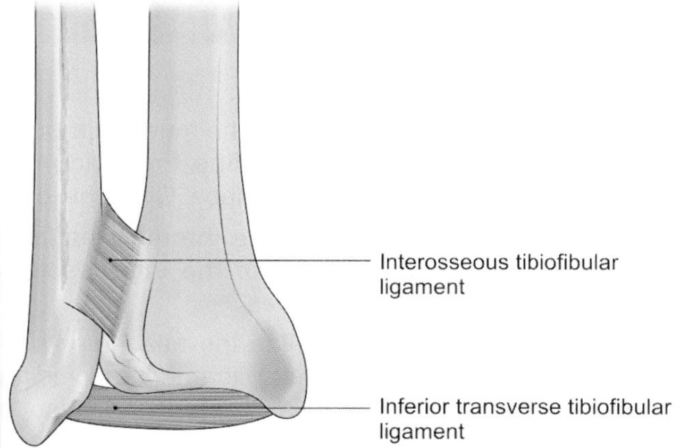

Fig. 12.18: Inferior tibiofibular joint

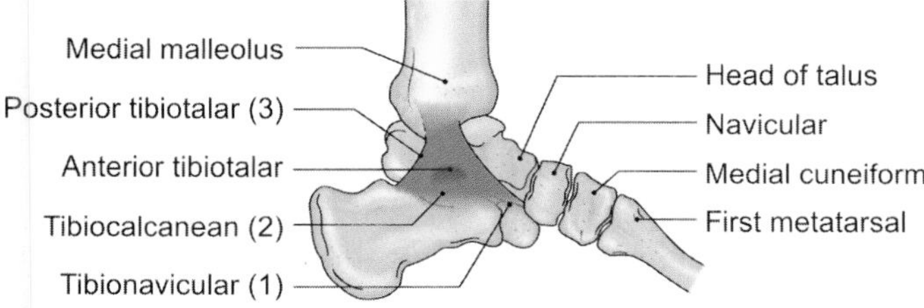

Fig. 12.19: Medial side of the ankle joint showing the parts of deltoid ligament

into a superficial and a deep part. Both parts have a common attachment above to the apex and margins of the medial malleolus. The lower attachment is indicated by the name of the fibres (Fig. 12.19).

Superficial part

1 Anterior fibres or *tibionavicular* are attached to the tuberosity of the navicular bone and to the medial margin of the spring ligament.
2 The middle fibres or *tibiocalcanean* are attached to the whole length of the sustentaculum tali.
3 The posterior fibres or *posterior tibiotalar* are attached to the medial tubercle and to the adjoining part of the medial surface of the talus.

Deep part or *anterior tibiotalar* is attached to the anterior part of the medial surface of the talus.

The deltoid ligament is crossed by the tendons of the tibialis posterior and flexor digitorum longus.

The deltoid ligament is a very strong ligament and excessive tensile forces on the ligament result in an avulsion fracture rather than a tear of the ligament. The ligament is prone to injuries in inversion.

Lateral Ligament

This ligament consists of three bands as follows.

1 The *anterior talofibular ligament* is a flat band which passes from the anterior margin of the lateral malleolus to the neck of the talus, just in front of the fibular facet (Fig. 12.20).

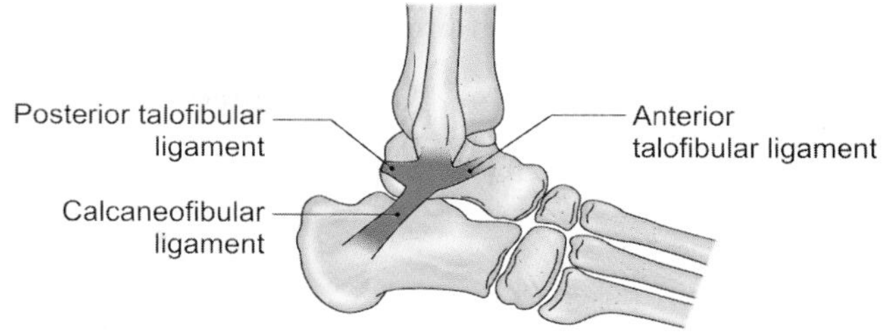

Fig. 12.20: Lateral side of the ankle joint showing the lateral ligament

2 The *posterior talofibular ligament* passes from the lower part of the malleolar fossa of the fibula to the lateral tubercle of the talus.
3 The *calcaneofibular ligament* is a long rounded cord which passes from the notch on the lower border of the lateral malleolus to the tubercle on the lateral surface of the calcaneum. It is crossed by the tendons of the peroneus longus and brevis.
4 The interosseous tibiofibular ligament, inferior extensor retinaculum and inferior and superior peroneal retinacula also contribute to the stability of the ankle joint (*see* Figs 8.4 and 8.9).

Relations of the Ankle Joint

Anteriorly, from medial to lateral side, there are the tibialis anterior, the extensor hallucis longus, the anterior tibial vessels, the deep peroneal nerve, the extensor digitorum longus, and the peroneus tertius (Fig. 12.17).

Posteromedially, from medial to lateral side, there are the tibialis posterior, the flexor digitorum longus, the posterior tibial vessels, the tibial nerve, the flexor hallucis longus.

Posterolaterally the peroneus longus, and the peroneus brevis (Fig. 12.17).

Movements

Active movements are dorsiflexion and plantar flexion (Table 12.3).

1 In *dorsiflexion* the forefoot is raised, and the angle between the front of the leg and the dorsum of the foot is diminished. It is a close-pack position with maximum congruence of the joint surfaces. The wider anterior trochlear surface of the talus fits into lower end of narrow posterior part of the lower end of tibia. There are no chances of dislocation in dorsiflexion (*see* Fig. 11.13).
2 In *plantar flexion,* the forefoot is depressed, and the angle between the leg and the foot is increased. The narrow posterior part of trochlear surface of talus loosely fits into the wide anterior part of the lower end of tibia. High heels cause plantar flexion of ankle joint and its dislocations (*see* Fig. 9.10).

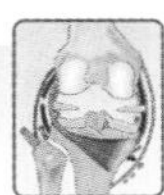

Table 12.3: Muscles producing movements		
Movement	*Principal muscles*	*Accessory muscles*
A. Dorsiflexion	Tibialis anterior	1. Extensor digitorum longus 2. Extensor hallucis longus 3. Peroneus tertius
B. Plantar flexion	1. Gastrocnemius 2. Soleus	1. Plantaris 2. Tibialis posterior 3. Flexor hallucis longus 4. Flexor digitorum longus

Blood Supply

From anterior tibial, posterior tibial, and peroneal arteries.

Nerve Supply

From deep peroneal and tibial nerves.

CLINICAL ANATOMY

- The *sprains of the ankle* are almost always abduction sprains of the subtalar joints, although a few fibres of the deltoid ligament are also torn. True sprains of the ankle joint are caused by forced plantar flexion, which leads to tearing of the anterior fibres of the capsule. The joint is unstable during plantar flexion.
- *Dislocations of the ankle* are rare because joint is very stable due to the presence of deep tibiofibular socket. Whenever dislocation occurs, it is accompanied by fracture of one of the malleoli.
- Acute sprains of lateral ankle occur when the foot is plantar flexed and excessively inverted. The lateral ligaments of ankle joint are torn giving rise to pain and swelling.
- Acute sprains of medial ankle occur in excessive eversion, leading to tear of strong deltoid ligament. These cases are less common.
- The *optimal position* of the ankle to avoid ankylosis is one of slight plantar flexion.
- For injections into the ankle joint, the needle is introduced between tendons of extensor hallucis longus and tibialis anterior with the ankle partially plantar flexed.
- During walking, the plantar flexors raise the heel from the ground. When the limb is moved forwards the dorsiflexors help the foot in clearing the ground. The value of the ankle joint resides in this hinge action, in this to and fro movement of the joint during walking.

TIBIOFIBULAR JOINTS

DISSECTION

Superior tibiofibular joint: Remove the muscles around the superior tibiofibular joint. Define the tendon of popliteus muscle on its posterior surface. Open the joint.

Middle tibiofibular joint: Remove the muscles from anterior and posterior surface of the interosseous membrane and define its surfaces.

Inferior tibiofibular joint: Define the attachments of anterior and posterior tibiofibular ligaments including inferior transverse tibiofibular ligament. Divide these to expose the strong interosseous tibiofibular ligament. Use dry bones and articulated foot to understand the attachments of the ligaments.

The tibia and fibula articulate at three joints, the superior, middle and inferior tibiofibular joints.

Superior Tibiofibular Joint

This is a small synovial joint of the plane variety. It is formed by articulation of small, rounded, flat facets present on the head of the fibula, and on the lateral condyle of the tibia. The joint permits slight gliding or rotatory movements that help in adjustment of the lateral malleolus during movements at the ankle joint.

The bones are united by a fibrous capsule which is strengthened by anterior and posterior ligaments. These ligaments are directed forwards and laterally. The cavity of the joint may communicate with the knee joint through the popliteal bursa. The joint is supplied by the nerve to the popliteus, and by the recurrent genicular nerve (*see* Fig. 6.7).

Middle Tibiofibular Joint

This is a fibrous joint formed by the interosseous membrane connecting the shafts of the tibia and the fibula. The interosseous membrane is attached to the interosseous borders of the two bones. Its fibres are directed downwards and laterally. It is wide above and narrow below where it is continuous with the interosseous ligament of the inferior tibiofibular joint. It presents a large opening at the upper end for the passage of the anterior tibial vessels, and a much smaller opening near its lower end for the passage of the perforating branch of the peroneal artery (*see* Fig. 2.24).

Relations

Anteriorly

Tibialis anterior, extensor digitorum longus, anterior tibial vessels, deep peroneal nerve extensor hallucis longus and peroneus tertius (*see* Fig. 8.5).

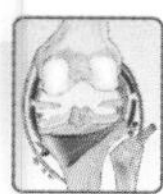

Posteriorly

Tibialis posterior and flexor hallucis longus (*see* Fig. 9.4).

Nerve Supply

Nerve to popliteus.

Functions

1 The membrane provides additional surface for attachment of muscles.
2 Binds the tibia and the fibula.
3 Resists the downward pull exerted on the fibula by the powerful muscles attached to the bone. Note that the biceps femoris is the only muscle that pulls the fibula upwards.

Inferior Tibiofibular Joint

This is a syndesmosis uniting the lower ends of the tibia and the fibula (Fig. 12.18). The bony surfaces are connected by a very strong *interosseous ligament*, which forms the chief bond of union between the lower ends of these bones.

The interosseous ligament is concealed both in front and behind by the *anterior* and *posterior tibiofibular ligaments*, whose fibres are directed downwards and laterally.

The posterior tibiofibular ligament is stronger than the anterior. Its lower and deep portion forms the *inferior transverse tibiofibular ligament*, which is a strong thick band of yellowish fibres passing transversely from the upper part of the malleolar fossa of the fibula to the posterior border of the articular surface of the tibia, reaching up to the medial malleolus (Fig. 12.18).

Blood Supply

Perforating branch of the peroneal artery; and the malleolar branches of the anterior and posterior tibial arteries (*see* Fig. 9.7).

Nerve Supply

Deep peroneal, tibial and saphenous nerves.

The joint permits slight movements, so that the lateral malleolus can rotate laterally during dorsiflexion of the ankle.

CLINICAL ANATOMY

- The inferior tibiofibular joint is strong. The strength of the ligaments uniting the lower ends of the tibia and fibula is an important factor in maintaining the integrity of the ankle joint.
- The slight movements of the lateral malleolus taking place at this joint provide suppleness to the ankle joint.

JOINTS OF THE FOOT

DISSECTION

Remove all the tendons, muscles from both dorsal and plantar aspects of the tarsal, metatarsal and phalanges. Define, identify the ligaments joining the various bones. Ligaments are stronger on the plantar aspect than the dorsal aspect.

Subtalar joint

Divide the ligaments which unite the talus and calcaneus together at the talocalcanean, talocalcaneonavicular joints. Study these joints carefully to understand the movements of inversion and eversion.

On the lateral side of foot, define the attachments of long plantar ligament. Reflect this ligament from its proximal attachment to see the deeper plantar calcaneo-cuboid ligament.

Classification

The joints of the foot are numerous. They can be classified as:

1 Intertarsal (Fig. 12.21),
2 Tarsometatarsal,
3 Intermetatarsal,
4 Metatarsophalangeal, (*see* Fig. 2.44)
5 Interphalangeal.

The main intertarsal joints are the subtalar or talocalcanean joint, the talocalcaneonavicular joint and the calcaneocuboid joint. Smaller intertarsal joints include the cuneonavicular, cuboidonavicular, intercuneiform and cuneocuboid joints.

The movements permitted at these joints are as follows.

a. The intertarsal, tarsometatarsal and intermetatarsal joints permit gliding and rotatory movements,

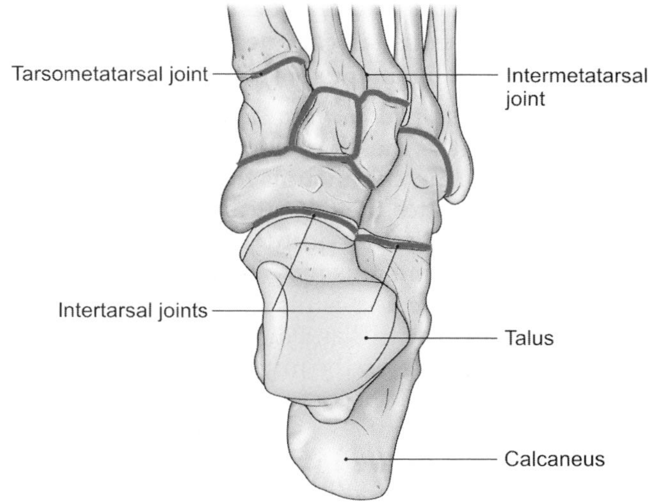

Fig. 12.21: Some joints of the foot

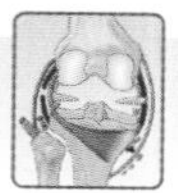

which jointly bring about inversion, eversion, of the foot. Pronation is a component of eversion, while supination is a component of inversion.

b. The metatarsophalangeal joints permit flexion, extension, adduction and abduction of the toes.

c. The interphalangeal joints of hinge variety permit flexion and extension of the distal phalanges.

A brief description of the relevant joints is given below.

SUBTALAR OR TALOCALCANEAN JOINT

There are three joints, posterior, anterior and medial between the talus and the calcaneum. The posterior joint is named the talocalcanean or subtalar joint where concave undersurface of body of talus articulates with convex posterior facet of the calcaneum.

The anterior joints are parts of the talocalcaneonavicular joint. On the anterior and medial side of undersurface of head of talus, the surfaces are convex and articulate with concave articulating surfaces of calcaneum.

Since the three joints form a single functional unit, clinicians often include these joints under the term subtalar joint. However, the sinus tarsi separates the posterior articulations from the anterior and medial articulations. The greater part of the talocalcaneonavicular joint lies in front of the head of the talus and not below it (Figs 12.22a and b).

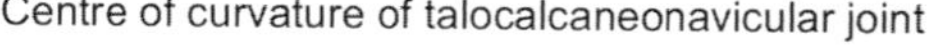

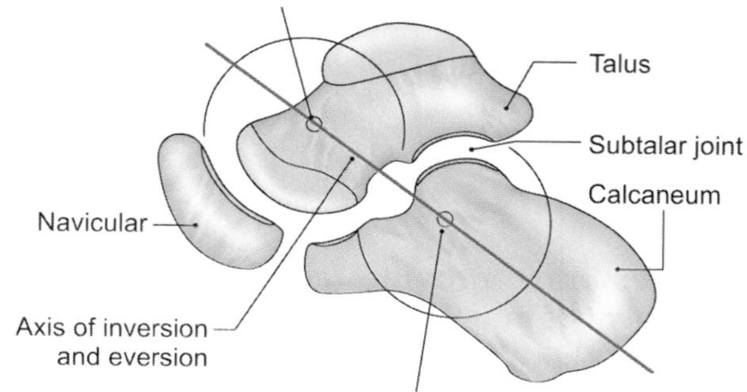

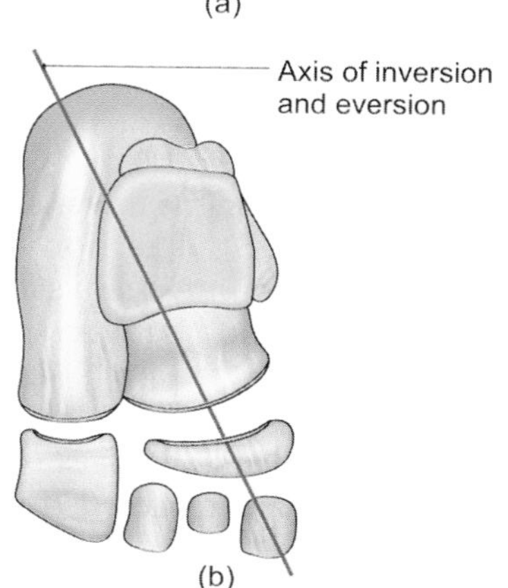

Figs 12.22a and b: Axis of movements of inversion and eversion at subtalar joint: (a) Side view, and (b) superior view

Talocalcanean Joint

The *talocalcanean joint* is a plane synovial joint between the concave facet on the inferior surface of the body of the talus and the convex facet on the middle one-third of the superior surface of the calcaneum.

The bones are connected by:

a. A fibrous capsule,
b. The lateral and medial talocalcanean ligaments,
c. The interosseous talocalcanean ligament, and
d. The cervical ligament:

The *interosseous talocalcanean ligament* is thick and very strong. It is the chief bond of union between the talus and the calcaneum. It occupies the sinus tarsi, and separates the talocalcanean joint from the talocalcaneonavicular joint. It becomes taut in eversion, and limits this movement.

The *cervical ligament* is placed lateral to the sinus tarsi. It passes upwards and medially, and is attached above to a tubercle on the inferolateral aspect of the neck of the talus. It becomes taut in inversion, and limits this movement.

In addition to the interosseous and cervical ligament, the collateral ligaments of the ankle joint also provide stability to the talocalcanean joint.

Movements

The joint participates in the movements of inversion and eversion of the foot described at the end of chapter.

Talocalcaneonavicular Joint

The joint has some of the features of a ball and socket joint. The head of the talus fits into a socket formed partly by the navicular bone, and partly by the calcaneum. Two ligaments also take part in forming the socket: these are the spring ligament medially, and the medial limb of the bifurcate ligament laterally (Figs 12.22a and b).

The bones taking part in forming the joint are connected by a fibrous capsule. The capsule is supported posteriorly by the interosseous talocalcanean ligament; dorsally by the dorsal talonavicular ligament; ventromedially by the spring ligament; and laterally by the medial limb of the bifurcate ligament. The spring ligament is described below. The bifurcate ligament is described with the calcaneocuboid joint.

Movements

The movements permitted at this joint are those of inversion and eversion. They are described below.

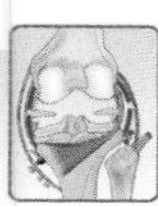

The *spring ligament* or *plantar calcaneonavicular ligament* is powerful. It is attached posteriorly to the anterior margin of the sustentaculum tali, and anteriorly to the plantar surface of the navicular bone between its tuberosity and articular margin. The head of the talus rests directly on the upper surface of the ligament, which is covered by fibrocartilage. The plantar surface of the ligament is supported by the tendon of tibialis posterior medially, and by the tendons of flexor hallucis longus and flexor digitorum longus, laterally.

The spring ligament is the most important ligament for maintaining the medial longitudinal arch of the foot.

CALCANEOCUBOID JOINT

This is a saddle joint. The opposed articular surfaces of the calcaneum and the cuboid are concavoconvex. On account of the shape of articular surfaces, medial movement of the forefoot is accompanied by its lateral rotation and adduction or inversion. Lateral movement of the forefoot is accompanied by medial rotation and abduction or eversion. The bones are connected by:

1 A fibrous capsule,
2 The lateral limb of the bifurcate ligament,
3 The long plantar ligament (Fig. 12.23) and
4 The short plantar ligament.

The *bifurcate ligament* is Y-shaped. Its stem is attached to the anterolateral part of the sulcus calcanei; the medial limb or calcaneonavicular ligament, to the dorsolateral surface of the navicular bone; and the lateral limb or calcaneocuboid ligament, to the dorsomedial surface of the cuboid bone. Thus each limb of the ligament strengthens a separate joint.

The *long plantar ligament* (Fig. 12.23) is a long and strong ligament whose importance in maintaining the arches of foot is surpassed only by the spring ligament.

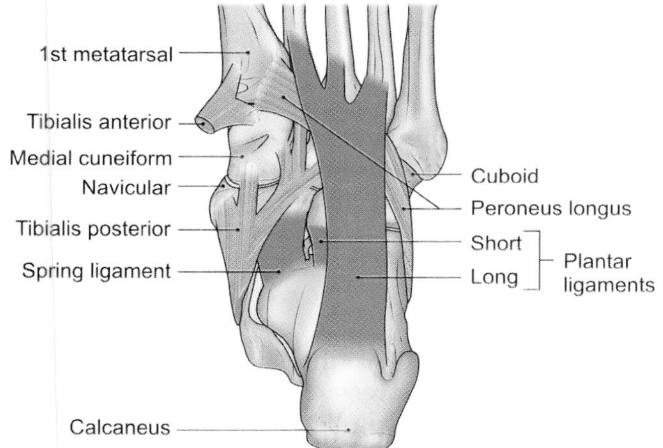

Fig. 12.23: Some ligaments of the foot with the tendons of peroneus longus

It is attached posteriorly to the plantar surface of the calcaneum, and anteriorly to the lips of the groove on the cuboid bone, and to the bases of the middle three metatarsals. It converts the groove on the plantar surface of the cuboid into a tunnel for the tendon of the peroneus longus. Morphologically, it represents the divorced tendon of the gastrocnemius.

The *short plantar ligament* or *plantar calcaneocuboid ligament* lies deep to the long plantar ligament. It is broad and strong ligament extending from the anterior tubercle of the calcaneum to the plantar surface of the cuboid, behind its ridge.

TRANSVERSE TARSAL OR MIDTARSAL JOINT

This includes the calcaneocuboid and the talonavicular joints (Fig. 12.21). The talonavicular joint is a part of the talocalcaneonavicular joint, and hence the transverse tarsal joint may be said to be made up of only one and a half joints. These joints are grouped together only by virtue of being placed in nearly the same transverse plane. In any case, the two joints do not form a functional unit. They have different axes of movements. It demarcates the forefoot from the hindfoot. Its movements help in inversion and eversion of the foot.

Inversion and Eversion of the Foot

Inversion is a movement in which the medial border of the foot is elevated, so that the sole faces medially.

Eversion is a movement in which the lateral border of the foot is elevated, so that the sole faces laterally. These movements can be performed voluntarily only when the foot is off the ground. When the foot is on the ground these movements help to adjust the foot to uneven ground.

In inversion and eversion, the entire part of the foot below the talus moves together. The movement takes place mainly at the subtalar and talocalcaneonavicular joints and partly at the transverse tarsal joint. The calcaneum and the navicular bone, move medially or laterally round the talus carrying the forefoot with them. Inversion is accompanied by plantar flexion of the foot and adduction of the forefoot. Eversion is accompanied by dorsiflexion of the foot and abduction of the forefoot.

Joints Taking Part

Main

1 Subtalar (talocalcanean).
2 Talocalcaneonavicular.

Accessory

Transverse tarsal which includes calcaneocuboid and talonavicular joints.

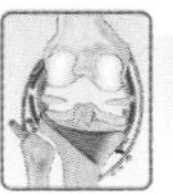

Axis of Movements

Inversion and eversion take place around an oblique axis which runs forwards, upwards and medially, passing from the back of the calcaneum, through the sinus tarsi, to emerge at the superomedial aspect of the neck of the talus. The obliquity of the axis partly accounts for adduction, abduction, plantar flexion and dorsiflexion which are associated with these movements (Fig. 12.22).

Range of Movements

1 Inversion is much more free than eversion.
2 The range of movements is appreciably increased in plantar flexion of the foot because, in this position, the narrow posterior part of the trochlear surface of the talus occupies the tibiofibular socket. In this position slight side to side movements of the talus are permitted.

Muscles Producing Movements

Inversion is produced by the actions of the tibialis anterior and the tibialis posterior, helped by the flexor hallucis longus and the flexor digitorum longus (Table 12.4).

Table 12.4: Muscles producing movements of inversion and eversion

Movement	*Principal muscles*
A. Inversion	Tibialis anterior Tibialis posterior
B. Eversion	Peroneus longus Peroneus brevis

Mechanism: During inversion the forepart of foot is adducted at mid tarsal joint followed by lateral rotation of foot at subtalar jont. During eversion the reverse of this occurs.

Pronation and Supination of the Foot

These are really components of the movements of inversion and eversion. In pronation and supination, the forefoot (i.e. the distal part of the tarsus and metatarsus) moves on the calcaneum and talus. The medial border or the forefoot is elevated in supination (which is thus a part of inversion), while the reverse occurs in pronation (and the eversion). These movements take place chiefly at the transverse tarsal joint and partly at smaller intertarsal, tarsometatarsal and intermetatarsal joints.

There are differences when supination and pronation occur in weight bearing and nonweight bearing situations. In weight bearing supination and pronation, the calcaneum is not free to move in all directions and the motions are thus completed by compensatory movements of the talus.

Limiting Factors

Inversion is limited by:
1 Tension of peronei
2 Tension of cervical ligament.

Eversion is limited by:
1 Tension of tibialis anterior
2 Tension of tibialis posterior
3 Tension of deltoid ligament.

Functional Significance

Inversion and eversion greatly help the foot in adjusting to uneven and slippery ground. When feet are supporting the body weight, these movements occur in a modified form called supination and pronation, which are forced on the foot by the body weight.

SMALLER JOINTS OF FOREFOOT

DISSECTION

Cut across the cuneocuboid, cuneonavicular and intercuneiform joints to expose the articulating surfaces.

With a strong knife cut through tarsometatarsal and intermetatarsal joints. Try to separate the bones to see interosseous ligaments.

Detach abductor hallucis, flexor hallucis brevis, adductor hallucis from the sesamoid bones of the big toe.

Cut the deep transverse metatarsal ligaments on each side of the third toe. Now the tendons of dorsal and plantar interossei can be seen till their insertion. Identify the distal attachments of the lumbrical muscles as well.

Identify the extensor expansion on the dorsum of digits and see its continuity with the collateral ligaments. Study these joints from the text provided.

Features

These are plane joints between the navicular, the cuneiform, the cuboid and the metatarsal bones. They permit small gliding movements, which allow elevation and depression of the heads of the metatarsals, as well as pronation and supination of the foot.

Joint Cavities of Foot

There are only six joint cavities in the proximal part of the foot. These are intertarsal, tarsometatarsal and intermetatarsal joints (Fig. 12.24). The cavities are:
1 Talocalcanean
2 Talocalcaneonavicular
3 Calcaneocuboid

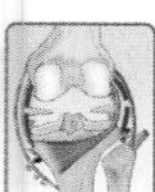

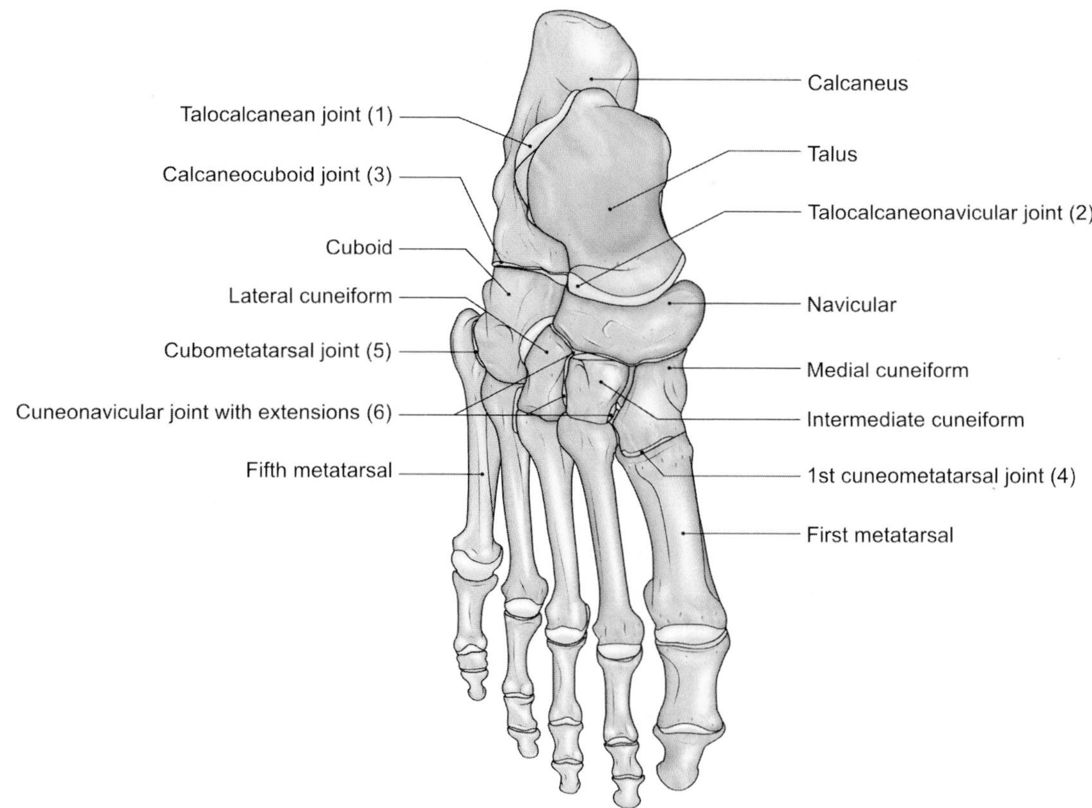

Fig. 12.24: Joint cavities in the proximal part of the foot

4 First cuneometatarsal
5 Cubometatarsal
6 Cuneonavicular with extensions (Fig. 12.21), i.e. navicular with three cuneiforms and second and third cuneometatarsal joints.

Metatarsophalangeal and Interphalangeal Joints

The structure of these joints is similar to the corresponding joints of the hand, with two exceptions.

1 The deep transverse ligaments of the foot connect all the five toes instead of only four fingers in the hand.
2 The toes are adducted and abducted with reference to the second toe and not the third finger as in the hand.

GAIT WALKING

Gait is a motion which carries the body forwards. There are two phases: Swing and stance (Figs 12.25a to d).

Swing Phase

1 Flexion of hip, flexion of knee and plantar flexion of ankle.
2 Flexion of hip, extension of knee and dorsiflexion of ankle.

Stance Phase

1 Flexion of hip, extension of knee and foot on the ground.
2 Extension of hip, extension of knee and foot on the ground.

CLINICAL ANATOMY

- Females wearing high heels (more than 5 cm), put stress on their back and lower limbs. The spine is pushed forwards, knees are excessively bent, resulting in too much pull on some muscles and ligaments. High heels result in shift in position of centre of gravity. The problems caused by high heels are "fashionable diseases". The sprains of the medial and lateral ligaments of ankle joint are almost always due to high heels (*see* Fig. 9.10).
- Joints of the foot lead to various deformities like mallet toe, hammer toe and claw toe (Fig. 12.26).
- *Arthroscopy:* One can look into the joints by special instruments called the arthroscopes.

  For hip joint, the instrument is introduced 4 cm lateral to the femoral pulse and 4 cm below inguinal ligament.

  For knee joint, the arthroscope is introduced from the front of the semiflexed knee joint.

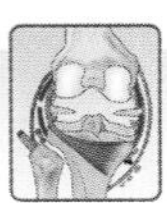

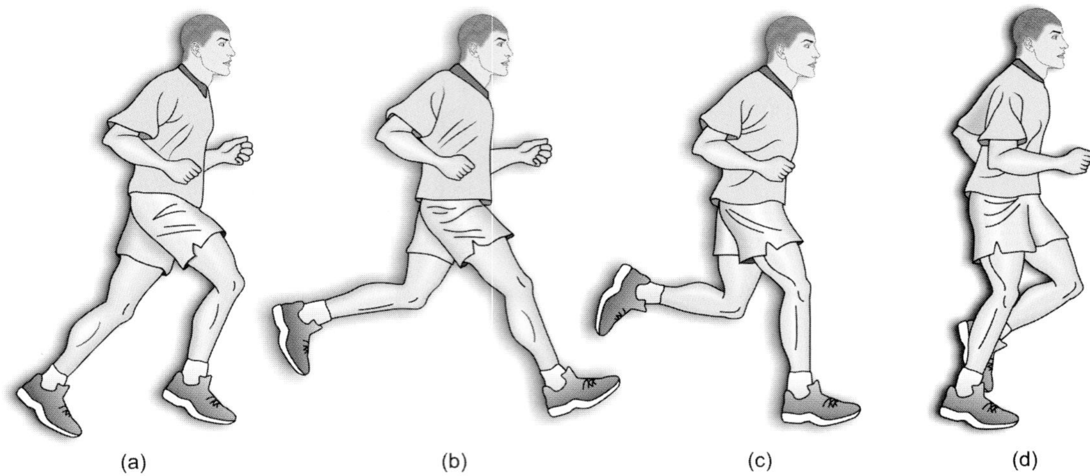

Figs 12.25a to d: Phases of gait: (a) and (b) Swing phase, (c) and (d) stance phase

For ankle joint, the instrument is introduced medial to the tendon of tibialis anterior muscle. One needs to be careful of the great saphenous vein.

- *Hallux valgus:* Due to ill-fitting shoes great toe gets pushed laterally, even dislocating the sesamoid bone. Head of 1st metatarsal points medially and adventitious bursa develops there. Toes may be deformed at their joints resulting in claw toe.
- Fractured toe is bandaged with the adjacent toe, this is called buddy splint (Fig. 12.27).

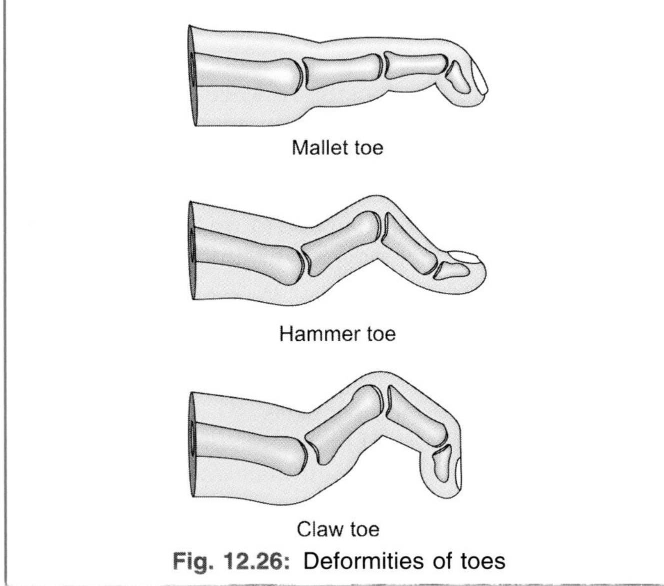

Fig. 12.26: Deformities of toes

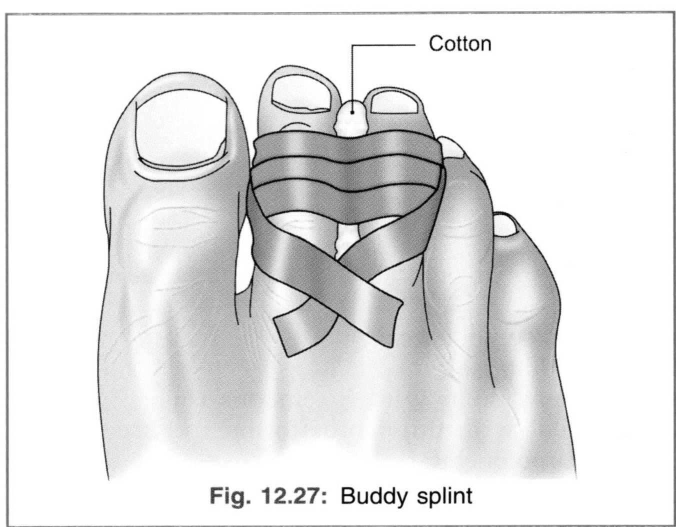

Fig. 12.27: Buddy splint

Morphologic Significance

In intrauterine life and early infancy, the soles of the feet are turned inwards, so that they face each others. As growth proceeds, the feet are gradually everted to allow a plantigrade posture. Such eversion does not occur in apes.

Mnemonics of Locking and Unlocking

L M F T T E

Locking is **m**edial rotation of **f**emur on **t**ibia at **t**erminal stages of **e**xtension when foot is on the ground.

U L F T I F

Unlocking is **l**ateral rotation of **f**emur on **t**ibia at **i**nitial stages of **f**lexion when foot in on the ground.

L L T F T E

Locking is **l**ateral rotation of **t**ibia on **f**emur at **t**erminal stages of **e**xtension when foot in off the ground.

U M T F I F

Unlocking is **m**edial rotation of **t**ibia on **f**emur at **i**nitial stages of **f**lexion when foot is off the ground.

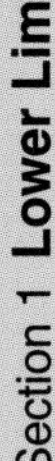

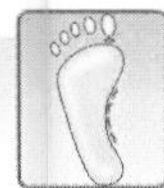

1 Shape of the bones concerned.
2 *Intersegmental ties/staples* or ligaments (and muscles) that hold the different segments of the arch together.
3 *Tie beams* or *bowstrings* that connect the two ends of the arch.
4 *Slings* that keep the summit of the arch pulled up.
5 Suspension

Each of these factors is considered below.

Bony Factor

The posterior transverse arch is formed, and maintained mainly because of the fact that many of the tarsal bones involved (e.g. the cuneiform bones), and the bases of the metatarsal bones, are wedge-shaped, the apex of the wedge pointing downwards.

The bony factor is not very important in the case of the other arches.

Intersegmental Ties

All arches are supported by the ligaments uniting the bones concerned. The most important of these are as follows:

1 The spring ligament for the medial longitudinal arch (Fig. 13.5).
2 The long and short plantar ligaments for the lateral longitudinal arch (*see* Fig. 12.23).
3 In the case of the transverse arch, the metatarsal bones are held together by the interosseous muscles also.

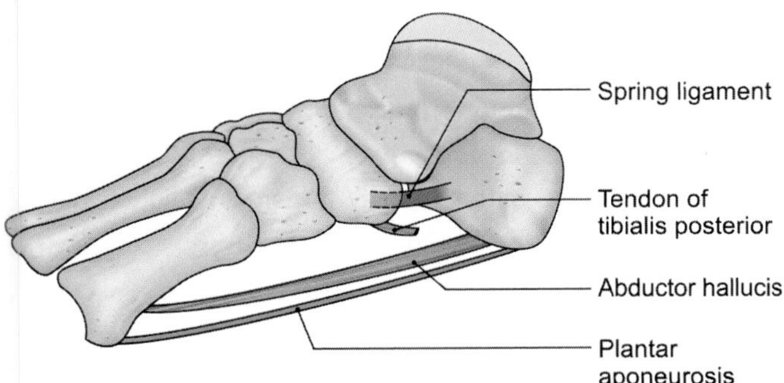

Fig. 13.5: Scheme showing some factors maintaining the medial longitudinal arch of the foot

Tie Beams

The longitudinal arches are prevented from flattening by the plantar aponeurosis, and by the muscles of the first layer of the sole. These structures keep the anterior and posterior ends of these arches pulled together. In the case of the transverse arch, the adductor hallucis acts as a tie beam (*see* Figs 10.4a and 10.6a).

Slings

1 The summit of the medial longitudinal arch is pulled upwards by tendons passing from the posterior compartment of the leg into the sole, i.e. tibialis posterior, flexor hallucis longus, flexor digitorum longus (Fig. 13.7).
2 The summit of the lateral longitudinal arch is pulled upwards by the peroneus longus and peroneus brevis (Fig. 13.6).
3 The tendons of tibialis anterior and peroneus longus together form a sling (stirrup) which keeps the middle of the foot pulled upwards, thus supporting the longitudinal arches.
4 As the tendon of the peroneus longus runs transversely across the sole, it pulls the medial and lateral margins of the sole closer together, thus maintaining the transverse arches. The transverse arch is also supported by tibialis posterior which grips many of the bones of the sole through its slips (Fig. 13.7).

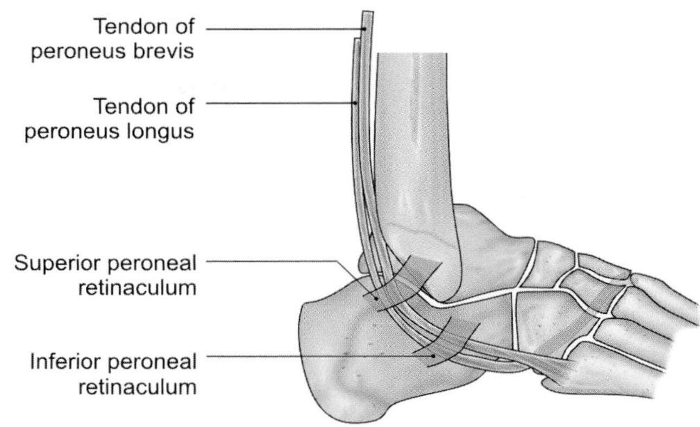

Fig. 13.6: Peroneal tendons helping to support the lateral longitudinal arch of the foot

Suspension

1 Medial longitudinal arch—Tibialis anterior
2 Lateral longitudinal arch—Peroneus longus.

FUNCTIONS OF ARCHES

1 The arches of the foot distribute body weight to the weight-bearing areas of the sole, mainly the heel and the toes. Out of the latter, weight is borne mainly on the first and fifth toes. The lateral border of the foot bears some weight, but this is reduced due to the presence of the lateral longitudinal arch.
2 The arches act as springs (chiefly the medial longitudinal arch) which are of great help in walking and running.
3 They also act as shock absorbers in stepping and particularly in jumping.
4 The concavity of the arches protects the soft tissues of the sole against pressure.
5 The character of medial longitudinal arch is resiliency and that of lateral longitudinal arch is rigidity.

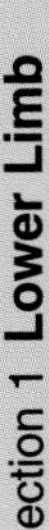

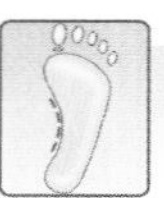

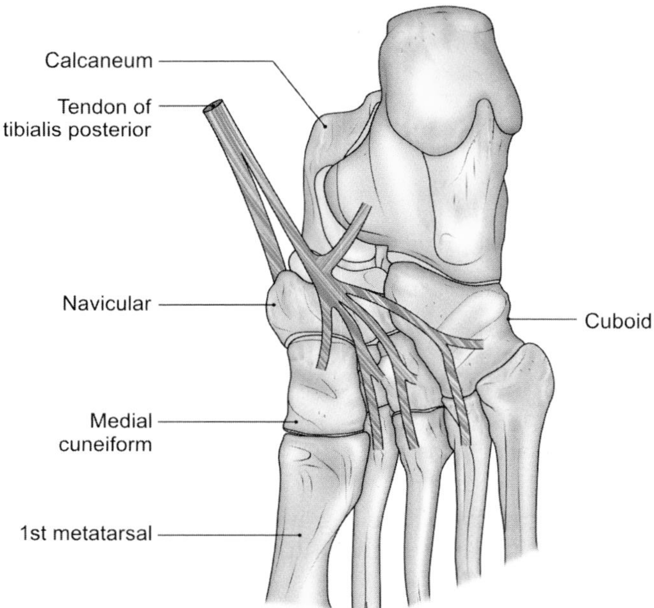

Fig. 13.7: Insertion of the tibialis posterior. Note the slips passing to all tarsal bones (except the talus) and to the middle three metatarsals

SUMMARY

The arches of the foot are well known features of the foot. There are two longitudinal arches, i.e. medial longitudinal arch and lateral longitudinal arch (Table 13.1).

In addition there are two transverse arches, i.e. posterior transverse arch and an anterior transverse arch (Table 13.2).

The medial longitudinal arch is the most important and is primarily affected in pes planus and pes cavus.

This arch is formed by the calcaneus, navicular, three cuneiforms and medial three metatarsals.

Flattening of the arch is common and is assessed clinically.

The medial arch is supported by:

- Spring ligament which supports the head of the talus.
- Plantar aponeurosis: Acts as a tie beam.
- Abductor hallucis and flexor digitorum brevis which act as spring ties.
- Tibialis anterior which lifts the centre of the arch. This muscle also forms a stirrup like support with the help of peroneus longus muscle.
- Tibialis posterior adducts the mid-tarsal joint and supports the spring ligament.
- Flexor hallucis longus extending between the anterior and posterior ends also supports the head of talus.

The lateral longitudinal arch is formed by calcaneum, cuboid, 4th and 5th metatarsals. It is rather shallow and gets flattened on weight bearing.

- This arch is supported by long plantar ligament, short plantar ligament. Plantar aponeurosis acts as a tie beam.
- Flexor digitorum brevis, flexor digiti minimi and abductor digiti minimi act as tie beams.
- Peroneus longus, peroneus brevis and peroneus tertius support this arch.

Table 13.1: Comparison of medial longitudinal arch and lateral longitudinal arch

	Medial longitudinal arch	*Lateral longitudinal arch*
Features	Higher, more mobile, resilient and shock absorber	Lower, limited mobility transmits weight, rigid
Anterior end	Heads of 1st, 2nd, 3rd metatarsal bones	Heads of 4th, 5th metatarsals
Posterior end	Medial tubercle of calcaneum	Lateral tubercle of calcaneum
Summit	Superior articular surface of talus	Articular facet on superior surface of calcaneum at level of subtalar joint
Anterior pillar	Talus, navicular, 3 cuneiforms and 1–3 metatarsals	Cuboid and 4th, 5th metatarsals
Posterior pillar	Medial half of calcaneum	Lateral half of calcaneum
Main joint	Talocalcaneonavicular joint	Calcaneocuboid joint
Bony factor	Wedge-shaped	Wedge-shaped
Intersegmental ties	Spring ligament	Long plantar ligament Short plantar ligament
Tie beams	Plantar aponeurosis (medial part) Abductor hallucis Medial part of flexor digitorum brevis	Plantar aponeurosis (lateral part) Abductor digiti minimi Lateral part of flexor digitorum brevis
Slings	Tibialis posterior Flexor hallucis longus Flexor digitorum longus	Peroneus longus Peroneus brevis
Suspension	Sling formed by tibialis anterior and peroneus longus	Sling formed by tibialis anterior and peroneus longus

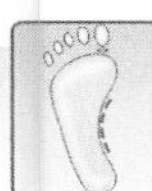

Table 13.2: Comparison of anterior transverse arch and posterior transverse arch

	Anterior transverse arch	*Posterior transverse arch*
Formation	Heads of 1st to 5th metatarsals	Navicular, 3 cuneiforms, bases and shafts of metatarsals
Features	Complete arch	Incomplete. Arch is half dome raised medially
Bony factor	Round-shaped	Wedge-shaped
Intersegmental ties	Dorsal interosseous muscles	Dorsal interosseous muscles
Tie beams	Adductor hallucis Deep transverse metatarsal ligaments	Flexor hallucis brevis Intertarsal and tarsometatarsal ligaments
Slings	Peroneus longus Tibialis posterior	Peroneus longus Tibialis posterior

Posterior transverse arch is formed by three cuneiforms and cuboid. This arch extends across the sole in a coronal plane. It is only a half arch, the other half gets completed by the other foot. This arch is supported by the ligaments binding the bones. It gets specific support from the tendon of peroneus longus as it extends from the lateral side to the medial side of the sole

Anterior transverse arch also lies in coronal plane. It is formed by the heads of five metatarsals. During weight bearing, the metatarsal heads flatten out.

This arch is supported by intermetatarsal ligaments and the intrinsic muscles of the sole. The transverse head of adductor hallucis holds the heads of metatarsals together (*see* Fig. 10.6a).

CLINICAL ANATOMY

- Absence or collapse of the arches leads to flat foot (pes planus), which may be congenital or acquired. The effects of a flat foot are as follows.
  a. Loss of spring in the foot leads to a clumsy, shuffling gait.
  b. Loss of shock absorbing function makes the foot more liable to trauma and osteoarthritis.
  c. Loss of the concavity of the sole leads to compression of the nerves and vessels of the sole. Compression of the communication between the lateral and medial plantar nerves causes neuralgic pain in the forefoot (metatarsalgia). Compression of blood vessels may cause vascular disturbances in the toes.
- Exaggeration of the longitudinal arches of the foot is known as *pes cavus*. This is usually a result of contracture (plantar flexion) at the transverse tarsal joint. When dorsiflexion of the metatarso-phalangeal joints, and plantar flexion of the interphalangeal joints (due to atrophy of lumbricals and interossei) are superadded, the condition is known as *claw-foot*. The common causes of pes cavus and claw-foot are spina bifida and poliomyelitis (Figs 13.8a to d and 13.9).
- Other deformities of the foot are as follows.
  a. *Talipes equinus* in which the patient walks on toes, with the heel raised.
  b. *Talipes calcaneus* in which the patient walks on heel, with the forefoot raised.
  c. *Talipes varus* in which the patient walks on the outer border of foot which is inverted and adducted (*see* Fig. 10.13).
  d. *Talipes valgus* in which the patient walks on inner border of foot which is everted and abducted.
  e. Commonest deformity of the foot is *talipes equinovarus* (*club foot*). In this condition the foot is inverted, adducted and plantar flexed. The condition may be associated with spina bifida.
- Talipes (club foot) may be of two types: Talipes calcaneovalgus—foot is dorsiflexed at ankle joint, everted at midtarsal joints.
- Talipes equinovarus—foot is plantar flexed at ankle joint and inverted at midtarsal joints (Fig. 13.10).

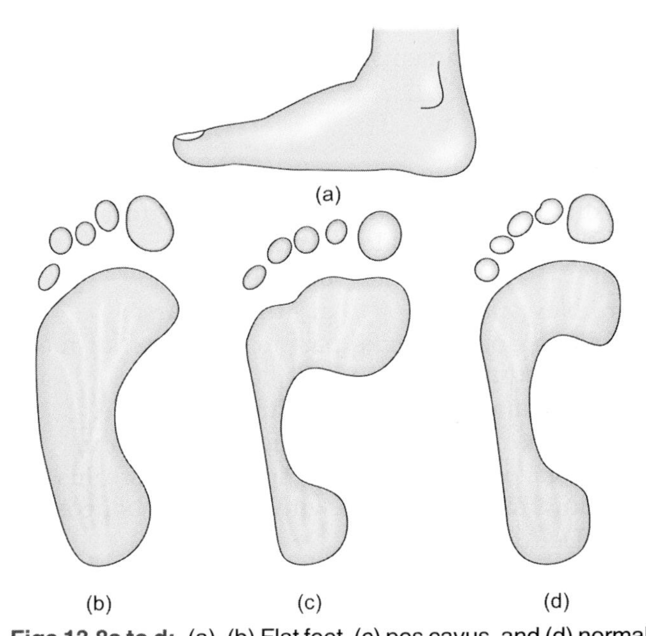

Figs 13.8a to d: (a), (b) Flat feet, (c) pes cavus, and (d) normal

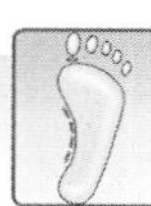

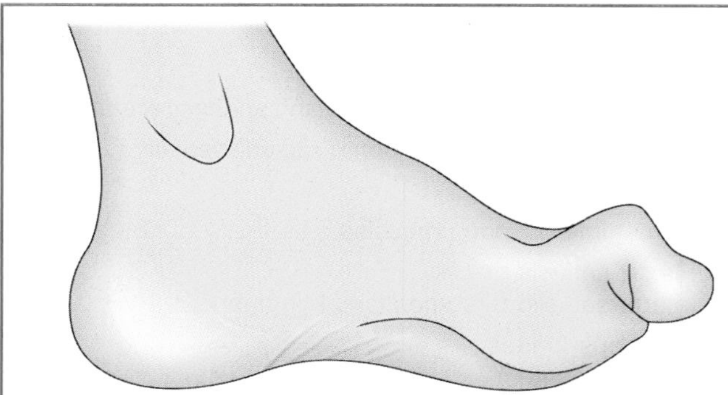

Fig. 13.9: Claw-foot/pes cavus

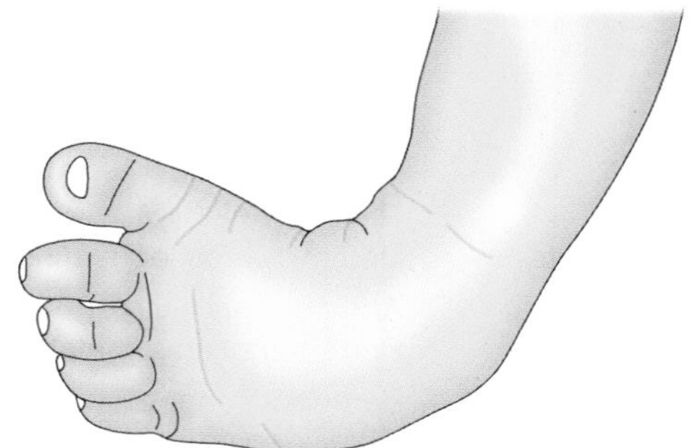

Fig. 13.10: Club foot/talipes equinovarus

FACTS TO REMEMBER

- Talus is the summit of medial longitudinal arch of the foot.
- Important joint of medial longitudinal arch is talocalcaneonavicular joint
- Main supports of this arch are tibialis posterior, tibialis anterior and peroneus longus muscles
- Important ligaments of the arch are spring or plantar calcaneonavicular, interosseous talocalcanean
- Arches distribute the weight evenly to the ground
- Great toe through its two sesamoid bones transfers double the weight of the other toes.
- Important joint of lateral longitudinal arch is calcaneocuboid joint. Its main supports are tendon of peroneus longus, long plantar and short plantar ligaments.
- Posterior transverse arch is supported by tendon of peroneus longus muscle.
- Anterior transverse arch is supported by deep metatarsal ligaments and dorsal interossei muscles.

CLINICOANATOMICAL PROBLEM

A young adult was disqualified in his medical examination of the army due to his flat feet

- What are flat feet?
- Name the factors maintaining the medial longitudinal arch of the foot

Ans: When the feet do not show the upward concavity along the medial border of foot, the foot is called "flat foot". If such a person puts his wet feet on the ground, there will be impression of the whole foot. Flat foot persons cannot run as fast as arched foot persons. The in army persons are required to run fast, so a flat foot person may be disqualified.

Factors maintaining medial longitudinal arch of the foot are:

1. Proper shape of the bones, e.g. talus, calcaneum.
2. Ligaments like spring ligament, deltoid ligaments
3. Short muscles like abductor hallucis, flexor hallucis brevis, dorsal interossei
4. Long tendons like flexor hallucis longus, tibialis posterior, peroneus longus, tibialis anterior.

MULTIPLE CHOICE QUESTIONS

1. All of following bones takes part is formation of lateral longitudinal arch *except*:
   a. Calcaneum b. Cuboid
   c. Navicular d. 4th metatarsal
2. Which does not take part in formation of medial longitudinal arch of foot?
   a. Calcaneum b. Cuboid
   c. Talus d. Medial cuneiform
3. The major ligament that supports head of talus from below, as it articulates with navicular bone is:
   a. Deltoid
   b. Plantar calcaneonavicular
   c. Anterior talofibular
   d. Posterior talofibular
4. Main muscular support of medial longitudinal arch is the following *except*:
   a. Tibialis posterior b. Flexor hallucis longus
   c. Peroneus brevis d. Flexor digitorum longus
5. Main muscular support of lateral longitudinal arch is following *except*:
   a. Peroneus longus b. Peroneus brevis
   c. Peroneus tertius d. Extensor digitorum brevis

ANSWERS

1. c **2.** b **3.** b **4.** c **5.** d

14

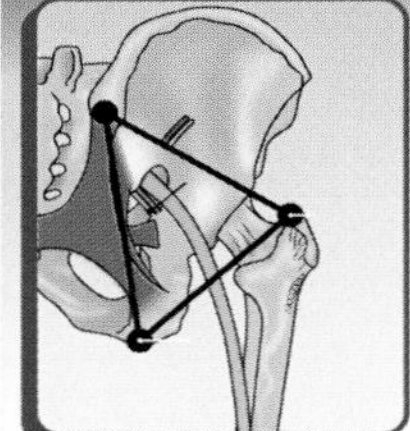

Surface and Radiological Anatomy

God gave you a gift of 86,400 seconds today. Have you used one to say, Thank You?
—WA Ward

SURFACE MARKING OF ARTERIES

Femoral Artery

It corresponds to the upper two-thirds of a line joining the following two points.

- *Midinguinal point:* A point midway between the anterior superior iliac spine and the pubic symphysis (Fig. 14.1).
- *Adductor tubercle*: It lies at the lower end of the cord-like tendon of the adductor magnus. The tendon can be felt in a shallow groove just behind the prominence of the vastus medialis *when the thigh is semiflexed, abducted and laterally rotated.*

The upper one-third of the line represents the upper half of the artery lying in the femoral triangle. The middle one-third of the line represents the lower half of the artery lying in the adductor canal. The lower one-third of the line represents the descending genicular and saphenous branches of the artery.

Fig. 14.1: Femoral vessels, profunda femoris artery, femoral nerve, femoral ring and saphenous opening in the thigh

Profunda Femoris Artery

First mark the femoral artery. The profunda artery is then marked by joining the following two points on the femoral artery (Fig. 14.1).

- *First point:* 3.5 cm below the midinguinal point.
- *Second point:* 10 cm below the midinguinal point.

The artery is slightly convex laterally in its upper part.

Popliteal Artery

It is marked by joining the following points.

- *First point:* At the junction of the middle and lower thirds of the thigh, 2.5 cm medial to the midline on the back of the limb (Fig. 14.2).
- *Second point:* On the midline of the back of the knee.
- *Third point:* On the midline of the back of leg at the level of the tibial tuberosity.

Superior Gluteal Artery

Mark the following points.

- *First point:* At the posterior superior iliac spine.
- *Second point:* At the apex of the greater trochanter (Fig. 14.3).

The superior gluteal artery enters the gluteal region at the junction of the upper and middle thirds of the line joining points (1st) and (2nd).

Inferior Gluteal Artery

Mark the following points.

- *First point:* Posterior superior iliac spine.
- *Second point:* Ischial tuberosity.

Then mark a third point 2.5 cm lateral to the midpoint of the line joining 1st and 2nd points. The sciatic nerve

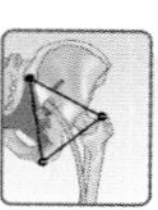

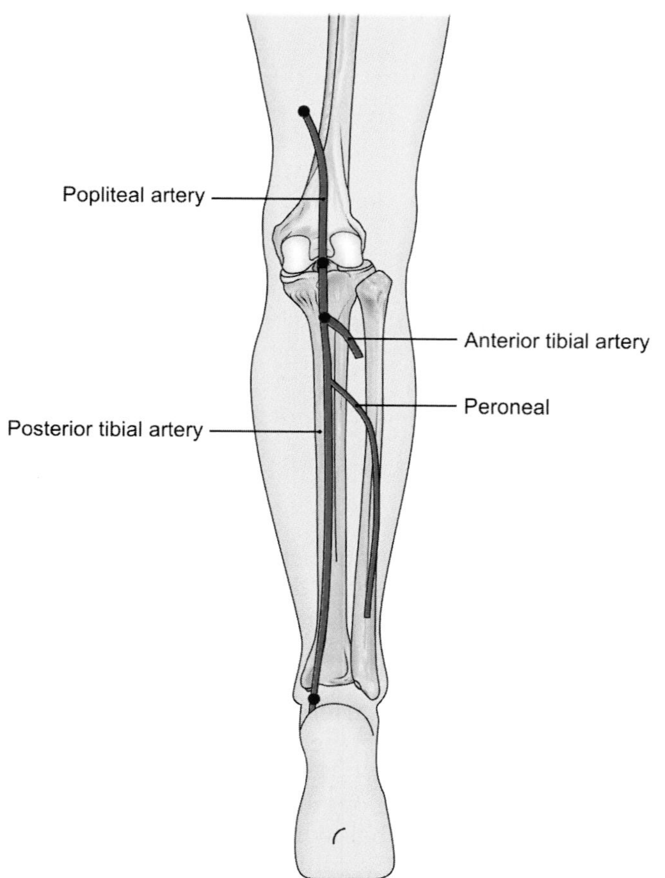

Fig. 14.2: Surface marking of popliteal, posterior tibial

enters the gluteal region at this point. The inferior gluteal artery appears just medial to the entry of the sciatic nerve (Fig. 14.3).

Anterior Tibial Artery

It is marked by joining the following two points.

- *First point:* 2.5 cm below the medial side of the head of the fibula (Fig. 14.4).
- *Second point*: Midway between the two malleoli. The artery passes downwards and slightly medially.

Posterior Tibial Artery

It is marked by joining the following two points.

- *First point:* On the midline of the back of the leg at the level of the tibial tuberosity.
- *Second point:* Midway between the medial malleolus and the tendocalcaneus (Fig. 14.2).

Dorsalis Pedis Artery

It is marked by joining the following two points.

- *First point:* Midway between the two malleoli.
- *Second point:* At the proximal end of the first intermetatarsal space (Fig. 14.4).

Medial Plantar Artery

It is marked by joining the following two points.

- *First point:* Midway between the medial malleolus and the prominence of the heel.
- *Second point:* On the navicular bone which lies midway between the back of the heel and the root of

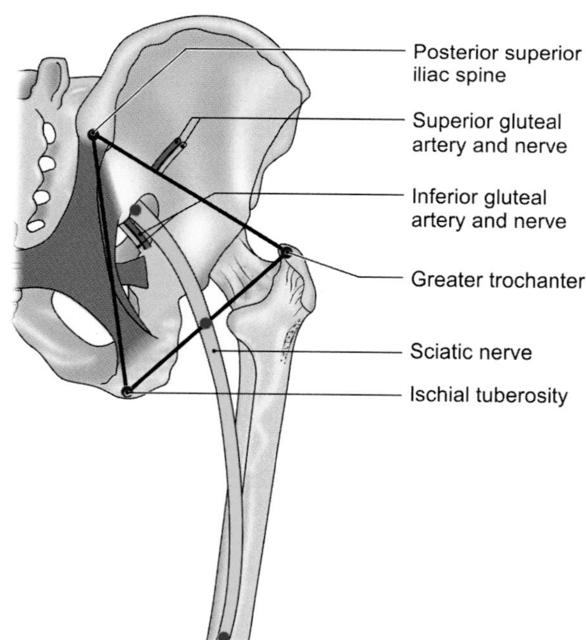

Fig. 14.3: Surface marking of sciatic nerve gluteal arteries and nerves

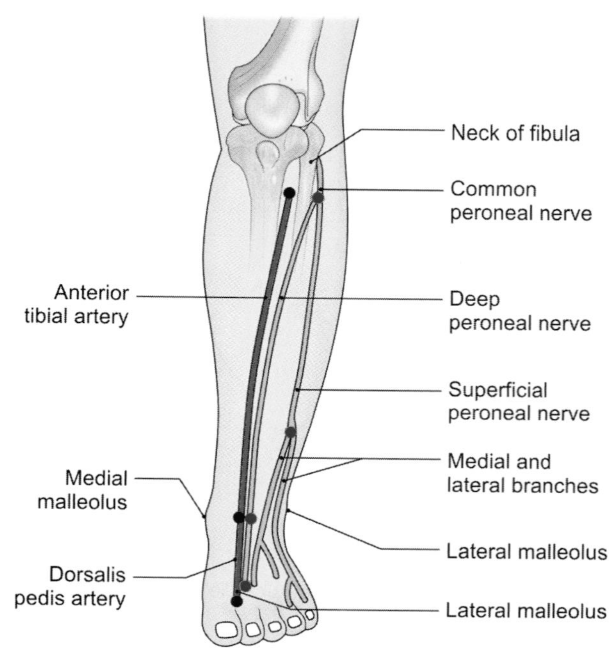

Fig. 14.4: Surface marking of anterior tibial, dorsalis pedis arteries; deep and superficial peroneal nerves

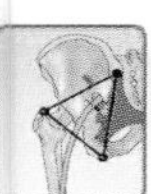

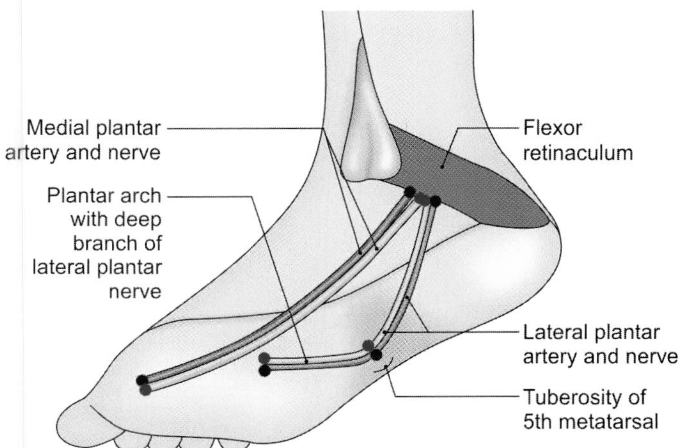

Fig. 14.5: Surface marking of medial and lateral plantar nerves and vessels, including the plantar arch

the big toe. The artery runs in the direction of the first interdigital cleft (Fig. 14.5).

Lateral Plantar Artery

It is marked by joining the following two points.

- *First point:* Midway between the medial malleolus and the prominence of the heel.
- *Second point:* 2.5 cm medial to the tuberosity of the fifth metatarsal bone (Fig. 14.5).

Plantar Arch

It is marked by joining the following two points.

- *First point:* 2.5 cm medial to the tuberosity of the fifth metatarsal bone.
- *Second point:* At the proximal end of the first intermetatarsal space, 2.5 cm distal to the tuberosity of the navicular bone (Fig. 14.5).

The arch is slightly curved with its convexity directed forwards.

VEINS

Femoral Vein

Its marking is same as that of the femoral artery, except that the upper point is taken 1 cm medial to the midinguinal point, and the lower point 1 cm lateral to the adductor tubercle. The vein is medial to the artery at the upper end, posterior to it in the middle, and lateral to it at the lower end (Fig. 14.1).

Great Saphenous Vein

It can be marked by joining the following points, although it is easily visible in living subjects.

1. *First point:* On the dorsum of the foot at the medial end of the dorsal venous arch.
2. *Second point:* On the anterior surface of the medial malleolus.
3. *Third point:* On the medial border of the tibia at the junction of the upper two-thirds and lower one-third of the leg.
4. *Fourth point:* At the adductor tubercle.
5. *Fifth point:* Just below the centre of the saphenous opening (Fig. 14.6).

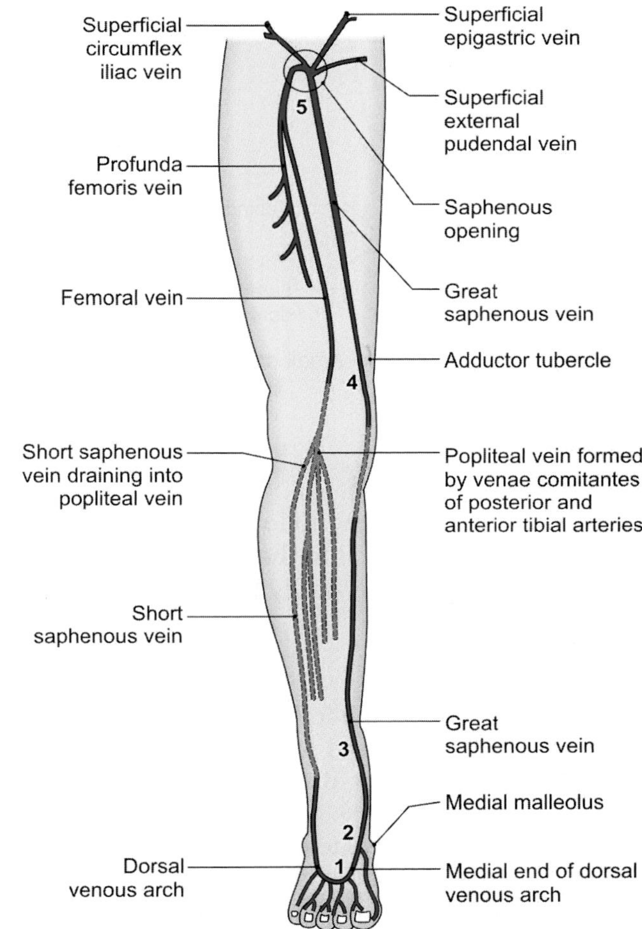

Fig. 14.6: Scheme to show the arrangement of the veins of the lower limb (*see* text)

Small Saphenous Vein

It can be marked by joining the following points, although this vein is also easily visible in its lower part (Fig. 14.7).

1. *First point:* On the dorsum of the foot at the lateral end of the dorsal venous arch.
2. *Second point:* Behind the lateral malleolus.
3. *Third point:* Just lateral to the tendocalcaneus above the lateral malleolus.
4. *Fourth point:* At the centre of the popliteal fossa.

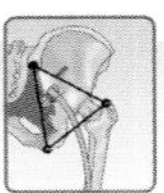

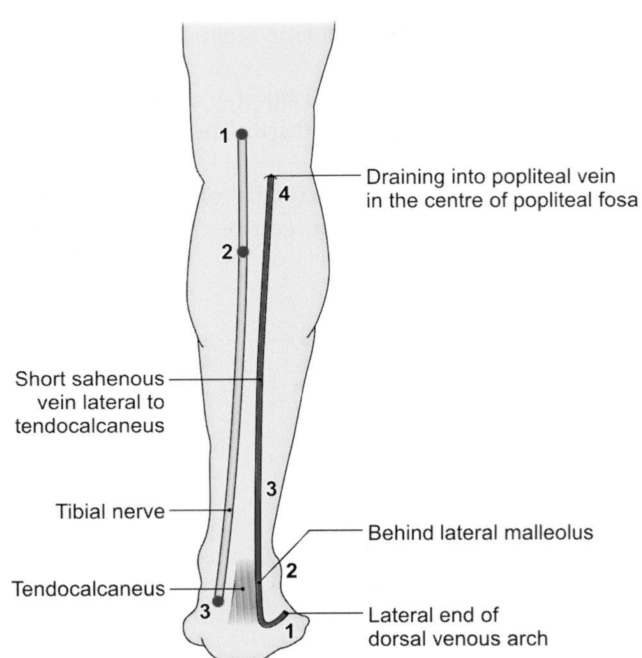

Fig. 14.7: Surface marking of small saphenous vein (*see* text)

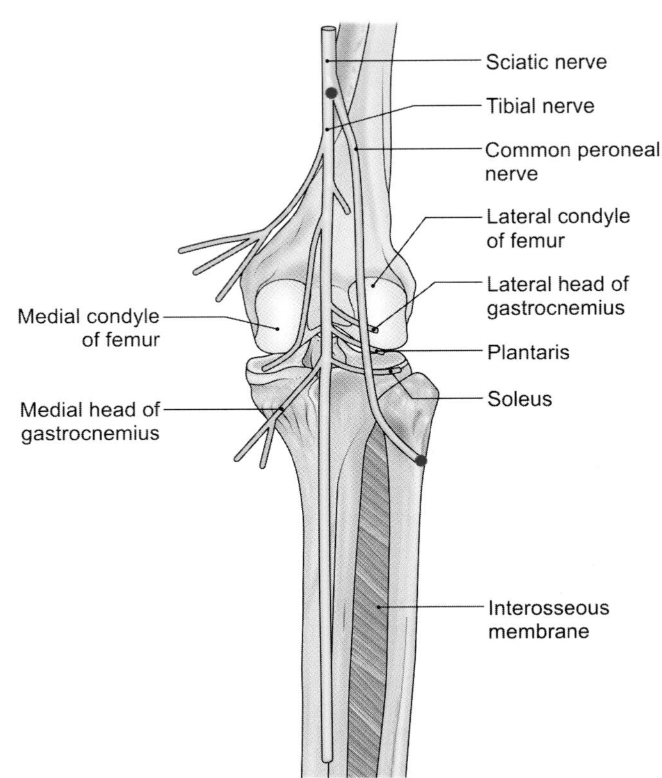

Fig. 14.8: Tibial and common peroneal nerves

NERVES

Femoral Nerve

It is marked by joining the following two points.

- *First point:* 1.2 cm lateral to the midinguinal point.
- *Second point:* 2.5 cm vertically below the first point (Fig. 14.1).

Sciatic Nerve

It is marked by joining the following points.

- *First point:* 2.5 cm lateral to the midpoint between the posterior superior iliac spine and the ischial tuberosity (Fig. 14.3).
- *Second point:* Just medial to the midpoint between the ischial tuberosity and the greater trochanter.
- *The third point:* In the midline of the back of the thigh at the junction of its upper two-thirds and lower one-third, i.e. at the apex of the popliteal fossa.

Tibial Nerve

Mark the following points.

- *First point:* In the midline of back of the thigh at the junction of its upper two-thirds and lower one-third, i.e. at the apex of the popliteal fossa.
- *Second point:* In the midline of back of the leg at the level of tibial tuberosity (Fig. 14.7).
- *Third point:* Midway between the medial malleolus and tendocalcaneus.

The line joining (1) and (2) represents the tibial nerve in the popliteal fossa, and the line joining (2) and (3) represents it in the back of the leg.

Common Peroneal Nerve

It is marked by joining the following two points.

- *First point:* At the apex of the popliteal fossa (Fig. 14.8).
- *Second point:* On the back of the neck of the fibula (*see* Fig. 7.7).

At the lower end the nerve turns forwards and ends deep to the upper fibres of the peroneus longus.

Deep Peroneal Nerve

It is marked by joining the following two points.

- *First point:* On the lateral aspect of the neck of the fibula (Fig. 14.4).
- *Second point:* In front of the ankle, midway between the two malleoli.
- *Third point:* First interosseous space

The nerve lies lateral to the anterior tibial artery in its upper and lower thirds, but anterior to the artery in its middle-third.

Superficial Peroneal Nerve

It is marked by joining the following two points.

- *First point:* On the lateral aspect of the neck of the fibula (Fig. 14.4).
- *Second point:* On the anterior border of the peroneus longus at the junction of the upper two-thirds and lower one-third of the leg.

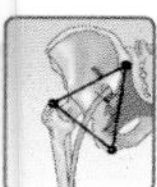

At the lower point the nerve pierces the deep fascia and divides into medial and lateral branches.

Medial Plantar Nerve

It is marked in a manner similar to the medial plantar artery (Fig. 14.5). Lies lateral to the artery.

Lateral Plantar Nerve

It is marked in a manner similar to that for the lateral plantar artery (Fig. 14.5). Lies medial to the artery.

MISCELLANEOUS STRUCTURES

Saphenous Opening

Its centre lies 4 cm below and 4 cm lateral to the pubic tubercle. It is about 2.5 cm long and 2 cm broad, with its long axis directed downwards and laterally (Fig. 14.1).

Femoral Ring

It is represented by a horizontal line 1.25 cm long over the inguinal ligament, 1.25 cm medial to the midinguinal point (Fig. 14.1).

Superior Extensor Retinaculum

The retinaculum is about 3 cm broad vertically. It is drawn from:

1 The anterior border of the triangular subcutaneous area of the fibula.
2 The lower part of the anterior border of the tibia, running medially and slightly upwards (Fig. 14.9).

Inferior Extensor Retinaculum

1 The *stem* is about 1.5 cm broad. It extends from the anterior part of the upper surface of the calcaneum to a point medial to the tendon of the extensor digitorum longus on the dorsum of the foot.
2 The *upper band* is about 1 cm wide, and extends from the medial end of the stem to the anterior border of the medial malleolus (Fig. 14.9).
3 The *lower band* is also about 1 cm wide. It extends from the medial end of the stem to the medial side of the foot, extending into the sole.

Flexor Retinaculum

It is about 2.5 cm broad, and extends from:

1 The medial malleolus
2 The medial side of the heel, running downwards and backwards (Fig. 14.10).

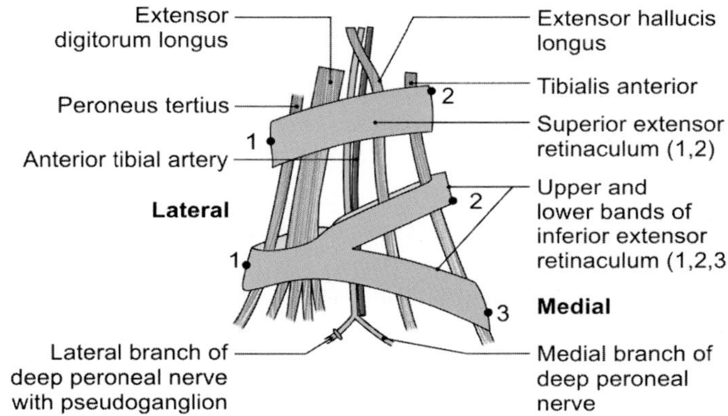

Fig. 14.9: Superior and inferior extensor retinacula of the ankle, surface view

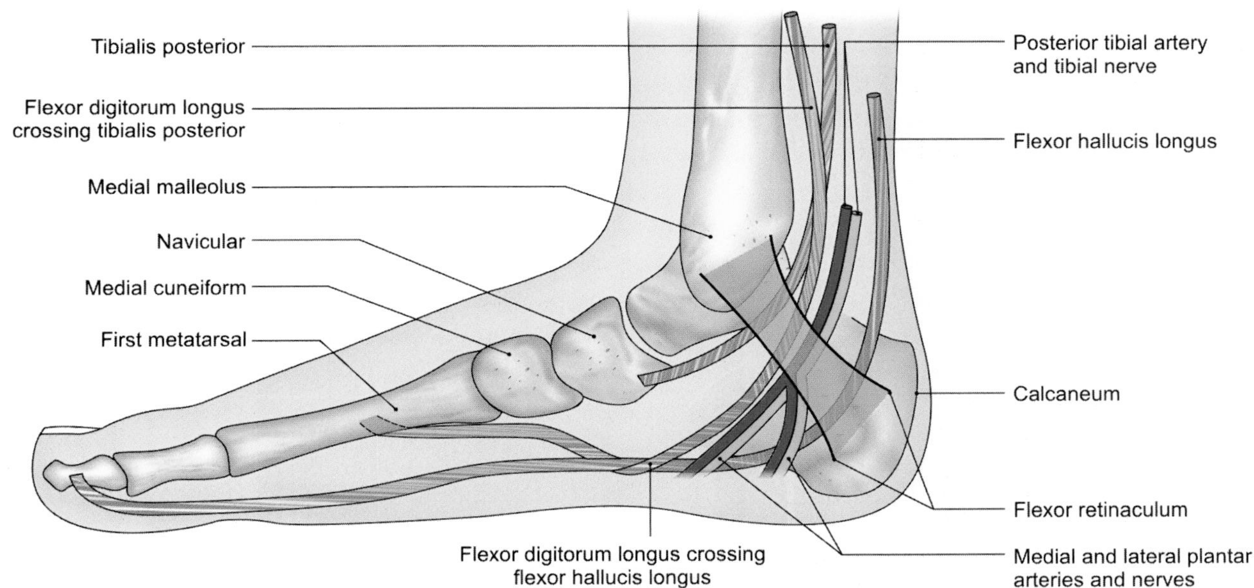

Fig. 14.10: Flexor retinaculum of the ankle, and the structures passing deep to it

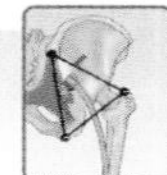

RADIOLOGICAL ANATOMY

In the study of plain skiagrams of the limbs, the following points should be noted.

1 View of the radiograph.
2 Identification of all bones visible.
3 Normal relations of the bones forming joints and the radiological 'joint space'.
4 The presence of epiphyses in the young bones.

Briefly, such skiagrams are helpful in the diagnosis of the following.

a. Fractures.
b. Dislocations.
c. Diseases.
   i. Infective (osteomyelitis),
   ii. Degenerative (osteoarthritis),
   iii. Neoplastic (benign and malignant),
   iv. Deficiency (rickets and scurvy).
d. Developmental defects.
e. The age below 25 years.

HIP

Identify the Following Bones in AP View

1 *Hip bone,* including ilium, pubis, ischium and acetabulum.
2 *Upper end of femur,* including the head, neck, greater trochanter, lesser trochanter, and upper part of shaft. The *neck-shaft angle* is about 125 degrees in adults, being more in children (140°) and less in females. In the head, a dense wedge or triangle of cancellous bone is known as *Ward's triangle.* It represents the epiphyseal scar.

Give X-ray photo

Calcar femorale is a dense plate of compact bone forming a buttress to strengthen the concavity of the neck-shaft angle in front of the lesser trochanter. It transmits weight from the head of femur to the linea aspera.

Cervical torus is a thickened band or ridge of compact bone on the upper part of the neck between the head and the greater trochanter.

3 The *lumbosacral spine* may have been included.

Study the Normal Appearance of the Following Joints

1 *Hip joint:* Normal relation of the head of femur with the acetabulum is indicated by the *Shenton's line,* which is a continuous curve formed by the upper border of obturator foramen and the lower border of the neck of femur (Fig. 14.11).
2 *Pubic symphysis*
3 *Sacroiliac joint.*

Note the epiphyses and other incomplete ossifications if any, and determine the age.

The ischiopubic rami fuse by 7–8 years, and the acetabulum is ossified by 17 years.

KNEE

Identify the Following Bones

1 *Lower end of femur,* including the two condyles (Figs 14.12 and 14.13).
2 *Patella* is clearly seen only in the lateral views; in AP views it overlaps the lower end of femur. It lies about 1 cm above the knee joint.

Bilateral separation of the superolateral angles of the patellae is known as *bipartite patella.* The small fragment may be further subdivided to form the multipartite

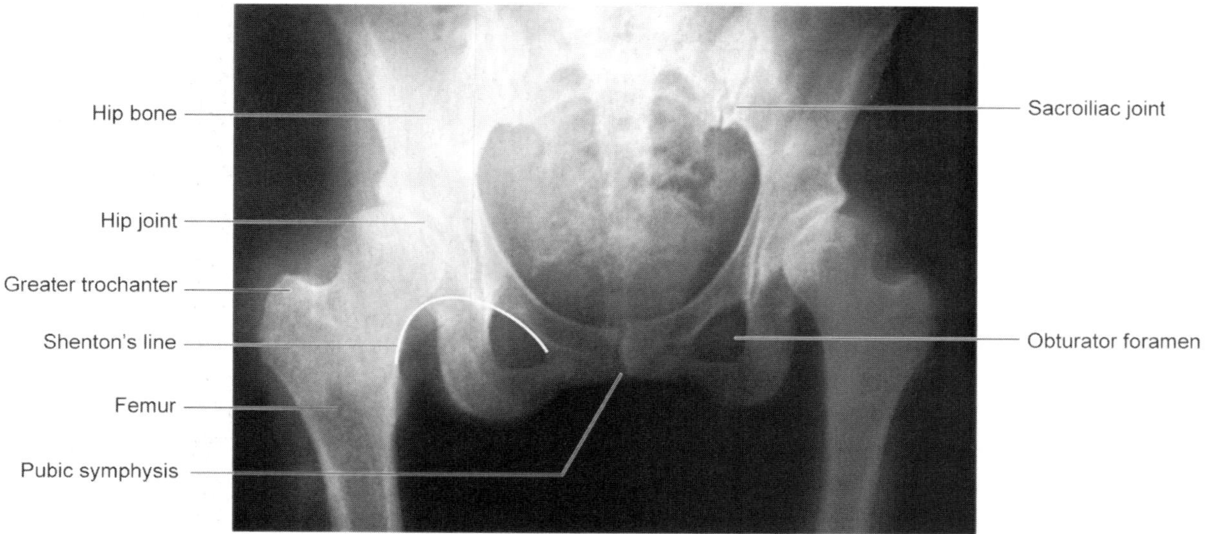

Fig. 14.11: Anteroposterior view of the female pelvis

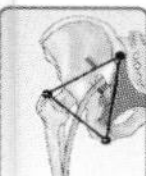

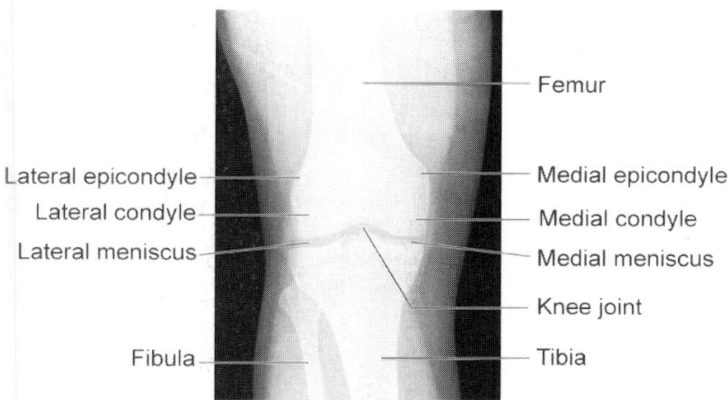

Fig. 14.12: Anteroposterior view of the knee joint

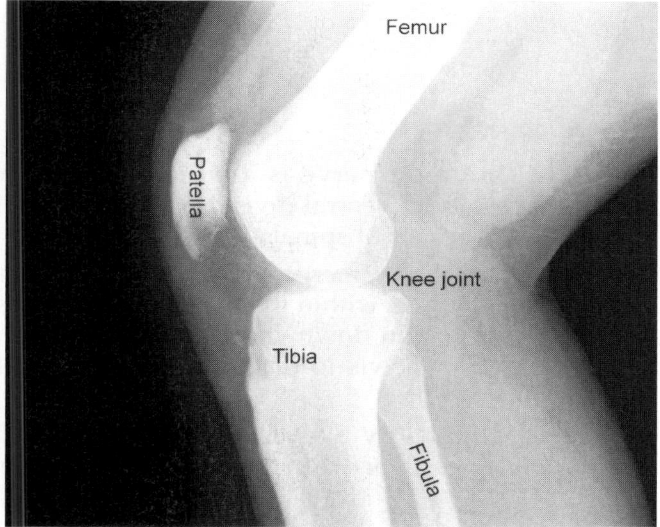

Fig. 14.13: Lateral view of the knee joint

patella. This is due to failure of the ossific centers to fuse.

In *emargination of patella*, its outer margin is concave. The concavity is bounded by a tubercle above and a spine below. This reflects the mode of attachment of the vastus lateralis.

3 *Upper end of tibia*, including the two condyles, intercondylar eminence and tibial tuberosity.
4 *Upper end of fibula*, including the head, neck and upper part of shaft.
5 *Fabella:* It is a small, rounded sesamoid bone in the lateral head of gastrocnemius. It articulates with the posterior surface of the lateral condyle of femur. It measures 1–1.5 cm in diameter, and is present in about 15% individuals. As a rule it is bilateral, and appears at 12–15 years of age.

Study the Normal Appearance of the Following Joints

1 *Knee joint*: The joint space varies inversely with the age. In young adults, it is about 5 mm. It is entirely due to articular cartilage and not due to menisci.
2 *Superior tibiofibular joint.*

Note the epiphyses if any, and determine the age with the help of ossification studied

FOOT

Identify the Following Bones

1 *Talus* and *calcaneum* are better seen in lateral view.
2 *Navicular* and *cuboid* are seen clearly in almost all the views (Fig. 14.14).
3 *Cuneiform bones* are seen separately in dorsoplantar views; they overlap each other in a lateral view.
4 *Metatarsals* and *phalanges* are seen separately in dorsoplantar views, but overlap each other in lateral views.
5 Sesamoid and accessory bones should be distinguished from fractures.

The common *sesamoids* are found on the plantar surface of the head of first metatarsal bone. They may also be present in the tendons of tibialis anterior, tibialis posterior and peroneus longus.

Accessory bones are separate small pieces of bone which have not fused with the main bone. For example, os trigonum (lateral tubercle of talus) and os vesalianum (tuberosity of fifth metatarsal bone).

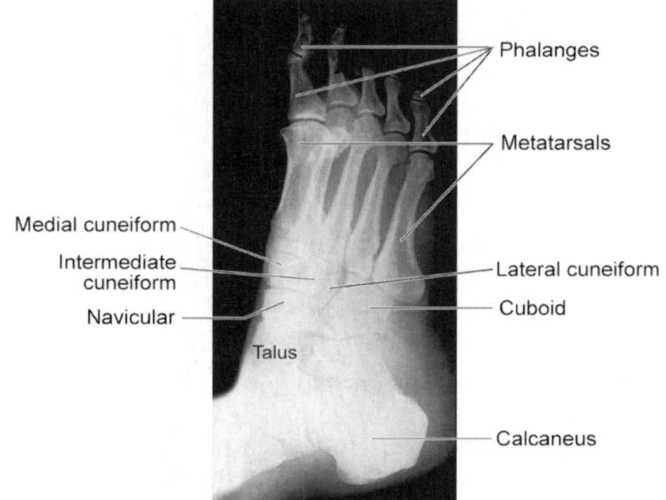

Fig. 14.14: Dorsoplantar view of the ankle and foot

Study the Normal Appearance of the Following Joints

1 Ankle joint.
2 Subtalar, talocalcaneonavicular and transverse tarsal joints.
3 Tarsometatarsal, intermetatarsal, metatarsophalangeal, and interphalangeal joints.

Note the epiphyses and other incomplete ossification if any, and determine the age.

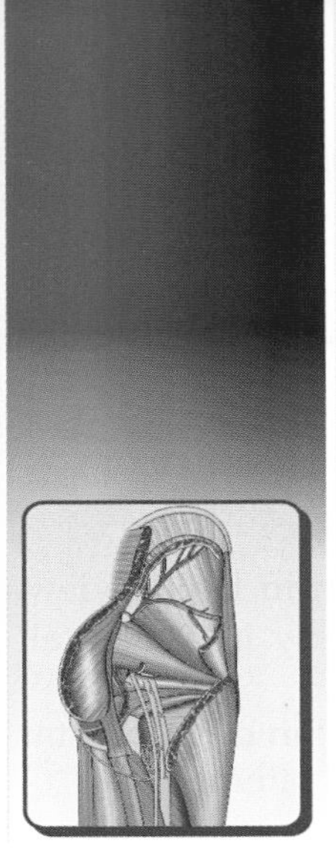

Appendix 1

The chief function of your body is to carry your brain around
—Thomas Alva Edison

NERVES OF LOWER LIMB

FEMORAL NERVE

Femoral nerve is the nerve of anterior compartment of thigh. Its cutaneous branch, the saphenous nerve extends to the medial side of leg and medial border of foot till the ball of the big toe.

Root value: Dorsal division of ventral rami of L2, L3, L4 segments of spinal cord (*see* Figs 3.3 and 3.11).

Beginning and course: It emerges at the lateral border of psoas major muscle in abdomen. It passes downwards between psoas major and iliacus muscles. The nerve enters the thigh behind the inguinal ligament, lateral to femoral sheath. It is not a content of femoral sheath as its formation is behind fascia iliaca.

Termination: It ends by dividing into two divisions 2.5 cm below the inguinal ligament. Both these divisions end in a number of branches. In between the two divisions, lateral circumflex femoral artery is present.

Branches: In *abdomen*, femoral nerve supplies iliacus muscle. Just above the inguinal ligament, it gives a branch to pectineus muscle, which passes behind the femoral sheath to reach the muscle. Its branches in the thigh are shown in Table A1.1.

OBTURATOR NERVE

Root value: Obturator nerve is a branch of lumbar plexus. It arises from ventral division of ventral rami of L2, L3, L4 segments of spinal cord (*see* Fig. 4.4).

Beginning and course: It emerges on the medial border of psoas major muscle within the abdomen. It crosses the pelvic brim to run downwards and forwards on the lateral wall of pelvis to reach the upper part of obturator foramen.

Termination: It ends by dividing into anterior and posterior divisions. In between the divisions, adductor brevis is seen.

Anterior division: It passes downwards in front of obturator externus. Then it lies between pectineus and adductor longus anteriorly and adductor brevis posteriorly. It gives muscular, articular and vascular branches.

Posterior division: It pierces the obturator externus and passes behind adductor brevis and in front of adductor magnus. It also ends by giving muscular, articular and vascular branches.

The branches are shown in Table A1.2.

ACCESSORY OBTURATOR NERVE

It is present in 30% subjects (*see* Fig. 4.6).

Table A1.1: Branches of femoral nerve in thigh

	Anterior/ Superficial division	*Posterior / Deep division*
Muscular	Sartorius	Vastus medialis Vastus intermedius Vastus lateralis Rectus femoris
Cutaneous	Medial cutaneous nerve of thigh Intermediate cutaneous nerve of thigh	Saphenous (for medial side of leg and medial border of foot till ball of big toe)
Articular and vascular	Sympathetic fibres to femoral artery	Knee joint from branches to vasti Hip joint from branch to rectus femoris

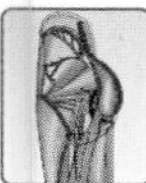

Table A1.2: Branches of obturator nerve		
	Anterior division	*Posterior division*
Muscular	Pectineus, adductor longus, adductor brevis, gracilis	Obturator externus, adductor magnus (adductor part)
Articular	Hip joint	Knee joint
Vascular and cutaneous	Femoral artery—Medial side of thigh	Popliteal artery

Root value: Ventral division of ventral rami of L3, L4 nerves.

Course: Runs along medial border of psoas major, crosses superior ramus of pubis behind pectineus muscle.

Branches: Deep surface of pectineus, hip joint and communicating branch to anterior division of obturator nerve (*see* Fig. 4.6).

SUPERIOR GLUTEAL NERVE

Root value: L4, L5, S1.

Course: Enters the gluteal region through greater sciatic notch above piriformis muscle. Runs between gluteus medius and gluteus minimus to end in tensor fasciae latae (*see* Fig. 5.14).

Branches: It supplies gluteus medius, gluteus minimus and tensor fasciae latae.

INFERIOR GLUTEAL NERVE

Root value: L5, S1, S2.

Course: Enters the gluteal region through greater sciatic notch below piriformis muscle (*see* Fig. 5.14).

Branches: It gives a number of branches to the gluteus maximus muscle only. It is the sole supply to the large antigravity, postural muscle with red fibres, responsible for extending the hip joint.

NERVE TO QUADRATUS FEMORIS

Root value: L4, L5, S1.

Branches: It supplies quadratus femoris, inferior gemellus and hip joint.

NERVE TO OBTURATOR INTERNUS

Root value: L5, S1, S2.

Branches: It supplies obturator internus and superior gemellus.

SCIATIC NERVE

Sciatic nerve is the thickest nerve of the body. It is the terminal branch of the lumbosacral plexus.

Root value: Ventral rami of L4, L5, S1, S2, S3. It consists of two parts (*see* Figs 5.6 and 5.14).

Tibial part: Its root value is ventral division of ventral rami of L4, L5, S1, S2, S3, segments of spinal cord (*see* Fig. 7.6).

Common peroneal part: Its root value is dorsal division of ventral rami of L4, L5, S1, S2 segments of spinal cord.

Course: Sciatic nerve arises in the pelvis. Leaves the pelvis by passing through greater sciatic foramen below the piriformis to enter the gluteal region (*see* Fig. 7.7).

In the gluteal region, it lies deep to the gluteus maximus muscle, and crosses superior gemellus, obturator internus, inferior gemellus, quadratus femoris to enter the back of thigh. During its short course, it lies between ischial tuberosity and greater trochanter with a convexity to the lateral side. It gives no branches in the gluteal region.

In the back of thigh, it lies deep to long head of biceps femoris and superficial to adductor magnus (*see* Fig. 7.7).

Termination: It ends by dividing into its two terminal branches in the back of thigh.

Branches: The branches of sciatic nerve are shown in Table A1.3.

TIBIAL NERVE

Root value: Ventral division of ventral rami of L4, L5, S1, S2, S3, segments of spinal cord.

Beginning: It begins as the larger subdivision of sciatic nerve in the back of thigh (*see* Fig. 6.7).

Course: It has a long course first in the popliteal fossa and then in the back of leg.

Popliteal fossa: The nerve descends vertically in the popliteal fossa from its upper angle to the lower angle.

Table A1.3: Branches of sciatic nerve			
	Gluteal region	*Back of thigh; from tibial part*	*From common peroneal part*
Muscular	Nil	Long head of biceps femoris, semitendinosus, semimembranosus, ischial part of adductor magnus	Short head of biceps femoris
Articular	Nil	Hip joint	—
Terminal	Nil	Tibial and common peroneal nerves	—

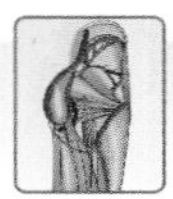

It lies superficial to the popliteal vessels. It continues in the back of leg beyond the distal border of popliteus muscle (*see* Fig. 6.7).

In back of leg: The nerve descends as the neurovascular bundle with posterior tibial vessels. It lies superficial to tibialis posterior and deep to flexor digitorum longus. Lastly it passes deep to the flexor retinaculum of ankle (*see* Figs 9.2 and 9.7).

Branches: Its branches are shown in Table A1.4.

Termination: The tibial nerve terminates by dividing into medial plantar and lateral plantar nerves as it lies deep to the flexor retinaculum.

COMMON PERONEAL NERVE

This is the smaller terminal branch of sciatic nerve. Its root value is dorsal division of ventral rami of L4, L5, S1, S2 segments of spinal cord.

Beginning: It begins in the back of thigh as a smaller subdivision of the sciatic nerve.

Course: It lies in the upper lateral part of popliteal fossa, along the medial border of biceps femoris muscle. It turns around the lateral surface of fibula. Then it lies in the substance of peroneus longus muscle (*see* Fig. 6.4).

Branches: Its branches are shown in Table A1.5.

Termination: Ends by dividing into two terminal branches, i.e. superficial peroneal and deep peroneal nerves (*see* Fig. 8.9).

DEEP PERONEAL NERVE

The deep peroneal nerve is the nerve of the anterior compartment of the leg and the dorsum of the foot. It corresponds to the posterior interosseous nerve of the forearm. This is one of the two terminal branches of the common peroneal nerve given off between the neck of the fibula and the peroneus longus muscle.

Course and relations: The deep peroneal nerve begins on the lateral side of the neck of fibula under cover of the upper fibres of peroneus longus. It enters the anterior compartment of leg by piercing the anterior intermuscular septum. It then pierces the extensor digitorum longus and comes to lie next to the anterior tibial vessels (*see* Fig. 14.4).

In the leg, it accompanies the anterior tibial artery and has similar relations. The nerve lies lateral to the artery in the upper and lower third of the leg, and anterior to the artery in the middle one-third.

The nerve ends on the dorsum of the foot, close to the ankle joint, by dividing into the lateral and medial terminal branches (*see* Fig. 8.4).

The lateral terminal branch turns laterally and ends in a pseudoganglion deep to the extensor digitorum brevis. Branches arise from the pseudoganglion and supply the extensor digitorum brevis and the tarsal joints.

The medial terminal branch ends by supplying the skin adjoining the first interdigital cleft and the proximal joints of the big toe.

Branches and distribution of the deep peroneal nerve:

Muscular branches: The muscular branches supply the following muscles.

1. Muscles of the anterior compartment of the leg. These include:
   a. Tibialis anterior
   b. Extensor hallucis longus

Table A1.5: Branches of common peroneal nerve in popliteal fossa

Muscular	— Short head of biceps femoris
Cutaneous and vascular	— Lateral cutaneous nerve of calf — Sural communicating
Articular	— Superior lateral genicular — Inferior lateral genicular — Recurrent genicular
Terminal	— Deep peroneal — Superficial peroneal

Table A1.4: Branches of tibial nerve

	Popliteal fossa	*Back of leg*
Muscular	— Medial head of gastrocnemius — Lateral head of gastrocnemius — Plantaris — Soleus — Popliteus. These are given in lower part of fossa	Soleus Flexor digitorum longus Flexor hallucis longus Tibialis posterior
Cutaneous and vascular	Sural nerve. This is given in middle of fossa	Medial calcanean branches and branch to posterior tibial artery
Articular	— Superior medial genicular — Middle genicular — Inferior medial genicular. These are given in upper part of fossa	Ankle joint
Terminal	—	Medial plantar and lateral plantar nerves

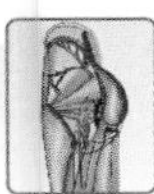

c. Extensor digitorum longus
d. Peroneus tertius.

2 The extensor digitorum brevis (on the dorsum of foot) is supplied by the lateral terminal branch of the deep peroneal nerve.

Cutaneous branches: The lateral terminal branch of the deep peroneal nerve ends by forming the dorsal digital nerves for the adjacent sides of the big toe and second toe (*see* Fig. 8.2).

Articular branches: These are given to the:

1 Ankle joint
2 Tarsal joints
3 Tarsometatarsal joint
4 Metatarsophalangeal joint of big toe.

SUPERFICIAL PERONEAL NERVE

It is the smaller terminal branch of the common peroneal nerve (*see* Fig. 8.9).

Origin: It arises in the substance of peroneus longus muscle, lateral to the neck of fibula.

Course: It descends in the lateral compartment of leg deep to peroneus longus. Then it lies between peroneus longus and peroneus brevis muscles and lastly between the peronei and extensor digitorum longus.

It pierces the deep fascia in distal one-third of leg and descends to the dorsum of foot.

Branches: It supplies both peroneus longus and peroneus brevis muscles.

It gives cutaneous branches (*see* Fig. 8.2) to most of the dorsum of foot including the digital branches to medial side of big toe, adjacent sides of 2nd and 3rd; 3rd and 4th and 4th and 5th toes. The nail beds are not supplied as these are supplied by medial plantar for medial 3½ and by lateral plantar for lateral 1½ toes. Adjacent sides of big and second toes are supplied by deep peroneal nerve. The medial border of foot is supplied by saphenous and lateral border by sural nerves.

PLANTAR NERVES

The medial and lateral plantar nerves are the terminal branches of the tibial nerve. These nerves begin deep to the flexor retinaculum.

Medial plantar nerve: It is the larger terminal branch of tibial nerve. Its distribution is similar to median nerve of the hand. It lies between abductor hallucis and flexor digitorum brevis and ends by giving muscular, cutaneous and articular branches (*see* Fig. 10.4b).

Branches: The branches of medial plantar nerve are shown in Table A1.6.

Lateral plantar nerve: It is the smaller terminal branch of tibial nerve, resembling the ulnar nerve of the hand in its distribution. It runs obliquely between the first and second layers of sole till the tuberosity of fifth metatarsal bone, where it divides into its superficial and deep branches (see Fig. 10.6b).

Branches: The structures supplied by the trunk, and its two branches are given in Table A1.7.

Table A1.6: Branches of medial plantar nerve

	Medial plantar nerve (S2, S3)	
Muscular	— Abductor hallucis	: 1st layer
	— Flexor digitorum brevis	: 1st layer
	— First lumbrical	: 2nd layer
	— Flexor hallucis brevis	: 3rd layer
Cutaneous	— Nail beds of medial 3½ toes	
and **vascular**	— Sympathetic branches to medial plantar artery	
Articular	— Tarsometatarsal, metatarsophalangeal and interphalangeal joints of medial 2/3rd of foot	

CLINICAL ANATOMY

- Femoral nerve supplying the quadriceps femoris through L2, L3, L4 segments of spinal cord is tested by doing the 'patellar jerk'. The ligamentum patellae is hit by the hammer and the contraction of the quadriceps is felt with extension of knee (*see* Fig. 3.30).
- Since obturator nerve supplies both the hip and knee joints, pain of one joint may be referred to the other joint.
- The paralysis of left superior gluteal nerve leads to paralysis of left gluteus medius and minimus

Table A1.7: Branches of lateral plantar nerve

	Trunk (S2, S3)	*Superficial branch*	*Deep branch*
Muscular	• Abductor digiti minimi: 1st layer • Flexor digitorum accessorius: 2nd layer	• Flexor digiti minimi brevis: 3rd layer • 3rd plantar interosseous: 4th layer • 4th dorsal interosseous: 4th layer	1st and 2nd plantar interossei: 4th layer 1st, 2nd, 3rd, dorsal interossei: 4th layer 2nd, 3rd, 4th lumbricals: 2nd layer Adductor hallucis: 3rd layer
Cutaneous and vascular	— —	Nail beds of lateral 1½ toes Sympathetic branches to lateral plantar artery	—
Articular	Tarsometatarsal	Interphalangeal	Metatarsophalangeal

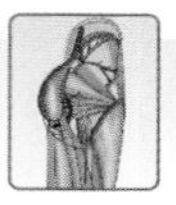

muscle. During walking when the body is supported on left foot, the right unsupported side of the pelvis droops, causing inability to walk with right foot. This is called *positive Trendelenburg's test* (*see* Fig. 5.12)

- *Sleeping foot:* Sometimes it happens that one is awake but the foot sleeps. Sciatic nerve lies on quadratus femoris and adductor magnus. Between the two muscles, the nerve lies on the hard femur. So the nerve gets pressed between the femur and the hard edge of table, chair or bed. There is numbness of the lower limb till the foot is hit against the ground a few times. The sensations come back (*see* Fig. 7.3).
- *Injury:* Injury to sciatic nerve leads to paralysis of hamstrings and all muscles of the leg and foot leading to "foot drop" (*see* Fig. 7.11).
- *Sciatica:* Is the name given when there is radiating pain in the back of lower limb. It may be due to slip disc.
- Common peroneal nerve is the commonest nerve to be paralysed. This is injured due to fracture of neck of fibula, 'lathi injury' on the lateral side of knee joint or due to plaster on the leg. In the last case, the nerve gets compressed between hard plaster and neck of fibula. To prevent this cotton must be placed on the upper lateral side of the leg (*see* Fig. 8.9).

  The effects of injury are:

  Motor loss: To dorsiflexors and evertors of foot. The typical position of the foot is "foot drop"; sensory loss is to the back of leg; lateral side of leg and most of dorsum of foot.

  Articular loss to the lateral side of knee joint.
- Paralysis of muscles of the anterior compartment of the leg results in loss of the power of dorsiflexion of the foot. As a result the foot is plantar flexed. The condition is called as "foot drop" (*see* Fig. 8.10).
- The motor and sensory loss in case of injury to the various nerves is shown in Table A1.8.
- Thus most of the muscles of the lower limb are supplied by sciatic nerve except the adductors of thigh and extensors of knee joint.
- Arterial occlusive disease of the lower limb: Occlusive disease causes ischaemia of the muscles of lower limb leading to cramp-like pain. The pain disappears with rest but comes back with activity. The condition is called 'intermittent claudication'.
- Palpation of dorsalis pedis artery and posterior tibial artery gives information about peripheral arterial diseases (*see* Fig. 8.11).
- Sympathetic innervation of the arteries: Thoracic 10–12 and L1–L3 segments provide sympathetic innervation to arteries of lower limb. Preganglionic fibres relay in the ganglia associated with these segments. Postganglionic fibres reach blood vessels via branches of lumbar and sacral plexuses.
- Femoral artery receives postganglionic fibres from femoral and obturator nerves.
- Arteries of the leg receive postganglionic fibres via the tibial and common peroneal nerves.
- Lumbar sympathectomy for occlusive arterial disease: Sympathectomy, i.e. removal of L2 and L3 ganglia with intervening sympathetic trunk is advised for this condition. This increases the collateral circulation. L1 ganglion is not removed as it is responsible for ejaculation.
- Blood supply to muscles of back of thigh reaches through a rich anastomosis (*see* Fig. 7.14) formed by:
  a. Superior gluteal artery
  b. Inferior gluteal artery
  c. Branches of femoral circumflex arteries
  d. Perforating arteries
  e. Branches of popliteal artery.
- Excessive fluid from knee joint can be aspirated by putting in a needle in the joint cavity from its lateral side.

Table A1.8: Injury to nerves and their effects

	Motor loss	*Sensory loss*
Femoral nerve	Quadriceps femoris	Anterior side of thigh, medial side of leg till ball of big toe
Sciatic nerve	Hamstring muscles; dorsiflexors and plantar flexors of ankle joint and evertors of foot Foot drop occurs	Back of leg, lateral side of leg, most of dorsum of foot, sole of foot
Common peroneal	Dorsiflexors of ankle, evertors of foot and foot drop occurs	Lateral and anterior sides of leg, most of dorsum of foot, most of digits
Tibial	Plantar flexors of ankle, intrinsic muscles of sole	Skin of sole. Later trophic ulcers develop
Obturator	Adductors of thigh except hamstring part of adductor magnus	Small area on the medial side of thigh

(*Contd...*)

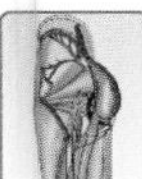

Table A1.8: Injury to nerves and their effects *(Contd...)*

	Motor loss	*Sensory loss*
Superior gluteal	Gluteal medius, gluteus minimus and tensor fascia latae	Nil
Inferior gluteal	Gluteus maximus	Nil
Pudendal nerve	Muscles of perineum	Skin of perineum
Deep peroneal	Muscles of anterior compartment of leg	1st interdigital cleft
Superficial peroneal	Peroneus longus and peroneus brevis	Lateral aspect of leg most of dorsum of foot
Medial plantar	Four intrinsic muscles of sole (Table A1.6)	Medial 2/3rd of sole and digital nerves to medial 3½ toes, including nail beds
Lateral plantar	Most of intrinsic muscles of sole (Table A1.7)	Lateral 1/3rd of sole and digital nerves to lateral 1½ toes, including nail beds

CLINICAL TERMS

Policeman's heel: Plantar aponeurosis is attached to posterior tubercle of calcaneus and to all five digits. In plantar fasciitis, there is pain in the heel. Since policeman has to stand for long hours, they often suffer from it.

Dipping gait: Gluteus medius and gluteus minimus support the opposite side of the pelvis, when the foot is raised during walking. If these two muscles get paralysed on right side, walking with left limb becomes difficult, as that limb dips down, while attempting to lift it. Walking with right leg is normal as this leg is supported by the normal left muscles (*see* Fig. 5.12).

Weaver's bottom: Inflammation of the bursa over the ischial tuberosity. Since weavers have to sit for a long time, they suffer from it more often.

Meralgia parasthetica: Lateral cutaneous nerve of thigh may pierce the inguinal ligament and it may get pressed and cause irritation over lateral side of upper thigh (*see* Fig. 3.20).

Housemaid knee: Inflammation of prepatellar bursa (*see* Fig. 3.6). It used to be common in housemaids as they had to sweep the floor with their knees bent acutely.

Clergyman's knee: Inflammation of subcutaneous infrapatellar bursa as he would sit for prayers with bent knees

Close-pack position of ankle joint: Dorsiflexed ankle joint when anterior wide trochlear area of talus fits tightly into posterior narrow articular area of lower end of tibia.

Inversion injuries more common than eversion injuries: Inversion is accompanied by plantar flexion. During plantar flexion the narrow posterior trochlear area of talus lies loosely in the anterior wide articular area of lower end of tibia. So inversion injuries are common.

Fresher's syndrome: Overexertion of the muscles of anterior compartment of leg causes oedema of leg as these are enclosed in tight compartment of deep fascia. This results in pain in the leg. Fresher's are students who are just admitted in the colleges. They are compelled to run by the senior students. So it occurs in them.

Sites of intramuscular injections: In upper lateral quadrant of gluteal region into the gluteus medius. Also into the vastus lateralis (*see* Fig. 5.9).

Sites of pulse palpation in lower limb: Femoral artery, popliteal artery, posterior tibial and dorsalis pedis arteries. Popliteal artery is used for auscultation to measure blood pressure in lower limb.

Cut open/venesection: A small cut given in great/long saphenous vein to insert a cannula for giving intravenous transfusions. Since position of this vein is constant, anterior to medial malleolus, the great saphenous vein is used for cut-open.

Tarsal tunnel syndrome: The syndrome occurs due to compression of tibial nerve within the fibro-osseous tunnel under the flexor retinaculum of ankle joint. This is associated with pain and parasthesia in the sole of the foot often worse at night.

Injury to medial meniscus: The medial meniscus is more vulnerable to injury than the lateral meniscus, because of its fixity to the capsule and tibial collateral ligament. The lateral meniscus is protected by the popliteus which pulls it backwards so that it is not crushed between the articular surfaces (*see* Fig. 2.18).

Cruciate ligaments: Tear of anterior cruciate ligament leads to abnormal anterior mobility while tear of posterior ligament leads to abnormal posterior mobility of tibia (*see* Fig. 12.15).

Pes planus: Absence or collapse of the arches leads to flat foot (pes planus) (*see* Fig.13.8).

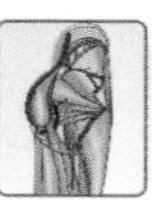

ARTERIES OF LOWER LIMB		
Artery	*Beginning, course and termination*	*Area of distribution*
Femoral artery (*see* Fig. 3.21)	It is the continuation of external iliac artery, begins behind the inguinal ligament at the midinguinal point Femoral artery. courses through femoral triangle and adductor canal. Then it passes through opening in adductor magnus to continue as the popliteal artery	In femoral triangle, femoral artery gives three superficial branches, e.g. superficial external pudendal, superficial epigastric and superficial circumflex iliac, and three deep branches, e.g. profunda femoris, deep external pudendal and muscular branches. In adductor canal, femoral artery gives muscular and descending genicular artery
Superficial external pudendal (*see* Fig. 3.11)	Superficial branch of femoral artery	Supplies skin of external genitalia
Superficial epigastric (*see* Fig. 3.11)	Superficial branch of femoral artery	Supplies skin of anterior abdominal wall as it passes towards epigastric region
Superficial circumflex iliac	Superficial branch of femoral artery	Supplies skin over the iliac crest
Profunda femoris (*see* Fig. 3.22)	Largest branch of femoral artery which descends posterior to femoral vessels, and ends as the fourth perforating artery	Branches are medial circumflex femoral, lateral circumflex femoral, 1st, 2nd and 3rd perforating. All these branches supply all muscles of thigh and muscles attached to trochanters
Deep external pudendal	Deep branch of femoral artery	Supplies deeper structures in the perineal region
Muscular branches	Deep branch of femoral artery	Supply muscles of thigh
Descending genicular	Deep branch of femoral artery	Supplies the knee joint
Popliteal artery (*see* Fig. 6.5)	It is the continuation of femoral artery and lies in the popliteal fossa. Popliteal artery ends by dividing into anterior tibial artery and posterior tibial artery at the distal border of popliteus muscle	Gives five genicular: • Superior medial genicular • Superior lateral genicular • Middle genicular • Inferior medial genicular • Inferior lateral genicular Cutaneous branches for skin of popliteal fossa Muscular branches for the muscles of the fossa
Anterior tibial artery (*see* Fig. 8.8)	Smaller terminal branch of popliteal artery reaches the front of leg through an opening in the interosseous membrane. Runs amongst muscles of front of leg till midway between medial and lateral malleoli, where it ends by changing its name to dorsalis pedis artery	Muscular to the muscles of anterior compartment of leg. Cutaneous to the skin of leg. Articular to the knee joint through anterior and posterior tibial recurrent branches. Also to the ankle joint through anterior medial and anterior lateral malleolar branches
Dorsalis pedis artery (*see* Fig. 8.8)	Continuation of anterior tibial artery. Runs along medial side of dorsum of foot to reach proximal end of 1st intermetatarsal space where it enters the sole. In the sole it completes the plantar arch	Two tarsal branches for the intertarsal joints. Arcuate artery runs over the bases of metatarsal bones and gives off 2nd, 3rd and 4th dorsal metatarsal arteries.1st dorsal metatarsal artery gives digital branches to big toe and medial side of 2nd toe
Posterior tibial artery (*see* Fig. 9.7)	It begins as the larger terminal branch of popliteal artery at the distal border of popliteus muscle. It descends down medially between the long flexor muscles to reach midway between medial malleolus and medial tubercle of calcaneus where it ends by dividing into medial plantar and lateral plantar arteries	Peroneal artery is the largest branch. Nutrient artery to tibia. Articular branches to the knee joint and ankle joint. Muscular branches to the neighbouring muscles
Peroneal artery (*see* Fig. 9.7)	Largest branch of popliteal artery given off 2.5 cm below lower border of popliteus	Muscular branches to muscles of posterior and lateral compartments. Cutaneous to skin of leg. Articular to ankle joint. Perforating branch enters

(*Contd...*)

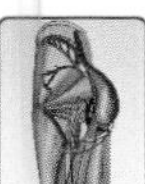

ARTERIES OF LOWER LIMB (*Contd...*)		
Artery	*Beginning, course and termination*	*Area of distribution*
		the front of leg through a hole in the interosseous membrane to assist the dorsalis pedis artery
Medial plantar artery (*see* Fig. 10.9)	The smaller terminal branch of posterior tibial artery given off under flexor retinaculum. Runs along the medial border of foot and ends by giving digital arteries	Muscular branches to muscles of medial side of foot. Cutaneous branches to medial side of sole and digital branches to medial 3½ digits. Also gives branches to the joints of foot
Lateral plantar artery (*see* Fig. 10.9)	The large terminal branch of posterior tibial artery given off under the flexor retinaculum. It runs laterally between muscles of 1st and 2nd layers of sole till the base of 5th metatarsal bone by becoming continuous with the plantar arch	Muscular branches to muscles of sole, cutaneous branches to skin and fasciae of lateral side of sole
Plantar arch (*see* Figs 10.9 and 10.10)	It is the direct continuation of lateral plantar artery and is completed medially by dorsalis pedis artery The arch lies between 3rd and 4th layers of muscles of sole. The deep branch of lateral plantar nerve lies in its concavity	Four plantar metatarsal arteries, each of them gives two digital branches for adjacent sides of two digits, including medial side of big toe and lateral side of little toe

MULTIPLE CHOICE QUESTIONS

A. Match the following on the left side with their appropriate answers on the right side.

1. Types of joints:

a. Hip joint	i. Saddle
b. Ankle joint	ii. Ball and socket
c. Inferior tibiofibular joint	iii. Syndesmosis
d. Calcaneocuboid joint	iv. Hinge

2. Characteristic features of tarsals:

a. Devoid of any muscular attachments	i. Cuboid
b. Forms the prominence of the heel	ii. Navicular
c. Boat-shaped	iii. Calcaneus
d. Has groove on inferior surface for the tendon of peroneus longus	iv. Talus

3. Muscles and their nerve supply:

a. Rectus femoris	i. Obturator
b. Short head of biceps femoris	ii. Femoral
c. Ischial part of adductor magnus	iii. Common peroneal
d. Gracilis	iv. Tibial part of sciatic

4. Movements at hip joint:

a. Extension	i. Gluteus medius
b. Flexion	ii. Iliacus
c. Abduction	iii. Obturator internus
d. Lateral rotation	iv. Gluteus maximus

5. Cutaneous innervation:

a. Medial aspect of leg	i. Deep peroneal
b. Lateral aspect of foot	ii. Superficial peroneal
c. Medial aspect of big toe	iii. Saphenous
d. Interdigital cleft between 1st and 2nd toes	iv. Sural

B. For each of the statements or questions below, one or more answers given is/are correct.

Select

A. If only a, b and c are correct
B. If only a, c are correct
C. If only b, d are correct
D. If only d is correct
E. If all are correct

1. The following structures pass through the saphenous opening:

a. Great saphenous vein
b. Lymph vessels connecting superficial inguinal lymph nodes with deep inguinal lymph nodes
c. Superficial epigastric artery
d. Superficial external pudendal vein

2. When the neck of femur is fractured:

a. There may be avascular necrosis of head of femur
b. Trendelenburg's test is positive
c. The distal fragment of the bone is rotated laterally
d. The affected limb is shortened

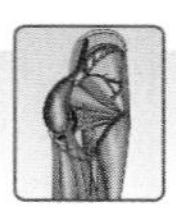

3. The following statement/s is/are true regarding sciatic nerve:
   a. It reaches gluteal region by passing through greater sciatic foramen above the piriformis muscle
   b. All the muscular branches arise from its lateral side
   c. At the back of the thigh it is crossed by semitendinosus
   d. Tibial nerve is its larger terminal branch
4. The common peroneal nerve:
   a. Conveys fibres from the dorsal divisions of ventral rami of L4, L5, S1 and S2
   b. May get injured in the fracture of neck of fibula
   c. Injury leads to foot drop
   d. Injury results in sensory loss on the whole of the dorsum of foot
5. Popliteus muscle:
   a. Has intracapsular origin
   b. Pulls the medial meniscus backwards and prevents it from being trapped at the beginning of flexion
   c. Initiates flexion of knee joint by unlocking the locked knee
   d. Is innervated by a branch from the common peroneal nerve

ANSWERS

A.	1. a – ii,	b – iv,	c – iii,	d – i	2. a – iv,	b – iii,	c – ii,	d – i
	3. a – ii,	b – iii,	c – iv,	d – i	4. a – iv,	b – ii,	c – i,	d – iii
	5. a – iii,	b – iv,	c – ii,	d – i				
B.	1. A	2. E	3. D	4. A	5. B			

FURTHER READING

- Crock HV. An atlas of the arterial supply of the head and neck of femur in man. *Clin orthop* 1980; 152:17–25.
- Eckhoff PG, Kramer RC, Watkins JJ, Alongi CA, Van Gerven DP. Variation in femoral anteversion. *Clin Anat* 1994; 7:72–5.
- Gardner E, Gray DJ. The innervation of the joints of the foot. *Anat Rec* 1968; 161:141–8.
- Gupte CM, Bull AMJ, Thomas RD, Amis AA. A review of the function and biomechanics of the meniscofemoral ligaments. *Arthroscopy* 2003; 19:161–71.
- Jayakumari S, Suri RK, Rath G, Arora S. Accessory tendon and tripartite insertion of pattern of fibularis longus muscle, A case report. *Int J Morphol* 2006; 24: 633–636.
- Joseph J. Movements at the hip joint. *Ann R Coll Surg Eng,* 1975; 56:192–201
- Kakar S, Garg K, Raheja S. Functional anatomy of human foot in relation to dimensions of the sesamoid bones, *Ann Natl Acad Med Sci (India)* 1998; 34 (3): 157–161.
- Neidre A, Macnab I 1983. Anomalies of the lumbosacral nerve roots. *Spine* 8:294–9.
- Raheja S, Choudhry R, Singh P, Tuli A, Kumar H. Morphological description of combined variation of distal attachments of fibulares in a foot. *Surg radiol Anat* 2005; 27: 158–160
- Rajendran K. Mechanism of locking at the knee joint. *J Anat* 1985; 143:189–94.
- Sarrafian SK. *Anatomy of the Foot and Ankle, Descriptive, Topographic, Functional,* 2nd edn. Philadelphia: Lippincott 1993.
- Watanabe M, Takedas S, Ikeuchi H. Atlas of Arthroscopy. Berlin: Springer–Verlag 1979.

Spots on Lower Limb are given on pages 453 and 454

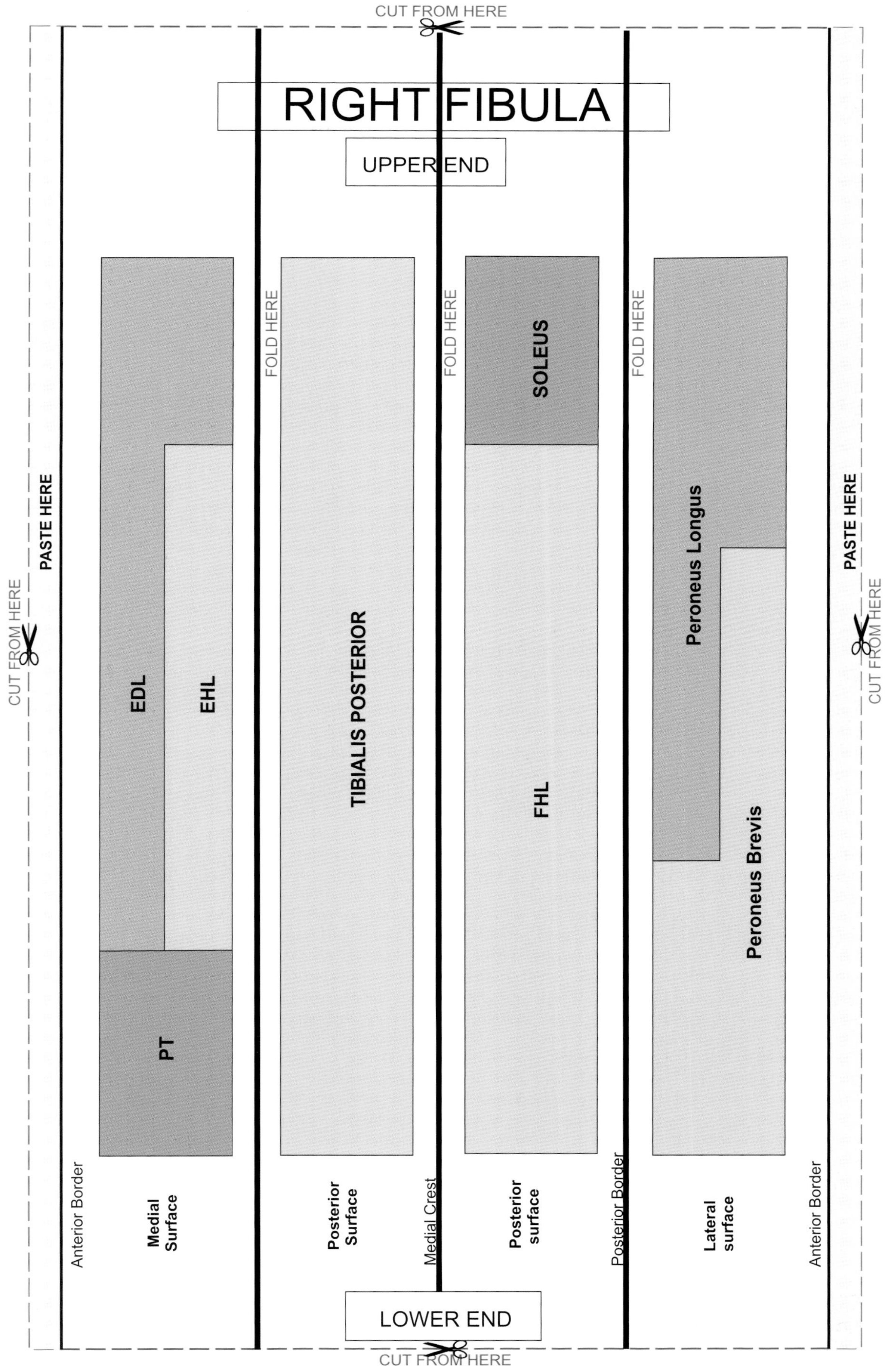

CUT FROM HERE

RIGHT FIBULA

UPPER END

PASTE HERE

CUT FROM HERE

EDL

EHL

PT

FOLD HERE

TIBIALIS POSTERIOR

FOLD HERE

SOLEUS

FHL

FOLD HERE

Peroneus Longus

Peroneus Brevis

PASTE HERE

CUT FROM HERE

Anterior Border

Medial Surface

Posterior Surface

Medial Crest

Posterior surface

Posterior Border

Lateral surface

Anterior Border

LOWER END

CUT FROM HERE

Section 2

Abdomen and Pelvis

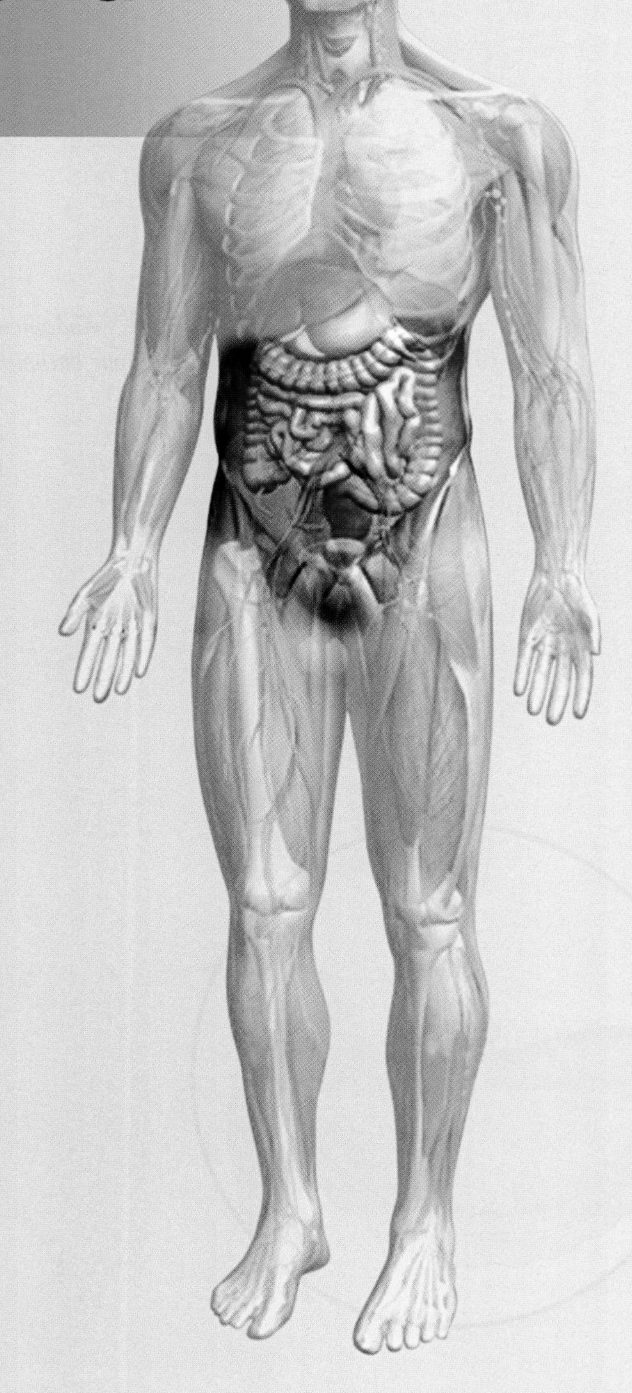

Anatomy Made Easy

Ichchak dana bichchak dana
dane upar dana, ichchak dana
Abdomen mai laita hai pancreas with spleen
Inke upar bathein hain kidney, suprarenal aur colon,
in sabke upar ek organ hai padhara
Usne jaldi se apne bed ko nihara
Poocha, kaisa laga mera aashiyana?
Lao yaar ab to kucch aabu-dana
Ichchak dana
Bolo kya—stomach,
Bolo kya—stomach

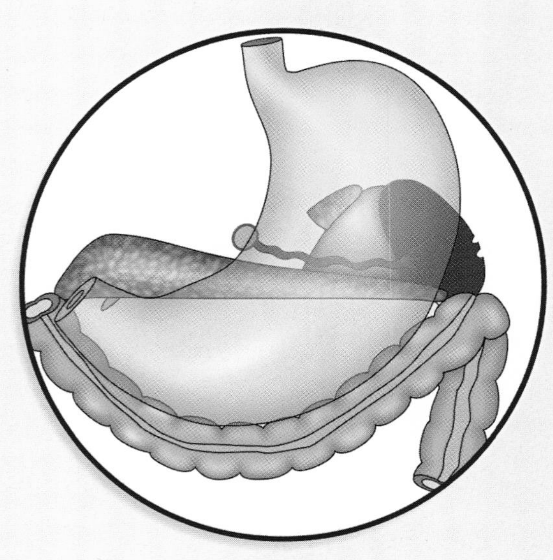

15

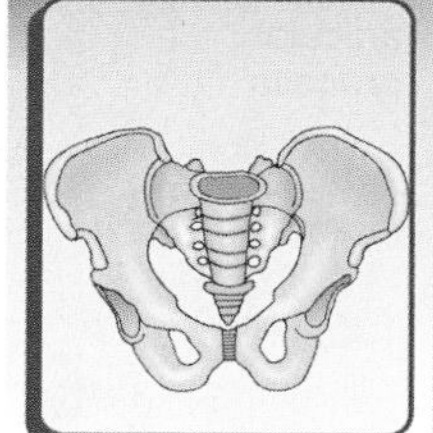

Introduction and Osteology

To know that we know what we know, and that we do not know what we do not know, that is true knowledge
—Confucius

INTRODUCTION TO ABDOMEN

The abdomen is the lower part of the trunk and lies below the diaphragm. It is divided by the plane of the pelvic inlet into a larger upper part, the abdomen proper, and a smaller lower part, the true or lesser pelvis and perineum. The abdomen is bounded to a large extent by muscles, which can easily adjust themselves to periodic changes in the capacity of the abdominal cavity. They can thin out to accommodate distensions of the abdomen imposed by *flatus* or gas, *fat*, *foetus* and *fluid*. The abdomen contains the greater parts of the digestive and urogenital systems. In addition, it also contains the spleen, the suprarenal glands, and numerous lymph nodes, vessels and nerves.

The abdominal wall is made up of the following six layers.

1 *Skin*,
2 *Superficial fascia*,
3 *Muscles* (and bones at places),
4 A continuous layer of fascia, named regionwise as the *diaphragmatic fascia*, *fascia transversalis*; *fascia iliaca*; *anterior layer of thoracolumbar fascia*, and *pelvic fascia*,
5 *Extraperitoneal connective tissue*, and
6 The *peritoneum* which provides a slippery surface for the movements of the abdominal viscera against one another.

The abdominal cavity is much more extensive than what it appears to be when seen from the outside. It projects upwards deep to the costal margin to reach the diaphragm. It also projects downwards as the pelvic cavity within the bony pelvis. Thus a considerable part of the abdominal cavity is overlapped by the thoracic bony cage above, and by the bony pelvis below.

The *importance of the abdomen* is manifold. To a physician, no examination is ever complete until he/she has thoroughly examined and auscultated the abdomen by the stethoscope (Greek *look at breast*) of the patient. In fact, the patient, irrespective of his complaints, is never satisfied without an examination of his/her abdomen. To an obstetrician and gynaecologist, the importance of the abdomen is obvious. The surgeon considers the abdomen as an enigma because in a good proportion of his/her cases, the cause of abdominal pain, or the nature of an abdominal lump, may not be decided in spite of all possible investigations. Laparotomy, i.e. opening up of the abdomen by a surgeon, may reveal the disease in many obscure cases, but not in all of them. In the course of evolution, adoption of the erect posture by man has necessitated a number of structural modifications in the abdominal wall and pelvis, some of which will be mentioned in the appropriate sections.

OSTEOLOGY

The various bones present in relation to the abdomen are the lumbar vertebrae, the sacrum, and the bony pelvis. These are described below. The lower ribs and costal cartilages are also closely related to the abdominal wall. These have already been considered along with the Thorax (Section 2) in Volume 1.

LUMBAR VERTEBRAE

There are five lumbar (Latin *loin*) vertebrae, of which the first four are typical, and the fifth is atypical. A lumbar vertebra is identified by (a) its large size, and (b) the absence of costal facets on the body (c) absence of foramen in transverse process.

Typical Lumbar Vertebra

1 The *body* is large, kidney shaped and is wider from side to side than from before backwards. The height of the body is slightly greater anteriorly than posteriorly; this difference contributes to the forward convexity of the lumbar spine (Figs 15.1a and b).

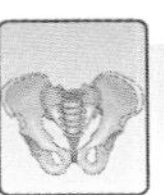

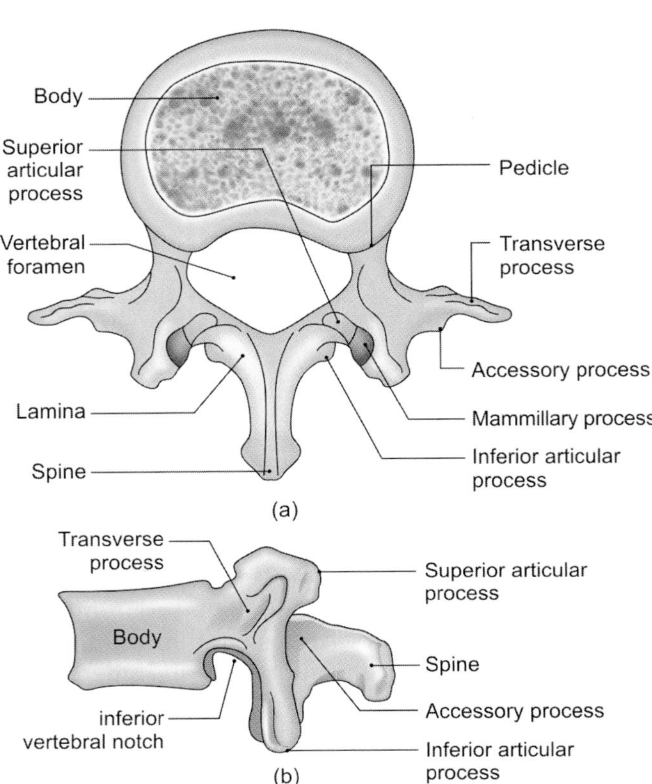

Figs 15.1a and b: Typical lumbar vertebra: (a) Seen from above, and (b) seen from the lateral side

2 The *vertebral foramen* is triangular in shape, and is larger than in the thoracic region; but is smaller than in the cervical region.
3 The *pedicles* are short and strong. They project backwards from the upper part of the body, so that the inferior vertebral notches are much deeper than the superior.
4 The *laminae* are short, thick and broad. They are directed backwards and medially to complete the vertebral foramen posteriorly. The overlapping between the laminae of the adjoining vertebrae is minimal.
5 The *spine* forms a vertical quadrilateral plate, directed almost backwards and only slightly downwards. It is thickened along its posterior and inferior borders.
6 The *transverse processes* are thin and tapering, and are directed laterally and slightly backwards. These develop from the costal element and are homologous with the ribs in the thoracic region. The postero-inferior aspect of the root of each transverse process is marked by a small, rough elevation, the accessory process, which represents the true transverse process of the vertebra as these develop from the transverse element of vertebra. The length of the transverse processes increases from vertebra L1 to L3 and, thereafter, it decreases (Fig. 15.1b).
7 The *superior articular processes* lie farther apart than the inferior. Each process bears a concave facet facing medially and backwards. The posterior border is marked by a rough elevation, the mammillary process.
8 The *inferior articular processes* lie nearer to each other than the superior. Each process bears a convex facet facing laterally and forwards.

Fifth Lumbar Vertebra

1 The most important distinguishing features are as follows.
   a. The *transverse processes* are thick, short and pyramidal in shape. Their base is attached to the whole thickness of the pedicle and encroaches on the side of the body (Fig. 15.2a).
   b. The distance between the *inferior articular processes* is equal to or more than the distance between the superior articular processes.
   c. The *spine* is small, short and rounded at the tip.
2 Other features of the fifth lumbar vertebra are as follows.
   a. The body is the largest of all lumbar vertebrae. Its anterior surface is much extensive than the posterior surface. This difference is responsible for the creation of the sharp lumbosacral angle or sacrovertebral angle and is 120° in an adult.

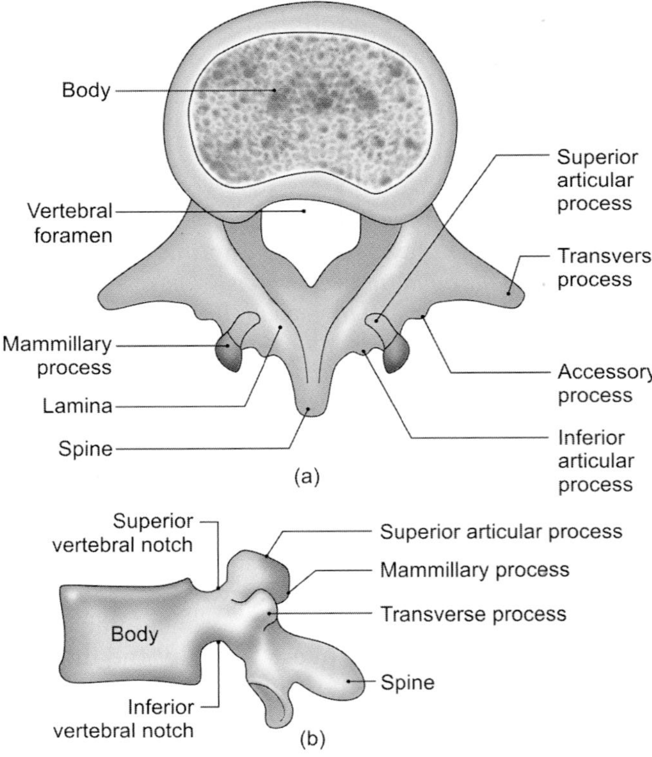

Figs 15.2a and b: Fifth lumbar vertebra: (a) Seen from above, and (b) seen from the lateral side

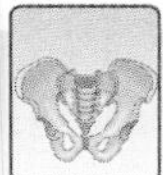

b. The pedicles are directed backwards and laterally.
c. The superior articular facets look more backwards than medially, and the inferior articular facets look more forwards than laterally, as compared to other lumbar vertebrae (Fig. 15.2b).

Attachments and Some Relations of Lumbar Vertebrae

Body

1 The upper and lower surfaces lie in contact with the *intervertebral discs.*
2 The upper and lower borders give attachment to the *anterior* and *posterior longitudinal ligaments* in front and behind, respectively.
3 Lateral to the anterior longitudinal ligament, the *right crus of the diaphragm* is attached to the upper three vertebrae, and the *left crus of the diaphragm* to the upper two vertebrae.
4 Behind the line of the crura, the upper and lower borders of all the lumbar vertebrae give origin to the psoas major (Fig. 15.3).
5 Across the constricted part of the body on either side *tendinous arches are attached. The lumbar vessels, and the grey ramus communicans from the sympathetic chain,* pass deep to each of these arches.

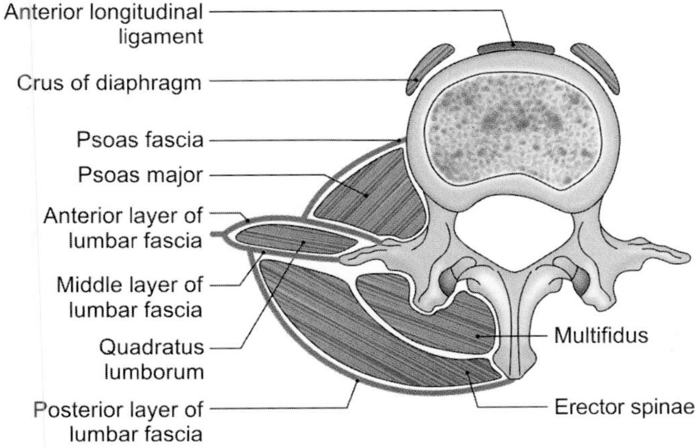

Fig. 15.3: Attachments of the lumbar vertebra

Vertebral Canal

The part of vertebral canal formed by the first lumbar vertebra contains the *conus medullaris*. The part formed by lower four vertebrae contains the *cauda equina*. The canal of all the lumbar vertebrae contains the *spinal meninges*.

Vertebral Arch

The *pedicles* are related above and below to spinal nerves.

The *laminae* provide attachment to the ligamentum flava.

The *spine* provides attachment to:
a. The posterior layer of the lumbar fascia (Fig. 15.3).
b. The interspinous and supraspinous ligaments.
c. The erector spinae, the multifidus and the interspinous muscles (EMI).

Transverse Processes

1 The tips of the transverse processes of all lumbar vertebrae give attachment to the *middle layer* of *the lumbar fascia*. In addition, the tip of the first process gives attachment to the *medial* and *lateral arcuate ligaments*, (*see* Fig. 26.1) and the tip of the fifth process to the *iliolumbar ligament* (*see* Fig. 34.7).
2 The faint vertical ridge on the anterior surface of each transverse process gives attachment to the *anterior layer of the lumbar fascia*. Medial to the ridge, the anterior surface gives origin to the *psoas major*, and lateral to the ridge to the *quadratus lumborum* (Fig. 15.3).
3 The posterior surface is covered by deep muscles of the back, and gives origin to the fibres of the *longissimus thoracis*. The *accessory process* gives attachment to the *medial intertransverse muscle*.
4 The upper and lower borders provide attachment to the *lateral intertransverse muscles*.

Articular Processes

1 The concave articular facets permit some rotation as well as flexion and extension.
2 The *mammillary process* gives attachment to the multifidus and to the *medial intertransverse muscles*.

OSSIFICATION

A lumbar vertebra ossifies from three primary centres—one for the body or centrum and one each for each half of the neural arch. These appear in the *third month of foetal life*. The two halves of the neural arch fuse with each other, posteriorly during the *first year*. Fusion of the neural arch with the centrum occurs during the sixth year. The posterolateral parts of the body develop from the centre for the neural arch.

There are seven secondary centres as follows:
1. An upper annular epiphysis for the upper surface of the body.
2. A similar epiphysis for the lower surface of the body.
3 and 4. One centre for the tip of each transverse process.
5 and 6. One centre for each mammillary process.
7. One centre for the tip of the spine.

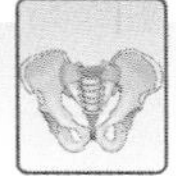

CLINICAL ANATOMY

- The lumbar region is a common site of a number of developmental deformities, causing symptoms ranging from simple backache to serious paralytic manifestations.

Sacralization of the fifth lumbar vertebra

- The *fifth lumbar vertebra* or its transverse process may be fused, on one or both sides, with the sacrum. Sometimes the transverse process may articulate with the ala of the sacrum or with the ilium. This may press on the fifth lumbar nerve.

  Sometimes the body ossifies from two primary centres, and if one centre fails to develop, it results in a *"hemivertebra"*.

Spina bifida

- The two halves of the neural arch may fail to fuse leaving a gap in the midline. This is called *spina bifida*. Meninges and spinal cord may herniate out through the gap.
- Protrusion of meninges alone results in the formation of a cystic swelling filled with cerebrospinal fluid. This swelling is called *meningocoele* (Fig. 15.4a). When the spinal cord is also present in the swelling the condition is called *meningomyelocoele* (Fig. 15.4b). The central canal of the herniated part of the cord may be dilated. This condition is called syringomyelocoele. At times the spinal cord may itself be open posteriorly. The condition is then called *myelocoele*. Sometimes a spina bifida is present, but there is no protrusion through it so that there is no swelling on the surface. This is referred to as *spina bifida occulta*.

Spondylolisthesis

- Sometimes the greater part of the fifth lumbar vertebra slips forwards over the sacrum. Normally the tendency to forward slipping is prevented by the fact that the inferior articular processes of the fifth lumbar vertebra lie behind the superior articular processes of the first sacral vertebra. At times, however, the inferior articular processes, spine and laminae of the fifth lumbar vertebra are separate from the rest of the vertebra (due to an anomaly in the mode of ossification). The body of the vertebra can now slip forwards leaving the separated parts behind (Fig. 15.5).
- Spondylolisthesis may be the cause of backache and of pain radiating along the course of the sciatic nerve known as *sciatica*.

Fracture-dislocation

- Fracture-dislocation of lumbar vertebrae results in the *cauda equina syndrome* (Fig. 15.6). It is characterized by:
  a. Flaccid paraplegia.
  b. Saddle-shaped area of anaesthesia, and analgesia.
  c. Sphincter disturbances in the form of incontinence of urine and faeces.
  d. Impotence.
- In the young adults, the discs are very strong and cannot be damaged alone. However, after the second decade, degenerative changes set in resulting in necrosis, with sequestration of nucleus pulposus, and softening and weakness of the annulus fibrosus. Such a disc is liable to internal or eccentric displacement or external derangements resulting in prolapse due to rupture of annulus fibrosus even after minor strains.
- Cauda equina syndrome described above.
- The unequal tension in the joint in internal derangement leads to muscle spasm and violent pain of acute lumbago.
- Disc prolapse is usually posterolateral (Fig. 15.7). This presses upon the adjacent nerve roots and gives rise to referred pain, such as sciatica. Disc prolapse occurs most commonly in lower lumbar region and is also common in lower cervical region (C5–C7). In sciatica, the pain is increased with rise of pressure in canal (as in sneezing); straight leg raising tests is positive; and the motor effects, with loss of power and reflexes, may follow.
- The spine of thoracic vertebrae may point to one side. The condition is scoliosis (Fig. 15.8).
- There may be projection of the spines posteriorly due to osteoporosis of the bodies of vertebrae leading to *kyphosis* (Fig. 15.9).
- Anterior convexity of lumbar vertebrae may get exaggerated, leading to *"lumbar lordosis"* (Fig. 15.10).

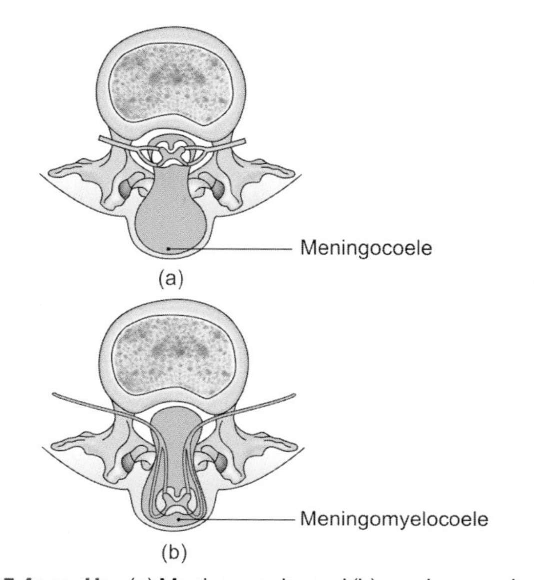

Figs 15.4a and b: (a) Meningocoele, and (b) meningomyelocoele

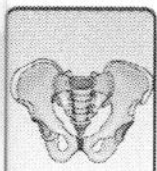

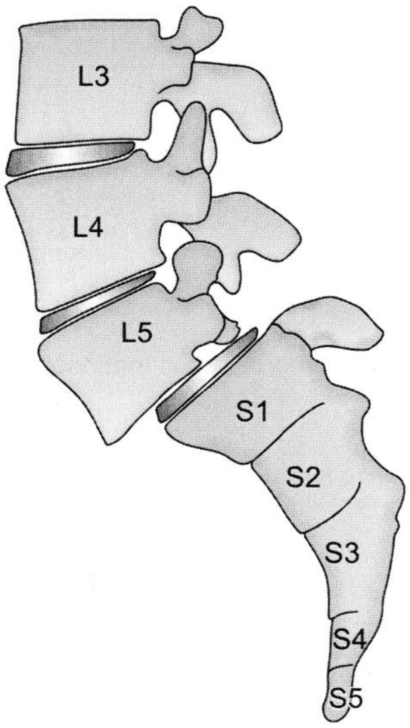

Fig. 15.5: Spondylolisthesis of fifth lumbar vertebra

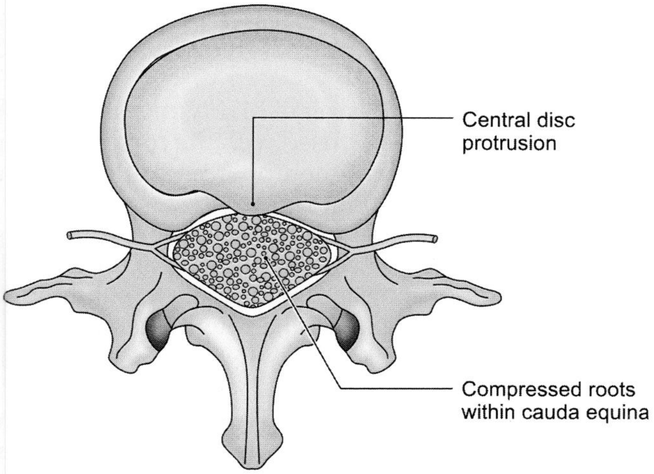

Fig. 15.6: Cauda equina syndrome

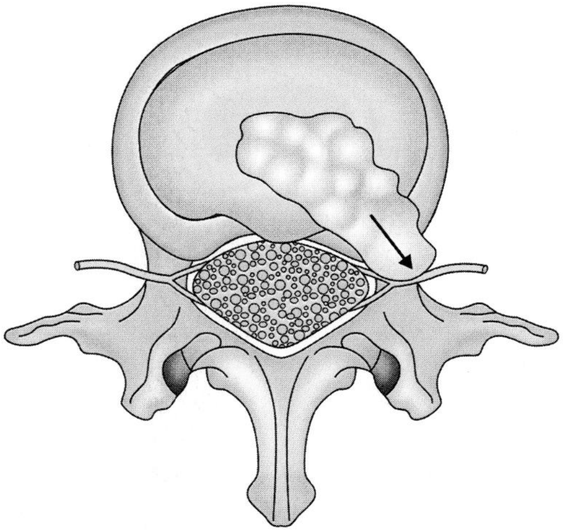

Fig. 15.7: Posterolateral disc prolapse

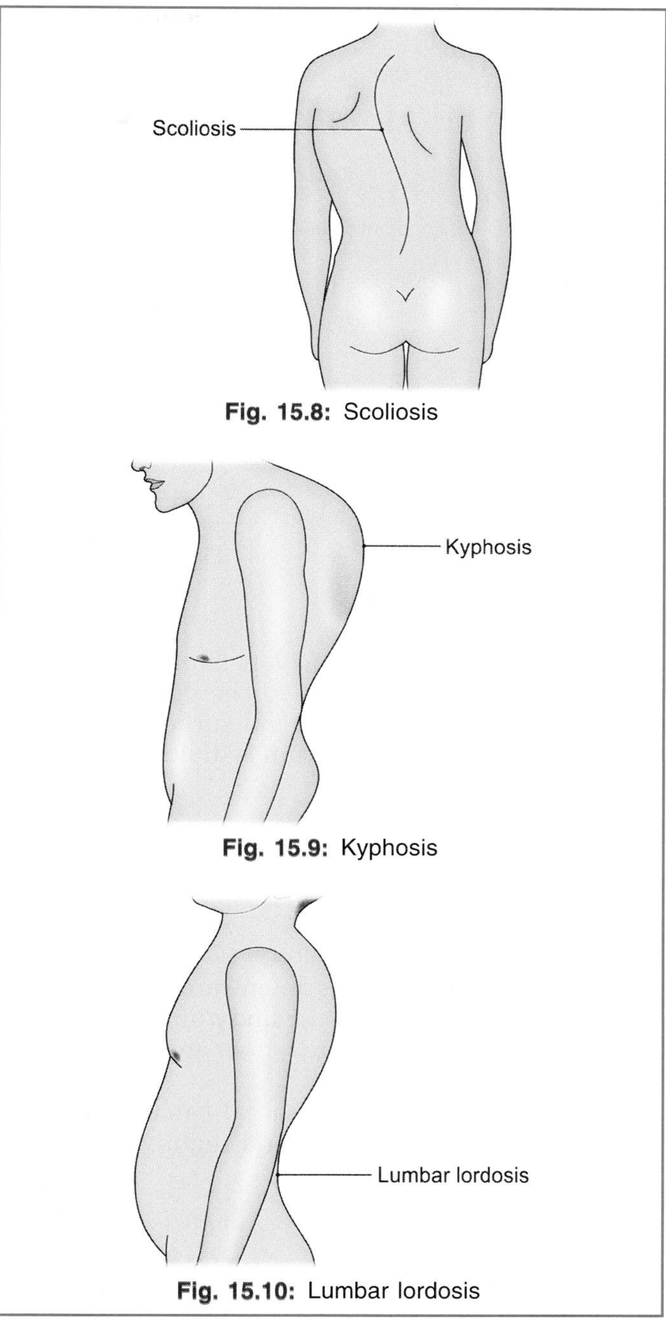

Fig. 15.8: Scoliosis

Fig. 15.9: Kyphosis

Fig. 15.10: Lumbar lordosis

THE SACRUM/VERTEBRA MAGNUM

The sacrum (Latin *sacred*) is a large, flattened, triangular bone formed by the fusion of five sacral vertebrae. It forms the posterosuperior part of the bony pelvis, articulating on either side with the corresponding hip bone at the sacroiliac joint. The upper part of the sacrum is massive because it supports the body weight and transmits it to the hip bones. The lower part is free from weight, and therefore tapers rapidly (Fig. 15.11).

Being triangular, the sacrum has a base or upper surface, an apex or lower end, and four surfaces—

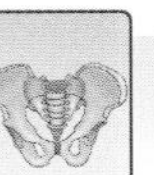

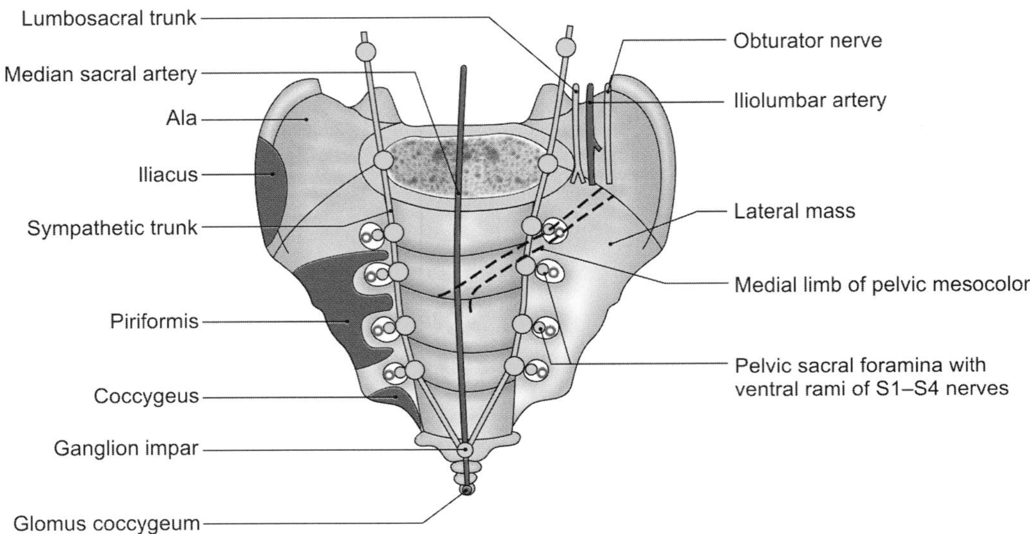

Fig. 15.11: Anterior (pelvic) view of the sacrum

pelvic, dorsal and right and left lateral. The pelvic surface is smooth and concave. The dorsal surface is irregular and convex. The lateral surface is irregular and partly articular. The sacrum is divided by rows of foramina into:

a. Median portion, traversed by the sacral canal.
b. A pair of *lateral masses* formed by fusion of the transverse processes posteriorly, and of the costal elements anteriorly.

When placed in the anatomical position:

a. The pelvic surface faces downwards and forwards.
b. The upper surface of the body of the first sacral vertebra slopes forwards at an angle of about 30 degrees.
c. The upper end of the sacral canal is directed almost directly upwards and slightly backwards.

Features

Base

The base is directed upwards and forwards. It is formed by the upper surface of the first sacral vertebra, and presents features of a typical vertebra in a modified form.

1 The body is lumbar in type. It articulates with vertebra L5 at the *lumbosacral joint*. The projecting anterior margin is called the *sacral promontory*. The surface slopes forwards at an angle of 30 degrees.
2 The vertebral foramen lies behind the body, and leads into the sacral canal. It is triangular in shape.
3 The pedicles are short and are directed backwards and laterally.
4 The laminae are oblique.
5 The spine forms the first spinous tubercle.
6 The superior articular processes project upwards. The facets on them are directed backwards and medially.
7 The transverse processes are highly modified. Each process is massive and fused with the corresponding costal element to form the upper part of the lateral mass of the sacrum (Fig. 15.11).

The base of the lateral mass, forms a broad sloping surface spreading fan wise from the side of the body. It is called the *ala* of the sacrum. The ala is subdivided into a smooth medial part and a rough lateral part.

Apex

The apex of the sacrum is formed by the inferior surface of the body of the fifth sacral vertebra. It bears an oval facet for articulation with the coccyx.

Pelvic Surface

This is concave and directed downwards and forwards. The median area is marked by four transverse ridges, which indicate the lines of fusion of the bodies of the five sacral vertebrae. These ridges end on either side at the *four pelvic sacral foramina*, which communicate with the sacral canal through the *intervertebral foramina*. The bony bars between the foramina represent the *costal elements*. Lateral to the foramina, the *costal elements* unite with each other and with the transverse processes to form the lateral mass of the sacrum (Fig. 15.11).

Dorsal Surface

The dorsal surface of the sacrum is rough, irregular and convex, and is directed backwards and upwards.

1 In the median plane, it is marked by the *median sacral crest* which bears 3 to 4 spinous tubercles, representing

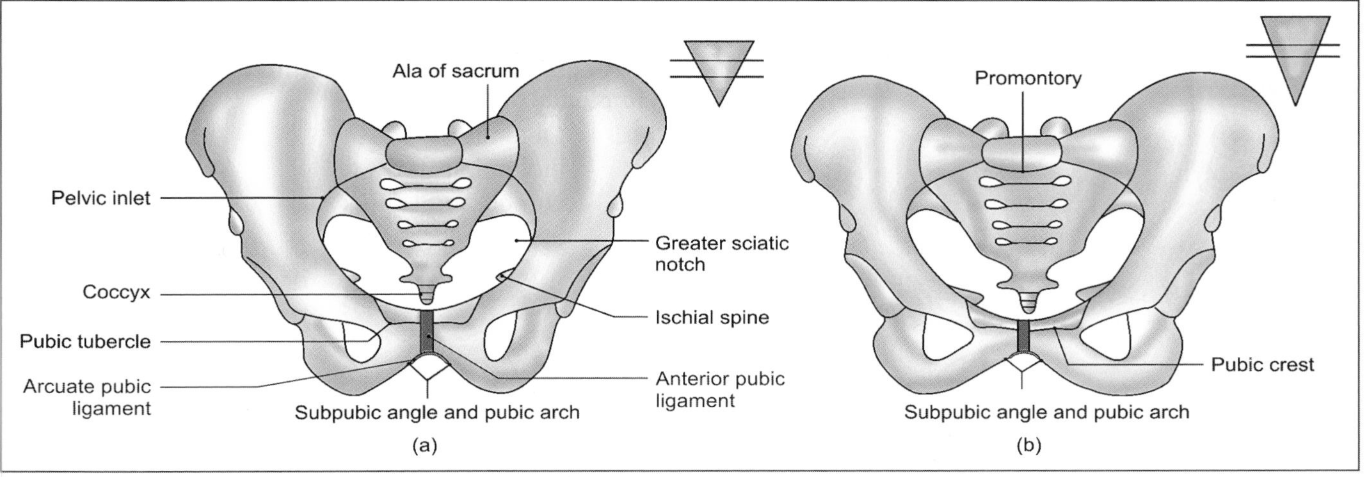

Figs 15.14a and b: Anterior view of (a) a male pelvis, and (b) a female pelvis

Anatomical Position of the Pelvis

When examining an isolated pelvis students generally do not orientate it as it is in the intact body. It can be correctly orientated keeping the following in mind.

In the anatomical position, i.e. with the person standing upright:

1 The anterior superior iliac spines and the pubic symphysis lie in the same vertical plane. A pelvis can be correctly oriented by placing these points against a wall.
2 The pelvic surface of the pubic symphysis faces backwards and upwards.
3 The plane of the pelvic inlet faces forwards and upwards at an angle of 50° to 60° with the horizontal.
4 The plane of the pelvic outlet makes an angle of 15° with the horizontal (*see* Fig. 29.6).
5 The upper end of the sacral canal is directed almost directly upwards.

INTERVERTEBRAL JOINTS

These joints include:

1 The joints between vertebral bodies.
2 The joints between vertebral arches.

The joints between vertebral bodies are *secondary cartilaginous* joints held by the intervertebral discs and two accessory ligaments, the anterior and posterior longitudinal ligaments. Intervertebral disc is described below.

Joints of the vertebral arches are formed by the articular processes of the adjacent vertebrae. These are plane synovial joints, permitting gliding movements. The accessory ligaments include:

a. Ligamenta flava,
b. Supraspinous,
c. Interspinous, and
d. Intertransverse ligaments.

The lumbar spine permits maximum of extension, considerable amount of flexion and lateral flexion, and least of rotation.

Intervertebral Disc

It is a fibrocartilaginous disc which binds the two adjacent vertebral bodies, from axis or second cervical vertebra to sacrum. Morphologically, it is a segmental structure as opposed to the vertebral body which is intersegmental (Figs 15.15a to c).

Shape

Its shape corresponds to that of the vertebral bodies between which it is placed.

Thickness

It varies in different regions of the column and in different parts of the same disc. In cervical and *lumbar* regions, the *discs* are *thicker in front* than behind, while in the thoracic region they are of uniform thickness. The discs are thinnest in the upper thoracic and thickest in the lumbar region.

The discs contribute about one-fifth of the length of vertebral column. Such contribution is greater in cervical and lumbar regions than in thoracic region.

Structure

Each disc is made up of the following three parts.

1 *Nucleus pulposus* is the central part of the disc which is soft and gelatinous at birth. Its water content is 90% in newborn and 70% in old age. It is kept under tension and acts as a hydraulic shock-absorber. It represents the remains of the notochord, and contains a few multinucleated notochordal cells during the first decade of life, after which there is a gradual replacement of the mucoid material by fibrocartilage, derived mainly from the cells of annulus fibrosus and partly from the cartilaginous

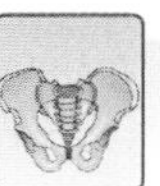

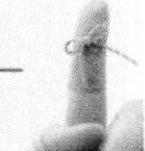

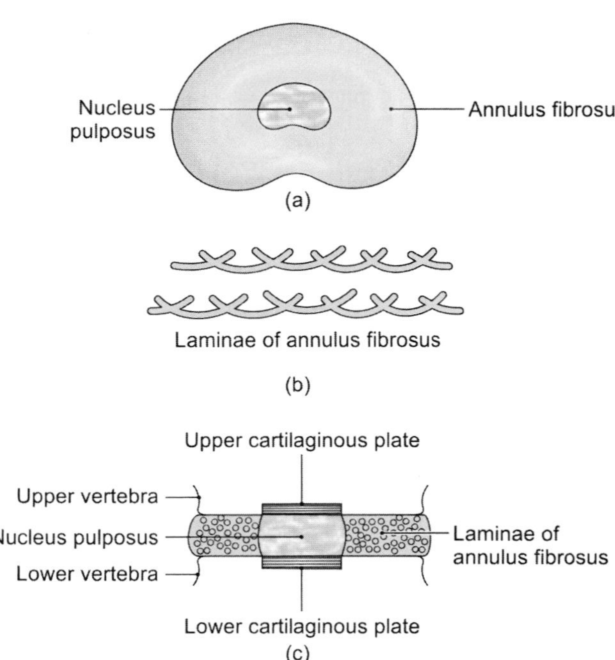

Figs 15.15a to c: The structure of an intervertebral disc: (a) Superior view showing its relations to the nerve roots and the longitudinal ligaments of vertebral column, (b) arrangement of laminae in the annulus fibrosus, and (c) a vertical section showing three parts of the disc

plates covering the upper and lower surfaces of the vertebrae. Thus with advancing age the disc becomes amorphous and difficult to differentiate from the annulus. Its water binding capacity and the elasticity are reduced.

2 *Annulus fibrosus* is the peripheral part of the disc made up of a narrower outer zone of collagenous fibres and a wider inner zone of fibrocartilage. The laminae form incomplete collars which are convex downwards and are connected by strong fibrous bands. They overlap or dovetail into one another at obtuse angles. The outer collagenous fibres blend with anterior and posterior longitudinal ligaments (Figs 15.15a to c).

3 *Two cartilaginous plates* lie one above and the other below the nucleus pulposus. Disc gains its nourishment from the vertebrae by diffusion through these plates (Figs 15.15a to c).

Functions

1 Intervertebral discs give shape to the vertebral column.

2 They act as a remarkable series of shock-absorbers or buffers. Each disc may be likened to a "coiled up spring". Should the confining walls be damaged the spring will bulge out at the weak area.

Mnemonics

Structures on the ala of sacrum from lateral to medial side OILS

- **O** – Obturator nerve
- **I** – Iliolumbar artery
- **L** – Lumbosacral trunk
- **S** – Sympathetic chain

FACTS TO REMEMBER

- Abdominal viscera occupy part of thoracic cavity and part of pelvic cavity. Abdominal cavity is the biggest cavity of the body.
- Transverse diameter is biggest at inlet of true pelvis. All the three diameters anteroposterior transverse and oblique are equal in pelvic cavity.
- Anteroposterior diameter is the biggest at the outlet of true pelvis.
- Subpubic angle is wider, i.e. 80°–85° in female while it is only 50°–60° in a male. Fifth lumbar vertebra is the largest and is atypical.
- Sacrum on its dorsal surface shows 5 crests. One median, two medial and two lateral. Median is formed by fusion of sacral spines. Medial ones are formed by fusion of articular processes and lateral ones by fusion of transverse processes.
- Abdominal cavity continues in downwards and backward direction with the pelvic cavity.
- Herniation of nucleus pulposus of the intervertebral disc is common in lumbar region. It presses upon the nerve roots causing severe pain in the area of cutaneous supply.
- Coccyx is a tail bone.

CLINICOANATOMICAL PROBLEM

A patient complained of chronic dull low backache. One day during sudden bending he developed radiating pain in the calf

- Give the reason for low backache.
- What triggered the radiating pain in the calf?

Ans: The low backache is likely due to "slipped intervertebral disc" in the lumbosacral region. The slip disc is mild in the beginning, so the pain is dull. During sudden bending and straightening the disc got herniated posterolaterally narrowing the intervertebral foramen between L5 and S1 vertebra, compressing one of the root of the sciatic nerve. This gives rise to shooting pain in the area of skin supplied by that root.

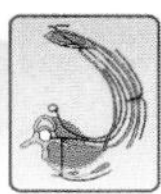

hernia may develop. *Infraumbilical median incisions* are safer because the close approximation of recti prevents formation of any ventral hernia. *Paramedian incisions* through the rectus sheath are more sound than median incisions. The rectus muscle is *retracted laterally* to protect the nerves supplying it from any injury. In these cases, the subsequent risk of weakness and of incisional or ventral hernia are minimal (Fig. 16.19).

- The nerves of anterior abdominal wall, T7–T12 and L1 supply skin, intercostal muscles and parietal pleura . In addition these supply skin, muscles of the abdominal wall and parietal peritoneum. Tubercular infection of lung and pleura may cause radiating pain in the abdominal wall. Peritonitis causes reflex contraction of the abdominal muscles.
- During repair of the wounds of anterior abdominal wall, the nerves T7–T12 need to be anaesthesised along the costal margin. Iliohypogastric and ilioinguinal nerves are anaesthesised by a needle above the anterior superior iliac spine on the spinoumbilical line.

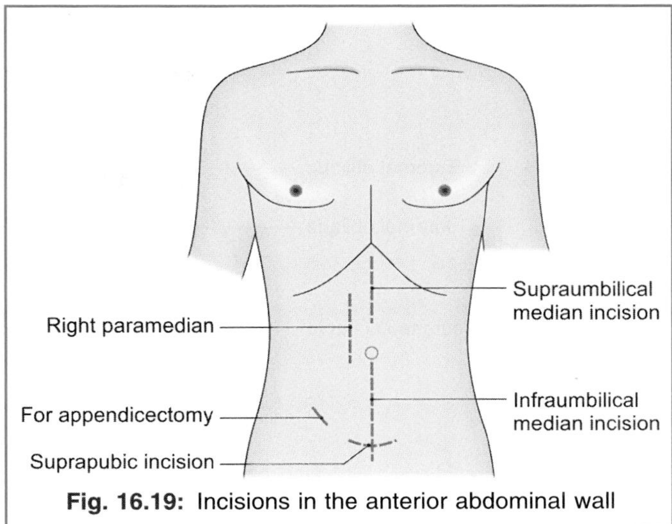

Fig. 16.19: Incisions in the anterior abdominal wall

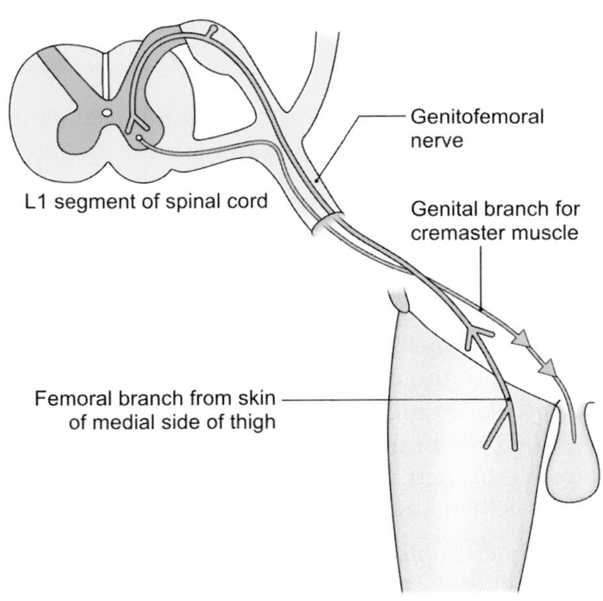

Fig. 16.18: Cremasteric reflex

PYRAMIDALIS

This is a small triangular muscle. It is rudimentary in human beings. It arises from the anterior surface of the body of the pubis. Its fibres pass upwards and medially to be inserted into the linea alba.

The muscle is supplied by the subcostal nerve (T12). It is said to be tensor of the linea alba, but the need for such action is not clear.

DEEP NERVES OF THE ANTERIOR ABDOMINAL WALL

The anterior abdominal wall is supplied by the lower six thoracic nerves or lower five intercostal, and subcostal; and by the first lumbar nerve through its iliohypogastric and ilioinguinal branches. These are the nerves which emerge as cutaneous nerves. Their deep course is described briefly with the cutaneous nerves in the beginning of this chapter (Figs 16.9 and 16.20).

DEEP ARTERIES OF ANTERIOR ABDOMINAL WALL

The anterior abdominal wall is supplied by:

1. Two large arteries from above, the *superior epigastric* and *musculophrenic* (Fig. 16.10).
2. Two large arteries from below, the *inferior epigastric* and the *deep circumflex iliac.*
3. Small branches of the intercostal, subcostal and lumbar arteries, which accompany the corresponding nerves (Fig. 16.21).

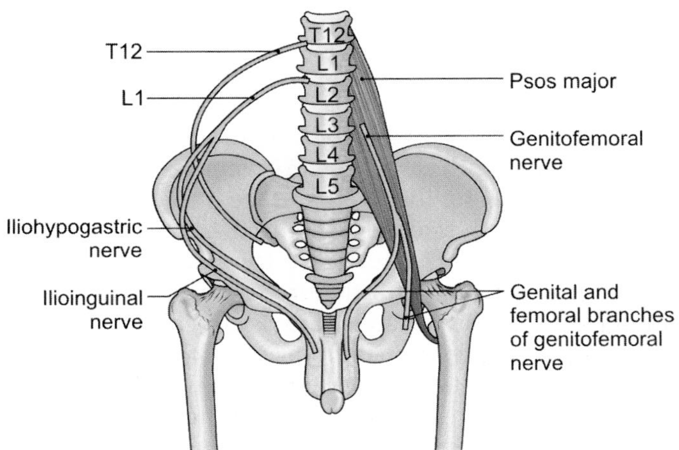

Fig. 16.20: Nerves of anterior abdominal wall

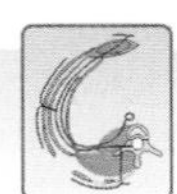

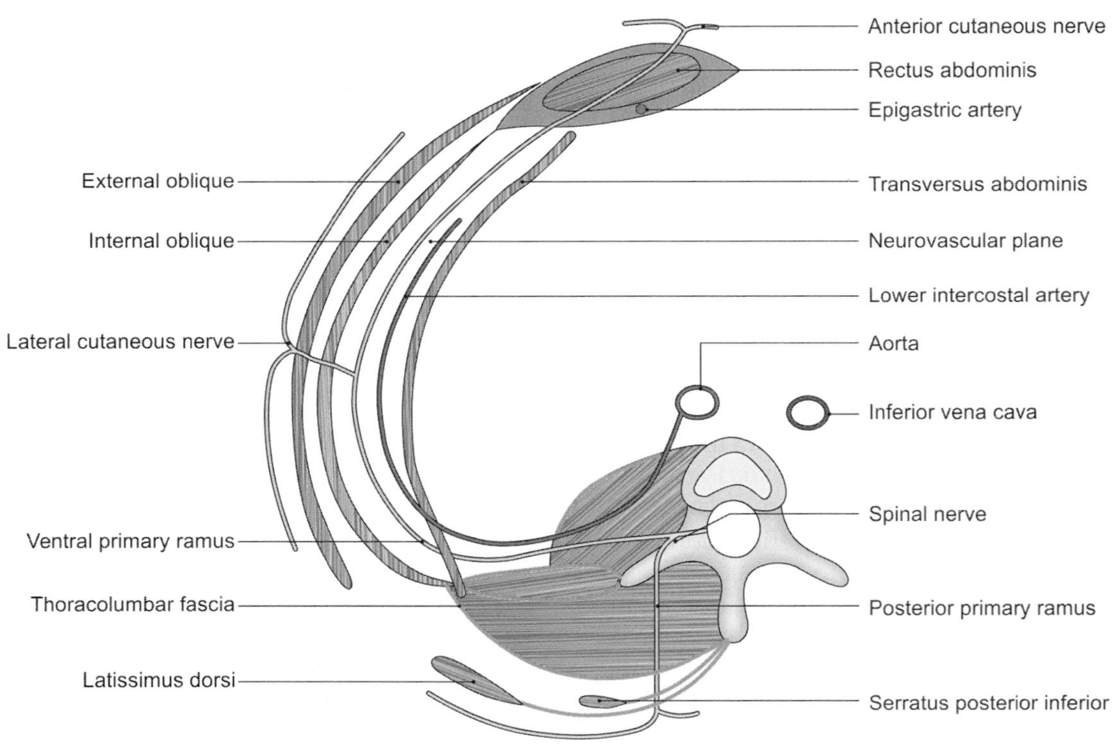

Fig. 16.21: A transverse section through the lumbar region showing the arrangement of the abdominal muscles and the neurovascular plane

The *superior epigastric artery* is one of the two terminal branches of the internal thoracic artery. It begins in the sixth intercostal space, and enters the abdomen by passing behind the seventh costal cartilage between the costal and xiphoid origins of the diaphragm. It enters the rectus sheath and runs vertically downwards, supplies the rectus muscle, and ends by anastomosing with the inferior epigastric artery. In addition to muscular and cutaneous branches, it gives a *hepatic branch* which runs in the *falciform ligament*, and an anastomotic branch, at the level of the xiphoid process, which anastomoses with the artery of the opposite side.

The *musculophrenic artery* is the other terminal branch of the internal thoracic artery. It runs downwards and laterally behind the seventh costal cartilage, and enters the abdomen by piercing the diaphragm between the seventh and eighth cartilages. It continues downwards and laterally along the deep surface of the diaphragm as far as the tenth intercostal space. It gives branches to the diaphragm, the anterior abdominal wall and the seventh, eighth and ninth intercostal spaces as the anterior intercostal arteries (Fig. 16.10).

The *inferior epigastric artery* arises from the external iliac artery near its lower end just above the inguinal ligament. It runs upwards and medially in the extraperitoneal connective tissue, passes just medial to the deep inguinal ring, pierces the fascia transversalis at the lateral border of the rectus abdominis and enters the rectus sheath by passing in front of the arcuate line (Fig. 16.10). Within the sheath it supplies the rectus muscle and ends by anastomosing with the superior epigastric artery. It gives off the following branches.

a. A *cremasteric branch* to the spermatic cord, in males or the artery of the round ligament in females.
b. A *pubic branch* which anastomoses with the pubic branch of the obturator artery.
c. *Muscular* branches to the rectus abdominis.
d. *Cutaneous* branches to the overlying skin. The pubic branch may replace the obturator artery, and is then known as the *abnormal obturator artery*.

The *deep circumflex iliac artery* is the other branch of the external iliac artery, given off from its lateral side opposite the origin of the inferior epigastric artery. It runs laterally and upwards behind the inguinal ligament, pierces the fascia transversalis, and continues along the iliac crest, up to its middle where it pierces the transversus abdominis to enter the interval between the transversus and the internal oblique muscles. At the anterior superior iliac spine it anastomoses with the superior gluteal, the lateral circumflex femoral and superficial circumflex iliac arteries. Just behind the anterior superior iliac spine it gives off an ascending branch which runs upwards in the neurovascular plane.

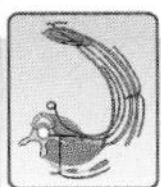

RECTUS SHEATH

DISSECTION

Identify the rectus abdominis muscle. At the lateral edge of the rectus abdominis, the aponeurosis of the internal oblique splits to pass partly posterior and partly anterior to the rectus abdominis; the anterior layer fusing with the aponeurosis of external oblique and the posterior layer with that of the transversus abdominis. This is how most of the rectus sheath is formed. Identify the arcuate line midway between umbilicus and pubic symphysis.

Define the origins of the transversus and follow its aponeurosis to fuse with that of the internal oblique, posterior to the rectus abdominis above the arcuate line and anteriorly to the unsplit aponeurosis of internal oblique below the line. See that aponeurosis of all three muscles pass anterior to rectus abdominis below the arcuate line.

Open the rectus sheath by a vertical incision along the middle of the muscle. Reflect the anterior layer of the sheath side ways, cutting its attachments to the tendinous intersections in the anterior part of the rectus muscle (Fig. 16.15).

Lift the rectus muscle and identify the 7–11 intercostal and subcostal nerves entering the sheath through its posterior lamina, piercing the muscle and leaving through its anterior wall.

Divide the rectus abdominis transversely at its middle. Identify its attachments and expose the posterior wall of the rectus sheath by reflecting its parts superiorly and inferiorly. Identify and trace the superior and inferior epigastric arteries.

Define the arcuate line on the posterior wall of the rectus sheath.

RECTUS SHEATH

Definition

This is an aponeurotic sheath covering the rectus abdominis. It has two walls, anterior and posterior.

Features

Anterior Wall

1 It is complete, covering the muscle from end to end.
2 Its composition is variable as described below.
3 It is firmly adherent to the tendinous intersections of the rectus muscle (Fig. 16.22).

Posterior Wall

1 It is incomplete, being deficient above the costal margin and below the arcuate line.
2 Its composition is variable as described below.
3 It is free from the rectus muscle (Fig. 16.19).

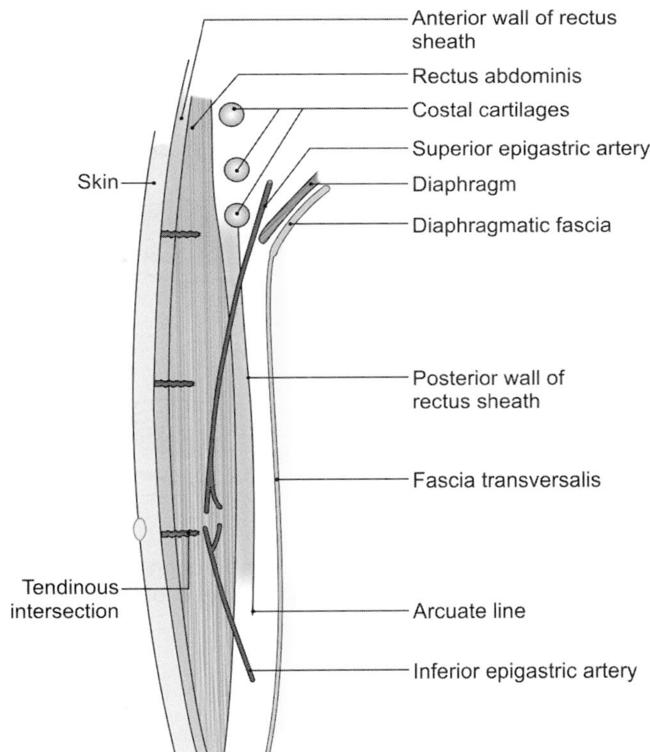

Fig. 16.22: Sagittal section through the rectus sheath

Medial Wall

Fusion of all the aponeuroses in the midline. It is called as linea alba.

Lateral Wall

It is called linea semilunaris, it extends from tip of 9th costal cartilage to pubic tubercle.

Formation

Details about the formation of the walls are as follows (Figs 16.23a and b).

Above the costal margin

Anterior wall: External oblique aponeurosis (Fig. 16.23a).

Posterior wall: It is deficient; the rectus muscle rests directly on the 5th, 6th and 7th costal cartilages.

Between the costal margin and the arcuate line

Anterior wall: External oblique aponeurosis and anterior lamina of the aponeurosis of the internal oblique.

Posterior wall: Posterior lamina of the aponeurosis of the internal oblique and aponeurosis of the transversus muscle (Fig. 16.23b).

Midway between the umbilicus and the pubic symphysis, the posterior wall of the rectus sheath ends in the arcuate line or *linea semicircularis* or *fold of Douglas*. The line is concave downwards.

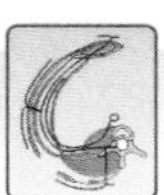

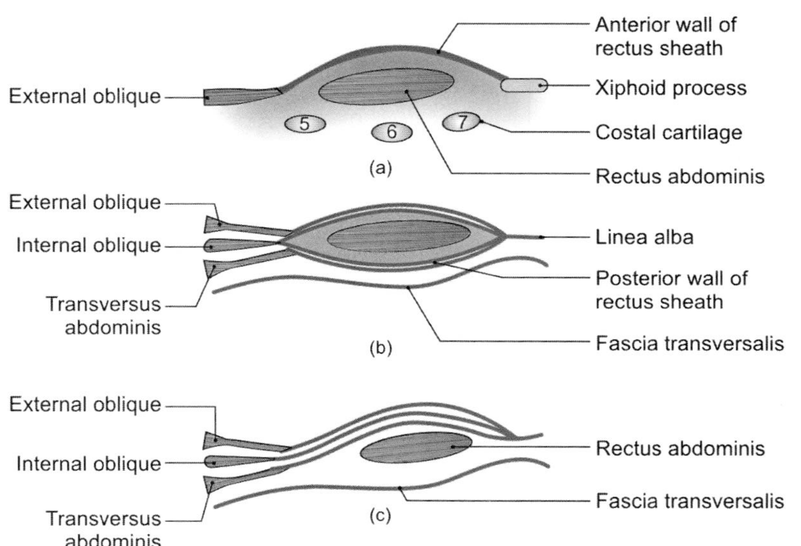

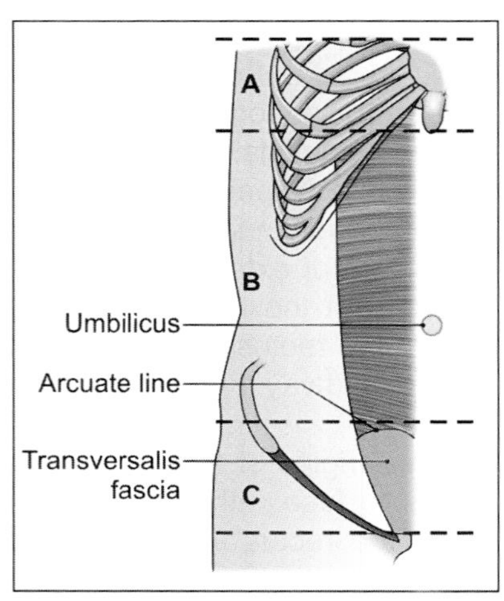

Figs 16.23a to c: Transverse sections through the rectus abdominis, and its sheath: (a) Above the costal margin, A of inset, (b) between costal margin and arcuate line, B of inset and (c) below arcuate line, C of inset

Below the arcuate line

Anterior wall: Aponeuroses of all the three flat muscles of the abdomen. The aponeuroses of the transversus and the internal oblique are fused, but the external oblique aponeurosis remains separate (Fig. 16.23c).

Posterior wall: It is deficient. The rectus muscle rests on the fascia transversalis.

Contents

Muscles

1 The *rectus abdominis* is the chief and largest content.
2 The *pyramidalis (if present)* lies in front of the lower part of the rectus abdominis.

Arteries

1 The *superior epigastric artery* enters the sheath by passing between the costal and xiphoid origins of the diaphragm. It crosses the upper border of the transversus abdominis behind the seventh costal cartilage. It supplies the rectus abdominis muscle and anastomoses with the inferior epigastric artery (Fig. 16.22).
2 The *inferior epigastric artery* enters the sheath by passing in front of the arcuate line.

Veins

1 The *superior epigastric vena comitantes* accompany its artery and join the vena comitantes of internal thoracic vein.
2 The *inferior epigastric vena comitantes* accompany its artery and join the external iliac vein.

Nerves

These are the terminal parts of the lower six thoracic nerves, including the *lower five intercostal nerves* and the *subcostal nerves* (Fig. 16.21).

Functions

1 It checks bowing of rectus muscle during its contraction and thus increases the efficiency of the muscle.
2 It maintains the strength of the anterior abdominal wall.

NEW CONCEPT OF RECTUS SHEATH

Rectus sheath is formed by decussating fibres from three abdominal muscles of each side. Each forms a bilaminar aponeurosis at their medial borders. Fibres from all three anterior leaves run obliquely upwards, while the posterior fibers run obliquely downwards at right angles to anterior leaves.

Anterior Sheath of Rectus

Both leaves of external oblique aponeurosis and anterior leaf of internal oblique aponeurosis.

Posterior Sheath

Posterior leaf of aponeurosis of internal oblique and both leaves of aponeurosis of transversus abdominis.

Fibres of each layer decussate to the opposite side of the sheath. Fibres also decussate between anterior and posterior sheaths.

The three lateral abdominal muscles may be said to be digastric with a central tendon in the form of linea alba.

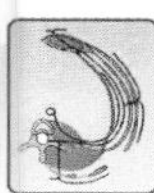

Coverings of medial direct inguinal hernia:

i. Extraperitoneal tissue
ii. Fascia transversalis
iii. Conjoint tendon
iv. External spermatic fascia
v. Skin

Epigastric hernia: It occurs through the upper part of wide linea alba (Fig. 16.36).

Divarication of recti: Occurs in multiparous female with weak anterolateral abdominal muscles. Loop of intestine protrude during coughing, but returns back (Fig. 16.36).

Incisional hernia: Occurs through the anterolateral abdominal wall when some incisions were made for the surgery, involving cutting of the spinal nerves.

Lumbar hernia: Occurs through the lumbar triangle in the posterior part of the abdominal wall. It is bounded by the iliac crest, anterior border of latissimus dorsi and posterior border of external oblique muscle.

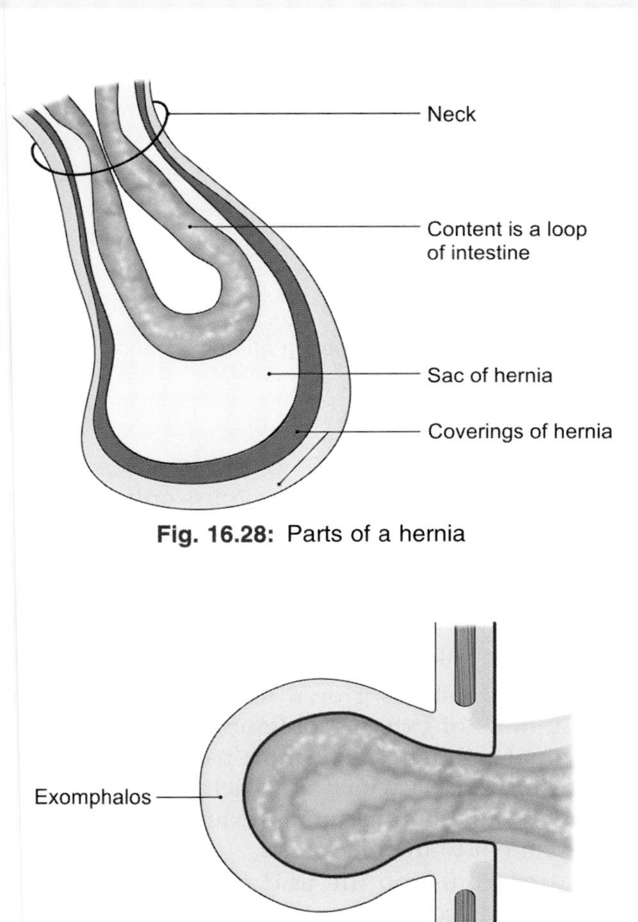

Fig. 16.28: Parts of a hernia

Exophalos figure:

Fig. 16.29: Exomphalos

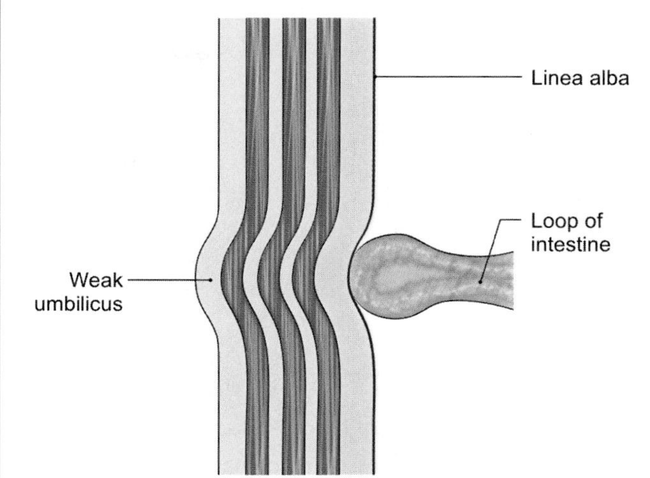

Fig. 16.30: Infantile umbilical hernia

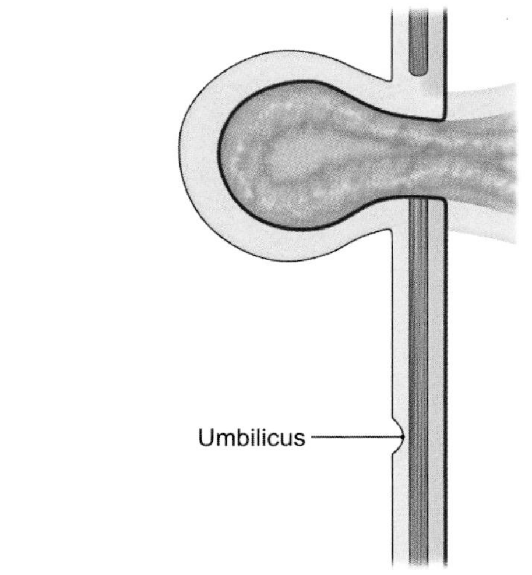

Fig. 16.31: Paraumbilical hernia

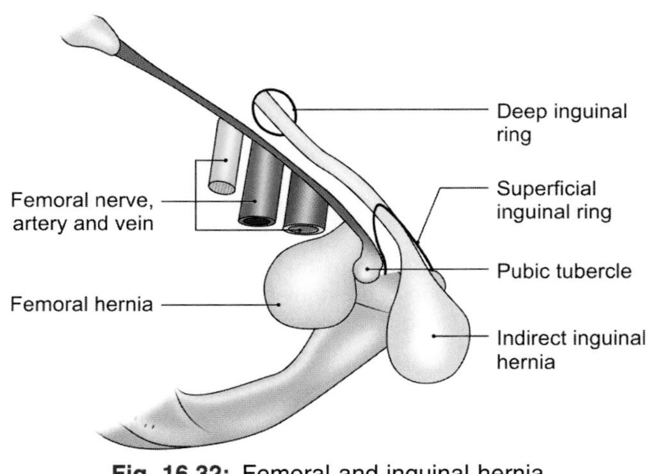

Fig. 16.32: Femoral and inguinal hernia

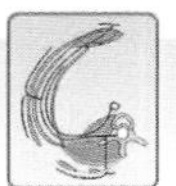

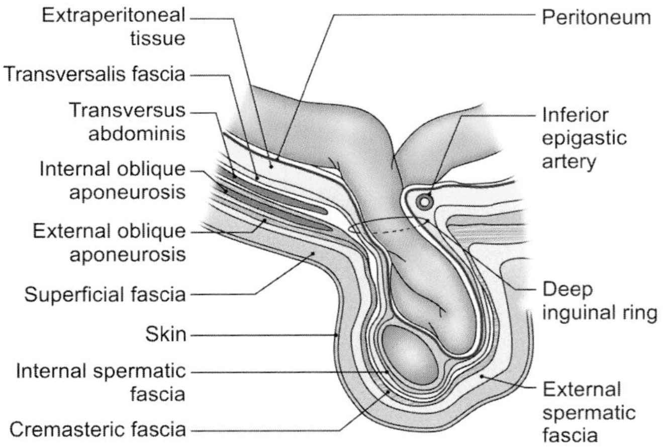

Fig. 16.33: Indirect inguinal hernia

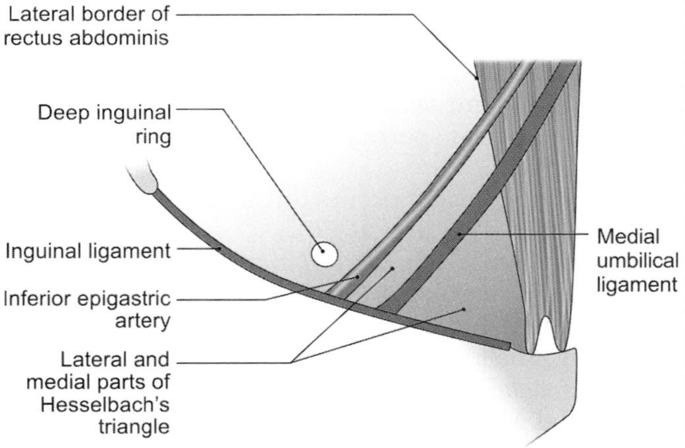

Fig. 16.34: Hesselbach's triangle

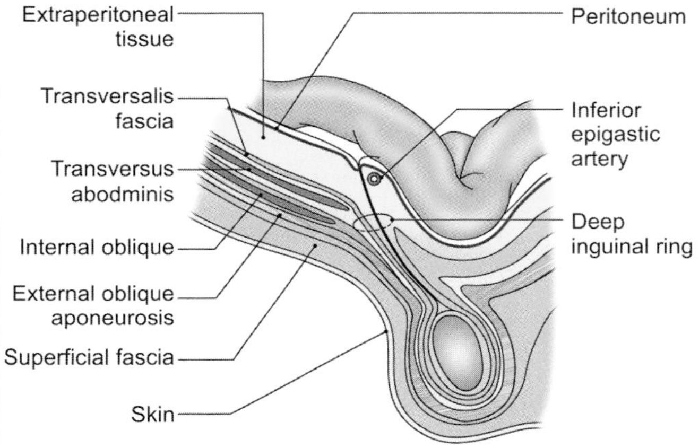

Fig. 16.35: Direct inguinal hernia

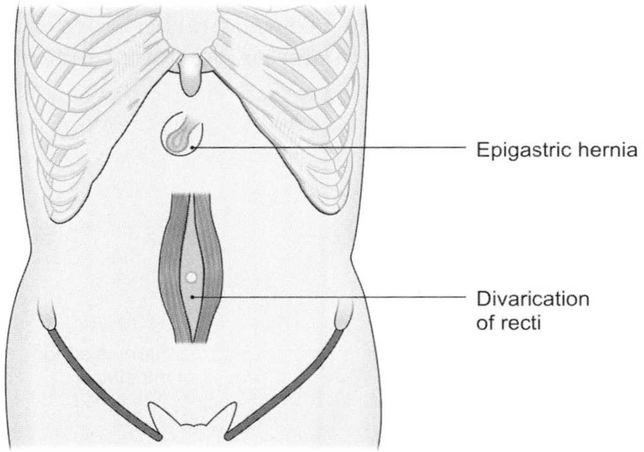

Fig. 16.36: Epigastric hernia and divarication of recti

Table 16.1: Differences between indirect and direct inguinal hernia

	Indirect inguinal hernia	*Direct inguinal hernia*
1. Aetiology	Preformed sac	Weakness of posterior wall of inguinal canal
2. Precipitating factors	—	Chronic bronchitis, enlarged prostate
3. On standing	Does not come out	Comes out
4. Direction of the sac	Sac comes through the deep inguinal ring	It comes out of Hesselbach's triangle
5. Obstruction	Common, as neck is narrow	Not common because neck is wide
6. Internal ring occlusion test	Not seen	The swelling is seen

Morphologically

The inguinal hernia peculiarly occurs only in man and not in any other mammal. This predisposition of man to hernia is due to the evolutionary changes that have taken place in the inguinal region as a result of his upright posture. He has to pay a heavy price for being upright. The important changes are as follows.

1 The iliac crest has grown forwards into the lower digitations of external oblique muscle, so that the inguinal ligament can no more be operated by fleshy fibres of muscle which now helps in balancing the body. In all other mammals, external oblique has no attachment to the iliac crest.
2 The internal oblique and transversus initially originated from the anterior border of ilium and the sheath of iliopsoas, and acted as a powerful sphincter of the inguinal canal. The shift of their origin to the inguinal ligament and iliac crest has minimised their role.

3 Due to peculiar growth of hip bones and pelvis, the crural passage (between hip bone and inguinal ligament) in man has become much wider than any other mammal. This predisposes to femoral hernia.

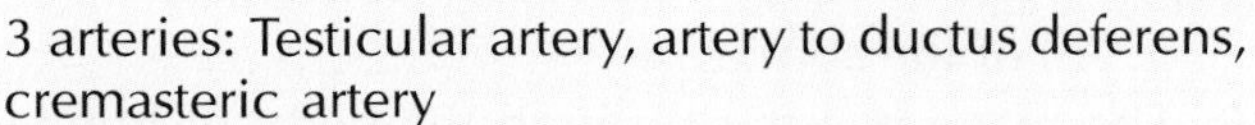

Mnemonics

Spermatic cord contents "3-3-3"

3 arteries: Testicular artery, artery to ductus deferens, cremasteric artery

3 nerves: Genital branch of the genitofemoral, ilioinguinal, autonomic nerves

3 other things: Ductus deferens, pampiniform plexus, remains of processus vaginalis

FACTS TO REMEMBER

- Transpyloric plane is an important landmark in the abdominal cavity.
- Umbilicus is normally a region of "water shed" for the lymphatic and venous drainage. It is an important landmark.
- At umbilicus three systems meet. These are digestive (vitellointestinal duct), the excretory (urachus) and vascular (umbilical vessels).
- Thoracic 10 spinal nerve supplies the region of umbilicus.
- External oblique is the largest and most superficial muscle of anterior abdominal wall.
- Internal oblique forms anterior wall, roof and posterior wall of the inguinal canal. It forms rectus sheath differently in upper and lower parts of abdominal wall. It also forms the cremaster muscle and conjoint tendon.
- Rectus abdominis is the largest content of rectus sheath.
- Transversus abdominis interdigitates with the fibres of thoracoabdominal diaphragm.
- Inguinal ligament forms the boundary between abdomen and lower limb.
- Cremasteric reflex indicates that L1 segment of spinal cord is intact
- Inguinal hernia lies above and medial to pubic tubercle. Femoral hernia lies below and lateral to pubic tubercle.
- Femoral hernia is never congenital.
- Femoral hernia is common in females because of the larger pelvis, bigger femoral canal and smaller femoral artery.
- Indirect inguinal hernia is more liable to obstruction as the neck of such a hernia is narrow.
- Paramedian incision in the anterior abdominal wall is mostly preferred.

CLINICOANATOMICAL PROBLEM

In a case of intestinal obstruction an incision is to be made above the umbilicus.

- Which is an ideal site for the incision?
- Should the rectus muscle be retracted medially or laterally?

Ans: The ideal site is a paramedian incision. Though the median incision is relatively bloodless, it tends to leave a postoperative weakness through which a ventral hernia may develop. Paramedian incision through the rectus sheath is more sound than median incision. Rectus abdominis muscle is retracted laterally to the protect the thoracic nerves. The nerves enter the rectus muscle from lateral side.

MULTIPLE CHOICE QUESTIONS

1. The skin around the umbilicus is innervated by one of the following by the thoracic segments:
   a. T8 b. T9
   c. T10 d. T11
2. Which of the following does not contribute to the formation of the posterior wall of inguinal canal?
   a. Fascia transversalis
   b. Conjoint tendon
   c. Lacunar ligament
   d. Reflected part of inguinal ligament
3. Which is the most important landmark for distinguishing inguinal from femoral hernia?
   a. Superficial inguinal ring
   b. Pubic tubercle
   c. Midinguinal point
   d. Inguinal ligament
4. Hernia resulting due to non-return of the umbilical loop of midgut is:
   a. Acquired b. Congenital
   c. Infantile d. None of the above
5. Indirect inguinal hernia coming out at the superficial inguinal ring will have the following coverings:
   a. Cremasteric fascia
   b. Internal spermatic fascia
   c. External spermatic fascia
   d. All of the above

6. Which is the covering in all varieties of inguinal hernia?
   a. Fascia transversalis
   b. Internal spermatic fascia
   c. External spermatic fascia
   d. All of the above
7. Which type of hernia is commonest in young adults?
   a. Lateral direct inguinal
   b. Medial direct inguinal
   c. Oblique inguinal
   d. Umbilical
8. Transpyloric plane passes through all the following structures *except*:
   a. L1 vertebra b. Pylorus of stomach
   c. Tip of 10th rib d. Neck of pancreas
9. Which aponeurosis forms the inguinal ligament?
   a. Aponeurosis of internal oblique
   b. Aponeurosis of external oblique
   c. Aponeurosis of transversus abdominis
   d. All of the above
10. The plane passing through the body of lumbar 3 vertebra is:
   a. Subcostal b. Transpyloric
   c. Transumbilical d. Intertubercular

ANSWERS

1. c	**2.** c	**3.** b	**4.** b	**5.** d	**6.** d	**7.** c	**8.** c	**9.** b	**10.** a

17

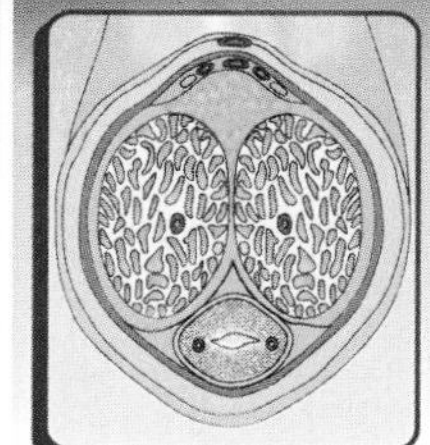

Male External Genital Organs

Commit the oldest sins, the newest kind of ways
—Shakespeare

INTRODUCTION

Male genital organs are situated both outside the pelvic cavity and within the pelvic cavity. As lower temperature is required for *spermatogenesis*, the *testes* are placed outside the pelvic cavity in the scrotal sac. Since urethra serves both the functions of urination and ejaculation, there is only one tube enclosed in the urogenital triangle.

DISSECTION

From the superficial inguinal ring, make a longitudinal incision downwards through the skin of the anterolateral aspects of the scrotum till its lower part. Reflect the skin alone if possible otherwise reflect skin, *dartos* and the other layers together till the testis enveloped in its *tunica vaginalis* is visualised.

Lift the testis and spermatic cord from the scrotum. Cut through the spermatic cord at the superficial inguinal ring and remove it together with the testis and put it in a tray of water.

Incise and reflect the coverings if any, e.g. remains of external spermatic fascia, cremaster muscle, cremasteric fascia and internal spermatic fascia. Separate the various structures of spermatic cord. Feel ductus deferens as the important constituent of spermatic cord. Make a transverse section through the testis to visualise its interior.

Identify the *epididymis* capping the superior pole and lateral surface of the testis. The slit-like *sinus of epididymis* formed by tucking-in of the visceral layer of peritoneum between the testis and the epididymis is seen on the anterolateral aspect of the testis.

Cut through and reflect the skin along the *dorsum of the penis* from the symphysis pubis to the end of the *prepuce*.

Find the extension of the membranous layer of the superficial fascia of the abdominal wall on to the penis (*fundiform ligament*). The *superficial dorsal vein* of the penis lies in the superficial fascia. Trace it proximally to drain into any of the superficial external pudendal veins of thigh.

Deep to this vein is the deep fascia and *suspensory ligament* of the penis. Divide the deep fascia in the same line as the skin incision. Reflect it to see the *deep dorsal vein* with the *dorsal arteries* and *nerves* on each side.

Make a transverse section through the body of the penis, but leave the two parts connected by the skin of urethral surface or ventral surface. Identify two *corpora cavernosa* and single *corpus spongiosum* traversed by the urethra.

ORGANS INCLUDED

1 Penis,
2 Scrotum,
3 Testes,
4 Epididymes, and
5 Spermatic cords.

The spermatic cord has been described in Chapter 16.

PENIS

The penis is the male organ of copulation. It is made up of: (a) A root or attached portion, and (b) a body or free portion (Fig. 17.1a).

Root of Penis

The root of the penis is situated in the *superficial perineal pouch*. It is composed of three masses of erectile tissue, namely the two crura and one bulb. Each *crus* (Latin *leg*) is firmly attached to the margins of the pubic arch, and is covered by the ischiocavernosus. The *bulb* is attached to the perineal membrane in between the two crura. It is covered by the *bulbospongiosus*. Its deep

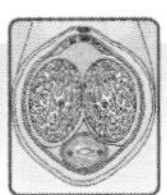

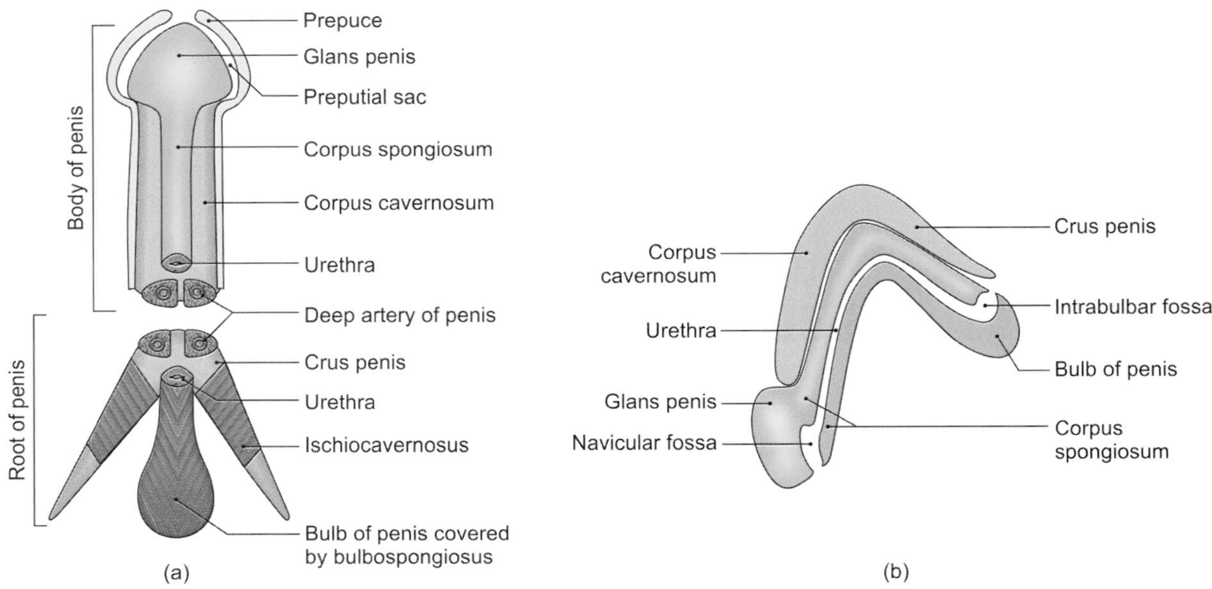

Figs 17.1a and b: Parts of the penis: (a) Ventral view, and (b) sagittal section

surface is pierced (above its centre) by the urethra, which traverses its substance to reach the corpus spongiosum (located in the body). This part of the urethra within the bulb shows a dilatation in its floor, called the *intrabulbar fossa* (Fig. 17.1b).

Body of Penis

The free portion of the penis is completely enveloped by skin. It is continuous with the root in front of the lower part of the pubic symphysis. It is composed of three elongated masses of erectile tissue. During erection of the penis these masses become engorged with blood leading to considerable enlargement. These masses are the right and left corpora cavernosa, and a median corpus spongiosum (Fig. 17.2).

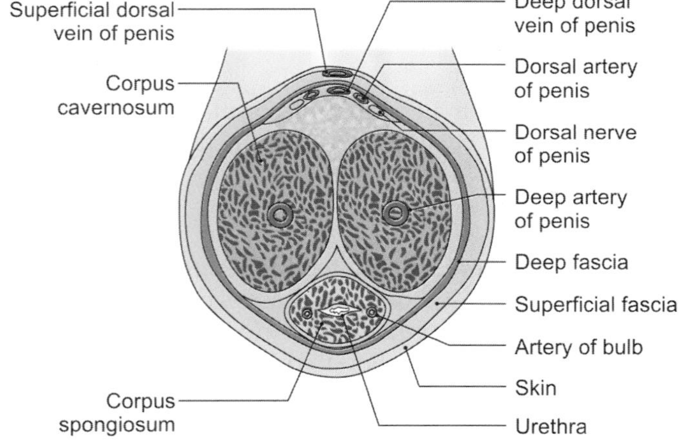

Fig. 17.2: Transverse section through the body of the penis

The penis has a ventral surface that faces backwards and downwards, and a dorsal surface that faces forwards and upwards.

The two *corpora cavernosa* (Latin *hollow*) are the forward continuations of the crura. They are in close apposition with each other throughout their length. The corpora cavernosa do not reach the end of the penis. Each of them terminates under cover of the *glans penis* in a blunt conical extremity. They are surrounded by a strong fibrous envelope called the *tunica albuginea*. The tunica albuginea has superficial longitudinal fibres enclosing both the corpora, and deep circular fibres that enclose each corpus separately, and also form a median septum.

The *corpus spongiosum* is the forward continuation of the bulb of the penis. Its terminal part is expanded to form a conical enlargement, called the *glans penis*. Throughout its whole length it is traversed by the urethra. Like the corpora, it is also surrounded by a fibrous sheath (Fig. 17.2).

The base of the *glans* (Latin *acron*) *penis* has a projecting margin, the *corona* (Latin *crown*) *glandis*, which overhangs an obliquely grooved constriction, known as the *neck of the penis*. Within the glans the urethra shows a dilatation (in its roof) called the *navicular fossa*.

The *skin* covering the penis is very thin and dark in colour. It is loosely connected with the fascial sheath of the organ. At the neck it is folded to form the *prepuce* (Latin *before penis*) or *foreskin* which covers the glans to a varying extent and can be retracted backwards to expose the glans. On the undersurface of the glans there is a median fold of skin called the *frenulum* (Latin *bridle*).

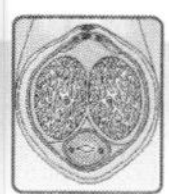

The potential space between the glans and the prepuce is known as the *preputial sac*. On the corona glandis and on the neck of the penis there are numerous small preputial or sebaceous glands which secrete a sebaceous material called the *smegma*, which collects in the preputial sac (Fig. 17.1a).

The *superficial fascia of the penis* consists of very loosely arranged areolar tissue, completely devoid of fat. It may contain a few muscle fibres. It is continuous with the membranous layer of superficial fascia of the abdomen above and of the perineum below. It contains the superficial dorsal vein of the penis.

The deep layer of superficial fascia is membranous and is called the *fascia of the penis* or *deep fascia of penis*, or Buck's fascia. It surrounds all three masses of erectile tissue, but does not extend into the glans. Deep to it there are the deep dorsal vein, the dorsal arteries and dorsal nerves of the penis. Proximally, it is continuous with the dartos and with the fascia of the urogenital triangle.

The supports of the body of penis are the following.

a. The *fundiform ligament* which extends downwards from the linea alba and splits to enclose the penis. It lies superficial to the suspensory ligament (*see* Fig. 16.8b).
b. The *suspensory ligament* lies deep to the fundiform ligament. It extends from the pubic symphysis and blends below with the fascia on each side of the penis.

Arteries of the Penis

1 The internal pudendal artery gives off three branches which supply the penis.
   a. The *deep artery of the penis* runs in the corpus cavernosum. It breaks up into arteries that follow a spiral course and are, therefore, called *helicine arteries*.
   b. The *dorsal artery of the penis* runs on the dorsum, deep to the deep fascia, and supplies the glans penis and the distal part of the corpus spongiosum, the prepuce and the frenulum.
   c. The *artery of the bulb of the penis* supplies the bulb and the proximal half of the corpus spongiosum.

2 The femoral artery gives off the *superficial external pudendal artery* which supplies the skin and fasciae of the penis.

Veins of the Penis

The dorsal veins, superficial and deep, are unpaired. Superficial dorsal vein drains the prepuce and penile skin. It runs back in subcutaneous tissue and inclines to right or left, before it opens into one of the external pudendal veins.

Deep dorsal vein lies deep to Buck's fascia. It receives blood from the glans penis and corpora cavernosa penis, and courses back in midline between paired dorsal arteries.

Near the root of the penis, it passes deep to the suspensory ligament and through a gap between the arcuate pubic ligament and anterior margin of perineal membrane, it divides into right and left branches which connect below the symphysis pubis with the internal pudendal veins and ultimately enters the prostatic plexus.

Nerve Supply of the Penis

1 The sensory nerve supply to the penis is derived from the dorsal nerve of the penis and the ilioinguinal nerve. The muscles of the root of the penis are supplied by the *perineal branch of the pudendal nerve.*

2 The autonomic nerves are derived from the pelvic plexus via the *prostatic plexus*. The *sympathetic nerves* are *vasoconstrictor*, and the *parasympathetic* nerves (S2, S3, S4) are *vasodilator*. The autonomic fibres are distributed through the branches of the *pudendal nerve*.

Lymphatic Drainage

Lymphatics from the glans drain into the deep inguinal nodes also called gland of Cloquet. Lymphatics from the rest of the penis drain into the superficial inguinal lymph nodes.

Mechanism of Erection of the Penis

Erection of the penis is a purely vascular phenomenon. The turgidity of the penis during its erection is contributed to by the following factors.

1 Dilatation of the *helicine* arteries pours an increased amount of arterial blood into the *cavernous spaces* of the corpora cavernosa. Blood is also poured in small amount into the corpus spongiosum and into the glans by their arteries. As the spaces within the *erectile tissue* fill up, the penis enlarges.

2 This enlargement presses on the veins preventing outflow of blood through them. Contraction of the ischiocavernosus muscles probably has the same effect.

3 Expansion of the corpora cavernosa, and to a lesser extent of the corpus spongiosum, stretches the deep fascia. This restricts enlargement of the penis. Further flow of blood increases the pressure within the erectile tissue and leads to rigidity of the penis.

4 Erection is controlled by parasympathetic nerves (nervi erigentes, S2, S3, S4).

SCROTUM

The scrotum (Latin *bag*) is a cutaneous bag containing the right and left testes, the epididymis and the lower parts of the spermatic cords.

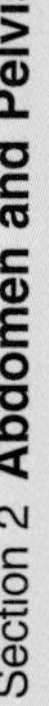

1 Externally, the scrotum is divided into right and left parts by a ridge or raphe which is continued forwards on to the undersurface of the penis and backwards along the middle of the perineum to the anus (Fig. 17.3).
2 The left half of the scrotum hangs a little lower than the right, in correspondence with the greater length of the left spermatic cord.
3 Under the influence of cold, and in young and robust persons, the scrotum is short, corrugated and closely applied to the testis. This is due to contraction of the subcutaneous muscle of scrotum, called the *dartos* (Greek *skinny*). However, under the influence of warmth, and in old and debilitated persons, the scrotum is elongated and flaccid due to relaxation of dartos. From this it appears that the dartos muscle helps in regulation of temperature within the scrotum.

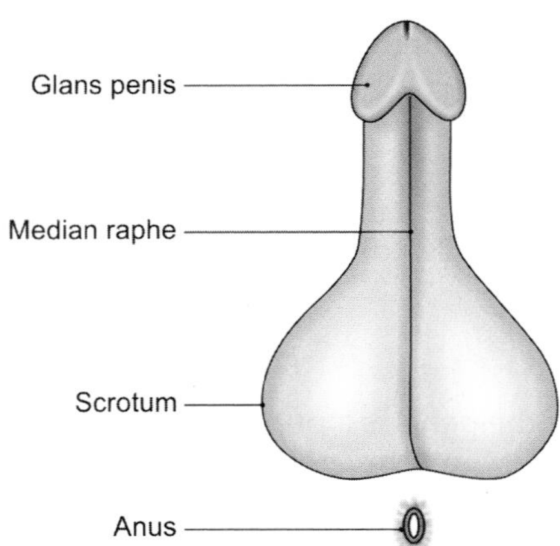

Fig. 17.3: Scrotum and penis viewed from below to show the median raphe

Layers of the Scrotum

The scrotum is made up of the following layers from outside inwards (Fig. 17.4).
1 Skin, continuation of abdominal skin.
2 Dartos muscle which replaces the superficial fascia. The dartos muscle is prolonged into a median vertical septum between the two halves of the scrotum.
3 The external spermatic fascia from external oblique muscle.
4 The cremasteric (Greek *to hang*) muscle and fascia from internal oblique muscle.
5 The internal spermatic fascia from fascia transversalis.

Blood Supply

The scrotum is supplied by the following arteries: Superficial external pudendal, deep external pudendal, scrotal branches of internal pudendal, and cremasteric branch of inferior epigastric.

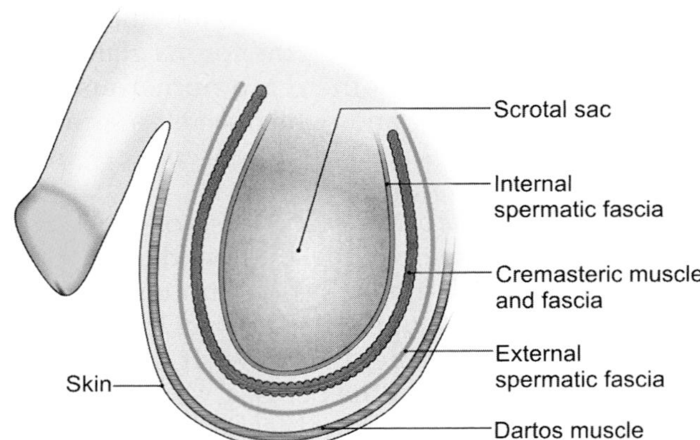

Fig. 17.4: Layers of the scrotum

Nerve Supply

The anterior one-third of the scrotum is supplied by segment L1 of the spinal cord through the *ilioinguinal nerve* and the *genital branch of the genitofemoral nerve* (Fig. 17.5).

The posterior two-thirds of the scrotum are supplied by *segment S3* of the spinal cord through the *posterior scrotal branches* of the pudendal nerve, and the perineal branch of the *posterior cutaneous nerve of the thigh*. The areas supplied by segments L1 and S3 are separated by the *ventral axial line*.

The dartos muscle is supplied by the *genital branch of the genitofemoral nerve*.

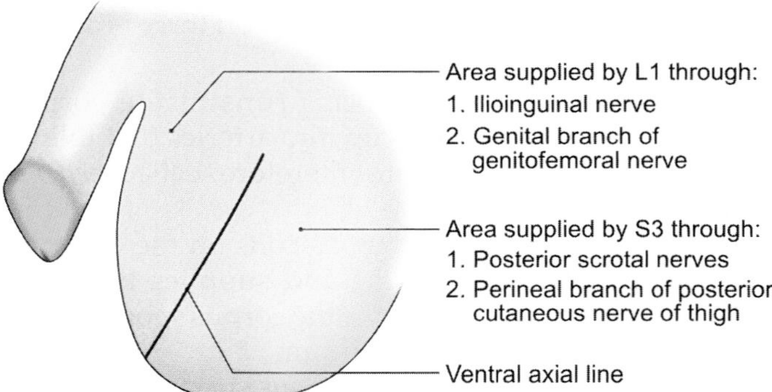

Fig. 17.5: Nerve supply of the scrotum

CLINICAL ANATOMY

- Due to laxity of skin and its dependent position, the scrotum is a *common site for oedema*. Abundance of hair and of sebaceous glands also makes it a *site of sebaceous cysts* (Fig. 17.6).
- As the scrotum is supplied by widely separated dermatomes (L1, S3) spinal anaesthesia of the whole scrotum is difficult to achieve (Fig. 17.5).
- The scrotum is *bifid* in male—*pseudohermaphroditism.*

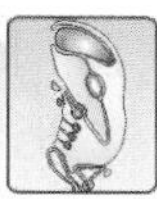

Two Curvatures

The *lesser curvature* is concave and forms the right border of the stomach. It provides attachment to the lesser omentum. The most dependent part of the curvature is marked by the *angular notch* or incisura angularis (Fig. 19.2).

The *greater curvature* is convex and forms the left border of the stomach (*see* Figs 18.9 and 18.18). It provides attachment to the greater omentum, the gastrosplenic ligament and the gastrophrenic ligament. At its upper end the greater curvature presents the *cardiac notch* which separates it from the oesophagus. It is 5 times longer than lesser curvature.

Two Surfaces

The *anterior* or *anterosuperior surface* faces forwards and upwards.

The *posterior* or *posteroinferior surface* faces backwards and downwards.

Two Parts Subdivided into Four

The stomach is divided into two parts. (i) Cardiac and (ii) Pyloric, by a line drawn downwards and to the left from the incisura angularis. The larger, cardiac part is further subdivided into the fundus and body, and the smaller, pyloric part is subdivided into the pyloric antrum and pyloric canal (Fig. 19.2).

Cardiac Part

1 The *fundus of the stomach* is the upper convex dome-shaped part situated above a horizontal line drawn at the level of the cardiac orifice. It is commonly distended with gas which is seen clearly in radiographic examination under the left dome of the diaphragm (*see* Fig. 20.14).

2 The *body of the stomach* lies between the fundus and the pyloric antrum. It can be distended enormously along the greater curvature. The gastric glands distributed in the fundus and body of stomach, contain all three types of secretory cells, namely:

   a. The mucous cells.

   b. The chief, peptic or zymogenic cells which secrete the digestive enzymes.

   c. The parietal or oxyntic cells which secrete HCl.

Pyloric Part

1 The *pyloric antrum* is separated from the pyloric canal by an inconstant sulcus, sulcus intermedius present on the greater curvature. It is about 7.5 cm long. The pyloric glands are richest in mucous cells.

2 The *pyloric canal* is about 2.5 cm long. It is narrow and tubular. At its right end it terminates at the pylorus.

Relations of Stomach

Peritoneal Relations

The stomach is lined by peritoneum on both its surfaces. At the lesser curvature the layers of peritoneum lining the anterior and posterior surfaces meet and become continuous with the *lesser omentum* (*see* Fig. 18.8).

Along the greater part of the greater curvature the two layers meet to form the *greater omentum*.

Near the fundus the two layers meet to form the gastrosplenic ligament.

Near the cardiac end the peritoneum on the posterior surface is reflected on to the diaphragm as the *gastrophrenic ligament* (*see* Fig. 18.8). Cranial to this ligament a small part of the posterior surface of the stomach is in direct contact with the diaphragm (left crus). This is the *bare area of the stomach*. The greater and lesser curvatures along the peritoneal reflections are also bare.

Visceral Relations

The anterior surface of the stomach is related to the liver, the diaphragm, transverse colon and the anterior abdominal wall. The areas of the stomach related to these structures are shown in Fig. 19.8. The diaphragm separates the stomach from the left pleura, the pericardium, and the sixth to ninth ribs. The costal cartilages are separated from the stomach by the transversus abdominis. Gastric nerves and vessels ramify deep to the peritoneum.

The space between left costal margin and lower edge of left lung on stomach is known as *Traube's space*. Normally, on percussion there is resonant note over this space; but in splenomegaly or pleural effusion, a dull note is felt at this site.

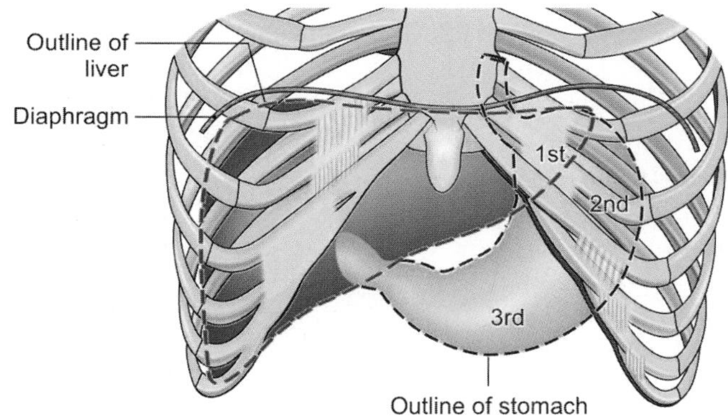

Fig. 19.8: Anterior relations of stomach. Area 1st is covered by the liver; area 2nd by the diaphragm; and area 3rd by the anterior abdominal wall

The posterior surface of the stomach is related to structures forming the stomach bed, *all of which are separated from the stomach by the cavity of the lesser sac.*

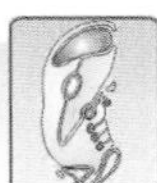

These structures are:

a. Diaphragm.
b. Left kidney.
c. Left suprarenal gland.
d. Pancreas (Fig. 19.9).
e. Transverse mesocolon.
f. Splenic flexure of the colon.
g. Splenic artery (Fig. 19.9). Sometimes the spleen is also included in the stomach bed, but it is separated from the stomach by the cavity of the greater sac (and not of the lesser sac). Gastric nerves and vessels ramify deep to the peritoneum (Figs 19.10 and 19.12).

Blood Supply

The stomach is supplied along

i. the lesser curvature by: The left gastric artery, a branch of the coeliac trunk and the right gastric artery, a branch of the proper hepatic artery.

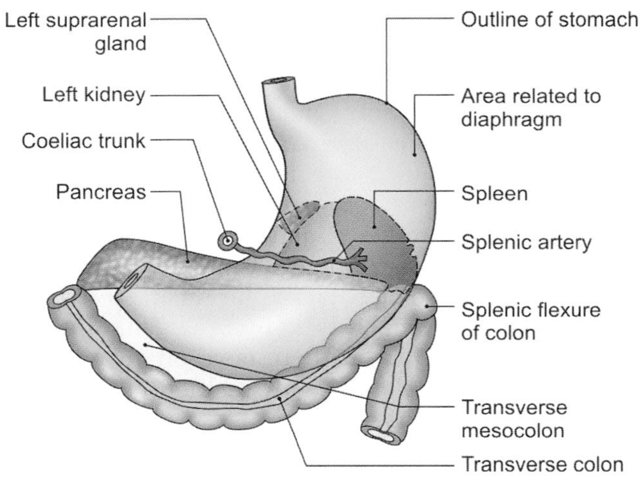

Fig. 19.9: The stomach bed

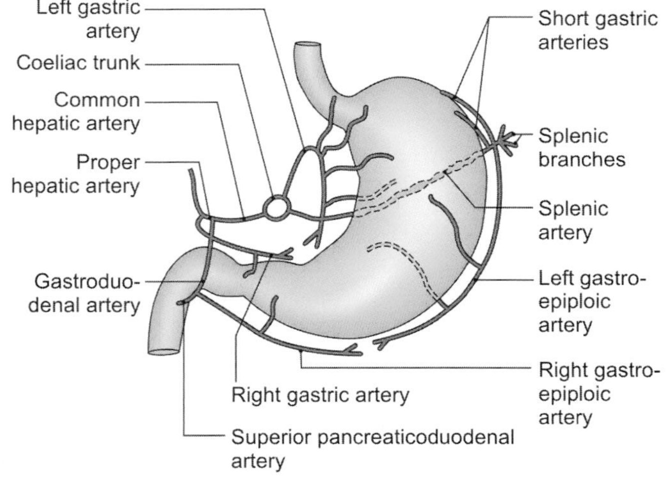

Fig. 19.10: Arteries supplying the stomach

ii. Along the greater curvature it is supplied by the right gastroepiploic artery, a branch of the gastroduodenal and the left gastroepiploic artery, a branch of the splenic.
iii. Fundus is supplied by 5 to 7 short gastric arteries, which are also branches of the splenic artery (Fig. 19.10).

The veins of the stomach drain into the portal, superior mesenteric and splenic veins.

Right and left gastric drain in the portal vein. Right gastroepiploic ends in superior mesenteric vein; while left gastroepiploic and short gastric veins terminate in splenic vein (Fig. 19.3).

LYMPHATIC DRAINAGE

The stomach can be divided into four lymphatic territories as shown in Fig. 19.11. The drainage of these areas is as follows.

Area (a) of Fig. 19.11, i.e. upper part of left 1/3rd drains into the *pancreaticosplenic nodes* lying along the splenic artery, i.e. on the back of the stomach. Lymph vessels from these nodes travel along the splenic artery to reach the coeliac nodes.

Area (b), i.e. right 2/3rd drains into the *left gastric nodes* lying along the artery of the same name. These nodes also drain the abdominal part of the oesophagus. Lymph from these nodes drains into the coeliac nodes.

Area (c), i.e. lower part of left 1/3rd drains into the right gastroepiploic nodes that lie along the artery of the same name. Lymph vessels arising in these nodes drain into the subpyloric nodes which lie in the angle between the first and second parts of the duodenum. From here the lymph is drained further into the hepatic nodes that lie along the hepatic artery; and finally into the coeliac nodes.

Lymph from *area* (d), i.e. pyloric part drains in different directions into the pyloric, hepatic, and left

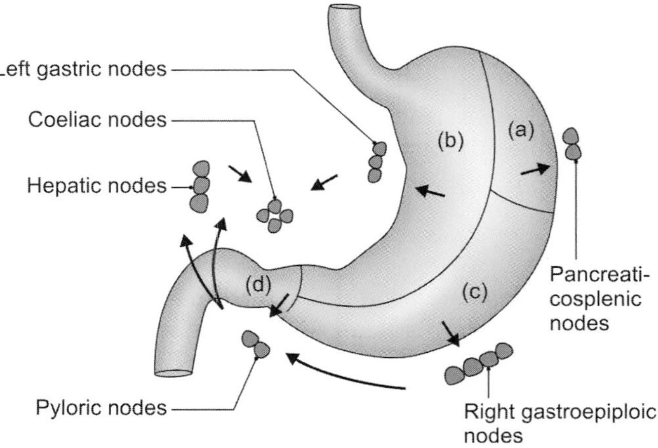

Fig. 19.11: Lymphatic drainage of the stomach. Note the manner in which the organ is subdivided into a to d different territories

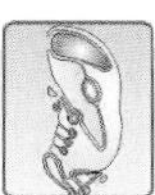

gastric nodes, and passes from all these nodes to the coeliac nodes.

Note that lymph from all areas of the stomach ultimately reaches the coeliac nodes. From here it passes through the *intestinal lymph trunk* to reach the *cisterna chyli*.

Nerve Supply

The stomach is supplied by sympathetic and parasympathetic nerves. The *sympathetic nerves* are derived from thoracic six to ten segments of the spinal cord, via the greater splanchnic nerves, coeliac and hepatic plexuses. They travel along the arteries supplying the stomach. These nerves are:

a. Vasomotor.
b. Motor to the pyloric sphincter, but inhibitory to the rest of the gastric musculature.
c. The chief pathway for pain sensations from the stomach.

The *parasympathetic nerves* (Figs 19.12a and b) are derived from the vagi, through the oesophageal plexus and gastric nerves. The anterior gastric nerve (made up of one or two trunks) contains mainly the left vagal fibres, and the posterior gastric nerve (again made up of one to two trunks) contains mainly the right vagal fibres.

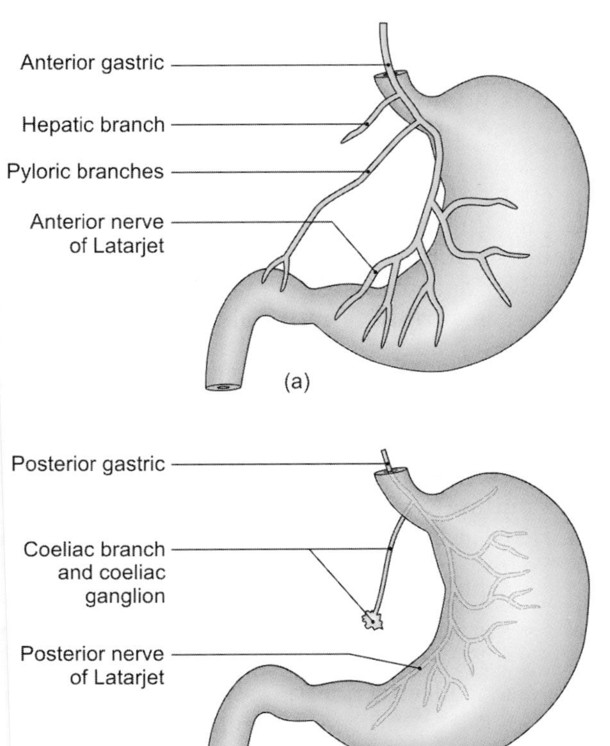

Figs 19.12a and b: Nerve supply of the stomach: (a) Anterior gastric nerve, and (b) posterior gastric nerve

The *anterior gastric nerve* divides into:

a. A number of gastric branches for the anterior surface of the fundus and body of the stomach.
b. Two pyloric branches, one for the pyloric antrum and another for the pylorus.

The *posterior gastric nerve* divides into:

a. Smaller, gastric branches for the posterior surface of the fundus, the body and the pyloric antrum.
b. Larger, coeliac branches for the coeliac plexus.

Parasympathetic nerves are motor and secretomotor to the stomach. Their stimulation causes increased motility of the stomach and secretion of gastric juice rich in pepsin and HCl. These are inhibitory to the pyloric sphincter.

INTERIOR OF STOMACH

DISSECTION

Open the stomach along the greater curvature and examine the mucous membrane with a hand lens.

Then strip the mucous membrane from one part and expose the internal muscle coat. Dissect the muscle coat, e.g. outer longitudinal, middle circular and inner oblique muscle fibres. Feel thickened pyloric sphincter.

Incise the beginning of duodenum and examine the duodenal and pyloric aspects of the pyloric sphincter.

Features

The stomach has to be opened to see its internal structure.

1 The *mucosa* of an empty stomach is thrown into folds termed as gastric rugae. The rugae are longitudinal along the lesser curvature and are irregular elsewhere. The rugae are flattened in a distended stomach. On the mucosal surface there are numerous small depressions that can be seen with a hand lens. These are the *gastric pits*. The gastric glands open into these pits.

The part of the lumen of the stomach that lies along the lesser curvature, and has longitudinal rugae, is called the *gastric canal* or *magenstrasse*. This canal allows rapid passage of swallowed liquids along the lesser curvature directly to the lower part before it spreads to the other part of stomach (Fig. 19.13).

Thus lesser curvature bears maximum insult of the swallowed liquids, which makes it vulnerable to peptic ulcer. *So, beware of your drinks.*

2 *Submucous coat* is made of connective tissue, arterioles and nerve plexus.

3 *Muscle coat* is arranged as under:

a. Longitudinal fibres are most superficial, mainly along the curvatures.
b. Inner circular fibres encircle the body and are thickened at pylorus to form pyloric sphincter (Fig. 19.14).

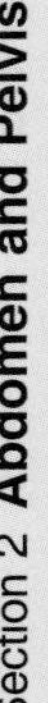

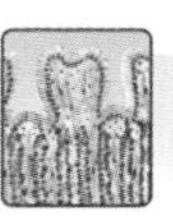

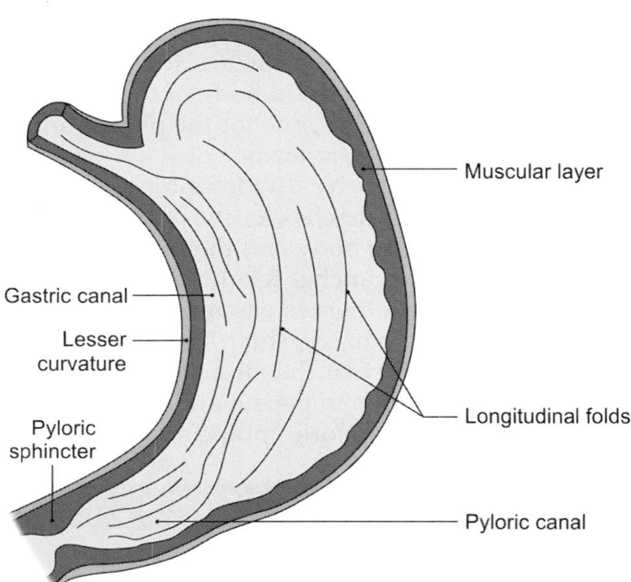

Fig. 19.13: Longitudinal folds of mucous membrane

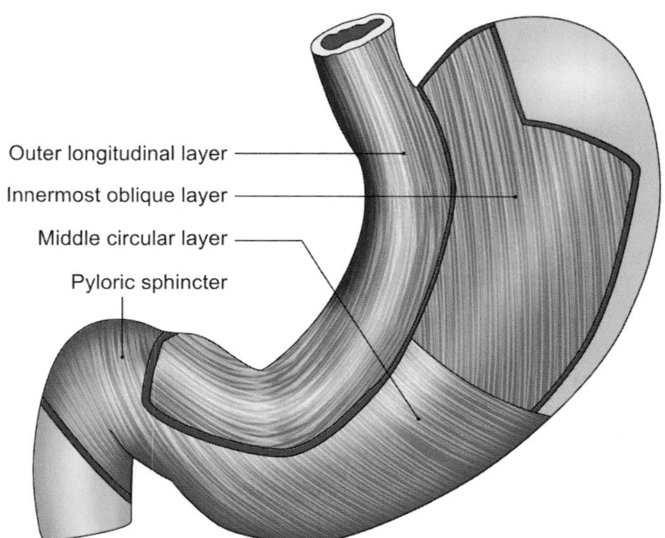

Fig. 19.14: Smooth muscle layers of the wall of stomach

c. The deepest layer consists of oblique fibres which loop over the cardiac notch. Some fibres spread in the fundus and body of stomach. Rest form a well-developed ridge on each side of the lesser curvature. These fibres on contraction form "gastric canal" for the passage of fluids.

4 *Serous coat* consists of the peritoneal covering.

Functions of Stomach

1 The stomach acts primarily as a reservoir of food. It also acts as a mixer of food.
2 By its peristaltic movements it softens and mixes the food with the gastric juice.
3 The gastric glands produce the gastric juice which contains enzymes that play an important role in digestion of food.
4 The gastric glands also produce hydrochloric acid which destroys many organisms present in food and drink.
5 The lining cells of the stomach produce abundant mucus which protects the gastric mucosa against the corrosive action of hydrochloric acid.
6 Some substances like alcohol, water, salt and few drugs are absorbed in the stomach.
7 Stomach produces the "intrinsic factor" of Castle which helps in the absorption of vitamin B_{12}.

CLINICAL ANATOMY

- Gastric pain is felt in the epigastrium because the stomach is supplied from segments T6 to T9 of the spinal cord, which also supply the upper part of the abdominal wall. Pain is produced either by spasm of muscle, or by over-distension. Ulcer pain is attributed to local spasm due to irritation (*see* Fig. 18.35).
- *Peptic ulcer* can occur in the sites of pepsin and hydrochloric acid, namely the stomach, first part of duodenum, lower end of oesophagus and Meckel's diverticulum. It is common in blood group 'O'.

  Gastric ulcer occurs typically along the lesser curvature (Fig. 19.13). This is possibly due to the following peculiarities of lesser curvature.

  a. It is homologous with the gastric trough of ruminants.
  b. Mucosa is not freely movable over the muscular coat.
  c. The epithelium is comparatively thin.
  d. Blood supply is less abundant and there are fewer anastomoses.
  e. Nerve supply is more abundant, with large ganglia.
  f. Because of the gastric canal, it receives most of the insult from irritating drinks.
  g. Being shorter in length the wave of contraction stays longer at a particular point, viz., the standing wave of incisura.
  h. *H. pylori* infection is also an important causative factor.

  Gastric ulcers are common in people who are always in "hurry", mostly "worry" about incidents and eat "spicy curry".

  Gastric ulcer is notoriously resistant to healing and persists for years together, causing great degree of morbidity. To promote healing the irritating effect of HCl can be minimised by antacids, partial gastrectomy or vagotomy.

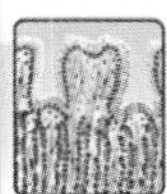

- *Gastric carcinoma* is common and occurs along the greater curvature. On this account the lymphatic drainage of stomach assumes importance. Metastasis can occur through the thoracic duct to the left supraclavicular lymph node (Troisier's sign). These lymph nodes are called as "signal nodes". It is common in blood group 'A'.
- *Pyloric obstruction* can be congenital or acquired. It causes visible peristalsis in the epigastrium, and vomiting after meals.
- *Hyposthenic stomach* is more prone for gastric ulcer, while hypersthenic stomach is prone for duodenal ulcer.

HISTOLOGY OF STOMACH

At the cardiac end of stomach the stratified epithelium of oesophagus *abruptly* changes to simple columnar epithelium of stomach.

Cardiac End

Mucous membrane: The epithelium is simple columnar with small tubular glands. Lower half of the gland is secretory and upper half is the conducting part. Muscularis mucosae consists of smooth muscle fibres.

Submucosa: It consists of loose connective tissue with Meissner's (German histologist 1829–1909) plexus.

Muscularis externa: It is made of outer longitudinal and inner circular layer including the myenteric plexus of nerves or Auerbach's plexus (German anatomist 1828–97).

Serosa: It is lined by single layer of squamous cells.

Fundus and Body of Stomach

Mucous membrane: It contains tall simple tubular gastric glands. Upper one-third is conducting, while lower two-thirds is secretory. The various cell types seen in the gland are chief or zymogenic, oxyntic or parietal and mucous neck cells (Fig. 19.15).

Muscularis mucosae and *submucosa* are same.

Muscularis externa: It contains an additional innermost oblique coat of muscle fibres.

Serosa is same as of cardiac end.

Pyloric Part

Mucous membrane: There are pyloric glands which consist of basal one-third as mucus secretory component and upper two-thirds as conducting part. Muscularis mucosae is made of two layers of fibres. Submucosa is same as in the cardiac end.

Muscularis externa comprises thick layer of circular fibres forming the pyloric sphincter. *Serosa* is same as of cardiac end.

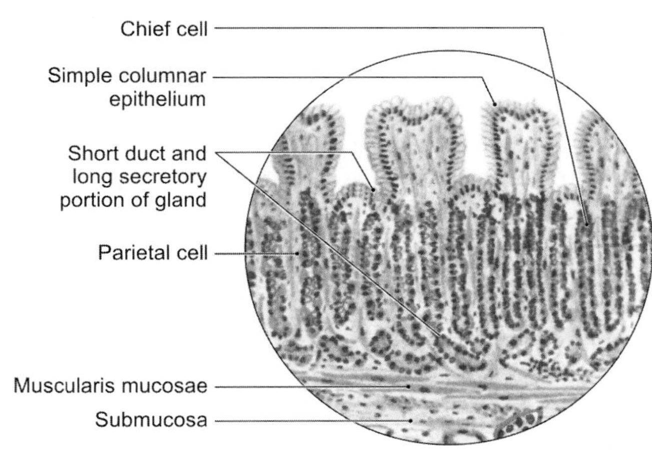

- All epithelial cells are simple columnar in type
- Parietal cells are large and pink, Chief cell are small and blue
- Duct is 1/3rd and secretory part is 2/3rd

Fig. 19.15: Body/fundic mucosa

DEVELOPMENT

Oesophagus

The posterior part of foregut forms the oesophagus. It is very small in the beginning, but it lengthens due to descent of lungs and heart. The muscle of upper one-third is striated, middle one-third, mixed, and lower one-third smooth. Nerve supply to upper two-thirds is from vagus and to lower one-third is from autonomic plexus. Epithelium of oesophagus is endodermal and rest of the layers are from splanchnic mesoderm.

Stomach

The caudal part of foregut shows a fusiform dilatation with anterior and posterior borders and left and right surfaces. This is the stomach. It rotates 90° clockwise, so that left surface faces anteriorly. Even the original posterior border of stomach grows faster, forming the greater curvature.

The stomach also rotates along anteroposterior axis, so that distal or pyloric part moves to right and proximal or cardiac part moves to left side.

The 90° rotation of stomach along the vertical axis pulls the dorsal mesogastrium to the left side creating the lessor sac or omental bursa.

Spleen appears as mesodermal condensation in the left leaf of dorsal mesogastrium.

Mnemonics

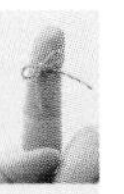

25 cm long

Oesophagus, stomach, duodenum and ureter

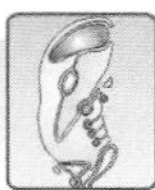

FACTS TO REMEMBER

- Abdominal part of oesophagus is the site of porto-systemic anastomoses. Some veins drain into hemiazygos → vena azygos → superior vena cava. Other veins drain into oesophageal veins → left gastric vein → portal vein.
- Stomach comprises:
  Two orifices: Cardiac and pyloric
  Two curvatures: Lesser and greater
  Two parts: Cardiac and pyloric
  Cardiac part: Fundus and body
  Pyloric part: Pyloric antrum, pyloric canal and pylorus.
- Anterior gastric nerve contains left vagal fibres and posterior gastric nerve contains right vagal fibres.
- Lesser curvature is the anterior border and greater curvature is the posterior border.
- Left and right gastric arteries run along lesser curvature.
- Left and right gastroepiploic arteries lie along greater curvature.
- Pylorus is identified by prepyloric vein
- Stomach bed is separated from the stomach by lesser sac.
- The gastric ulcer is common in people who "worry, hurry and eat hot curries". Gastric ulcer commonly occurs along lesser curvature.
- Gastric cancer mostly occurs along greater curvature. Lymph from cancer → thoracic duct → left supraclavicular node. It is called Virchow's node. This sign is called Troisier's sign.

CLINICOANATOMICAL PROBLEM

A young executive complained of pain in the abdomen, above the umbilicus. He was always in "hurry", gets 'worried' very often and loves to eat spicy "curries".

- What is the cause of pain?
- Why is pain referred to epigastric region?

Ans: The young man is suffering from gastric ulcer. The sympathetic nerves to the stomach are supplied by segments T6–T9 of the spinal cord, which also supply the upper part of the abdominal walls so the pain of gastric ulcer is referred to epigastric region. The pain of foregut derived areas is referred to epigastric region; those of midgut derived organs to periumbilical region while those of hindgut derived viscera to the suprapubic region.

A lifestyle change is recommended in such a case.

MULTIPLE CHOICE QUESTIONS

1. Following structures form part of the stomach bed *except*:
  a. Left suprarenal gland
  b. Coeliac trunk
  c. Splenic artery
  d. Pancreas

2. Which of the following is not present in the bed of stomach?
  a. Splenic artery
  b. Transverse mesocolon
  c. Transverse colon
  d. Fourth part of duodenum

3. A posteriorly perforating peptic ulcer will most likely produce peritonitis in the following:
  a. Greater sac b. Lesser sac
  c. Bare area of liver d. Morrison's pouch

4. Which of the following arteries supply the fundus of the stomach?
  a. Right gastric artery
  b. Splenic artery
  c. Short gastric arteries
  d. Gastroduodenal artery

5. Which cell of gastric gland gives it a beaded appearance?
  a. Zymogenic
  b. Oxyntic
  c. Mucus cells
  d. Columnar cell

6. Cardiac orifice of stomach lies behind one of the following costal cartilages:
  a. Left fifth b. Left seventh
  c. Left eighth d. Right eighth

ANSWERS

1. b **2.** d **3.** b **4.** c **5.** b **6.** b

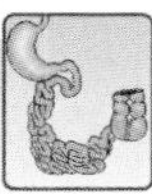

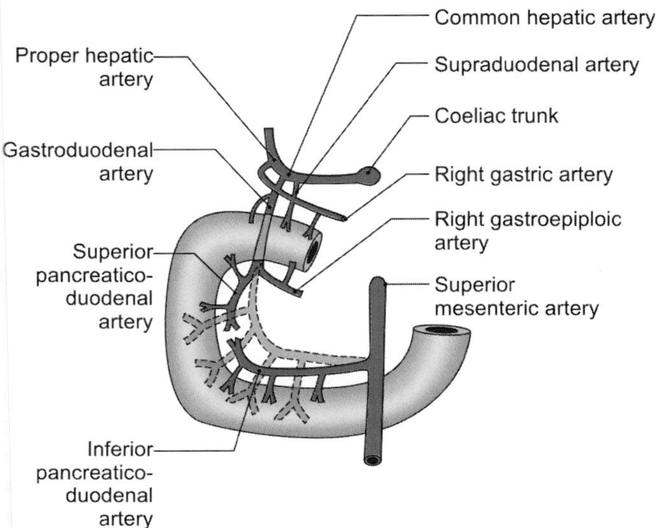

Fig. 20.13: Arterial supply of the duodenum

Venous Drainage

The veins of the duodenum drain into the splenic, superior mesenteric and portal veins.

Lymphatic Drainage

Most of the lymph vessels from the duodenum end in the *pancreaticoduodenal nodes* present along the inside of the curve of the duodenum, i.e. at the junction of the pancreas and the duodenum. From here the lymph passes partly to the *hepatic nodes*, and through them to the *coeliac nodes*; and partly to the superior mesenteric nodes and ultimately via *intestinal lymph trunk* into the *cisterna chyli*.

Some vessels from the first part of the duodenum drain into the pyloric nodes, and through them to the hepatic nodes. All the lymph reaching the hepatic nodes drains into the coeliac nodes.

Nerve Supply

Sympathetic nerves from thoracic ninth and tenth spinal segments and parasympathetic nerves from the vagus, pass through the coeliac plexus and reach the duodenum along its arteries.

HISTOLOGY

Mucous membrane: Shows evaginations in the form of *villi* and invaginations to form *crypts of Lieberkuhn*. Lining of villi is of columnar cells with microvilli. Muscularis mucosae comprises two layers.

Submucosa is full of mucus-secreting *Brunner's glands*.

The *muscularis externa* comprises outer longitudinal and inner circular layer of muscle fibres.

Outermost layer is mostly connective tissue.

CLINICAL ANATOMY

- In the skiagram taken after giving a barium meal, the first part of the duodenum is seen as a triangular shadow called the duodenal cap (Fig. 20.14).
- The first part of the duodenum is one of the commonest sites for peptic ulcer, possibly because of direct exposure of this part to the acidic contents reaching it from the stomach.

  The patient is usually an over busy young person with a tense temperament. The ulcer pain located at the right half of epigastrium is relieved by meals and reappears on an empty stomach.
- The first part of duodenum is overlapped by the liver and gallbladder, either of which may become adherent to, or even ulcerated by a duodenal ulcer. Other clinically important relations of duodenum are the right kidney and transverse colon (Fig. 20.9).
- Duodenal diverticula are fairly frequent. They are seen along its concave border, generally at points where arteries enter the duodenal wall.
- Congenital stenosis and obstruction of the second part of the duodenum may occur at the site of the opening of the bile duct. Other causes of obstruction are:
  a. An annular pancreas.
  b. Pressure by the superior mesenteric artery (Fig. 20.15) on the third part of duodenum.
  c. Contraction of the suspensory muscle of the duodenum (Fig. 20.12).
- Duodenal carcinoma

JEJUNUM AND ILEUM

DISSECTION

For examining the jejunum and ileum, tie a pair of ligatures around the jejunum close to the duodenojejunal flexure and a pair around the ileum close to the caecum. Cut through the small intestine between each pair of ligatures and remove it by dividing the mesentery close to the intestine.

Wash intestine with running tap water. Remove 10 cm each of jejunum and ileum and open it longitudinally. Remove the peritoneal coat to expose the longitudinal muscle layer.

Identify villi with a hand lens. Remove only the mucous membrane and submucosa to see the underlying circular muscle coat. Examine the differences between jejunum and ileum.

Features

The jejunum and ileum are suspended from the posterior abdominal wall by the mesentery and,

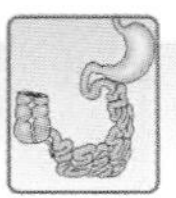

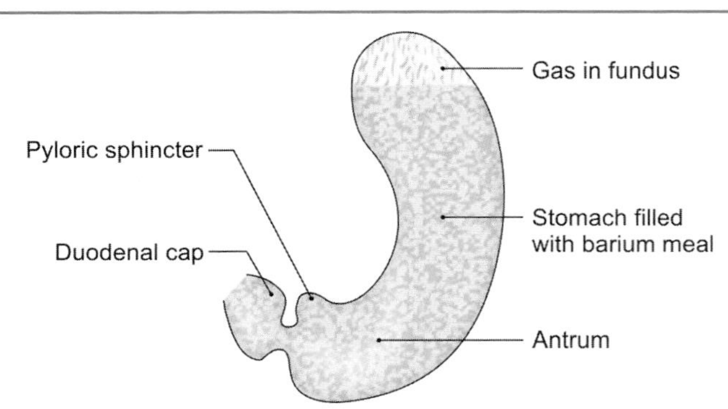

Fig. 20.14: Line drawing of radiograph of the stomach after barium meal

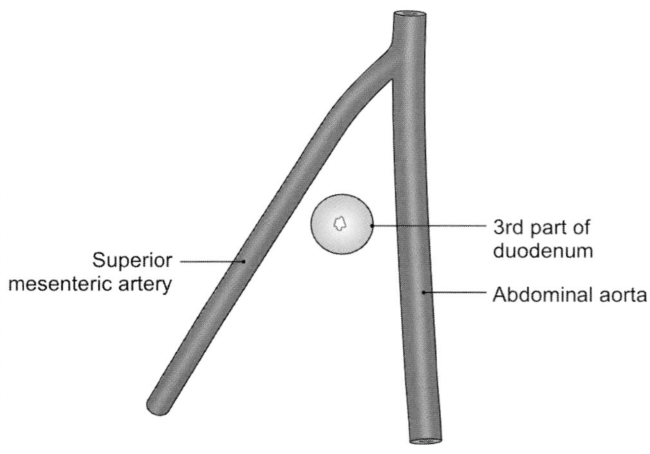

Fig. 20.15: Obstruction of third part of the duodenum between the two arteries

therefore, enjoy considerable mobility. The jejunum constitutes the upper two-fifths of the mobile part of the small intestine, while the ileum constitutes the lower three-fifths. The jejunum begins at the duodenojejunal flexure. The ileum terminates at the ileocaecal junction. The structure and functions of the jejunum and ileum correspond to the general description of the small intestine. The differences between the jejunum and the ileum are given in Table 20.1.

Blood Supply

The jejunum and ileum are supplied by branches from the superior mesenteric artery, and are drained by corresponding veins.

Lymphatic Drainage

Lymph from lacteals drains into plexuses in the wall of the gut. From there it passes into lymphatic vessels in the mesentery. Passing through numerous lymph nodes present in the mesentery, and along the superior mesenteric artery, it ultimately drains into nodes present in front of the aorta at the origin of the superior mesenteric artery.

Nerve Supply

Sympathetic nerves are from T9–T11 spinal segments and parasympathetic is from vagus.

HISTOLOGY

Jejunum

The *villi* here are tongue-shaped. No mucous glands or aggregated lymphoid follicles are present in the *submucosa*. *Muscularis externa* is same as in duodenum. Outermost is the serous layer.

Ileum

The *villi* are few, thin and finger-like. Collection of lymphocytes in the form of *Peyer's patches* in lamina propria extending into submucosa is a characteristic feature.

Rest is same as above.

Table 20.1: Differences between jejunum and ileum

Feature	*Jejunum*	*Ileum*
1. Location	Occupies upper and left parts of the intestinal area	Occupies lower and right parts of the intestinal area
2. Walls	Thicker and more vascular	Thinner and less vascular
3. Lumen	Wider and often empty	Narrower and often loaded
4. Mesentery	a. Windows present b. Fat less abundant c. Arterial arcades, 1 or 2 d. Vasa recta longer and fewer	a. No windows b. Fat more abundant c. Arterial arcades, 3 or 6 d. Vasa recta shorter and more numerous
5. Circular mucosal folds	Larger and more closely set	Smaller and sparse
6. Villi	Large, thick (leaf-like) and more abundant	Shorter, thinner (finger-like) and less abundant
7. Peyer's patches	Absent	Present
8. Solitary lymphatic follicles	Fewer	More numerous

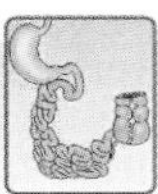

MECKEL'S DIVERTICULUM (DIVERTICULUM ILEI)

Meckel's diverticulum is the persistent proximal part of the vitellointestinal duct which is present in the embryo, and which normally disappears during the 6th week of intrauterine life. Some points of interest about it are as follows (Figs 20.16a and b).

1 It occurs in 2% subjects.
2 Usually it is 2 inches or 5 cm long.
3 It is situated about 2 feet or 60 cm proximal to the ileocaecal valve, attached to antimesenteric border of the ileum.
4 Its calibre is equal to that of the ileum.
5 Its apex may be free or may be attached to the umbilicus, to the mesentery, or to any other abdominal structure by a fibrous band.

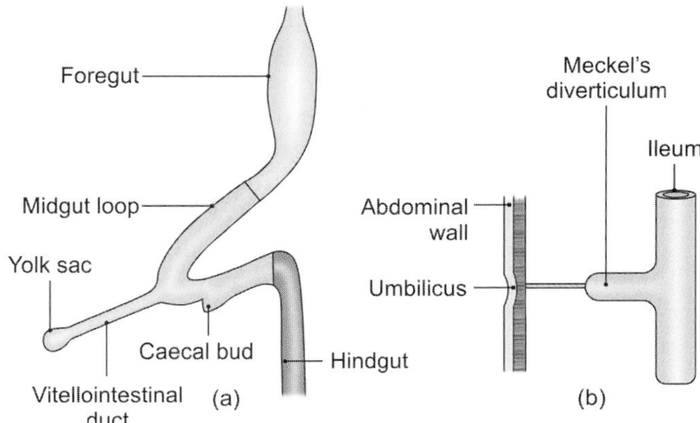

Figs 20.16a and b: Meckel's diverticulum: (a) Vitellointestinal duct in an early embryo, and (b) Meckel's diverticulum, the proximal persistent part of the vitellointestinal duct

CLINICAL ANATOMY

- Meckel's diverticulum may cause intestinal obstruction (Figs 20.16a and b).
- Occasionally it may have small regions of gastric mucosa/pancreatic tissue.
- Acute inflammation of the diverticulum may produce symptoms that resemble those of appendicitis.
- It may be involved in other diseases similar to those of the intestine.

LARGE INTESTINE

DISSECTION

Locate the various parts of large intestine, beginning from caecum, vermiform appendix, ascending, transverse, descending and sigmoid colons and ending with the rectum and anal canal. Identify the taenia, haustration and appendices epiploicae. Trace the taenia from the root of the vermiform appendix through the ascending to the transverse colon and note the change in their respective positions.

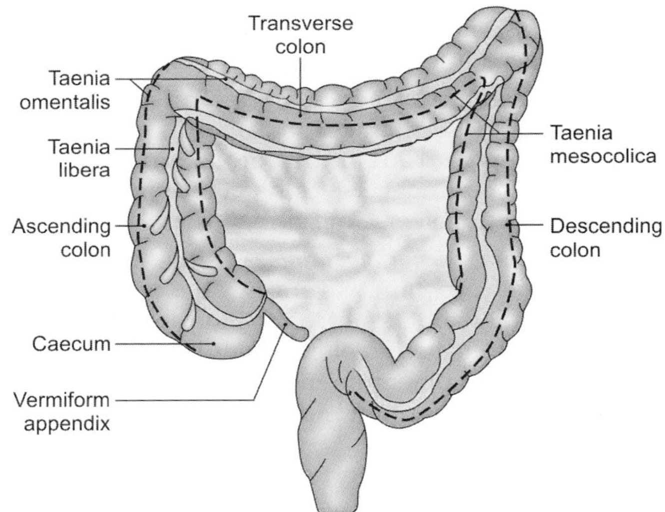

Fig. 20.17: Large intestine and the position of three taenia

Features

The large intestine extends from the ileocaecal junction to the anus. It is about blind 1.5 m long, and is divided into the caecum, (Latin *blind pouch*), the ascending colon, right colic flexure, the transverse colon, left colic flexure, the descending colon, the sigmoid colon, the rectum and the anal canal. In the angle between the caecum and the terminal part of the ileum there is a narrow diverticulum called the vermiform appendix (Latin *attachment*) (Fig. 20.17).

The general structure of large intestine is considered first followed by its parts one by one.

The structure of the large intestine is adapted for storage of matter reaching it from the small intestines, and for absorption of fluid and solutes from it. The epithelium is absorptive (columnar), but *villi are absent*. Adequate lubrication for passage of its contents is provided by numerous goblet cells scattered in the crypts as well as on the surface of the mucous membrane. The presence of numerous solitary lymphatic follicles provides protection against bacteria present in the lumen of the intestine.

Relevant Features

The relevant features of the large intestine are as follows:

1 The large intestine is *wider in calibre* than the small intestine. The calibre is greatest at its commencement, and gradually diminishes towards the rectum where it is dilated to form the rectal ampulla just above the anal canal.

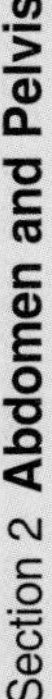

2 The greater part of the large intestine is *fixed*, except for the appendix, the transverse colon and the sigmoid colon.
3 The longitudinal muscle coat forms only a thin layer in this part of the gut. The greater part of it forms three ribbon-like bands, called the *taeniae coli*. Proximally the taeniae converge at the base of the appendix, and distally they spread out on the terminal part of the sigmoid colon to become continuous with the longitudinal muscle coat of the rectum. In the caecum, the ascending colon, the descending colon and sigmoid colon and sigmoid colon the positions of taeniae are anterior or taenia libera; posteromedial or taenia mesocolica and posterolateral or taenia omentalis but in the transverse colon the corresponding positions of taenia are inferior, posterior and superior.

   One taenia, *taenia libera,* is placed anteriorly in the caecum, ascending, descending and sigmoid colon, but is placed inferiorly in the transverse colon.

   Second taenia, *taenia mesocolica* is present on the posteromedial surface of caecum, ascending, descending and sigmoid colon, but is placed posteriorly on transverse colon at the site of attachment of the transverse mesocolon (Fig. 20.17).

   Third taenia, *taenia omentalis,* is situated posterolaterally in caecum, ascending, descending and sigmoid colon, but is situated on the anterosuperior surface of transverse colon where layers three and four of greater omentum meet the transverse colon. This change in position is due to twist in transverse colon.
4 Since the taeniae are shorter than the circular muscle coat, the colon is *puckered* and *sacculated*.
5 Small bags of peritoneum filled with fat, and called the *appendices epiploicae*, (Greek *to float on*) are scattered over the surface of the large intestine, except for the appendix, the caecum and the rectum. These are most numerous on the sides of the sigmoid colon and on the posterior surface of the transverse colon.

   The differences between the small and large intestine are summarised in Table 20.2.
6 The *blood supply* to the colon is derived from the marginal artery of Drummond. It is formed by colic branches of superior and inferior mesenteric arteries (*see* Fig. 21.11). Terminal branches from the marginal artery are distributed to the intestine as long and short vessels, *vasa longa* and *vasa brevia*. The long arteries divide into anterior and posterior branches close to the mesocolic taenia to pass between the serous and muscular coats and reach the amesocolic taeniae. They gradually pierce the muscular coat and reach the submucosa. The anastomosis between the two amesocolic taeniae is extremely poor. So longitudinal incisions should be made along this line.

Short branches arise either from the marginal artery or from the long branches, and the majority of them at once sink into the bowel wall at the mesocolic border. The short and long branches together thus provide the mesocolic region of the wall with abundant blood supply. It is only the amesocolic region which has scanty blood supply.

Subserous coat of long branches is intimately related to appendices epiploicae, to which they contribute branches. During removal of these appendages care must be taken not to pull on them in order to avoid traction on the subjacent vessel.

Bowel wall is weakened where it is pierced by the vessels and at the sites of attachment of appendices epiploicae. Mucosa may herniate in these situations

Table 20.2: Differences between the small intestine and the large intestine

Feature	*Small intestine*	*Large intestine*
1. Appendices epiploicae	Absent	Present
2. Taeniae coli	Absent	Present
3. Sacculations	Absent	Present
4. Distensibility and diameter	Less distensibility and less diameter	More distensibility and more diameter
5. Fixity	Greater part is freely mobile	Greater part is fixed
6. Villi	Present	Absent
7. Transverse mucosal folds	Permanent	Obliterated when longitudinal muscle coat relaxes
8. Peyer's patches	Present in ileum	Absent
9. Common site for	a. Intestinal worms b. Typhoid c. Tuberculosis	a. *Entamoeba histolytica* b. Dysentery organisms c. Carcinoma
10. Effects of infection and irritation	Diarrhoea	Dysentery (Greek *bad intestine*)

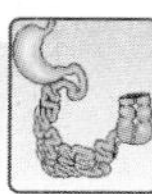

causing diverticulosis, with associated dangers of diverticulitis, fibrosis and stricture.

7 *Lymph* from the large intestine passes through four sets of lymph nodes.
   a. *Epicolic lymph nodes,* lying on the wall of the gut (Fig. 20.26).
   b. *Paracolic nodes,* on the medial side of the ascending and descending colon and near the mesocolic border of the transverse and sigmoid colon.
   c. *Intermediate nodes,* on the main branches of the vessels.
   d. *Terminal nodes,* on the superior and inferior mesenteric vessels.

   In carcinoma of the colon, the related paracolic and intermediate lymph nodes have to be removed. Their removal is possible only after the ligature of the main branch of the superior or inferior mesenteric artery along which the involved lymph nodes lie. It is necessary, therefore, to remove a large segment of the bowel than is actually required by the extent of the disease, in order to avoid gangrene as a result of interference with the blood supply. It is always wise to remove the whole portion of the bowel supplied by the ligated vessel.

8 The *nerve supply* of the large intestine, barring the lower half of the anal canal, is both sympathetic and parasympathetic. The midgut territory receives its sympathetic supply from the coeliac and superior mesenteric ganglia (T11 to L1), and its parasympathetic supply from the vagus. Both types of nerves are distributed to the gut through the superior mesenteric plexus.

The hindgut territory receives its sympathetic supply from the lumbar sympathetic chain (L1, L2), and its parasympathetic supply from the pelvic splanchnic nerve (*nervi erigentes*), both via the superior hypogastric and inferior mesenteric plexuses. Some parasympathetic fibres reach the colon along the posterior abdominal wall. The ultimate distribution of nerves in the gut is similar to that in the wall of the small intestine.

The parasympathetic nerves are motor to the large intestine and inhibitory to the internal anal sphincter. The sympathetic nerves are largely vasomotor, but also motor to the internal anal sphincter, and inhibitory to colon. Pain impulses from the gut up to the descending colon travel through the sympathetic nerves, and from the sigmoid colon and rectum through the pelvic splanchnic nerves.

Functions of Colon

The functions of the colon are as follows.

1 Lubrication of faeces by mucus.
2 Absorption of the water, salts and the other solutes.
3 Bacterial flora of colon synthesises vitamin B.
4 Mucoid secretion of colon is rich in antibodies of IgA group, which protect it from invasion by micro-organisms.
5 The microvilli (apical tufts) of some columnar cells serve a sensory function.

CLINICAL ANATOMY

- Large intestine can be directly viewed by a procedure called *colonoscopy.*
- Diverticulum is a small evagination of mucous membrane of colon at the entry point of the arteries. Its inflammation is called diverticulitis (Fig. 20.18).

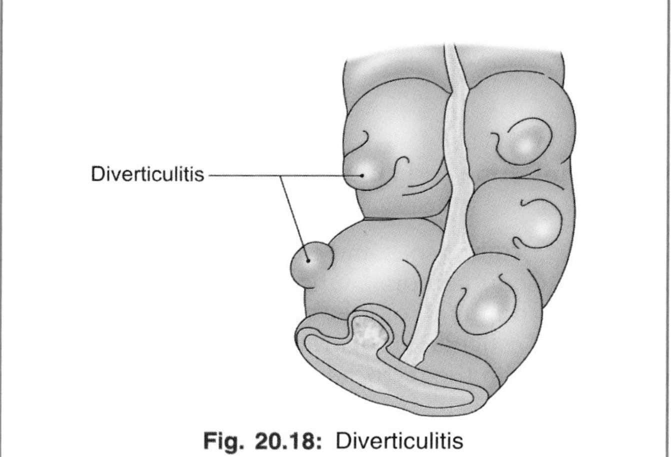

Fig. 20.18: Diverticulitis

CAECUM

DISSECTION

Turn the caecum upwards and identify its posterior relations.

Incise the lateral wall of the caecum and locate the ileocaecal orifice and its associated valve. Below the ileocaecal valve identify the orifice of the vermiform appendix.

Features

Caecum is a large blind sac (Latin *blind*) forming the commencement of the large intestine. It is situated in the right iliac fossa, above the lateral half of inguinal ligament. It communicates superiorly with ascending colon, medially at the level of caecocolic junction with ileum, and posteromedially with the appendix (Fig. 20.19).

Dimensions

It is 6 cm long and 7.5 cm broad. It is one of those organs of the body that have greater width than the length. The other examples are the prostate, pons and pituitary.

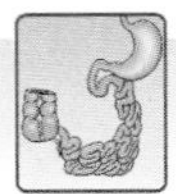

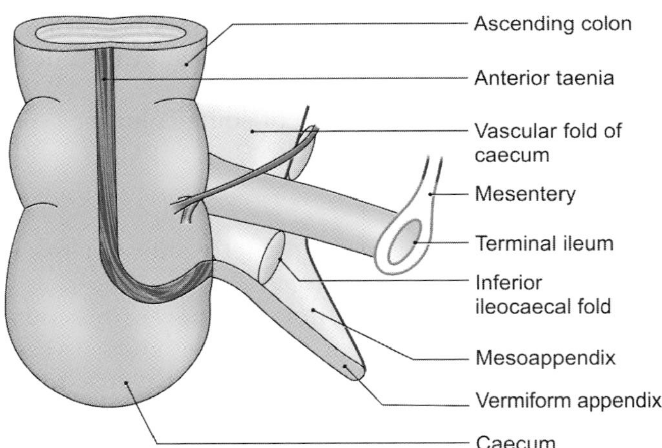

Fig. 20.19: Anterior view of the ileocaecal region

Relations

Anterior

Coils of intestine and anterior abdominal wall.

Posterior

1. *Muscles:* Right psoas and iliacus (Fig. 20.20).
2. *Nerves:* Genitofemoral, femoral and lateral cutaneous nerve of thigh (all of the right side).
3. *Vessels:* Testicular or ovarian.
4. Appendix in the retrocaecal recess.

Vessels and Nerves

The arterial supply of the caecum is derived from the caecal branches of the ileocolic artery. The veins drain into the superior mesenteric vein. The nerve supply is same as that of the midgut (thoracic 11 to lumbar 1; parasympathetic, vagus).

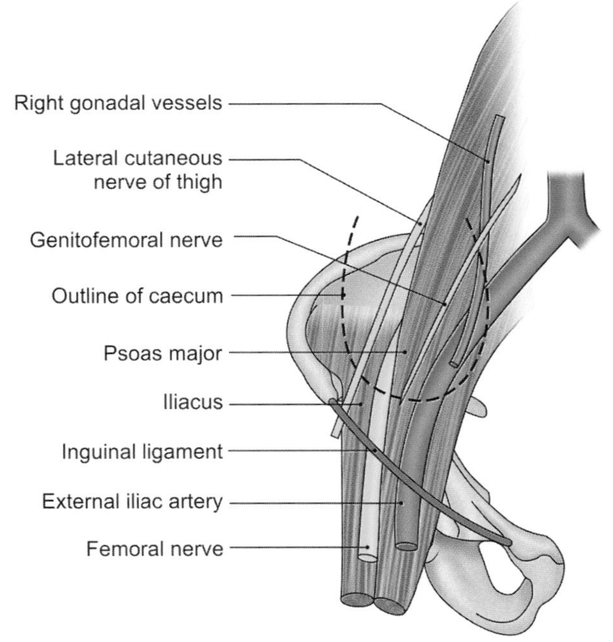

Fig. 20.20: Relations of caecum

DEVELOPMENT

The caecum and appendix develop from the caecal bud arising from the *postarterial segment* of the midgut loop. The proximal part of the bud dilates to form the caecum. The distal part remains narrow to form the appendix. Thus initially the appendix arises from the apex of the caecum. However, due to rapid growth of the lateral wall of the caecum, the attachment of the appendix shifts medially (Fig. 20.21).

ILEOCAECAL VALVE

The lower end of the ileum opens on the posteromedial aspect of the caecocolic junction. The ileocaecal opening is guarded by the ileocaecal valve (Fig. 20.22).

Structure

The valve has two lips and two frenula.

1. The *upper lip* is horizontal and lies at the ileocolic junction.

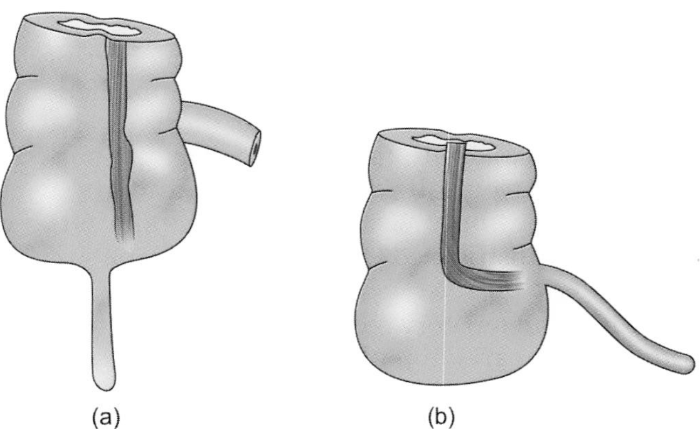

Figs 20.21a and b: Development of the caecum: (a) Early stage, and (b) later stage

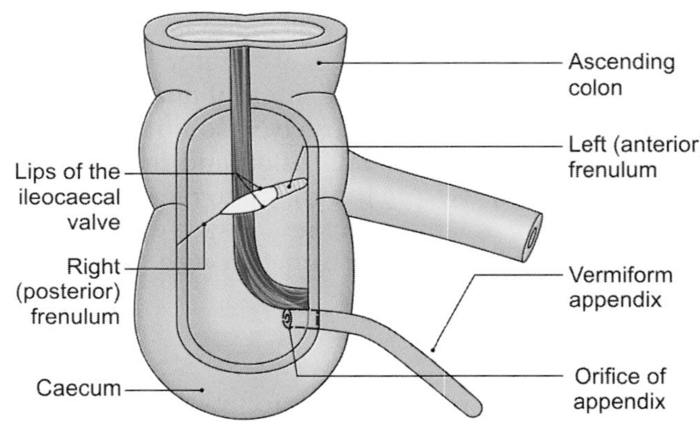

Fig. 20.22: The ileocaecal valve seen after removal of the anterior walls of the caecum and of the lower part of the ascending colon

it becomes the rectum. It forms a sinuous loop, and hangs down in pelvis over the bladder and uterus. Occasionally, it is very short, and takes a straight course. It is suspended by the sigmoid mesocolon and is covered by coils of small intestine.

The rectum and the anal canal are described later.

HISTOLOGY OF COLON

Mucous Membrane

It shows only invagination to form deep crypts of Lieberkuhn. Lining epithelium is of columnar cells with intervening goblet cells. Muscularis mucosae is well defined.

Submucosa

Contains solitary lymphoid follicles with the Meissner's plexus of nerves.

Muscularis Externa

Outer longitudinal coat is thickened at three places to form taenia coli. Inner coat is of circular fibres. *Outermost layer* is serous/adventitia.

DEVELOPMENT

Duodenum

During rotation of stomach, the C-shaped duodenum falls to the right. At the same time it lies against posterior abdominal wall and gets retroperitoneal. Duodenum develops partly from foregut and partly from midgut. Till the origin of hepatic bud it develops from foregut, i.e. first and upper half of second part. The remaining two and a half parts arise from midgut.

Duodenum is supplied both by branches of coeliac axis (artery of foregut) and by branches of superior mesenteric artery (artery of midgut).

Midgut

It gives rise to the part of duodenum distal to the opening of bile duct, jejunum, ileum, caecum, vermiform appendix, ascending colon, hepatic flexure and right two-thirds of transverse colon.

Midgut is in the form of primary intestinal loop. At the apex of the loop it is connected to the yolk sac and grows very rapidly during 6th week, so much so that it protrudes into the umbilical cord. This is called *physiological herniation*. After an interval of 4 weeks, i.e. at 10th week it returns back into the enlarged abdominal cavity. During this herniation and return the midgut loop rotates by 270° in a counter clockwise direction.

Hindgut

Its cranial part gives rise to left one-third of transverse colon, descending colon, pelvic colon, proximal part of rectum. The distal part of hindgut is dilated to form the cloaca, which gets separated by urorectal septum into a posterior part—the anorectal canal and an anterior part—the primitive urogenital sinus. The anorectal canal forms distal part of rectum and proximal part of anal canal. Distal or terminal part of anal canal is formed from an invagination of surface ectoderm called the proctodeum.

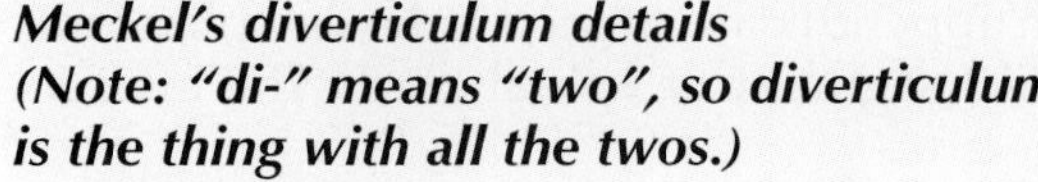

Mnemonics

Meckel's diverticulum details
(Note: "di-" means "two", so diverticulum is the thing with all the twos.)

2 inches long
2 feet from end of ileum
2 times more common in men
2% occurrence in population
2 types of tissues may be present

FACTS TO REMEMBER

- Small intestine is characterized by the evaginations called the *villi*.
- Most of the duodenum is fixed and retroperitoneal
- 2nd part of duodenum contains the openings of bile and pancreatic ducts
- 3rd part of duodenum is crossed anteriorly by superior mesenteric vessels
- Duodenal cap is triangular shadow of its first part seen in Ba meal (X-ray). Transverse colon is the most mobile part of large intestine.
- Meckel's diverticulum is the proximal persistent part of vitellointestinal duct.
- Caecum is broader than longer.
- The commonest position of vermiform appendix is retrocaecal.
- Pain of early appendicitis is referred to the region of umbilicus. The visceral peritoneum of appendix receives supply from lesser splanchnic nerve, arising from T10 sympathetic ganglion and T10 segment of spinal cord. Same segment receives sensation from the umbilical area. Later appendicitis pain is localized to right iliac fossa.
- McBurney's point is a point at the junction of medial 2/3rd and lateral 1/3rd of a line joining umbilicus to the right anterior superior iliac spine.
- Ileocaecal junction is the commonest site of TB of intestines.
- Cancer of colon mostly occurs at rectosigmoid junction.

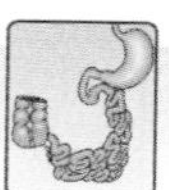

CLINICOANATOMICAL PROBLEM

A young male felt pain in the region of umbilicus. He also had nausea, temperature and increased pulse rate with leucocytosis. Later on the pain was localised in right iliac fossa.

- Discuss the referred pain of appendicitis?
- Where is his appendix likely to be located?
- What is McBurney's point?

Ans: Initially the pain of acute appendicitis is referred to the skin in the region of umbilicus. Afferent nerve fibres from appendix are carried in lesser splanchnic nerve to T10 segment of spinal cord. The afferent impulses from the skin of umbilicus also reach T10 segment through 10th intercostal nerve. Since both the somatic and visceral impulses reach the same segment, and somatic impulses being appreciated better by brain, the pain is referred to the skin of the umbilicus. The most common position of appendix is retrocaecal, and since the patient's pain is in right iliac fossa, the position of the appendix is likely to be retrocaecal.

McBurney's point lies at the junction of lateral one-third and medial two-thirds of a line joining anterior superior iliac spine to the umbilicus.

MULTIPLE CHOICE QUESTIONS

1. Which of the following is not a characteristic feature of large intestine?
a. Sacculations b. Villi
c. Taenia coli d. Appendices epiploicae

2. Which of the following is true about Meckel's diverticulum?
a. Length is about 5 cm
b. Occurs in 2% subjects
c. 2 feet proximal to ileocaecal value
d. Attached to mesenteric border of the ileum

3. Peyer's patches are present in:
a. Duodenum b. Jejunum
c. Ileum d. Transverse colon

4. Appendices epiploicae are seen in:
a. Stomach b. Ileum
c. Duodenum d. Colon

5. False fact regarding vermiform appendix is:
a. Is covered by peritoneum
b. Commonest site is retrocaecal
c. Supplied by appendicular artery
d. Superior to caecum

6. Most common position of vermiform appendix is:
a. Pelvic b. Retrocaecal
c. Preileal d. Postileal

7. First 2.5 cm of 1st part of duodenum is not supplied by:
a. Superior pancreaticoduodenal artery
b. Right gastroepiploic artery
c. Right gastric artery
d. Hepatic artery

8. Meckel's diverticulum is a remnant of:
a. Mullerian duct b. Wolfian duct
c. Mesonephric duct d. Vitellointestinal duct

9. Mesentery of small intestine crosses following structures *except*:
a. Inferior vena cava
b. Right psoas major
c. Abdominal aorta
d. Right kidney

10. Which part of intestine contains Brunner's glands?
a. Ileum b. Duodenum
c. Jejunum d. Colon

ANSWERS

1. b **2.** d **3.** c **4.** d **5.** d **6.** b **7.** d **8.** d **9.** d **10.** b

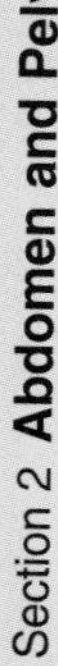

21

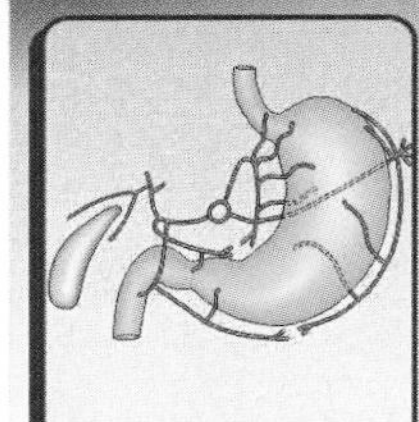

Large Blood Vessels of the Gut

Give me blood, I will give you Azadi
—Netaji Subhash Chandra Bose

INTRODUCTION

The three ventral branches of the abdominal aorta are coeliac trunk, superior mesenteric and inferior mesenteric arteries. These are the arteries of the foregut, midgut and hindgut, respectively. There is anastomoses between the branches of these three main arteries.

In this chapter the coeliac trunk, the superior and inferior mesenteric vessels, and the portal vein will be studied.

BLOOD VESSELS

DISSECTION

Identify the short trunk of coeliac axis artery at the level of the intervertebral disc between T12 and L1 vertebrae arising from the aorta. Dissect its relations especially with the coeliac ganglion and identify its three branches and their further divisions.

Clean the superior mesenteric vessels with its branches both from its right and left surfaces. Dissect these branches and trace them till the organs of their supply.

Identify the inferior mesenteric artery arising at the L3 vertebra. Trace its course and branches.

Identify the large portal vein formed by the union of superior mesenteric and splenic vein posterior to the neck of pancreas. Trace it upwards towards the remains of free margin of lesser omentum till the porta hepatis where it divides into two branches. Identify the veins taking part in portosystemic anastomoses.

COELIAC TRUNK

The coeliac trunk is the artery of the foregut (Figs 21.1 and 21.2). It supplies all derivatives of the foregut that lie in the abdomen namely:

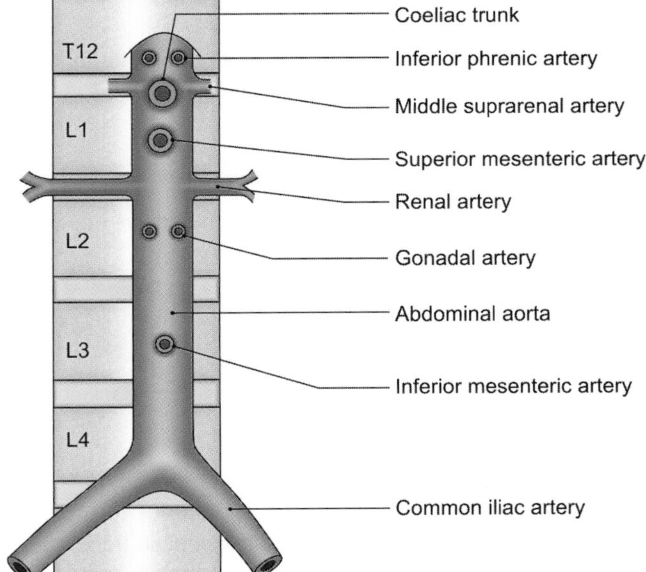

Fig. 21.1: Ventral and lateral branches of the abdominal aorta with their levels of origin

1. The lower end of the oesophagus, the stomach and upper part of the duodenum up to the opening of the bile duct.
2. Liver
3. Spleen
4. Greater part of the pancreas.

Origin and Length

The coeliac trunk arises from the front of the abdominal aorta just below the aortic opening of the diaphragm at the level of the disc between thoracic twelve and first lumbar vertebrae . The trunk is only about 1.25 cm long. It ends by dividing into its three terminal branches, namely the left gastric, common hepatic and splenic arteries (Figs 21.3 to 21.5).

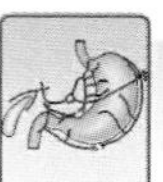

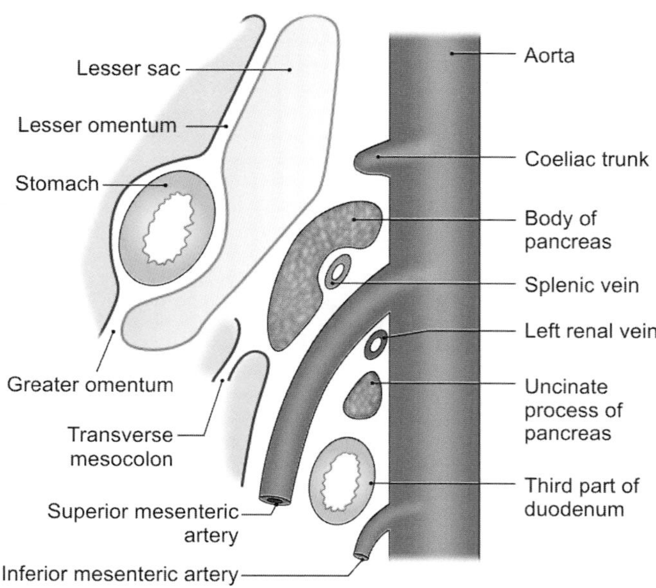

Fig. 21.2: Left view of a sagittal section through the abdominal aorta showing the origin of its three ventral branches

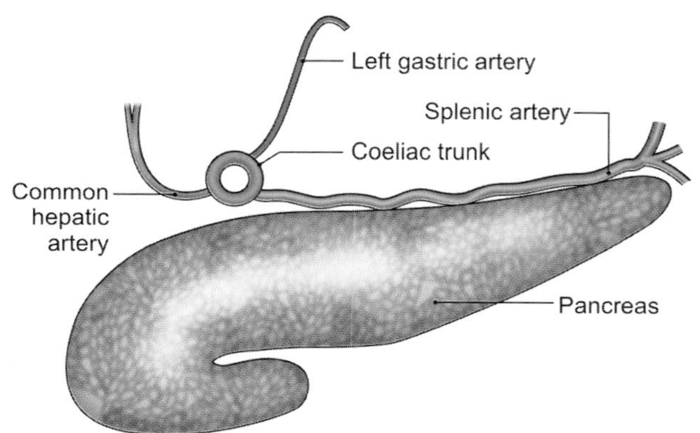

Fig. 21.3: Three branches of the coeliac trunk

Relations

1 It is surrounded by the coeliac plexus of nerves (*see* Fig. 27.6).
2 Anteriorly, it is related to the lesser sac and to the lesser omentum (Fig. 21.2).
3 To its right, there are the right crus of the diaphragm, the right coeliac ganglion and the caudate process of the liver.
4 To its left, there are the left crus of the diaphragm, the left coeliac ganglion and the cardiac end of the stomach.
5 Inferiorly, it is related to the body of the pancreas and to the splenic vein (Fig. 21.2).

Branches

Left Gastric Artery

The *left gastric artery* is the smallest of the three branches of the coeliac trunk. It runs upwards to the left behind the lesser sac to reach the cardiac end of the stomach where it turns forwards and enters the lesser omentum to run downwards along the lesser curvature of the stomach. It ends by anastomosing with the right gastric artery.

It gives off:

a. Two or three *oesophageal branches* at the cardiac end of the stomach.
b. Numerous *gastric branches* along the lesser curvature of the stomach (Fig. 21.4).

Common Hepatic Artery

The *common hepatic artery* runs downwards, forwards and to the right, behind the lesser sac to reach the upper border of the duodenum. Here it enters the lesser omentum. It then run upwards as proper hepatic artery in the right free margin of the lesser omentum, in front of the portal vein, and to the left of the bile duct (*see* Figs 18.10 and 21.3). Reaching the porta hepatis it terminates by dividing into right and left hepatic branches.

Branches

1 The *gastroduodenal artery* is a large branch which arises at the upper border of the first part of the duodenum. The part of the hepatic artery till the origin of the gastroduodenal artery is called the *common hepatic artery*. The part distal to it is the *proper hepatic artery*.

The gastroduodenal artery runs downwards behind the first part of the duodenum and divides at its lower border into the right gastroepiploic and superior pancreaticoduodenal arteries.

The *right gastroepiploic artery* enters the greater omentum, follows the greater curvature of the stomach, and anastomoses with the left gastro-epiploic artery.

The *superior pancreaticoduodenal artery* (often represented by two arteries anterior and posterior) runs downwards in the pancreaticoduodenal groove, and ends by anastomosing with the inferior pancreaticoduodenal artery, a branch of the superior mesenteric.

2 The *right gastric artery* is a small branch which arises from the proper hepatic artery close to the gastroduodenal artery. It runs to the left along the lesser curvature and ends by anastomosing with the left gastric artery.

3 The *cystic artery* is a branch of the right hepatic artery. It passes behind the common hepatic and cystic ducts to reach the upper surface of the neck of the gall bladder where it divides into superficial and deep branches for the inferior and superior surfaces of the gallbladder, respectively.

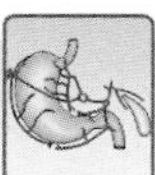

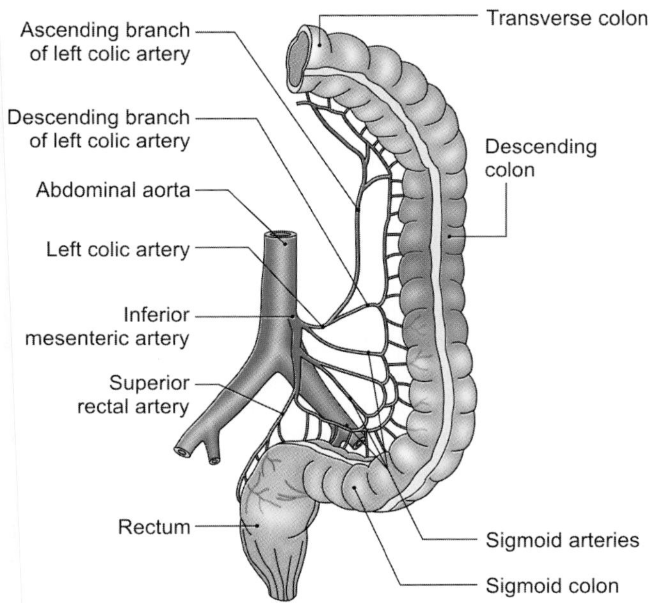

Fig. 21.10: Branches of the inferior mesenteric artery

other to form the lower part of the marginal artery. The uppermost branch anastomoses with the descending branch of the left colic artery, whereas the lowest sigmoid artery sends a branch to anastomose with the superior rectal artery. They supply the descending colon in the iliac fossa and the sigmoid colon.

Superior Rectal Artery

Superior rectal artery is the continuation of the inferior mesenteric artery beyond the root of the sigmoid mesocolon, i.e. over the left common iliac vessels. It descends in the sigmoid mesocolon to reach the rectum. Opposite third sacral vertebra it divides into right and left branches which descend one on each side of the rectum. They pierce the muscular coat of the rectum and divide into several branches, which anastomose with one another at the level of the anal sphincter to form loops around the lower end of the rectum. These branches communicate with the middle and inferior rectal arteries in the submucosa of the anal canal (Figs 21.10 and 21.16).

INFERIOR MESENTERIC VEIN

1 The inferior mesenteric vein drains blood from the rectum, the anal canal, the sigmoid colon and the descending colon.

2 It begins as the *superior rectal vein* from the upper part of the internal rectal venous plexus. In the plexus it communicates with the middle and inferior rectal veins. The superior rectal vein crosses the left common iliac vessels medial to the left ureter and continues upwards as the inferior mesenteric vein. This vein lies lateral to the inferior mesenteric artery. The vein ascends behind the peritoneum, passes lateral to the duodenojejunal flexure and behind the body of the pancreas. It opens into the splenic vein (Fig. 21.9).

3 Its *tributaries* correspond to the branches of the inferior mesenteric artery.

CLINICAL ANATOMY

Inferior mesenteric vein lies in the free margin of paraduodenal fold before draining into splenic vein. In case of strangulated internal hernia in duodenojejunal recess these folds may be cut to enlarge the space. One needs to remember that inferior mesenteric vein (not the artery) lies in the fold, and it needs to be ligated (*see* Fig. 18.32).

MARGINAL ARTERY OF DRUMMOND

Marginal artery was described by von Haller in 1803 and its present name was given by Sudeck in 1907. The marginal artery is an arterial arcade situated along the concavity of the colon. It is formed by anastomoses between the main arteries supplying the colon, namely the ileocolic, right colic, middle colic, left colic and sigmoid arteries. It lies at a distance of 2.5 to 3.8 cm from the colon. It is closest to the colon in its descending and sigmoid parts. Vasa recta arise from the marginal artery and supply the colon (Fig. 21.11).

The marginal artery is capable of supplying the colon even in the absence of one of the main feeding trunks. This fact is utilized in surgery. However, at the junctional points between the main vessels, there may be variations in the competence of the anastomoses.

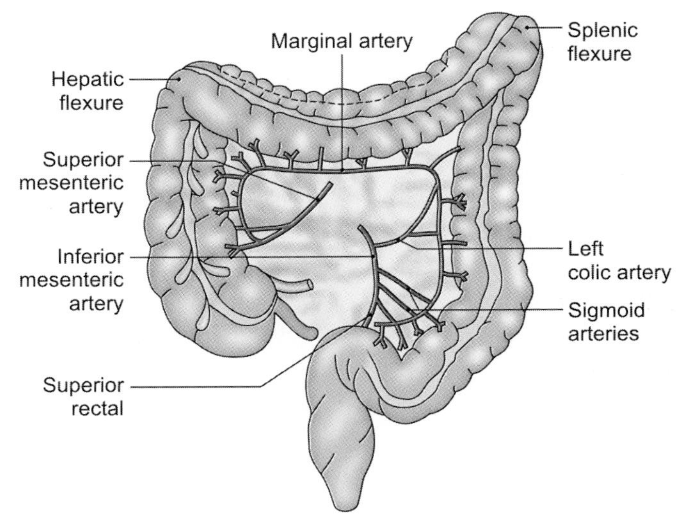

Fig. 21.11: The marginal artery

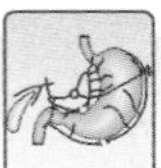

PORTAL VEIN

Portal vein is a large vein which collects blood from:

1 The abdominal part of the alimentary tract
2 The gallbladder
3 The pancreas
4 The spleen, and conveys it to the liver. In the liver, the portal vein breaks up into sinusoids which are drained by the hepatic veins to the inferior vena cava (Figs 21.12 and 21.13).

It is called the portal vein because its main tributary, the superior mesenteric vein, begins in one set of capillaries (in the gut) and the portal vein ends in another set of capillaries in the liver.

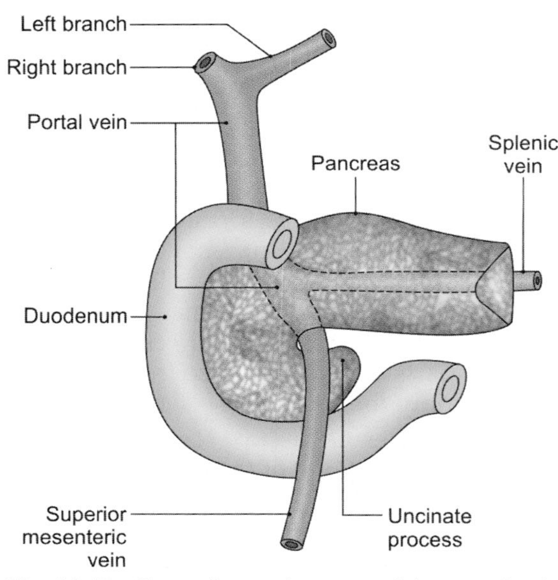

Fig. 21.12: Formation and course of the portal vein

Formation

The portal vein is about 8 cm long. It is formed by the union of the superior mesenteric and splenic veins behind the neck of the pancreas at the level of second lumbar vertebra. Inferior mesenteric vein drains into splenic vein.

Course

It runs upwards and a little to the right, first behind the neck of the pancreas, next behind the first part of the duodenum, and lastly in the right free margin of the lesser omentum.

The blood flow in portal vein is slow. Blood of superior mesenteric vein drains into right lobe. Blood of splenic and inferior mesenteric vein drains into left lobe. This is called "streamline flow".

The portal vein can thus be divided into infraduodenal, retroduodenal and supraduodenal parts.

Termination

The vein ends at the right end of the porta hepatis by dividing into right and left branches which enter the liver.

Relations

Infraduodenal Part

Anteriorly: Neck of pancreas.

Posteriorly: Inferior vena cava (*see* Figs 20.8a and 21.14).

Retroduodenal Part

Anteriorly

1 First part of duodenum
2 Bile duct
3 Gastroduodenal artery.

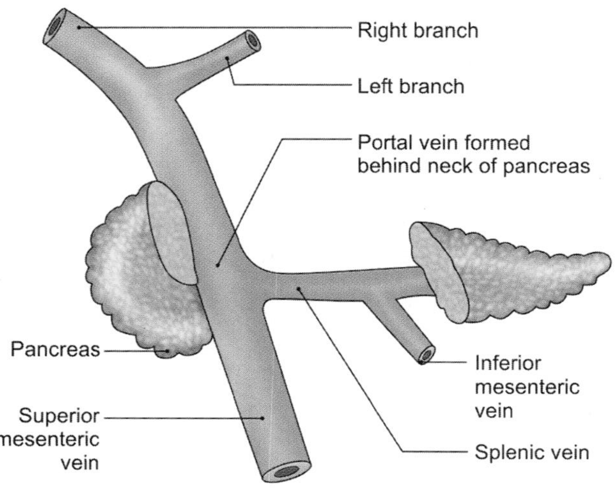

Fig. 21.13: Formation of portal vein

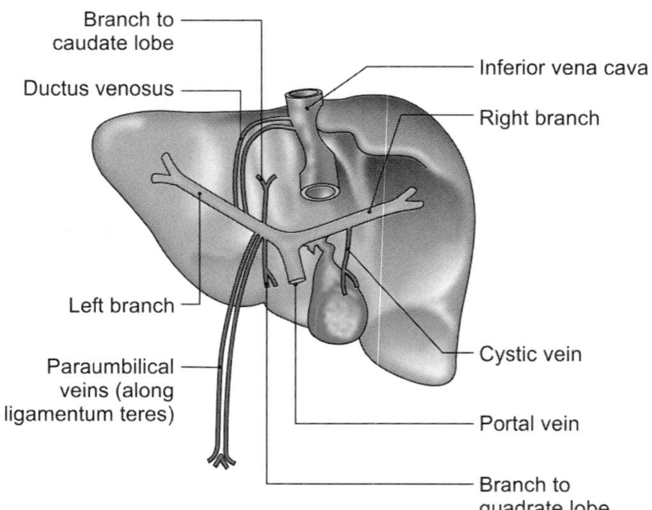

Fig. 21.14: The portal vein, its communications and branches

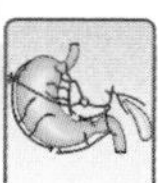

Posteriorly
Inferior vena cava (*see* Fig. 20.8b).

Supraduodenal Part

Anteriorly
1 Hepatic artery
2 Bile duct (within free margin of the lesser omentum).

Posteriorly
Inferior vena cava, separated by epiploic foramen (*see* Fig. 18.10).

Intrahepatic Course

After entering the liver, each branch divides and redivides along with the hepatic artery to end ultimately in the hepatic sinusoids, where the portal venous blood mixes with the hepatic arterial blood.

Branches

1 The *right branch* is shorter and wider than the left branch. After receiving the cystic vein, it enters the right lobe of the liver (Fig. 21.16).
2 The left branch is longer and narrower than the right branch. It traverses the porta hepatis from its right end to the left end, and furnishes branches to the caudate and quadrate lobes. Just before entering the left lobe of the liver, it receives:
   a. Paraumbilical veins along the ligamentum teres.
   b. Ligamentum venosum.

Tributaries

Portal vein receives the following veins.
1 Left gastric
2 Right gastric (Fig. 21.15)
3 Superior pancreaticoduodenal
4 Cystic vein in its right branch
5 Paraumbilical veins in its left branch

The left gastric vein accompanies the corresponding artery. At the cardiac end of the stomach it receives a few oesophageal veins. The right gastric vein accompanies the corresponding artery. It receives the prepyloric vein.

The paraumbilical veins are small veins that run in the falciform ligament, along the ligamentum teres, and establish anastomoses between the veins of the anterior abdominal wall present around the umbilicus and the portal vein (Fig. 21.16).

PORTOSYSTEMIC COMMUNICATIONS (PORTOCAVAL ANASTOMOSES)

These communications form important routes of collateral circulation in portal obstruction. The tributaries of portal and systemic system are put in Table 21.1. Various sites of portosystemic anastomoses are put in Table 21.2 and Fig. 21.17.

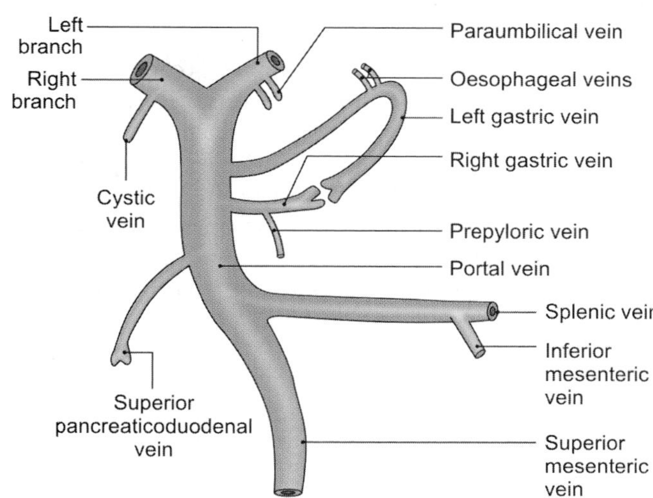

Fig. 21.15: Tributaries of the portal vein

CLINICAL ANATOMY

- *Portal pressure:* Normal pressure in the portal vein is about 5–15 mm Hg. It is usually measured by splenic puncture and recording the intrasplenic pressure.
- *Portal hypertension* (pressure above 40 mm Hg): It can be caused by the following.
  a. Cirrhosis of liver, in which the vascular bed of liver is markedly obliterated.
  b. Banti's disease
  c. Thrombosis of portal vein.

  The effects of portal hypertension are as follows.
  a. Congestive splenomegaly
  b. Ascites
  c. Collateral circulation through the portosystemic communications. It forms
     i. Caput medusae around the umbilicus, which is of diagnostic value to the clinician (*see* Fig. 16.5b).
     ii. Oesophageal varices at the lower end of oesophagus which may rupture and cause dangerous or even fatal haematemesis (*see* Fig. 19.4).
     iii. Haemorrhoids in the anal canal may be responsible for repeated bleeding felt per rectum (*see* Fig. 33.9).

  In cases of cirrhosis of liver, sometimes a shunt operation is done, where one of the main portal channels (splenic, superior mesenteric, or portal vein) is directly anastomosed with either inferior vena cava or the left renal vein (Fig. 21.18).
- Since the blood flow in portal vein is slow, and streamlined, the toxic infective substances absorbed from small intestine pass via the superior mesenteric vein into the right lobe of liver leading

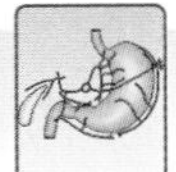

to toxic changes or amoebic abscess in right lobe. The blood lacking in amino acids, etc. which is absorbed via the inferior mesenteric vein affect the left lobe, leading to its fibrosis or cirrhosis (Fig. 21.19).

- The lower end oesophagus is one of the sites of portocaval anastomoses. Some oesophageal veins drain into left gastric vein and then into portal vein. Other oesophageal veins drain into hemiazygos and then into vena azygos and superior vena cava. In liver cirrhosis portal vein pressure is raised, leading to oesophageal varices, which may rupture leading to haematemesis (*see* Fig. 19.4).

DEVELOPMENT

Portal vein develops from the following sources.

1 Infraduodenal part, from a part of the left vitelline vein distal to the dorsal anastomosis.
2 Retroduodenal part, from the dorsal anastomosis between the two vitelline veins.
3 Supraduodenal part, from the cranial part of the right vitelline vein.

FACTS TO REMEMBER

- Coeliac trunk is the first short unpaired ventral visceral branch of the abdominal aorta which supplies structures derived from the foregut.
- Superior mesenteric and inferior mesenteric arteries supply structures derived from midgut and hindgut respectively.
- Inferior mesenteric vein lies in the free margin of paraduodenal recess and is not accompanied by its artery in this region.
- Branches of portal vein anastomose with the branches of systemic circulation at few places.
- Portal vein supplies 80% blood to liver, while hepatic artery gives 20%.

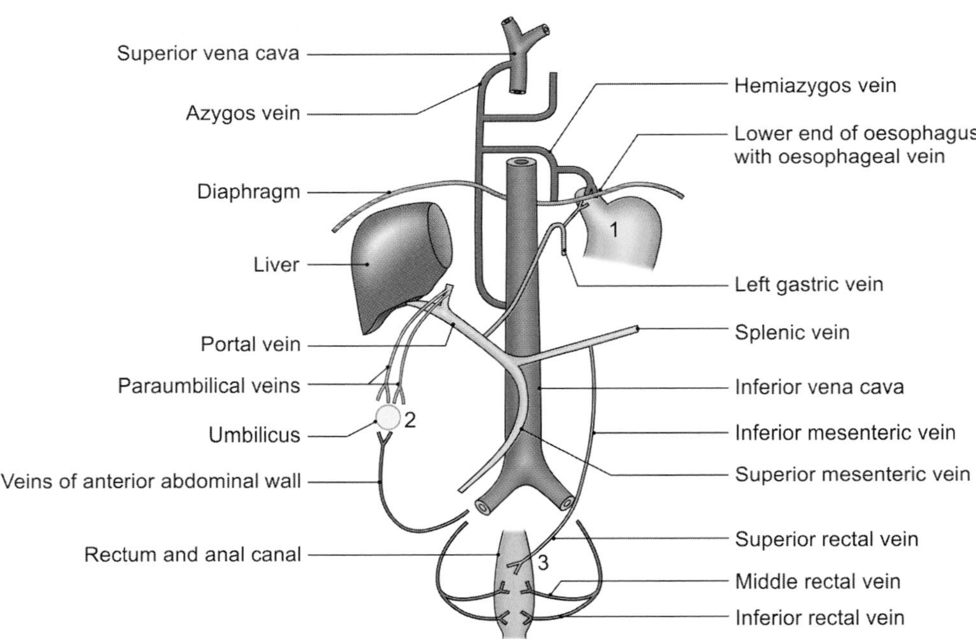

Fig. 21.16: Important sites of communication of portal and systemic veins: (1) Lower end of oesophagus, (2) around umbilicus, and (3) anal canal

Table 21.1: Tributaries of portal and systemic system

S.no.	*Tributaries*	*Clinical conditions*
1. Abdominal part of oesophagus	Some oesophageal veins drain via left gastric vein into the portal vein. Some oesophageal veins drain into hemiazygos →vena azygos →superior vena cava.	In liver cirrhosis, these tributaries anastomose, giving rise to *oesophageal varices*. These varices my rupture to cause haematemesis (*see* Fig. 19.4).

(Contd...)

Table 21.1: Tributaries of portal and systemic system *(Contd...)*

S.no.	*Tributaries*	*Clinical conditions*
2. Umbilicus	Few paraumbilical veins run along ligamentum teres and left branch of portal vein (Fig. 21.16). Veins around umbilicus drain via superior and inferior epigastric veins into superior and inferior vena cava respectively.	In liver cirrhosis the paraumbilical veins open up to transfer portal venous blood into systemic circulation. It result in caput medusae (*see* Fig. 16.5b)
3. Anal canal	Superior rectal vein continues up as inferior mesenteric vein which drains into portal vein. The middle and inferior rectal veins drain into inferior vena cava (Figs 21.16 and 21.17).	Liver cirrhosis causes anastomoses between superior rectal and other rectal veins. These anastomosing veins result in piles or haemorrhoids
4. Bare area of liver	Central veins and sublobular veins are part of portal circulation. Intercostal veins and phrenic veins end in systemic circulation.	There is some anastomoses between portal vein and systemic veins. No significance.
5. Veins of ascending and descending colon	Veins of colon end in the portal circulation. Veins of posterior abdominal wall end up in systemic veins	There is some anastomoses between these 2 sets of tributaries. These may get injured in procedures done in these areas
6. Patent ductus venosus of liver	It joins left branch of portal vein to inferior vena cava.	It may be accompanied by other congenital anomalies.

Table 21.2: Sites of portocaval/portosystemic anastomoses

S.no Position	*Portal vein*	*Systemic vein*
1. Lower end of oesophagus	Left gastric	Oesophageal veins
2. Lower end of rectum	Superior rectal	Middle and inferior rectal veins
3. Umbilicus	Paraumbilical	Above – Superior epigastric lateral thoracic Below – Superficial epigastric inferior epigastric Sides – Posterior intercostal and lumbar
4. Posterior abdominal wall	Splenic	Left renal vein
5. Bare area of liver	Portal radicles	Diaphragmatic
6. Falciform ligament	Paraumbilical	Diaphragmatic
7. Ligamentum venosum	Left branch of portal	Inferior vena cava

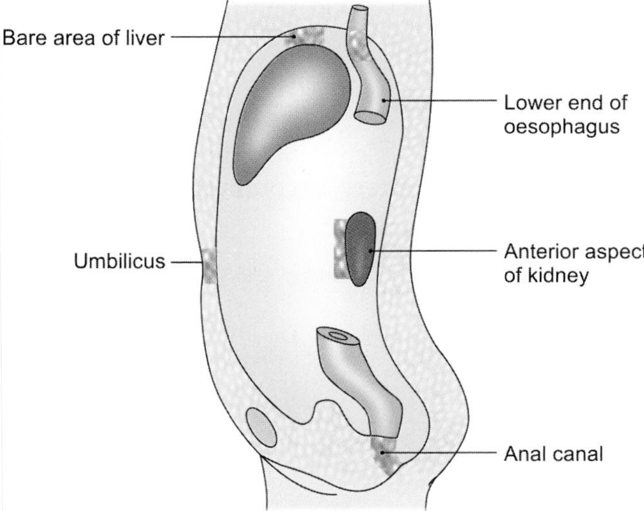

Fig. 21.17: Sites of portosystemic anastomoses

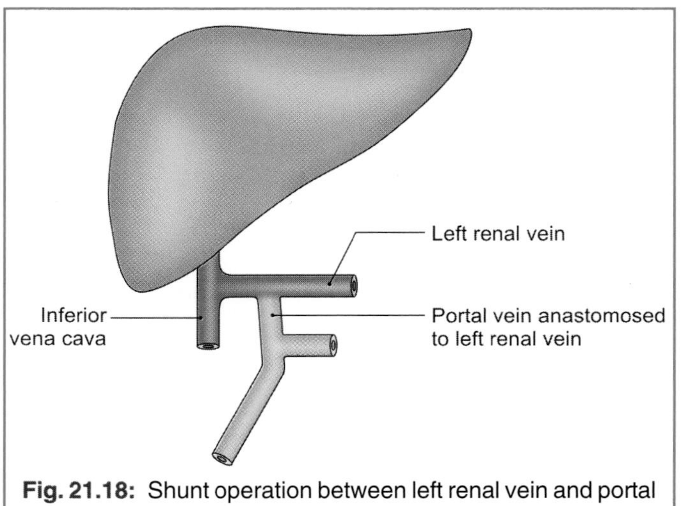

Fig. 21.18: Shunt operation between left renal vein and portal vein

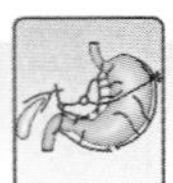

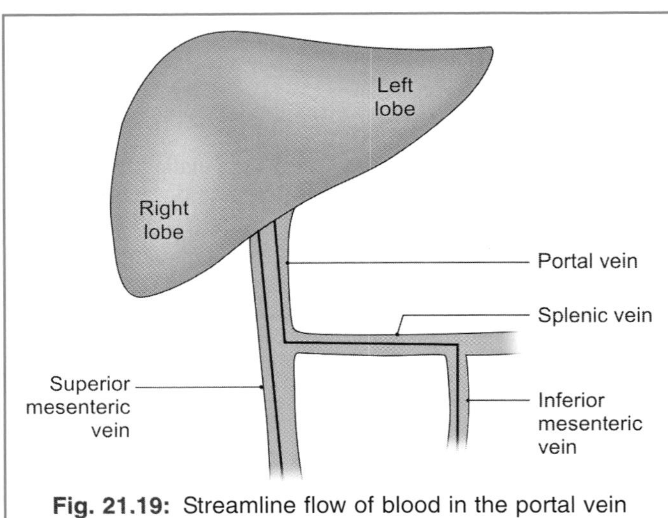

Fig. 21.19: Streamline flow of blood in the portal vein

CLINICOANATOMICAL PROBLEM

A middle aged alcoholic patient complained of lot of blood in his vomit.

- What causes haematemesis?

Ans: The lower end of oesophagus is one of the sites of portocaval anastomoses. Some oesophageal veins drain into left gastric vein and then into portal vein. Other oesophageal veins drain into hemiazygos and then into vena azygos and superior vena cava.

In liver cirrhosis, portal vein pressure is raised, leading to oesophageal varices, which may rupture leading to blood in the vomit.

Normally the anastomoses between tributaries of portal vein and those of superior vena cava is very little. These anastomotic channels develop in an attempt to take portal blood into caval blood.

MULTIPLE CHOICE QUESTIONS

1. Inferior mesenteric vein opens into:
a. Portal vein b. Inferior vena cava
c. Splenic vein d. Superior mesenteric vein

2. Which of the following is not a direct branch of coeliac trunk?
a. Left gastric
b. Common hepatic
c. Splenic
d. Inferior pancreaticoduodenal

3. Cystic artery is a branch of:
a. Right hepatic b. Left hepatic
c. Coeliac trunk d. Common hepatic

4. Jejunal and ileal branches for small intestine arise from:
a. Coeliac trunk
b. Superior mesenteric artery
c. Inferior mesenteric artery
d. Abdominal aorta

5. Appendicular artery is a branch of:
a. Middle colic b. Right colic
c. Ileocolic d. Left colic

6. Portal vein is formed by union of which veins?
a. Union of inferior mesenteric and splenic
b. Union of superior mesenteric and splenic
c. Superior mesenteric and inferior mesenteric
d. Splenic, superior mesenteric and inferior mesenteric

7. Ligamentum venosum is attached to which vein?
a. Right branch of portal
b. Left branch of portal
c. Both the branches of portal
d. None of the above

8. Portocaval anastomoses occurs at the following sites *except*:
a. Umbilicus
b. Lower end of oesophagus
c. Stomach
d. The bare area of liver

9. Hepatic flexure is supplied by which artery?
a. Ileocolic
b. Middle colic
c. Right colic
d. Jejunal branches

10. Superior rectal artery is continuation of:
a. Superior mesenteric
b. Coeliac trunk
c. Inferior mesenteric
d. Abdominal aorta

ANSWERS

1. c **2.** d **3.** a **4.** b **5.** c **6.** b **7.** b **8.** c **9.** c **10.** c

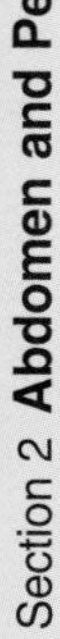

22

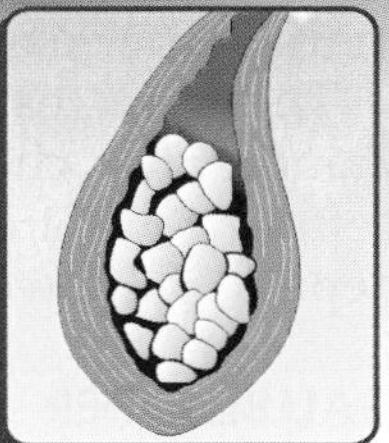

Extrahepatic Biliary Apparatus

Gallstones if threaded would make a beautiful emerald necklace

INTRODUCTION

The extrahepatic biliary apparatus collects bile from the liver, stores it in the gallbladder, and transmits it to the 2nd part of duodenum.

The apparatus consists of:

a. Right and left hepatic ducts,
b. Common hepatic duct,
c. Gallbladder,
d. Cystic duct, and
e. Bile duct (Fig. 22.1).

HEPATIC DUCTS

DISSECTION

Locate the porta hepatis on the inferior surface of liver. Look for two hepatic ducts there. Follow them till these join to form common hepatic duct. Identify cystic duct and usually green-coloured gallbladder.

See the point of junction of cystic duct with common hepatic duct and the formation of bile duct. Trace the bile duct in relation to the duodenum. Its opening has been seen in dissection of the duodenum.

Trace the cystic artery supplying gallbladder, cystic duct, hepatic ducts and upper part of bile duct.

RIGHT AND LEFT HEPATIC DUCTS

The right and left hepatic ducts emerge at the porta hepatis from the right and left lobes of the liver. The arrangement of structures at the porta hepatis from behind forwards is:

1 Branches of the portal vein,
2 Proper hepatic artery, and
3 Hepatic ducts (Fig. 22.2).

COMMON HEPATIC DUCT

It is formed by the union of the right and left hepatic ducts near the right end of the porta hepatis. It runs downwards for about 3 cm and is joined on its right side at an acute angle by the cystic duct to form the bile duct.

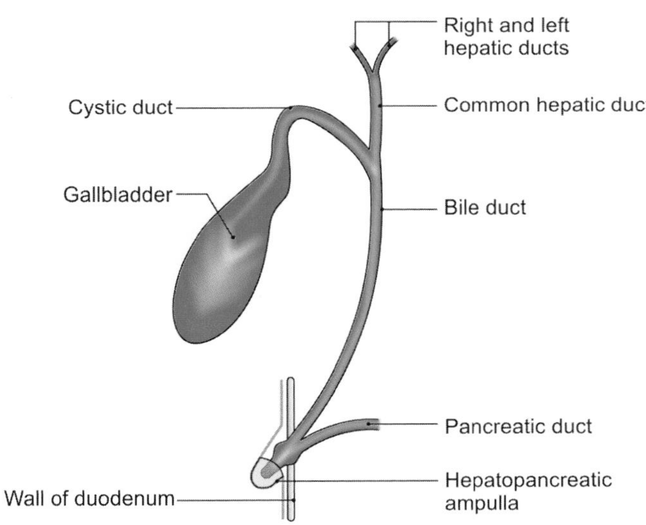

Fig. 22.1: Parts of the extrahepatic biliary apparatus

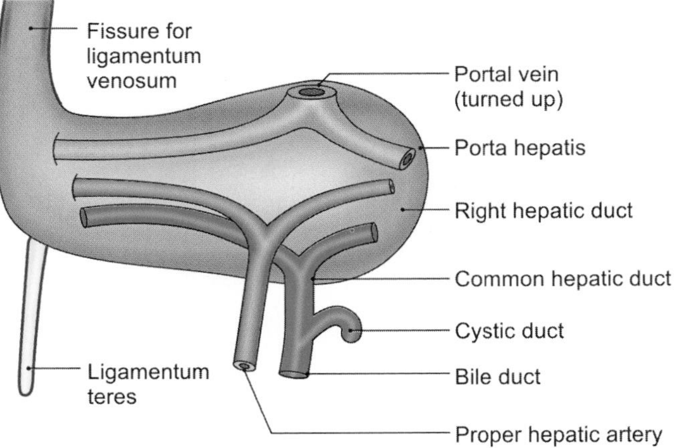

Fig. 22.2: Arrangement of structures in the porta hepatis

Accessory hepatic ducts are present in about 15% of subjects. They usually issue from the right lobe of the liver, and terminate either in the gallbladder, or in the common hepatic duct anywhere in its course, or even in the upper part of the bile duct (Fig. 22.3).

They are responsible for oozing of bile from the wound after cholecystectomy. Therefore, it is always better to use a drain to avoid retention of bile in the depths of the wound.

GALLBLADDER

Gallbladder is a pear-shaped reservoir of bile situated in a fossa on the inferior surface of the right lobe of the liver. The fossa for the gallbladder extends from the right end of the porta hepatis to the inferior border of the liver (Figs 22.1 and 22.4).

Dimensions and Capacity

The gallbladder is 7 to 10 cm long, 3 cm broad at its widest part, and about 30 to 50 ml in capacity.

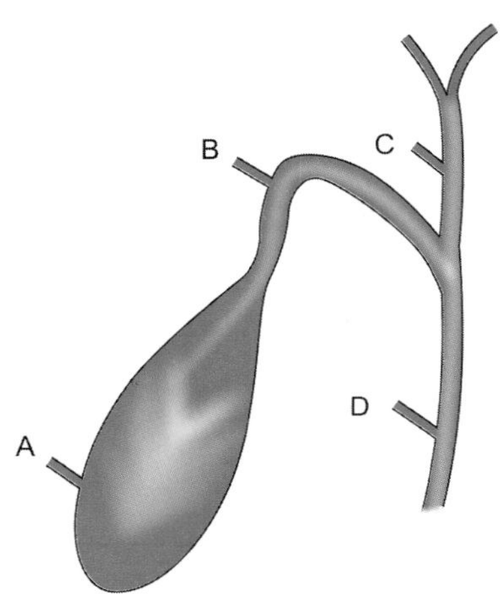

Fig. 22.3: The accessory hepatic ducts may open:
(A) directly into the gallbladder
(B) into the cystic duct
(C) into the common hepatic duct
(D) into the bile duct

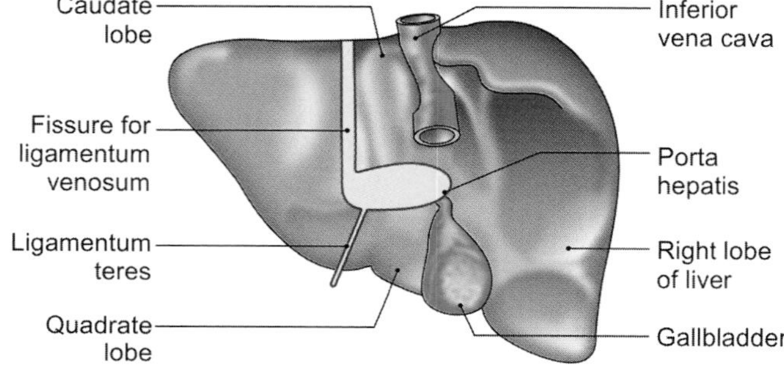

Fig. 22.4: Location of the gallbladder on the inferior surface of the right lobe of the liver

Parts

The gallbladder is divided into:
1 The fundus,
2 The body, and
3 The neck.

The *fundus* projects beyond the inferior border of the liver, in the angle between the lateral border of the right rectus abdominis and the ninth costal cartilage. It is entirely surrounded by peritoneum, and is related anteriorly to the anterior abdominal wall, and posteriorly to the beginning of the transverse colon.

The *body* lies in the fossa for the gallbladder on the liver. The upper narrow end of the body is continuous with the neck at the right end of the porta hepatis. The superior surface of the body is devoid of peritoneum, and is adherent to the liver. The inferior surface is covered with peritoneum, and is related to the beginning of the transverse colon and to the first and second parts of the duodenum (Fig. 22.5a).

The *neck* is the narrow upper end of the gallbladder. It is situated near the right end of the porta hepatis. It first curves anterosuperiorly and then posteroinferiorly to become continuous with the cystic duct. Its junction with the cystic duct is marked by a constriction (Fig. 22.5a).

Superiorly, the neck is attached to the liver by areolar tissue in which the cystic vessels are embedded. Inferiorly, it is related to the first part of the duodenum. The mucous membrane of the neck is folded spirally to prevent any obstruction to the inflow or outflow of bile. The posteromedial wall of the neck is dilated outwards to form a pouch called the *Hartmann's pouch* which is directed downwards and backwards. Gallstones may lodge in this pouch (Fig. 22.5b).

CYSTIC DUCT

Cystic duct is about 3 to 4 cm long. It begins at the neck of the gallbladder, runs downwards, backwards and to the left, and ends by joining the common hepatic duct at an acute angle to form the bile duct. The mucous membrane of the cystic duct forms a series of 5 to 12 crescentic folds, arranged spirally to form the so-called *spiral valve* of Heister. This is not a true valve (Fig. 22.6).

Functions of Gallbladder

1 Storage of bile, and its release into the duodenum when required.
2 Absorption of water, and concentration of bile. Bile may be concentrated as much as ten times.
3 The normal gallbladder also absorbs small amounts of a loose bile salt-cholesterol compound. When the gallbladder is inflamed, the concentration function becomes abnormal and the bile salts alone are absorbed leaving cholesterol behind. Bile salts have

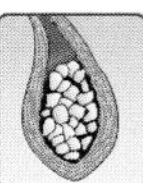

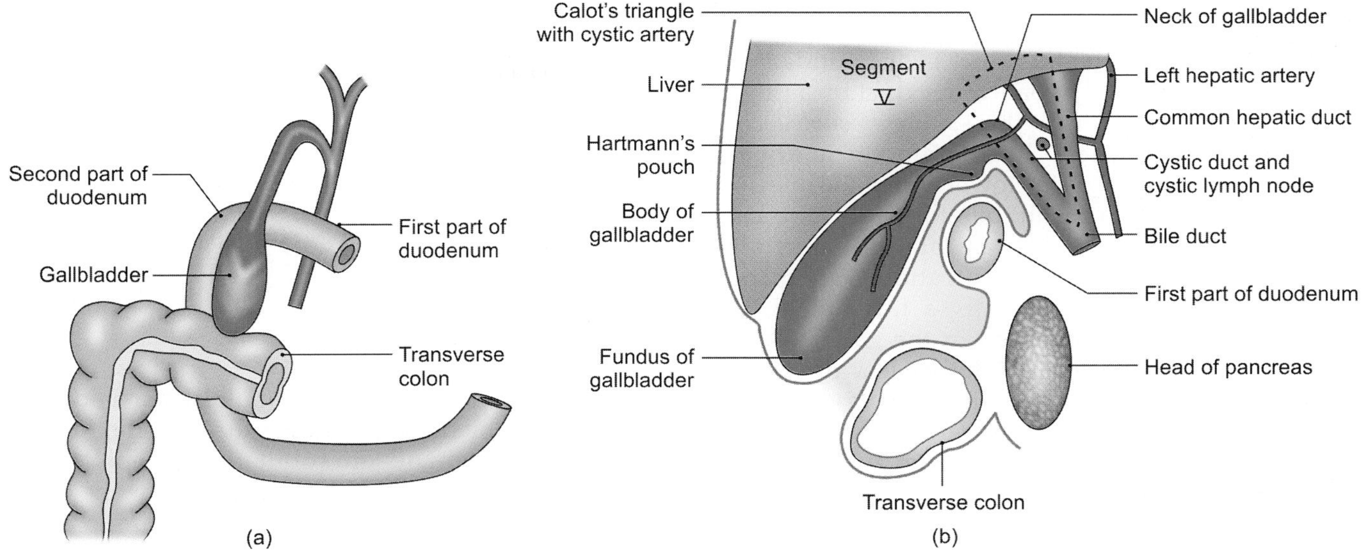

Figs 22.5a and b: Relations of the gallbladder: (a) Anterior view after removal of the liver, and (b) left view of sagittal section through the gallbladder fossa including the Calot's triangle

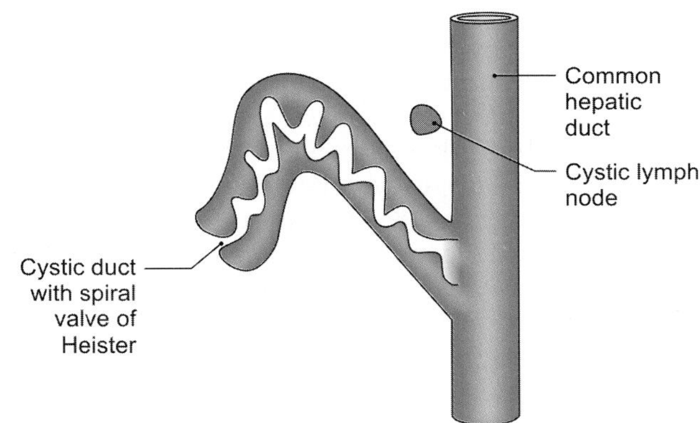

Fig. 22.6: The spiral valve of the cystic duct

a powerful solvent action on cholesterol which tends to be precipitated. This can lead to the formation of the gallstones.

4 It regulates pressure in the biliary system by appropriate dilatation or contraction. Thus the normal, choledocho-duodenal mechanism is maintained.

BILE DUCT

Bile duct is formed by the union of the cystic and common hepatic ducts near the porta hepatis. It is 8 cm long and has a diametre of about 6 mm.

Course

1 The bile duct runs downwards and backwards, first in the free margin of the lesser omentum, *supraduodenal part;*
2 Behind the first part of the duodenum the *retro-duodenal part;*
3 Then it lies behind, or embedded in, the head of pancreas *infraduodenal part;*
4 Near the middle of the left side of the second part of the duodenum it comes in contact with the pancreatic duct and accompanies it through the wall of the duodenum, the *intraduodenal part.*

Relations

Supraduodenal Part

Supraduodenal part in the free margin of lesser omentum.

1 *Anteriorly:* Liver.
2 *Posteriorly:* Portal vein and epiploic foramen.
3 *To the left:* Hepatic artery (Fig. 22.2).

Retroduodenal Part

1 *Anteriorly:* First part of duodenum (Fig. 22.5).
2 *Posteriorly:* Inferior vena cava.
3 *To the left:* Gastroduodenal artery.

Infraduodenal Part

1 *Anteriorly:* A groove in the upper and lateral parts of the posterior surface of the head of the pancreas.
2 *Posteriorly:* Inferior vena cava.

Intraduodenal Part

The course of the duct through the duodenal wall is very oblique. Within the wall the two ducts usually unite to form the *hepatopancreatic ampulla*, or *ampulla of Vater*. The distal constricted end of the ampulla opens at the summit of the *major duodenal papilla* 8 to 10 cm distal to the pylorus (*see* Fig. 23.16).

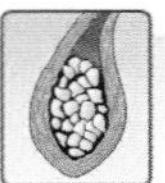

Sphincters Related to the Bile and Pancreatic Ducts

The terminal part of the bile duct is surrounded just above its junction with the pancreatic duct by a ring of smooth muscle that forms the *sphincter choledochus* (*choledochus* = bile duct). This sphincter is always present. It normally keeps the lower end of the bile duct closed (Fig. 22.7). As a result, bile formed in the liver keeps accumulating in the gallbladder and also undergoes considerable concentration. When food enters the duodenum, specially a fatty meal, the sphincter opens and bile stored in the gallbladder is poured into the duodenum. Another less developed sphincter, which is usually but not always present around the terminal part of the pancreatic duct is the *sphincter pancreaticus*. A third sphincter surrounds the hepatopancreatic ampulla and is called the *sphincter ampullae* or *sphincter of Oddi*.

Arteries Supplying the Biliary Apparatus

1 The cystic artery is the chief source of the blood supply, and is distributed to the gallbladder, the cystic duct, the hepatic ducts and the upper part of the bile duct (Fig. 22.8).

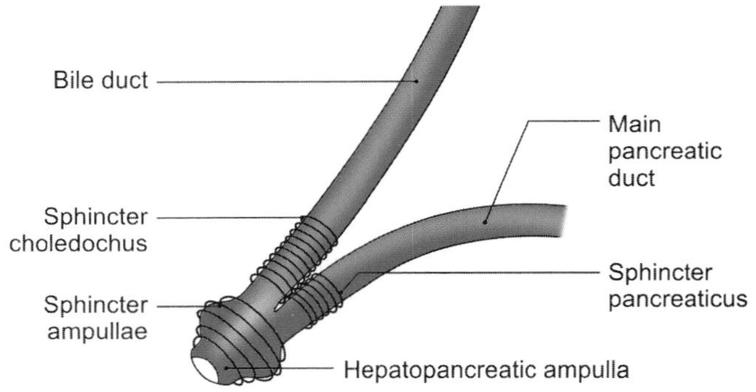

Fig. 22.7: Sphincters in the region of the junction of the bile duct and the main pancreatic duct with the duodenum

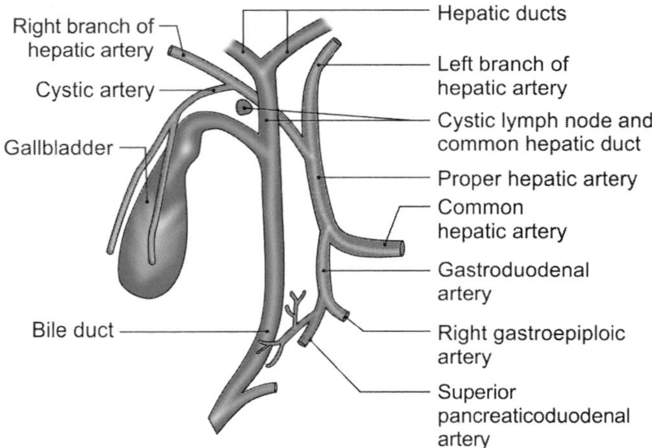

Fig. 22.8: Blood supply of the gallbladder and bile ducts

2 Several branches from the posterior superior pancreaticoduodenal artery supply the lower part of the bile duct.
3 The right hepatic artery forms a minor source of supply to the middle part of the bile duct.

The *cystic artery* usually arises from the right hepatic artery, passes behind the common hepatic and cystic ducts, and reaches the upper surface of the neck of the gallbladder, where it divides into superficial and deep branches.

Venous Drainage

1 The superior surface of the gallbladder is drained by veins which enter the liver through the fossa for the gallbladder and join tributaries of hepatic veins.
2 The rest of the gallbladder is drained by one or two cystic veins which open into the right branch of the portal vein (*see* Fig. 21.15).
3 The lower part of the bile duct drains into the portal vein.

Lymphatic Drainage

1 Lymphatics from the gallbladder, the cystic duct, the hepatic ducts and the upper part of the bile duct pass to the *cystic node and to the node of the anterior border of the epiploic* foramen. These are the most constant members of the upper hepatic nodes. The cystic node lies in the angle between the cystic and common hepatic ducts; it is constantly enlarged in cholecystitis (Fig. 22.5b).
2 The lower part of the bile duct drains into the *lower hepatic and upper pancreaticosplenic nodes*.

Nerve Supply

The *cystic plexus* of nerves, supplying the territory of the cystic artery, is derived from the hepatic plexus, which receives fibres from the coeliac plexus, the left and right vagi and the *right phrenic nerves*. The lower part of the bile duct is supplied by the nerve plexus over the superior pancreaticoduodenal artery.

Parasympathetic nerves are motor to the musculature of the gallbladder and bile ducts, but inhibitory to the sphincters. *Sympathetic nerves* from thoracic seven to nine are vasomotor and motor to the sphincters.

Pain from the gallbladder may travel along the vagus, the sympathetic nerves, or along the phrenic nerves. It may be referred to different sites through these nerves as follows.

a. Through vagus to the stomach (epigastrium).
b. Through the sympathetic nerves to the inferior angle of the right scapula. Lateral horn of thoracic 7 segment of spinal cord gives sympathetic fibres to coeliac ganglion through greater splanchnic nerve. T7 segment receives pain fibres from skin

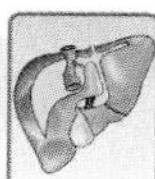

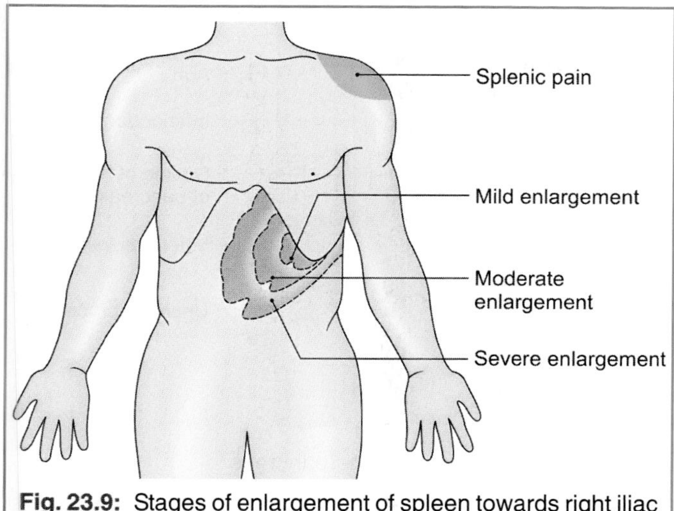

Fig. 23.9: Stages of enlargement of spleen towards right iliac fossa

Location

The pancreas lies more or less transversely across the posterior abdominal wall, at the level of first and second lumbar vertebrae.

Size and Shape

It is J-shaped or retort-shaped, set obliquely. The bowl of the retort represents its head, and the stem of the retort, its neck, body and tail. It is about 15–20 cm long, 2.5–3.8 cm broad and 1.2–1.8 cm thick and weighs about 90 g (Fig. 23.10).

The pancreas is divided (from right to left) into head, neck, body and the tail. The head is enlarged and lies within the concavity of the duodenum. The tail reaches the hilum of the spleen (Fig. 23.11). The entire organ lies posterior to the stomach separated from it by the lesser sac (*see* Figs 18.17 and 18.18).

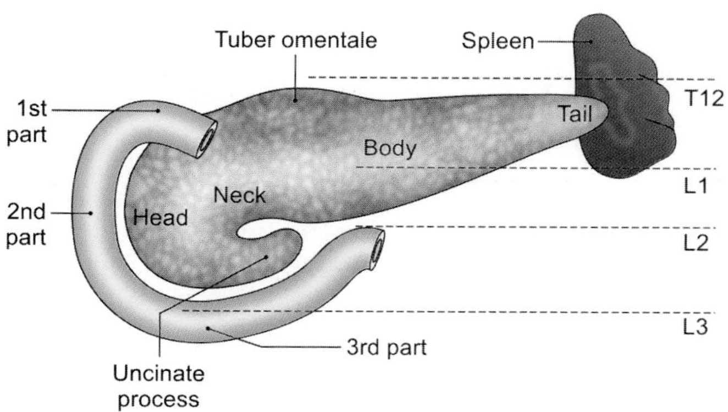

Fig. 23.11: Location of the pancreas and parts of pancreas

HEAD OF THE PANCREAS

Head is the enlarged flattened right end of pancreas, situated within the "C-shaped" curve of the duodenum.

External Features

The head has three *borders,* superior, inferior and right lateral; two *surfaces,* anterior and posterior; and one *process,* called the uncinate process, which projects from the lower and left part of the head towards the left (Fig. 23.11).

Relations

Three Borders

The *superior border* is overlapped by the first part of the duodenum and is related to the superior pancreaticoduodenal artery (Fig. 23.11). The *inferior border* is related to the third part of the duodenum and to the inferior pancreaticoduodenal artery. The *right lateral border* is related to the second part of the duodenum, the terminal part of the bile duct and the anastomosis between the two pancreaticoduodenal arteries.

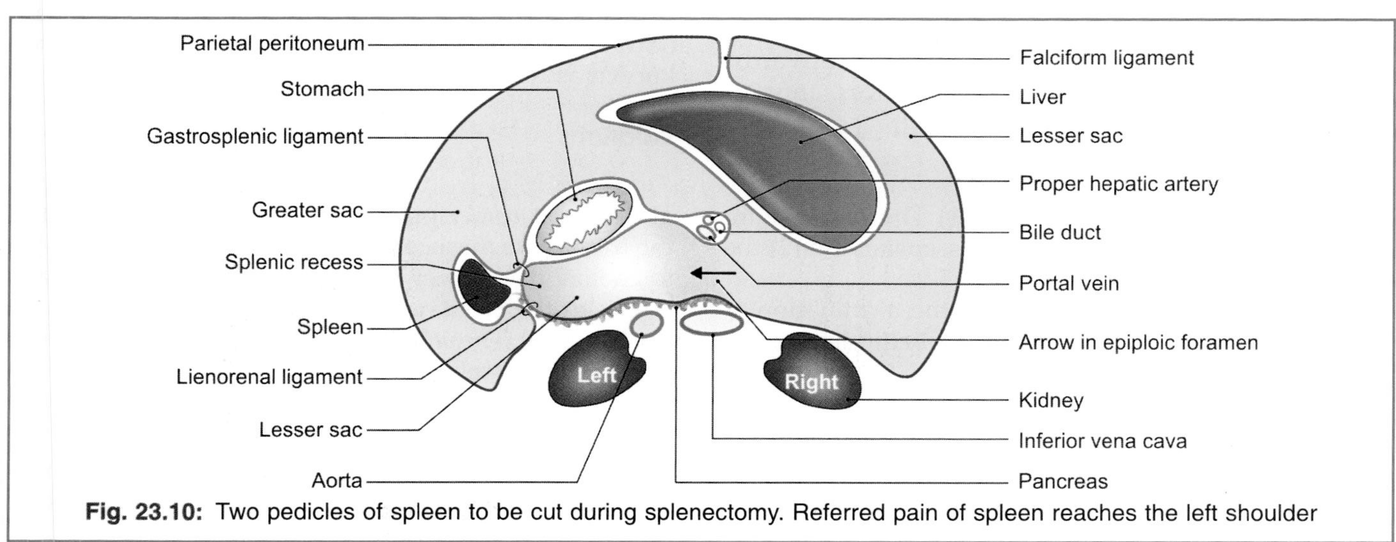

Fig. 23.10: Two pedicles of spleen to be cut during splenectomy. Referred pain of spleen reaches the left shoulder

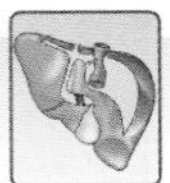

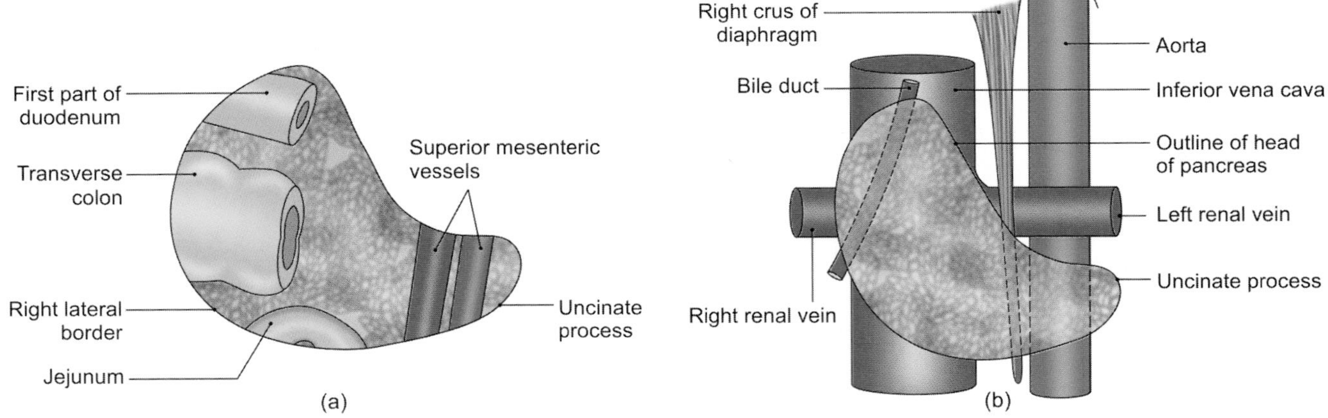

Figs 23.12a and b: (a) Anterior, and (b) posterior relations of the head of the pancreas

Two Surfaces

The *anterior surface* is related, from above downwards, to:

1 The first part of duodenum.
2 Transverse colon.
3 Jejunum which is separated from it by peritoneum (Fig. 23.12a).

The *posterior surface* is related to:

1 Inferior vena cava.
2 Terminal parts of the renal veins.
3 Right crus of the diaphragm.
4 Bile duct which runs downwards and to the right and is often embedded in the substance of pancreas (Fig. 23.12b).

Uncinate Process

It is related anteriorly to the superior mesenteric vessels, and posteriorly to the aorta (Fig. 23.12a).

NECK OF THE PANCREAS

This is the slightly constricted part of the pancreas between its head and body. It is directed forwards, upwards and to the left. It has two surfaces, anterior and posterior.

Relations

The *anterior surface* is related to: (1) The peritoneum covering the posterior wall of the lesser sac, and (2) the pylorus (Fig. 23.13a).

The *posterior surface* is related to the termination of the superior mesenteric vein and the beginning of the portal vein (Fig. 23.13b).

BODY OF THE PANCREAS

The body of the pancreas is elongated. It extends from its neck to the tail. It passes towards the left with a slight upward and backward inclination.

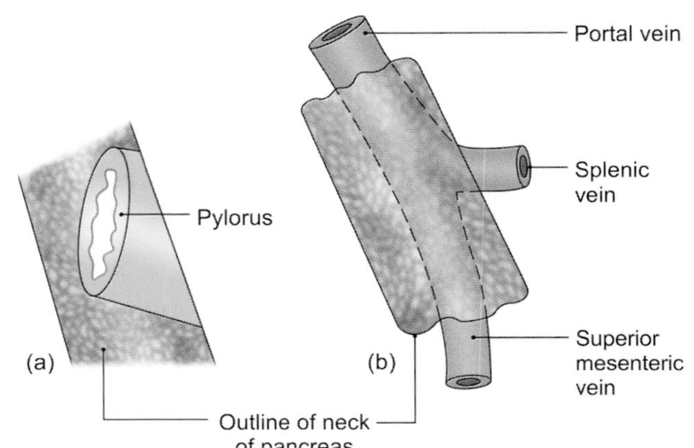

Figs 23.13a and b: Relations of the neck of the pancreas: (a) Anterior, and (b) posterior relations

External Features

It is triangular on cross-section, and has three *borders* (anterior, superior and inferior). A part of the body projects upwards beyond the rest of the superior border, a little to the left of the neck. This projection is known as the *tuber omentale.*

Relations

Three Borders

The *anterior border* provides attachment to the root of the transverse mesocolon. The *superior border* is related to coeliac trunk over the tuber omentale, the hepatic artery to the right, and the splenic artery to the left (*see* Fig. 21.3). The *inferior border* is related to the superior mesenteric vessels at its right end (Fig. 23.14).

Three Surfaces

The *anterior surface* is concave and is directed forwards and upwards. It is covered by peritoneum, and is related to the lesser sac and to the stomach.

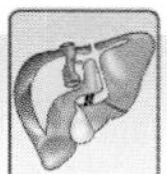

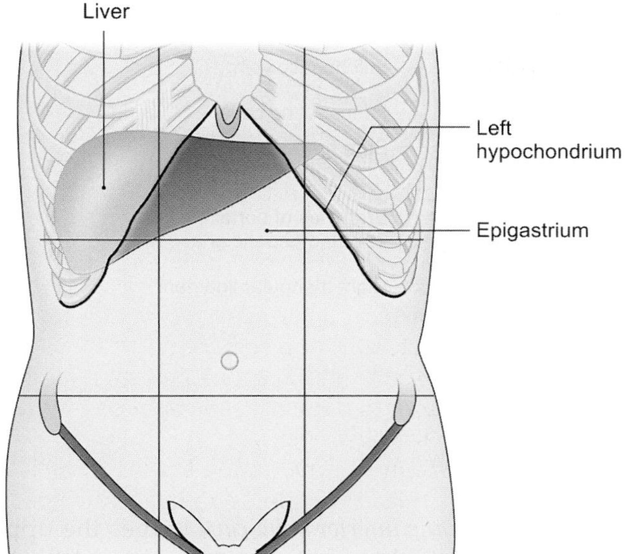

Fig. 23.21: Location of the liver

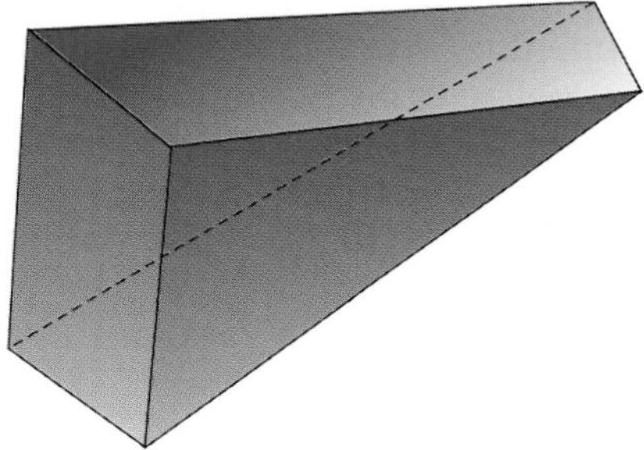

Fig. 23.22: Comparison of the orientation of the surfaces of the liver to those of a four-sided pyramid

4 Inferior, and
5 Right.

Out of these the inferior surface is well defined because it is demarcated, anteriorly, by a sharp inferior border. The other surfaces are more or less continuous with each other and are imperfectly separated from one another by ill-defined, rounded borders.

One Prominent Border

The *inferior border* is sharp anteriorly where it separates the anterior surface from the inferior surface. It is somewhat rounded laterally where it separates the right surface from the inferior surface. The sharp anterior part is marked by:

a. An *interlobar notch* or the notch for the ligamentum teres.
b. A *cystic notch* for the fundus of the gallbladder (Fig. 23.23).

In the epigastrium, the inferior border extends from the left 8th costal cartilage to the right 9th costal cartilage.

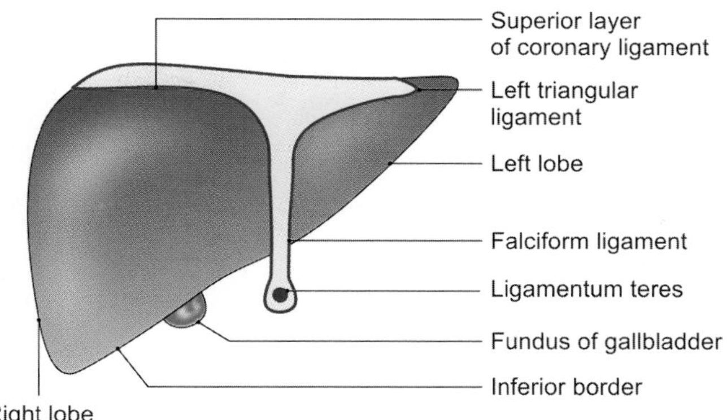

Fig. 23.23: Liver seen from the front

Two Lobes

The liver is divided into right and left lobes by the attachment of the *falciform ligament* anteriorly and superiorly; by the *fissure for the ligamentum teres* inferiorly; and by the *fissure for the ligamentum venosum* posteriorly.

The *right lobe* is much larger than the left lobe, and forms five sixth of the liver. It contributes to all the five surfaces of the liver, and presents the caudate and quadrate lobes.

The *caudate lobe* is situated on the posterior surface. It is bounded on the right by the groove for the *inferior vena cava*, on the left by the fissure for the *ligamentum venosum*, and inferiorly by the *porta hepatis*. Above it is continuous with the superior surface. Below and to the right, just behind the porta hepatis, it is connected to the right lobe of the liver by the *caudate process* (Fig. 23.24). Below and to the left it presents a small rounded elevation called the *papillary process*.

The *quadrate lobe* is situated on the inferior surface, and is rectangular in shape. It is bounded anteriorly by the *inferior border*, posteriorly by the porta hepatis, on the right by the *fossa for the gallbladder*, and on the left by the *fissure for the ligamentum teres* (Fig. 23.24).

The *porta hepatis* is a deep, transverse fissure about 5 cm long, situated on the inferior surface of the right lobe of the liver. It lies between the caudate lobe above and the quadrate lobe below and in front. The *portal vein*, the *hepatic artery* and the *hepatic plexus of nerves* enter the liver through the porta hepatis, while the *right and left hepatic ducts* and a few lymphatics leave it. The relations within; the porta hepatis are from behind forwards are the portal vein, the hepatic artery and the hepatic ducts. The lips of the porta hepatis provide attachment to the lesser omentum (Fig. 23.24).

The *left lobe* of the liver is much smaller than the right lobe and forms only one-sixth of the liver. It is flattened from above downwards. Near the fissure for the ligamentum venosum, its inferior surface presents a rounded elevation, called the omental tuberosity or *tuber omentale*.

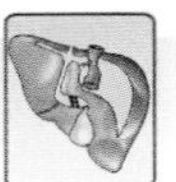

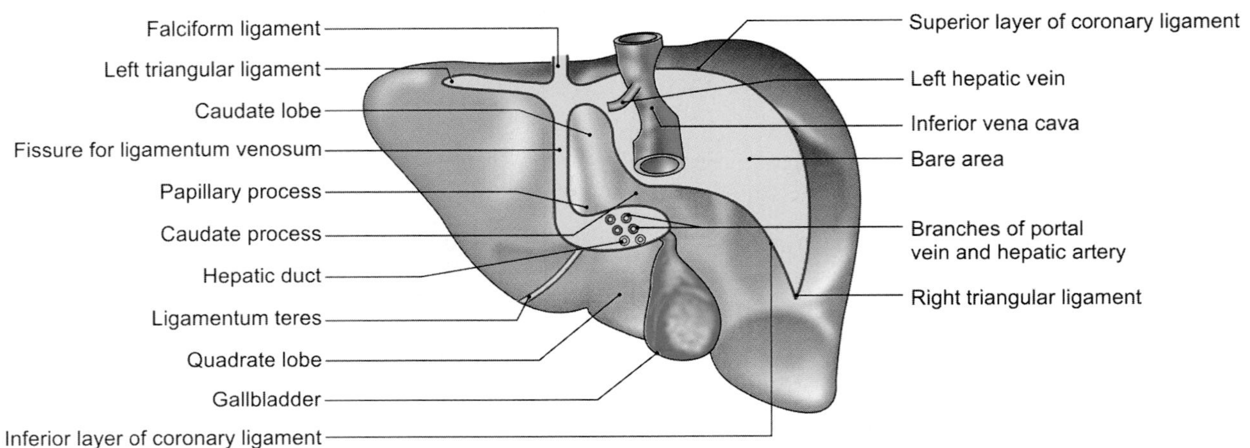

Fig. 23.24: Liver seen from behind and below

Relations

Peritoneal Relations

Most of the liver is covered by peritoneum. The areas not covered by peritoneum are as follows.

1 A triangular *bare area*, on the posterior surface of the right lobe, limited by the superior and inferior layers of the coronary ligament and by the right triangular ligament.
2 The *groove for the inferior vena cava*, on the posterior surface of the right lobe of the liver, between the caudate lobe and the bare area.
3 The *fossa for the gallbladder* which lies on the inferior surface of the right lobe to the right of the quadrate lobe.
4 The area of attachment of *lesser omentum* and the fissure for attachment of ligamentum venosum (Fig. 23.23).

Visceral Relations

Anterior Surface

The anterior surface is triangular and slightly convex. It is related to the xiphoid process and to the anterior abdominal wall in the median plane; and to diaphragm on each side. The diaphragm separates this surface from the pleura above the level of a line drawn from the xiphisternal joint to the 10th rib in the midaxillary line; and from the lung above the level of a line from the same joint to the 8th rib. The *falciform ligament* is attached to this surface a little to the right of the median plane (Figs 23.23 and 23.31).

Posterior Surface

The posterior surface is triangular. Its middle part shows a deep concavity for the vertebral column. Other relations are as follows.

1 The *bare area* is related to the diaphragm; and to the right suprarenal gland near the lower end of the groove for the inferior vena cava.
2 The *groove for the inferior vena cava* lodges the upper part of the vessel, and its floor is pierced by the hepatic veins.
3 The *caudate lobe* lies in the superior recess of the lesser sac. It is related to the crura of the diaphragm above the aortic opening, to the right inferior phrenic artery, and to the coeliac trunk.
4 The *fissure for the ligamentum venosum* is very deep and extends to the front of the caudate lobe. It contains two layers of the lesser omentum. The ligamentum venosum lies on its floor. The ligamentum venosum is a remnant of the ductus venosus of foetal life; it is connected below to the left branch of the portal vein, and above to the left hepatic vein near its entry into the inferior vena cava (Fig. 23.24).
5 The *posterior surface of the left lobe* is marked by the oesophageal impression (Fig. 23.25).

Superior Surface

The superior surface is quadrilateral and shows a concavity in the middle. This is the cardiac impression. On each side of the impression the surface is convex to fit the dome of the diaphragm. The diaphragm separates this surface from the pericardium and the heart in the middle; and from pleura and lung on each side (Fig. 23.30).

Inferior Surface

The inferior surface is quadrilateral and is directed downwards, backwards and to the left. It is marked by impressions for neighbouring viscera as follows.

1 On the inferior surface of the left lobe there is a large concave *gastric impression* (Fig. 23.25). The left lobe also bears a raised area that comes in contact with the lesser omentum: it is called the *omentale tuber*.
2 The *fissure for the ligamentum teres* passes from the inferior border to the left end of the porta hepatis.

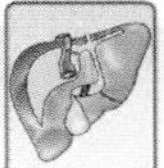

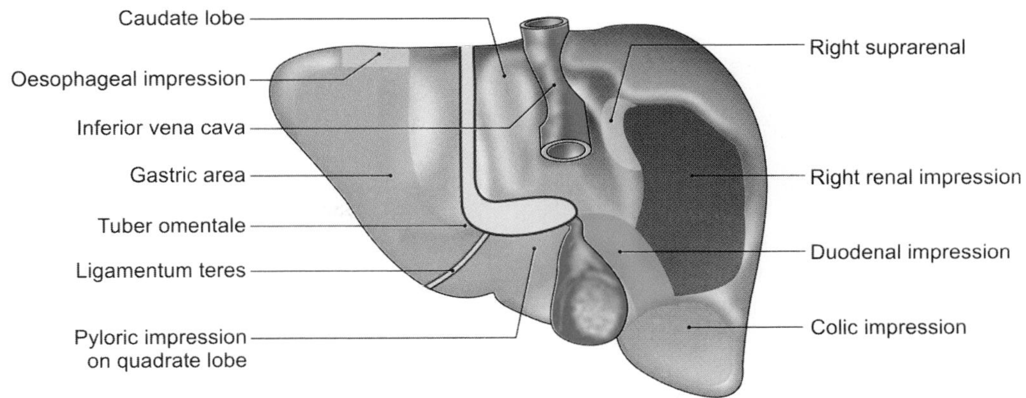

Fig. 23.25: Relations of the inferior surface of the liver

The ligamentum teres represents the obliterated left umbilical vein.

3 The *quadrate lobe* is related to the lesser omentum, the pylorus, and the first part of the duodenum. When the stomach is empty the quadrate lobe is related to the first part of the duodenum and to a part of the transverse colon.

4 The *fossa for the gallbladder* lies to the right of the quadrate lobe (Fig. 23.25).

5 To the right of this fossa the inferior surface of the right lobe bears the *colic impression* for the hepatic flexure of the colon, the renal impression for the right kidney, and the duodenal impression for the second part of the duodenum.

Right Surface

The right surface is quadrilateral and convex. It is related to the diaphragm opposite the 7th to 11th ribs in the midaxillary line. It is separated by the diaphragm from the pleura up to the 10th rib, and from the lung up to the 8th rib. Thus, the upper one-third of the surface is related to the diaphragm, the pleura and the lung; the middle one-third, to the diaphragm and the costodiaphragmatic recess of the pleura; and the lower one-third to the diaphragm alone (Fig. 23.30).

Blood Supply

The liver receives 20% of its blood supply through the hepatic artery, and 80% through the portal vein. Before entering the liver, both the hepatic artery and the portal vein divide into right and left branches. Within the liver, they redivide to form segmental vessels which further divide to form interlobular vessels which run in the portal canals. Further ramifications of the interlobular branches open into the hepatic sinusoids. Thus the hepatic arterial blood mixes with the portal venous blood in the sinusoids. There are no anastomoses between adjoining hepatic arterial territories and hence each branch is an end artery.

Venous Drainage

Hepatic sinusoids drain into interlobular veins, which join to form sublobular veins. These in turn unite to form the hepatic veins which drain directly into the inferior vena cava. These veins provide great support to the liver, besides the intra-abdominal pressure.

The *hepatic veins* are arranged in two groups, upper and lower. The *upper group* consists of three large veins right, left and middle, which emerge through the upper part of the groove for the inferior vena cava, and open directly into the vena cava. These veins keep the liver suspended. The *lower group* consists of a variable number of small veins from the right lobe and the caudate lobe which emerge through the lower part of the caval groove and open into the vena cava.

Microscopically the tributaries of hepatic veins, i.e. central veins are seen as separate channels from those of the portal radicles.

Lymphatic Drainage

The superficial lymphatics of the liver run on the surface of the organ beneath the peritoneum, and terminate in caval, hepatic, paracardial and coeliac lymph nodes. Some vessels from the coronary ligament may directly join the thoracic duct.

The deep lymphatics end partly in the nodes around the end of the inferior vena cava, and partly in the hepatic nodes.

Nerve Supply

The liver receives its nerve supply from the hepatic plexus which contains both sympathetic and parasympathetic or vagal fibres. Nerves also reach the liver through its various peritoneal ligaments.

HEPATIC SEGMENTS

On the basis of the intrahepatic distribution of the hepatic artery, the portal vein and the biliary ducts, the liver can be divided into the right and left functional

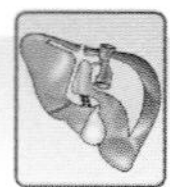

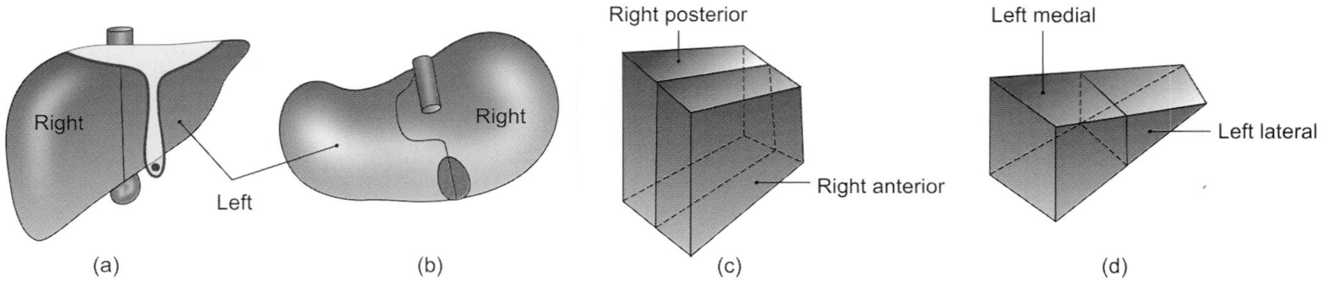

Figs 23.26a to d: The segments (physiological lobes) of the liver. (a) Anterior aspect, (b) inferior aspect, (c) scheme of the right lobe, and (d) scheme of the left lobe

lobes. These do not correspond to the anatomical lobes of the liver. The physiological lobes are separated by a plane passing on the anterosuperior surface along a line joining the cystic notch to the groove for the inferior vena cava. On the inferior surface the plane passes through the fossa for the gallbladder; and on the posterior surface it passes through the middle of the caudate lobe (Figs 23.26a to d).

The right lobe is subdivided into anterior and posterior segments, and the left lobe into medial and lateral segments. Thus there are four segments (Fig. 23.27) in the liver.

a. Right anterior (V and VIII),
b. Right posterior (VI and VII),
c. Left lateral (II and III) and
d. Left medial (I and IV).

The hepatic segments are of surgical importance. The hepatic veins tend to be intersegmental in their course.

FUNCTIONS

Liver is an indispensable gland of the body.

1 *Metabolism* of carbohydrates, fats and proteins;
2 *Synthesis* of bile and prothrombin;
3 *Excretion* of drugs, toxins, poisons, cholesterol, bile pigments and heavy metals;
4 *Protective* by conjugation, destruction, phagocytosis, antibody formation and excretion; and
5 *Storage* of glycogen, iron, fat, vitamin A and D.

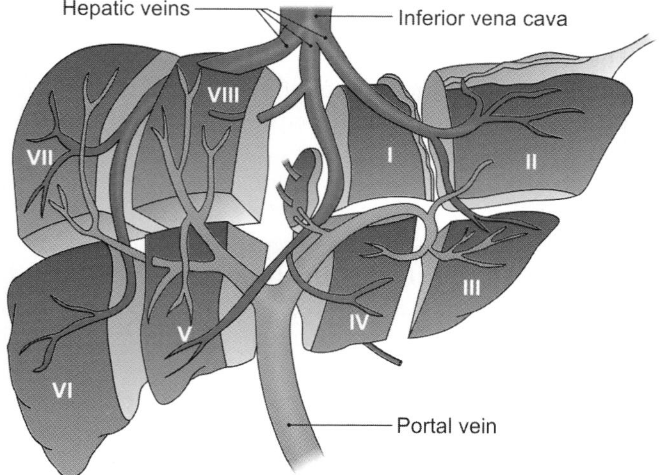

Fig. 23.27: The segments of liver

HISTOLOGY

Liver is covered by Glisson's capsule. In the pig there are hexagonal lobules with portal radicles at 3–5 corners. Each radicle contains bile ductule, branch each of portal vein and hepatic artery. Central vein lies in the centre and all around the central vein are the hepatocytes in form of laminae. On one side of the lamina is the sinusoid and on the other side is a bile canaliculus.

Portal lobule seen in human is triangular in shape with three central veins at the sides and portal tract in the centre.

The liver acinus is defined as the liver parenchyma around a preterminal branch of hepatic arteriole between two adjacent central veins. The liver acinus is the functional unit of liver. Blood reaches the acinus via branches of portal vein and hepatic artery to open into the sinusoids to reach the central vein. On the other hand, the flow of bile is along bile canaliculi, bile ductules and the interlobular bile ducts. Hepatocytes in zone I close to preterminal branch are better supplied by oxygen, nutrients and toxins. The liver cells in zone III close to central veins are relatively hypoxic while cells in zone II are intermediate in oxygen supply.

Histology of the liver can be studied by liver biopsy (Figs 23.28a and b) which is done from right lateral surface.

DEVELOPMENT

From the caudal end of foregut, an endodermal hepatic bud arises during 3rd week of development. The bud elongates cranially. It gives rise to a small bud on its right side. This is called *pars cystica* and the main part is *pars hepatica*. Pars cystica forms the gallbladder and the cystic duct which drains into common hepatic duct (CHD).

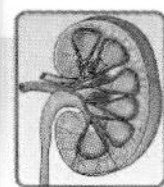

than the right kidney. On an average the kidney weighs 150 g in males and 135 g in females. The kidneys are reddish brown in colour.

The long axis of the kidney is directed downwards and laterally, so that the upper poles are nearer to the median plane than the lower poles (Fig. 24.2). The transverse axis is directed laterally and backwards.

In the foetus the kidney is lobulated and is made up of about 12 lobules. After birth the lobules gradually fuse, so that in adults the kidney is uniformly smooth. However, the evidence of foetal lobulation may persist.

EXTERNAL FEATURES

Each kidney is bean-shaped. It has upper and lower poles, medial and lateral borders, and anterior and posterior surfaces.

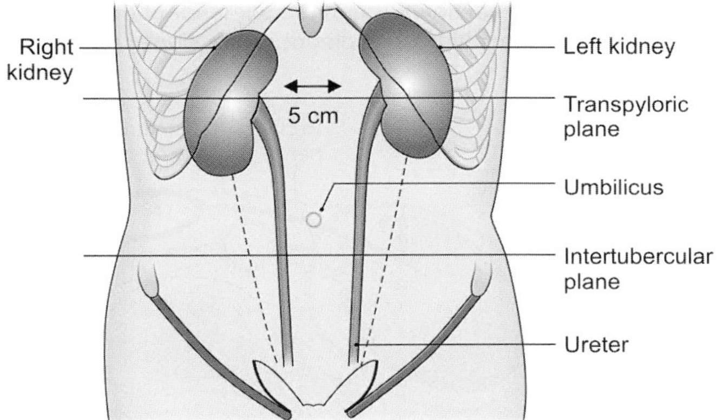

Fig. 24.2: Position of kidneys from anterior aspect

Two Poles of the Kidney

The upper pole is broad and is in close contact with the corresponding suprarenal gland. The lower pole is pointed.

Two Surfaces

The anterior surface is said to be irregular and the posterior surface flat, but it is often difficult to recognize the anterior and posterior aspects of the kidney by looking at the surfaces. The proper way to do this is to examine the structures present in the hilum as described below.

Two Borders

The lateral border is convex. The medial border is concave. Its middle part shows a depression, the hilus or hilum.

Hilum

The following structures are seen in the hilum from anterior to posterior side.

1 The renal vein
2 The renal artery, and
3 The renal pelvis, which is the expanded upper end of the ureter.

Examination of these structures enables the anterior and posterior aspects of the kidney to be distinguished from each other. As the pelvis is continuous inferiorly with the ureter, the superior and inferior poles of the kidney can also be distinguished by examining the hilum. So it is possible to determine the side to which a kidney belongs by examining the structures in the hilum. Commonly, one of the branches of the renal artery enters the hilus behind the renal pelvis, and a tributary of the renal vein may be found in the same plane.

RELATIONS OF THE KIDNEYS

The kidneys are retroperitoneal organs and are only partly covered by peritoneum anteriorly.

Relations Common to the Two Kidneys

1 The upper pole of each kidney is related to the corresponding suprarenal gland. The lower poles lie about 2.5 cm above the iliac crests.
2 The medial border of each kidney is related to:
   a. The suprarenal gland, above the hilus, and
   b. To the ureter below the hilus (Fig. 24.3).
3 Posterior relations: The posterior surfaces of both kidneys are related to the following.
   a. Diaphragm
   b. Medial and lateral arcuate ligaments
   c. Psoas major
   d. Quadratus lumborum
   e. Transversus abdominis
   f. Subcostal vessels; and
   g. Subcostal, iliohypogastric and ilioinguinal nerves (Fig. 24.4).

   In addition, the right kidney is related to twelfth rib, and the left kidney to eleventh and twelfth ribs.
4 The structures related to the hilum have been described earlier.

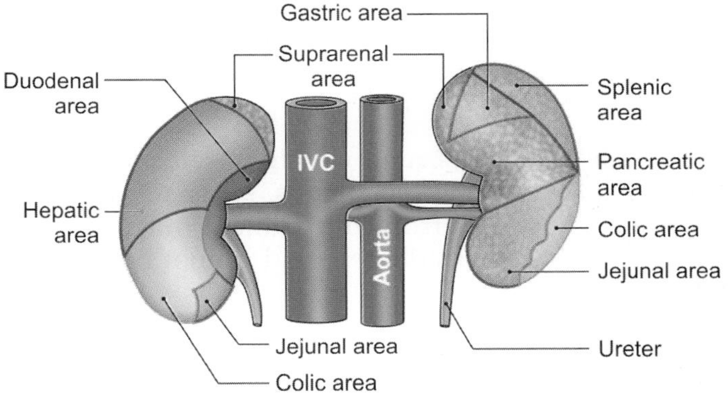

Fig. 24.3: Anterior relations of the kidneys. Areas covered by peritoneum are shaded

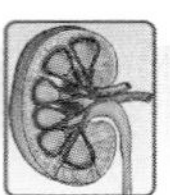

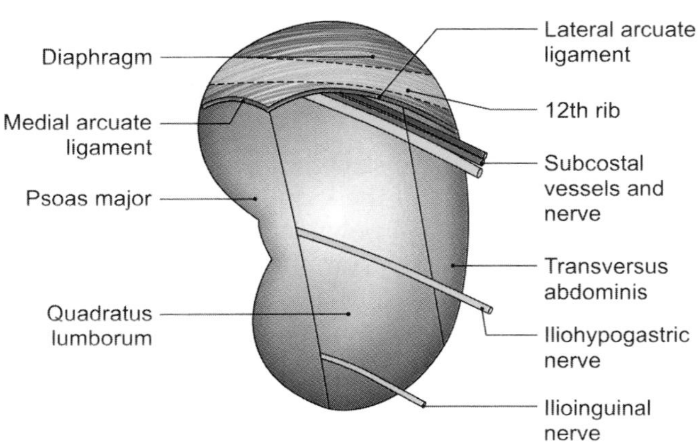

Fig. 24.4: Posterior relations of the right kidney

Other Relations of the Right Kidney

Anterior Relations

1 Right suprarenal gland
2 Liver
3 Second part of duodenum
4 Hepatic flexure of colon
5 Small intestine.

Out of these the hepatic and intestinal surfaces are covered by peritoneum.

The lateral border of the right kidney is related to the right lobe of the liver and to the hepatic flexure of the colon (Fig. 24.3).

Other Relations of the Left Kidney

Anterior Relations

1 Left suprarenal gland
2 Spleen
3 Stomach
4 Pancreas
5 Splenic vessels
6 Splenic flexure and descending colon
7 Jejunum.

Out of these the gastric, splenic and jejunal surfaces are covered by peritoneum.

The lateral border of the left kidney is related to the spleen and to the descending colon.

CAPSULES OR COVERINGS OF KIDNEY

The Fibrous Capsule

This is a thin membrane which closely invests the kidney and lines the renal sinus. Normally it can be easily stripped off from the kidney, but in certain diseases it becomes adherent and cannot be stripped (Figs 24.5 and 24.6).

Perirenal or Perinephric Fat

This is a layer of adipose tissue lying outside the fibrous capsule. It is thickest at the borders of the kidney and fills up the extra space in the renal sinus.

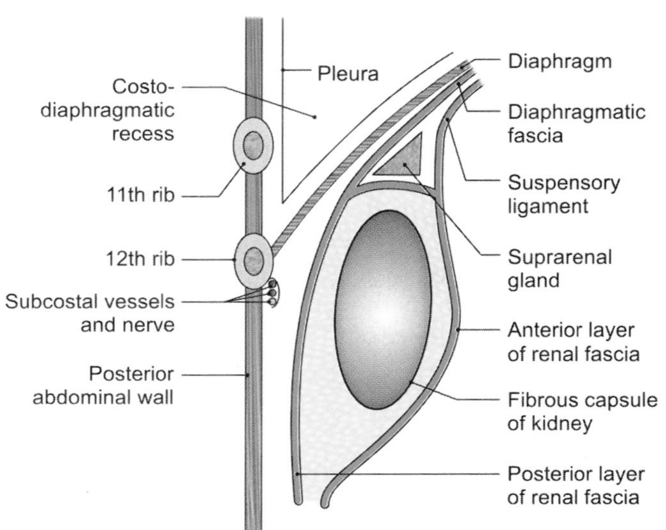

Fig. 24.5: Vertical section through the posterior abdominal wall showing the relationship of the pleura to the kidney

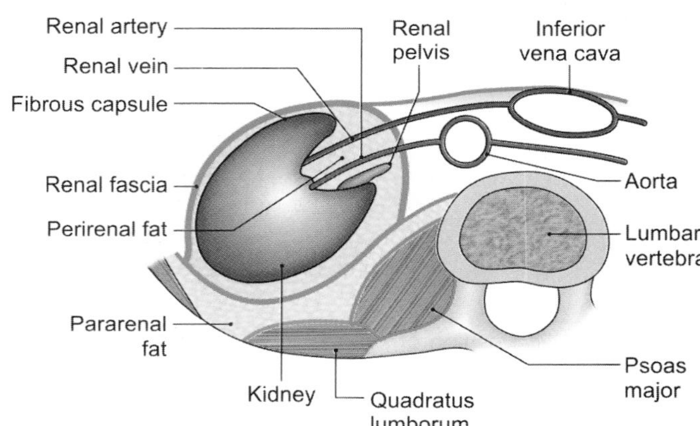

Fig. 24.6: Transverse section through the lumbar region showing the capsules of the kidney

Renal Fascia

The perirenal fascia was originally described as being made up of two separate layers.

Posterior layer was called fascia of Zuckerkandall and anterior layer as fascia of Gerota.

These two fasciae fused laterally to form lateral conal fascia. According to this view, lateral conal fascia continued anterolaterally behind colon to blend with parietal peritoneum.

But lately it has been researched that the fascia is not made up of fused fasciae, but of a single multi-laminated structure which is fused posteromedially with muscular fasciae of psoas major and quadratus lumborum muscles.

The fascia then extends anteromedially behind the kidney as bilaminated sheet, which divides at a variable point into thin layer which courses around the front of

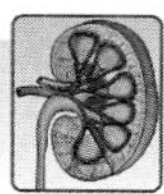

kidney as anterior perirenal fascia and a thicker posterior layer which continues anterolaterally as the lateral conal fascia.

It was believed earlier that above the suprarenal gland the anterior and posterior perirenal fasciae fuse with each other and then get fused to the diaphragmatic fascia, but research presently demonstrates that superior aspect of perirenal space is "open" and is in continuity to the bare area of liver on the right side and with subphrenic extraperitoneal space on the left side.

On the right side at the level of upper pole of kidney, anterior fascia blends with inferior coronary layer and bare area of liver.

On the left side, anterior layer fuses with gastrophrenic ligament.

Posterior layer on both right and left sides fuses with fasciae of muscles of posterior abdominal wall, i.e. psoas major and quadratus lumborum as well as with fascia on the inferior aspect of thoracoabdominal diaphragm.

Medially the anterior layer is continuous from one to the other kidney and the posterior layer is attached either side of vertebra.

Below both the layer extend along the ureter and fuse with iliac fascia.

Pararenal or Paranephric Body (Fat)

It consists of a variable amount of fat lying outside the renal fascia. It is more abundant posteriorly and towards the lower pole of the kidney. It fills up the paravertebral gutter and forms a cushion for the kidney.

STRUCTURE

Naked eye examination of a coronal section of the kidney shows:

1 An outer, reddish brown cortex.
2 An inner, pale medulla.
3 A space, the renal sinus (Fig. 24.7).

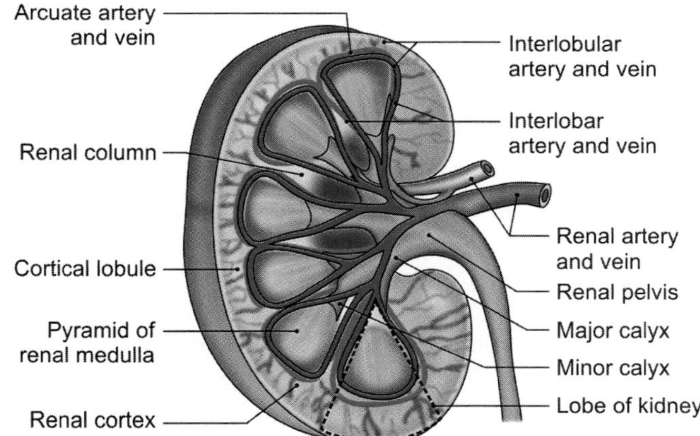

Fig. 24.7: A coronal section through the kidney showing the naked eye structure including the blood supply of the kidney

The *renal medulla* is made up of about 10 conical masses, called the *renal pyramids*. Their apices form the *renal papillae* which indent the minor calyces.

The *renal cortex* is divisible into two parts.

a. *Cortical arches* or *cortical lobules*, which form caps over the bases of the pyramids.
b. Renal columns, which dip in between the pyramids.

Each pyramid along with the overlying cortical arch forms a *lobe* of the kidney.

The *renal sinus* is a space that extends into the kidney from the hilus. It contains:

a. Branches of the renal artery.
b. Tributaries of the renal vein.
c. The renal pelvis. The pelvis divides into 2 to 3 major calyces, and these in their turn divide into 7 to 13 minor calyces. Each minor calyx (*kalyx* = cup of a flower) ends in an expansion which is indented by one to three renal papillae.

Structure of Uriniferous Tubule

Each kidney is composed of one to three million uriniferous tubules. Each tubule consists of two parts which are embryologically distinct from each other. These are as follows.

The *excretory part*, called the *nephron*, which elaborates urine. Nephron is the functional unit of the kidney, and comprises:

a. *Renal corpuscle* or *Malpighian corpuscle*, (for filtration of substances from the plasma) made up of glomerulus (Latin *ball*) a tuft of capillaries and Bowman's capsule (Fig. 24.8).
b. *Renal tubule*, (for selective resorption of substances from the glomerular filtrate) made up of the proximal convoluted tubule, loop of Henle with its descending and ascending limbs, and the distal convoluted tubule (Fig. 24.8).

The *collecting part* begins as a junctional tubule from the distal convoluted tubule. Many tubules unite together to form the ducts of Bellini which open into the minor calyces through the renal papillae.

Juxtaglomerular apparatus is formed at the vascular pole of glomerulus which is intimately related to its own ascending limb of the Henle's loop near the distal convoluted tubule. The apparatus consists of:

a. *Macula densa*, formed by altered cells of the tubule.
b. *Juxtaglomerular cells*, formed by the epithelioid cells in the media of the afferent arteriole.
c. *Some* agranular cells between macula densa and the glomerulus proper.

VASCULAR SEGMENTS

The renal artery gives 5 segmental branches, 4 from its anterior division and one from its posterior division (Fig. 24.9).

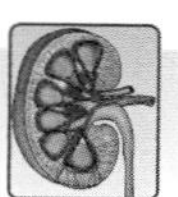

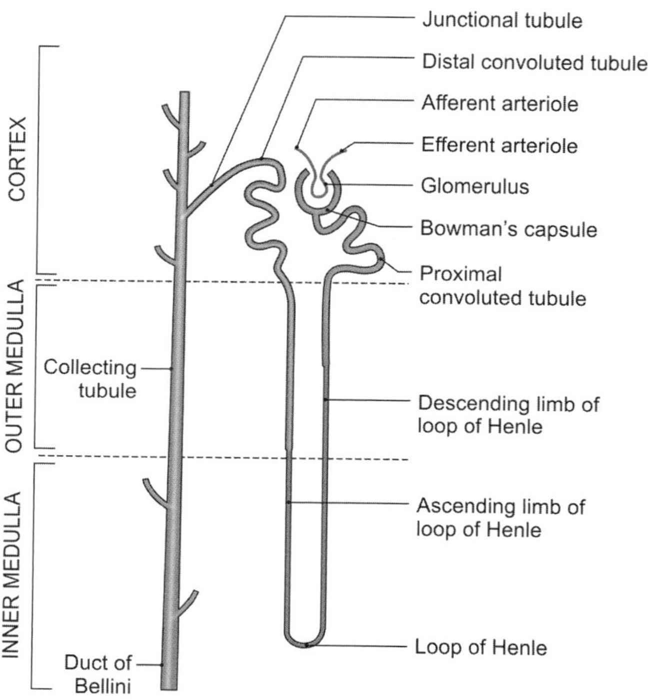

Fig. 24.8: Placement of the uriniferous tubule/nephron in various zones of kidney

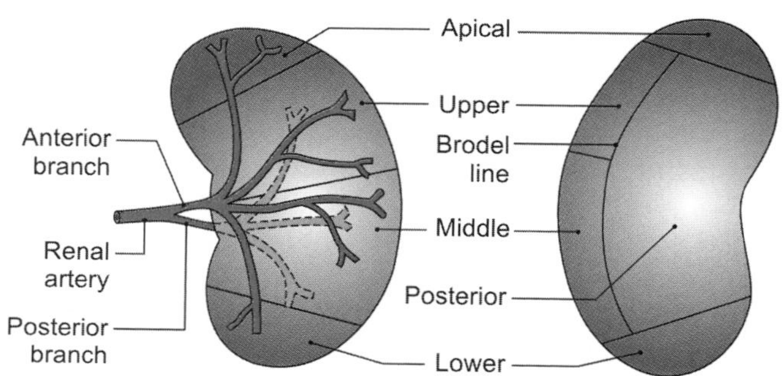

Fig. 24.9: Vascular segments of the kidney as seen in a sagittal section. Big anterior branch supplies four segments and posterior branch supplies only one segment

The segments are apical, upper, middle and lower on anterior aspect. On posterior aspect segments seen are posterior and parts of apical and lower segments.

Blood Supply of Kidney

The blood supply of kidney shown in Flow chart 24.1 and Figs 24.7 and 24.10.

Lymphatic Drainage

The lymphatics of the kidney drain into the lateral aortic nodes located at the level of origin of the renal arteries (L2).

Nerve Supply

The kidney is supplied by the renal plexus, an off shoot of the coeliac plexus. It contains sympathetic (T10–L1) fibres which are chiefly vasomotor. The afferent nerves of the kidney belong to segments T10 to T12.

Flow chart 24.1: Blood supply of kidney

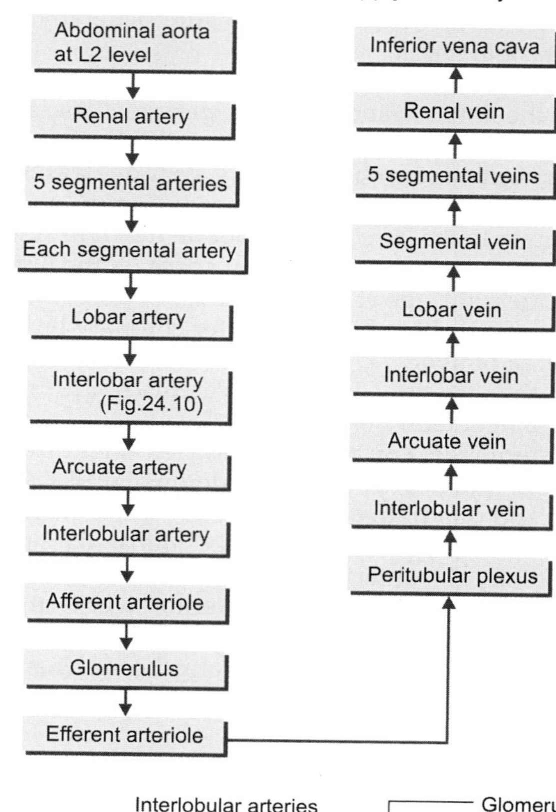

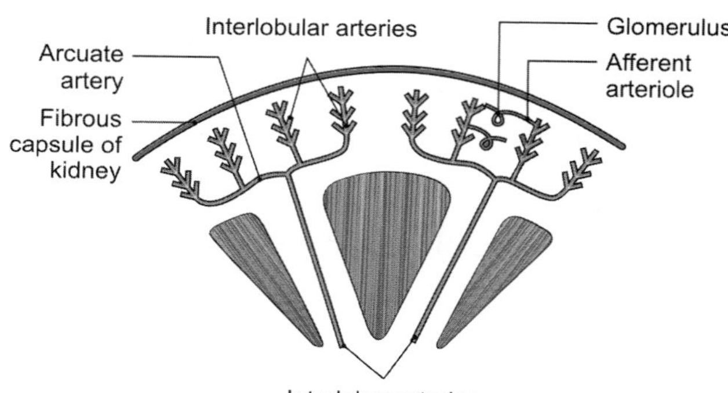

Fig. 24.10: Arrangement of the arteries in the kidney

EXPOSURE OF THE KIDNEY FROM BEHIND

In exposing the kidney from behind, the following layers have to be reflected one by one (Fig. 24.11).

1 Skin
2 Superficial fascia
3 Posterior layer of thoracolumbar fascia with latissimus dorsi and serratus posterior inferior
4 Erector spinae, which can be removed for convenience
5 Middle layer of thoracolumbar fascia
6 Quadratus lumborum
7 Anterior layer of thoracolumbar fascia in which the related nerves are embedded.

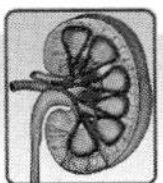

Nerve Supply

The ureter is supplied by sympathetic from T10–L1 segments and parasympathetic from S2–S4 nerves. They reach the ureter through the renal, aortic and hypogastric plexuses. All the nerves appear to be sensory in function.

Histology

Ureter is composed of:

1. The innermost mucous membrane.
2. Middle layer of well developed smooth muscle layer.
3. Outer tunica adventitia.

   The epithelial lining is of transitional epithelium. Muscle coat in upper two-thirds has inner longitudinal and outer circular fibres. Lower one-third comprises an additional outer longitudinal layer. Connective tissue forms the outer layer (Fig. 24.30).

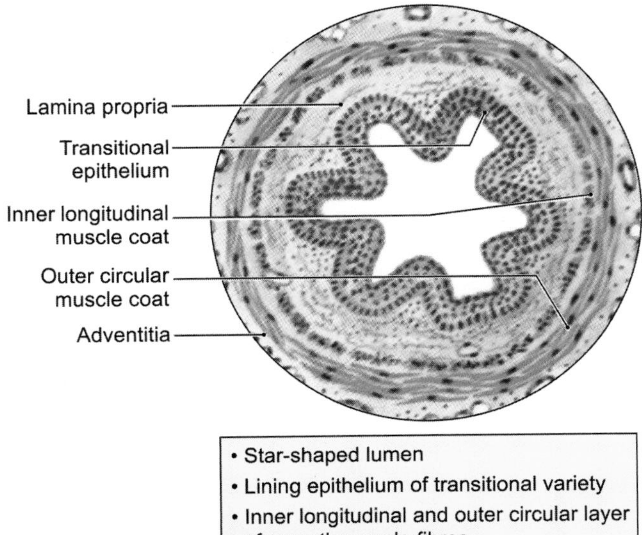

- Star-shaped lumen
- Lining epithelium of transitional variety
- Inner longitudinal and outer circular layer of smooth muscle fibres

Fig. 24.30: Histology of the ureter

DEVELOPMENT OF KIDNEY AND URETER

Kidney develops from metanephros, though pronephros and mesonephros appear to disappear. Only the duct of mesonephros, the mesonephric duct persists.

Thus the nephrons of the kidney arise from the metanephros. Parts of nephron formed are Bowman's capsule, proximal convoluted tubule, loop of Henle, distal convoluted tubule. Tuft of capillaries form the glomeruli.

Collecting part of kidney develops from ureteric bud, which is an outgrowth of the mesonephric duct. Ureteric bud gets capped by the metanephric tissue, the ureteric bud forms ureter. Soon it dilates to form renal pelvis and divides and subdivides to form major and minor calyces and 1–3 million collecting tubules.

Kidney starts developing in the sacral region, then it ascends to occupy its lumbar position (Figs 24.31a to e and 24.32a to e).

Anomalies of the Kidney and Ureter

1. Nonunion of the excretory and collecting parts of the kidney results in the formation of *congenital polycystic kidney.*
2. Fusion of the lower poles may occur, resulting in a *horseshoe kidney*. In these cases the ureters pass anterior to the isthmus of the kidney.
3. The early *pelvic position* of the kidney may persist. The renal artery then arises from the common iliac artery.
4. Unilateral *aplasia* or *hypoplasia* of the kidney may occur. Sometimes both kidneys may lie on any one side of the body.
5. The ureteric bud may divide into two, forming double ureter partly or completely.

CLINICAL ANATOMY

- *Ureteric colic:* This term is used for severe pain due to a ureteric stone or calculus which causes spasm of the ureter. The pain starts in the loin and radiates down the groin, the scrotum or the labium majus and the inner side of the thigh. Note that the pain is referred to the cutaneous areas innervated by segments, mainly T11 to L2, which also supply the ureter (Fig. 24.33).
- *Ureteric stone:* A ureteric stone is liable to become impacted at one of the sites of normal constriction of the ureter, e.g. pelviureteric junction, brim of the pelvis and intravesical course (Fig. 24.23).
- *Duplex ureter:* 2 ureters drain renal pelvis on one side called as duplex system.
- *Ectopic ureter:* Single ureter and longer ureter insert more caudally and medially than normal one.
- *Ureteroceles:* Cystic dilatation of lower end of ureter.
- *Blood supply:* Upper and middle parts of ureter are supplied by branches from its medial side. Pelvic part is supplied by branches from its lateral side.

Mnemonics

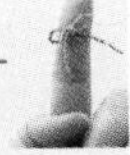

Ureter to uterine artery: "Water under the bridge"

The ureters (which carry **water**), are posterior to the **uterine artery**.

A common surgical error could be to ligate and cut ureter with uterine artery while removing uterus.

Structures at hilum of kidney

From anterior to posterior aspect—VAU

V – Renal **v**ein
A – Renal **a**rtery
U – Pelvis of **u**reter

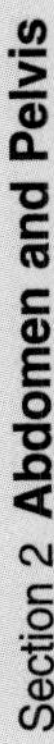

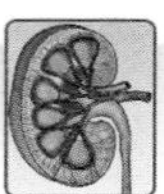

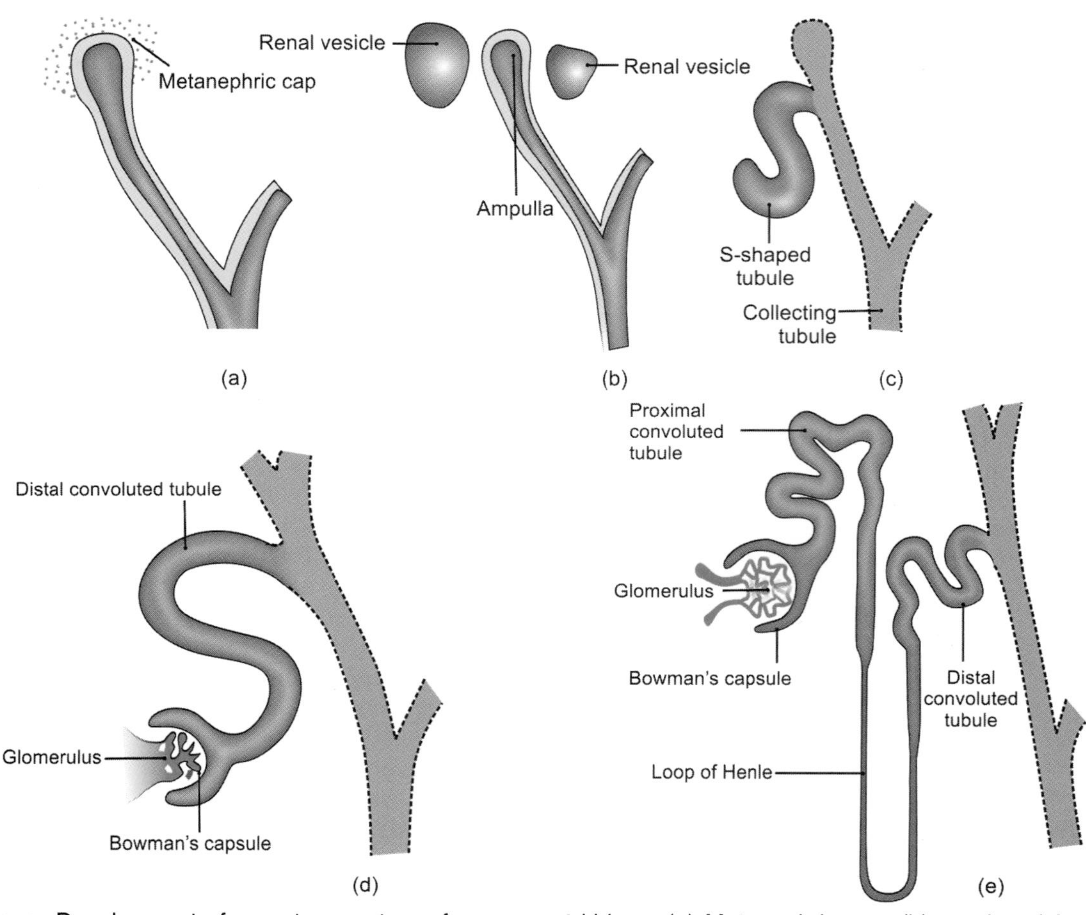

Figs 24.31a to e: Development of excretory system of permanent kidney: (a) Metanephric cap, (b) renal vesicles, (c) s-shaped tubule, (d) Bowman's capsule and glomerulus, and (e) differentiation and growth of parts of nephron, loop of Henle, proximal and distal convoluted tubules

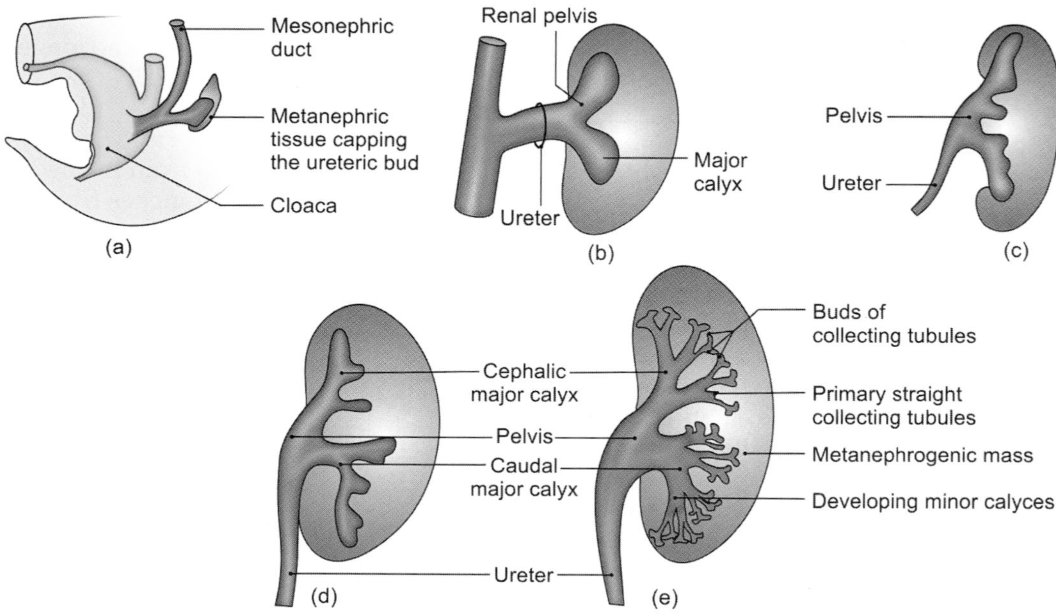

Figs 24.32a to e: Development of collecting system of permanent kidney: (a) Formation of ureteric buds, (b) capping of ureteric bud by metanephros, and (c to e) formation of ureter, renal pelvis, major calyces, minor calyces and collecting tubules

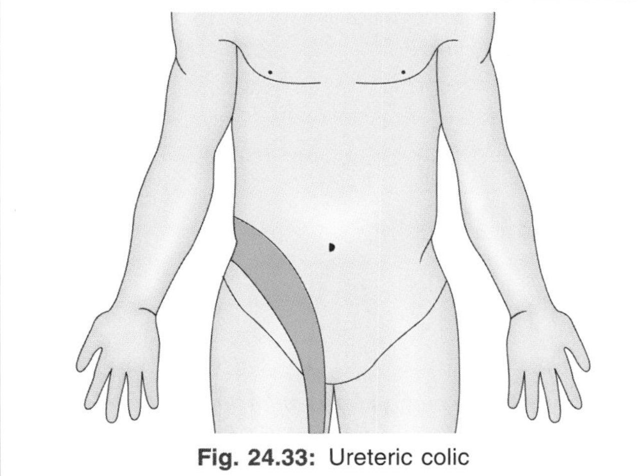

Fig. 24.33: Ureteric colic

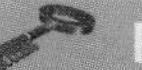

FACTS TO REMEMBER

- Order of structures at the hilum of kidney is renal vein, renal artery and pelvis of ureter from before backwards.
- Kidney is kept in position by intra-abdominal pressure, pararenal, fat, renal fascia, perirenal fat, renal capsule.
- There are 5 renal segments. These are apical, upper, middle, lower and posterior.
- Ureter shows 5 constrictions. These are at pelviureteric junction, at the brim of pelvis, at crossing with ductus deferens or broad ligament, intravesical course and at its termination at the trigone of the urinary bladder.
- Most of the renal stones are radiopaque while most of the gallstones non-radiopaque.
- Excretory part of kidney-develops from metanephros; collecting part of kidney develops from ureteric bud, arising from mesonephric duct.

CLINICOANATOMICAL PROBLEM

A patient of chronic renal failure needs a kidney transplant

- Where will the new kidney be put?
- Will the diseased kidney be removed?
- How will the new ureter and blood vessels be connected?

Ans: The new kidney is put in the right or left iliac fossa. The diseased kidney cut off from blood vessels and ureter is left within the patient's body

The new ureter is connected to the urinary bladder. The renal blood vessels are connected to internal iliac vessels. With proper precautions and medications, life gets sustained.

MULTIPLE CHOICE QUESTIONS

1. All of the following are related to the anterior surface of left kidney *except*:
a. Spleen b. Pancreas
c. Duodenum d. Left colic flexure

2. Which of the following muscles is not forming posterior relation of kidney?
a. Latissimus dorsi b. Transversus abdominis
c. Psoas major d. Quadratus lumborum

3. Structure not lying anterior to left ureter is:
a. Gonadal artery b. Left colic artery
c. Pelvic colon d. Internal iliac artery

4. All the following areas on the anterior surface of right kidney are not covered by peritoneum, *except*:
a. Suprarenal b. Hepatic
c. Duodenal d. Colic

5. Order of structures in the hila of kidney from before backwards is:
a. Pelvis, vein, artery
b. Vein, pelvis, artery
c. Vein, artery, pelvis
d. Artery, vein, pelvis

6. Number of minor calyces in a kidney is about:
a. 7–14 b. 14–24
c. 2–4 d. 25–28

7. Where is the perirenal fat thickest?
a. At the poles
b. Along the borders
c. Along posterior surface
d. Along anterior surface

8. What forms the lobe of the kidney?
a. Two renal pyramids with intervening renal column
b. Two renal columns with intervening pyramid
c. A renal pyramid with the cortex overlying it
d. Two renal columns plus the adjoining cortex

ANSWERS

1. c **2.** a **3.** d **4.** b **5.** c **6.** a **7.** b **8.** c

25

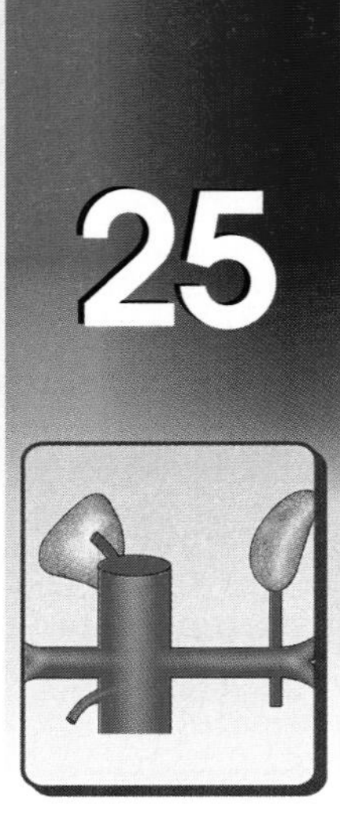

Suprarenal Gland and Chromaffin System

The two parts of the suprarenal gland are different from embryology and histology points of view, still these work in unison to keep up the body during adversity

INTRODUCTION

The suprarenal or adrenal glands are endocrine glands which help to maintain water and electrolyte balance. These also prepare the body for any emergency. These are subjected to hyper- or hypofunctioning. Lack of secretion of the cortical part leads to Addison's disease. Excessive secretion causes retention of salts and fluids.

Tumour of adrenal medulla or pheochromocytoma causes persistent severe hypertension.

SUPRARENAL GLAND

DISSECTION

Locate the suprarenal glands situated along the upper pole and medial border of the two kidneys. Identify the structures related to the right and left suprarenal glands.

Subdivisions

The suprarenal glands are a pair of important endocrine glands situated on the posterior abdominal wall over the upper pole of the kidneys behind the peritoneum (Fig. 25.1). They are made up of two parts.

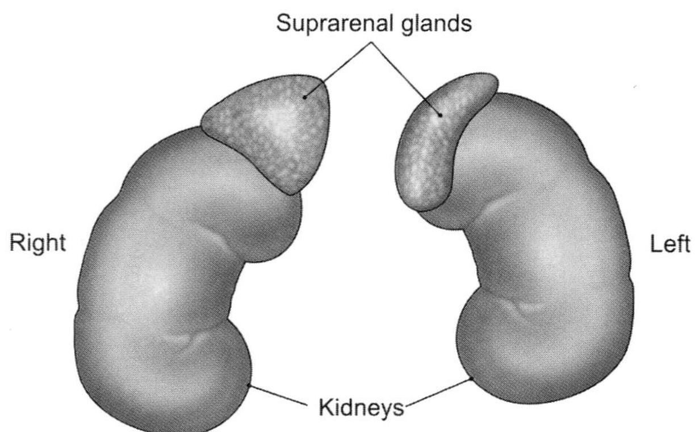

Fig. 25.1: The suprarenal glands

1. An outer cortex of mesodermal origin, which secretes a number of steroid hormones.
2. An inner medulla of neural crest origin, which is made up of chromaffin cells and secretes adrenaline and noradrenalin or catecholamines.

Location

Each gland lies in the epigastrium, at the upper pole of the kidney, in front of the crus of the diaphragm, opposite the vertebral end of the 11th intercostal space and the 12th rib.

Size, Shape and Weight

Each gland measures 50 mm in height, 30 mm in breadth and 10 mm in thickness. It is approximately one-third of the size of kidney at birth and about one-thirtieth of it in adults. It weighs about 5 g, the medulla forming one-tenth of the gland. Right suprarenal is triangular or pyramidal in shape and the left is semilunar in shape.

Sheaths

The suprarenal glands are immediately surrounded by areolar tissue containing considerable amount of fat.

Outside the fatty sheath, there is the perirenal fascia. Between the two layers lies the suprarenal gland (Fig. 25.2). The two layers are not fused above the suprarenal. The perirenal space is open and is in continuity with bare area of liver on the right side and with subphrenic extraperitoneal space on the left side.

The gland is separated from the kidney by a septum.

RIGHT SUPRARENAL GLAND

The right suprarenal gland is triangular to pyramidal in shape. It has:

1. An apex
2. A base

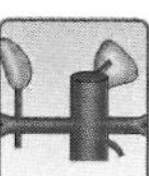

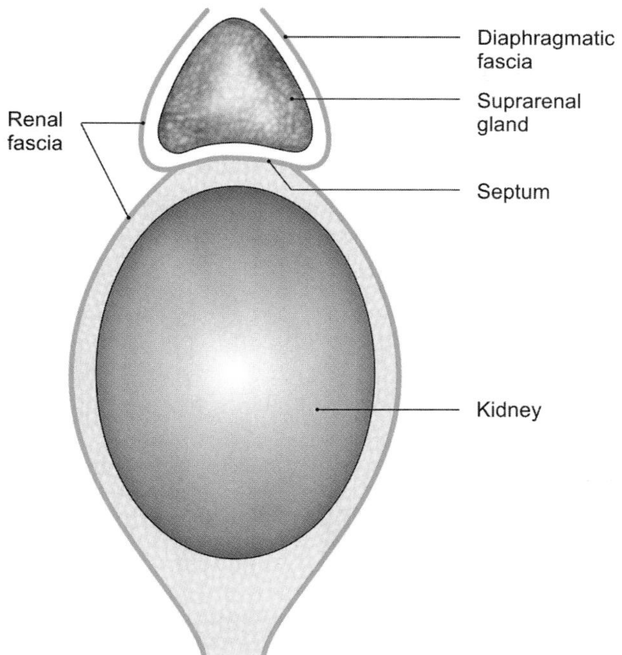

Fig. 25.2: The kidney and suprarenal glands enclosed in the renal fascia with a septum intervening

3. Two surfaces—anterior and posterior.
4. Three borders—anterior, medial and lateral (Figs 25.3a and d).

LEFT SUPRARENAL GLAND

The *left gland* is semilunar. It has:

1. Two ends—upper (narrow end) and lower (rounded end).
2. Two borders—medial convex and lateral concave.
3. Two surfaces—anterior and posterior (Figs 25.3b and c).

Comparison of right and left suprarenal glands is given in Table 25.1.

Structure and Function

Naked eye examination of a cross-section of the suprarenal gland shows an outer part, called the *cortex*, which forms the main mass of the gland, and a thin inner part, called the *medulla*, which forms only about one-tenth of the gland. The two parts are absolutely distinct from each other structurally, functionally and developmentally.

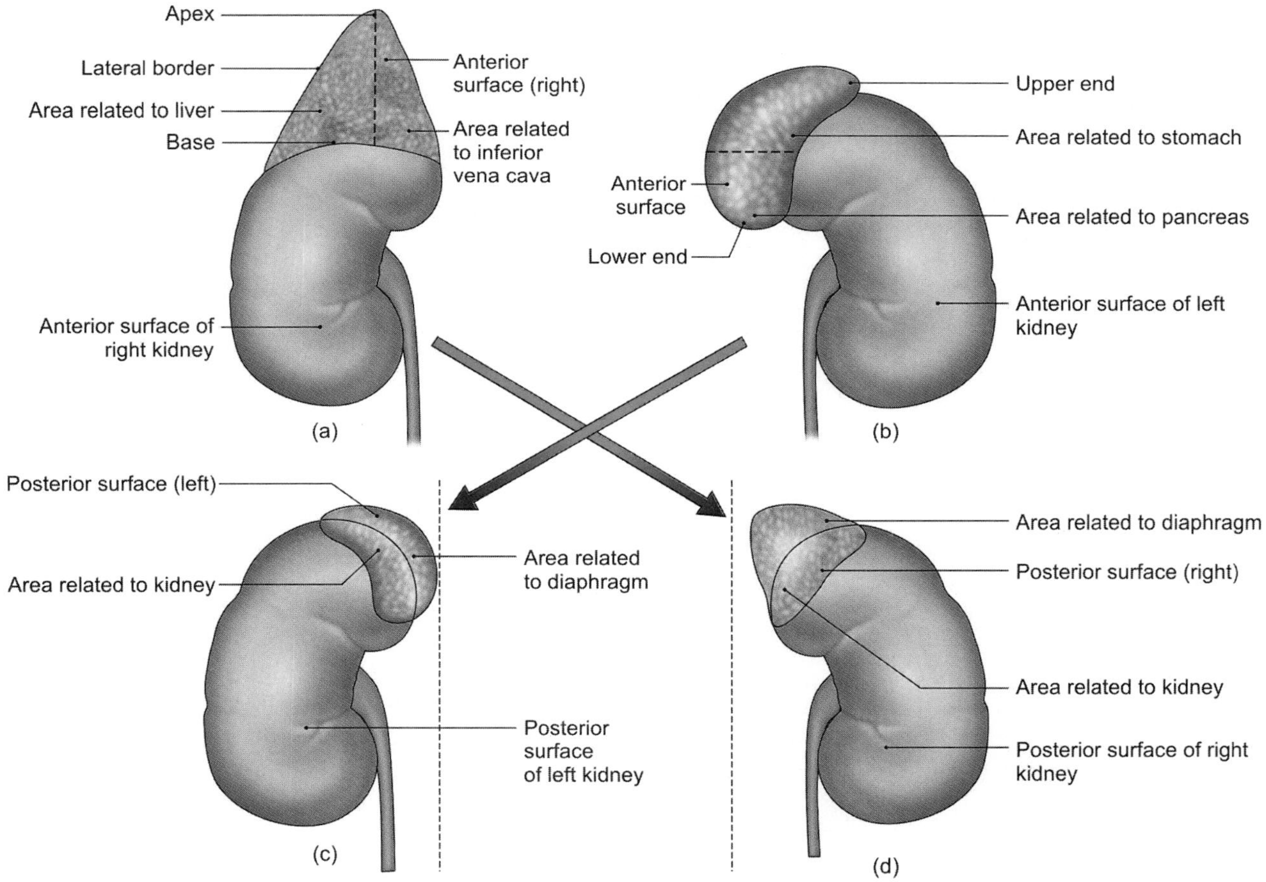

Figs 25.3a to d: Relations of the suprarenal glands: (a) Anterior view of right suprarenal gland, (b) anterior view of left suprarenal gland, (c) posterior view of left suprarenal gland, and (d) posterior view of right suprarenal gland

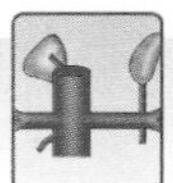

Table 25.1: Comparison of right and left suprarenal glands

	Right suprarenal gland	*Left suprarenal gland*
Shape	Pyramidal	Semilunar
Parts and relations	Apex: Bare area of liver Base: Upper pole of right kidney	Upper end: Close to spleen Lower end: Presents hilum, left vein emerges from here
Anterior surface	Inferior vena cava, bare area of liver	Cardiac end of stomach, pancreas with splenic artery
Posterior surface	Right crus of diaphragm, right kidney	Left crus of diaphragm, left kidney
Anterior border	Presents hilum, right vein emerges	—
Medial border	Coeliac ganglion	Coeliac ganglion
Lateral border	Liver	Stomach

The cortex is composed of three zones.

a. The outer, zona glomerulosa which produces mineralocorticoids that affect electrolyte and water balance of the body.
b. The middle, zona fasciculata which produces glucocorticoids.
c. The inner, zona reticularis which produces sex hormones.

The medulla is composed of chromaffin cells that secrete adrenaline and noradrenalin. It contains cells in groups with lots of capillaries. Autonomic ganglion cells are also seen.

Arterial Supply

Each gland is supplied by:

1 The *superior suprarenal artery*, a branch of the inferior phrenic artery.
2 The *middle suprarenal artery*, a branch of the abdominal aorta.
3 The *inferior suprarenal artery*, a branch of the renal artery (Fig. 25.4).

Venous Drainage

Each gland is drained by one vein (Fig. 25.5). The right suprarenal vein drains into the inferior vena cava, and the left suprarenal vein into the left renal vein.

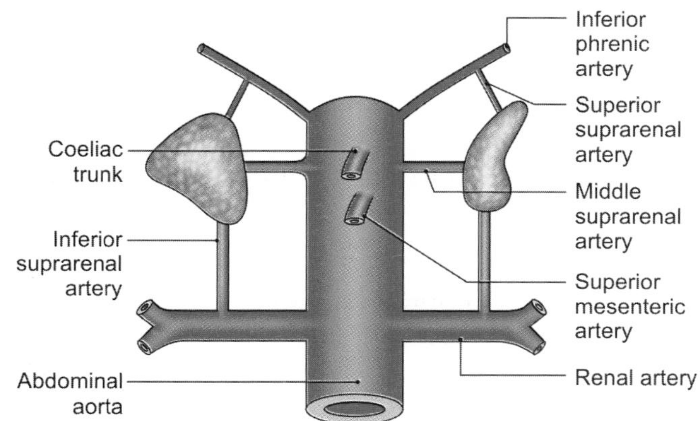

Fig. 25.4: Arterial supply of the suprarenal glands

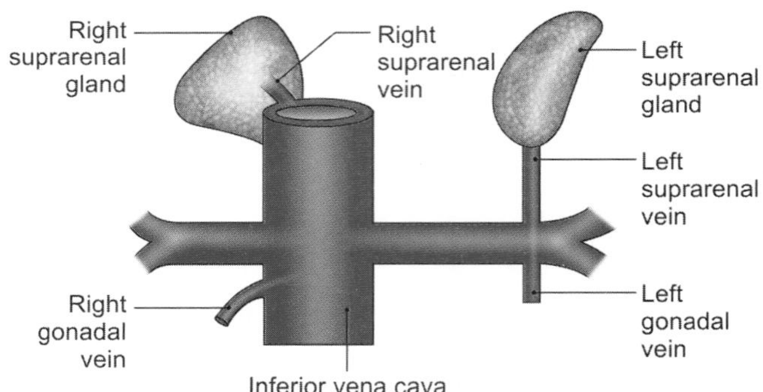

Fig. 25.5: Venous drainage of the suprarenal glands

Lymphatic Drainage

Lymphatics from the suprarenal glands drain into the lateral aortic nodes.

Nerve Supply

The suprarenal medulla has a rich nerve supply through myelinated *preganglionic* sympathetic fibres. The chromaffin cells in it are considered homologous with postganglionic sympathetic neurons.

Accessory Suprarenal Glands

These are small masses of cortical tissue often found in the areolar tissue around the main glands and sometimes in the spermatic cord, the epididymis, and the broad ligament of the uterus.

HISTOLOGY

Cortex: It consists of three zones. Outer zone is zona glomerulosa which contains groups of columnar cells with spherical nuclei. Middle zone or zona fasciculata has cells arranged in vertical rows. Cells have lots of vacuoles in the cytoplasm. The inner zone or zona reticularis contains cells in an anastomosing network. These cells are less vacuolated.

Medulla: It is composed of chromaffin cells, arranged in small groups, surrounded by capillaries. In between these cells are autonomic ganglion cells (Fig. 25.6).

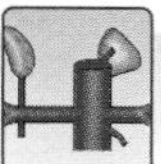

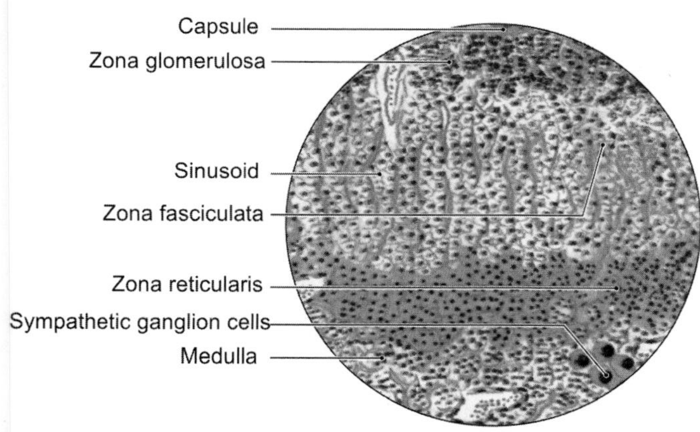

- Outer covering is the cortex and inside is the medulla
- Cortex comprises zona glomerulosa (outermost zone fasciculata (middle zone), and zona reticularis (innermost zone)
- Medulla comprises chromaffin cells and sympathetic ganglion cells

Fig. 25.6: Histology of suprarenal gland

DEVELOPMENT OF SUPRARENAL GLAND

The cortex of the gland develops from mesoderm of coelomic epithelium while the medulla is derived from the neural crest cells (neuroectoderm).

CHROMAFFIN SYSTEM

Chromaffin system is made up of cells which have an affinity for certain salt of chromic acid. Such cells are called chromaffin cells or pheochromocytes. These are situated close to sympathetic ganglia because both of them develop from the cells of the neural crest. Chromaffin cells secrete adrenaline and noradrenaline. This system includes the following groups of cells.

1 Suprarenal medulla (described above).
2 Paraganglia.
3 Para-aortic bodies.
4 Coccygeal body.
5 Small masses of chromaffin cells scattered irregularly amongst ganglia of sympathetic chain, splanchnic nerves, autonomic plexuses, and may be closely related to various organs like heart, liver, kidney, ureter, prostate, epididymis, etc.

PARAGANGLIA

These are rounded nodules of chromaffin tissue, about 2 mm in diameter, situated inside or closely related to the ganglia of the sympathetic chain. In adults they are generally represented by microscopic remnants only.

PARA-AORTIC BODIES

Two para-aortic bodies, each about 1 cm long, lie on each side of the origin of the inferior mesenteric artery. They are connected together above the artery to form an inverted horseshoe, or an H-shaped body. They develop during foetal life, attain their maximum size in the first three years of life, and gradually atrophy to disappear by the age of 14 years. The chromaffin cells of the para-aortic bodies secrete noradrenaline.

Other small chromaffin bodies are found in the foetus in all parts of the prevertebral sympathetic plexuses of the abdomen and pelvis. They reach their maximum size between the 5th and 8th months of foetal life. In adults, they can be made out only in the vicinity of the coeliac and superior mesenteric arteries.

COCCYGEAL BODY (GLOMUS COCCYGEUM)

Also known as glomus coccygeum, it is a small oval body about 2.5 cm in diameter situated in front of the coccyx. It is closely connected to the termination of the *median sacral artery* and to the *ganglion impar*. It is made up of epithelioid cells grouped around a sinusoidal capillary. Thus it does not clearly belong to the chromaffin system.

CLINICAL ANATOMY

- Suprarenal gland can be *demonstrated radiologically* by computerised tomography (CT scan).
- Insufficiency of cortical secretion due to atrophy or tuberculosis of the cortex results in *Addison's disease.* It is characterized by muscular weakness, low blood pressure, anaemia, pigmentation of skin and terminal circulatory and renal failure.
- Excessive cortical secretion due to hyperplasia of the cortex may produce various effects:
  a. In adults, hyperglucocorticism causes *Cushing's syndrome,* which is characterized by obesity, hirsutism, diabetes and hypogonadism.
  b. In women, excessive androgens may cause *masculinization (virilism).*
  c. In men, excessive oestrogens may cause *feminization* and breast enlargement.
  d. In children, excessive sex hormones cause *adrenogenital syndrome,* cortical hyperplasia. In female foetus excessive androgens cause *female pseudohermaphroditism;* in the male foetus, it causes excessive development of external genital organs.
- Bilateral removal of adrenal glands (*adrenalectomy*) is done as a treatment of some advanced and inoperable cases of disseminated carcinoma of the breast and prostate which do not respond to radiotherapy and which are considered to be dependent on hormonal control.
- Benign tumours of the suprarenal medulla (*pheochromocytoma*) cause attacks of hypertension associated with palpitation, headache, excessive sweating and pallor of skin.

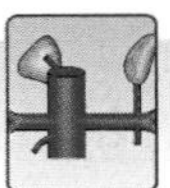

FACTS TO REMEMBER

- Suprarenal gland sustains the body during stress by its cortical and medullary hormones.
- Suprarenal is drained by one vein which ends in inferior vena cava on the right side and in left renal vein on the left side.
- Each suprarenal is supplied by 3 arteries.

CLINICOANATOMICAL PROBLEM

A patient has bouts of severe high blood pressure with headache and palpitation. The diagnosis is pheochromocytoma.

- How is the diagnosis finalised?
- Where does the blood supply to suprarenal gland come from?

Ans: The diagnosis is done by history, biochemical tests and CT scans.

There are three arteries supplying blood to the gland. These are superior suprarenal from inferior phrenic; middle suprarenal from abdominal aorta and inferior suprarenal from the renal artery.

Vein of suprarenal is only one. On the right side, the vein drains into inferior vena cava.

On the left side the suprarenal vein drains into the left suprarenal vein.

MULTIPLE CHOICE QUESTIONS

1. Right suprarenal vein drains into:
   a. Right renal vein b. Inferior vena cava
   c. Left renal vein d. Lumbar vein

2. Suprarenal gland does not receive blood supply from:
   a. Inferior phrenic artery
   b. Renal artery
   c. Superior mesenteric artery
   d. Abdominal aorta

3. Left suprarenal vein drains into:
   a. Left renal vein
   b. Right renal vein
   c. Inferior vena cava
   d. Lumbar vein

ANSWERS

1. b **2.** c **3.** a

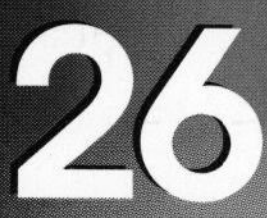

Diaphragm

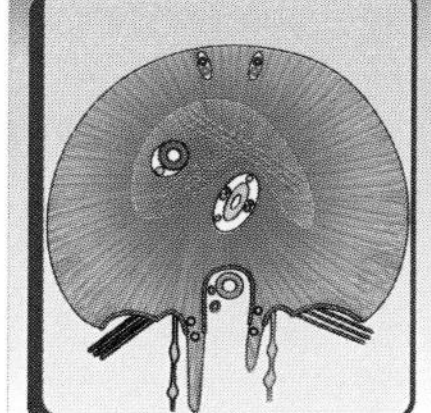

Nerves are most loyal. As the diaphragm descends from the neck to the thoraco-abdominal junction the phrenic nerve follows it

INTRODUCTION

The diaphragm is the chief muscle of quiet respiration. Though it separates the thoracic and abdominal cavities, it gives passage to a number of structures passing in both the directions. Since it develops in the region of the neck, it continues to be innervated by the same *loyal* nerve despite its descent to a much lower level.

During inspiration, the central tendon is pulled by the contracting muscle fibres, so that inferior vena caval opening is enlarged helping in venous return to the heart. This venous blood is pumped to the lungs. The air also gets into the lungs during inspiration. So both the venous blood in the capillaries and air in the alveoli *come close by* in the lung tissue, separated by the lining of the alveoli. The exchange of gases takes place, carbon dioxide is expelled in expiration and purified blood is returned to the left atrium.

GROSS ANATOMY

DISSECTION

Strip the peritoneum from the under aspect of the diaphragm and expose its crura on the anterior surfaces of the upper 2 or 3 lumbar vertebrae. Find the arcuate ligaments.

Expose the slips of diaphragm arising from the internal surfaces of the remaining costal cartilages and identify the intercostal vessels and nerves entering the abdominal wall between them.

Locate the main openings in the diaphragm and identify the structures passing through each one of them. Explore the other minor openings and the structures traversing these.

Definition

The diaphragm is a dome-shaped muscle forming the partition between the thoracic and abdominal cavities. It is the chief muscle of respiration.

Muscle fibres form the periphery of the partition. They arise from circumference of the thoracic outlet and are inserted into a central tendon (Fig. 26.1).

Origin

The muscle fibres may be grouped into three parts, sternal, costal and lumbar.

The *sternal part* arises by two fleshy slips from the back of the xiphoid process.

The *costal part* arises from the inner surfaces of the cartilages and the adjacent parts of the lower six ribs on each side, interdigitating with the transversus abdominis.

The *lumbar part* arises from the medial and lateral lumbocostal arches and from the lumbar vertebrae by right and left *crura*.

a. The *medial lumbocostal arch* or medial arcuate ligament is a tendinous arch in the fascia covering the upper part of the psoas major. Medially, it is attached to the side of the body of vertebra L1 and is continuous with the lateral margin of the corresponding crus. Laterally, it is attached to the front of the transverse process of vertebra L1.
b. The *lateral lumbocostal arch* or lateral arcuate ligament is a tendinous arch in the fascia covering the upper part of the quadratus lumborum. It is attached medially to the front of the transverse process of vertebra L1, and laterally to the lower border of the 12th rib.
c. The *right crus* is larger and stronger than the left crus, because it has to pull down the liver during

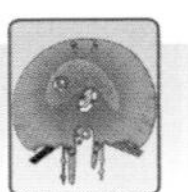

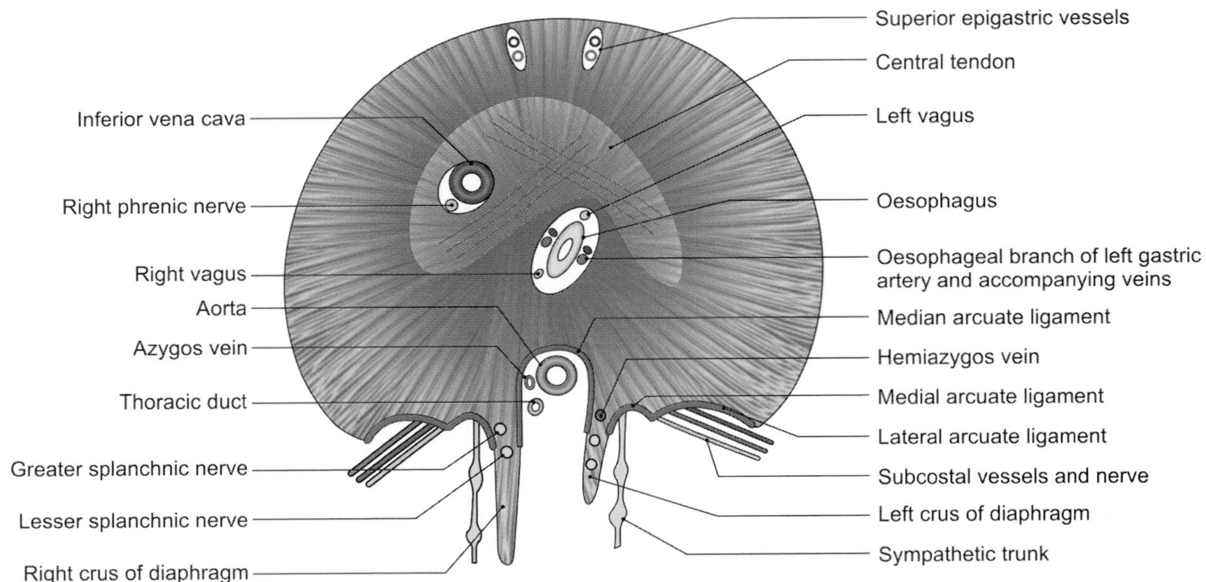

Fig. 26.1: The diaphragm as seen from below

each inspiration. It arises from the anterolateral surfaces of the bodies of the upper three lumbar vertebrae and the intervening intervertebral discs.

d. The *left crus* arises from the corresponding parts of the upper two lumbar vertebrae. The medial margins of the two crura form a tendinous arc across the front of the aorta, called the *median arcuate ligament*.

Muscle Fibres

1 From the circumferential origin described above, the fibres arch upwards and inwards to form the right and left domes. The right dome is higher than the left dome (Fig. 26.2a). In full expiration, it reaches the level of the fourth intercostal space. The left dome reaches the fifth rib. The central tendon lies at the level of the lower end of the sternum at 6th costal cartilage. The downward concavity of the dome is occupied by the liver on the right side and by the fundus of the stomach on the left side.

2 The medial fibres of the right crus run upwards and to the left, and encircle the oesophagus.

3 In general, all fibres converge towards the central tendon for their insertion (Fig. 26.2b).

Insertion

The *central tendon* of the diaphragm lies below the pericardium and is fused to the latter. The tendon is *trilobar* in shape, made up of three leaflets. The middle leaflet is triangular in shape with its apex directed towards the xiphoid process. The right and left leaflets are tongue-shaped and curve laterally and backwards, the left being a little narrower than the right. The central area consists of four well-marked *diagonal bands* which fan out from a central point of decussation located in front of the opening for the oesophagus (Fig. 26.1).

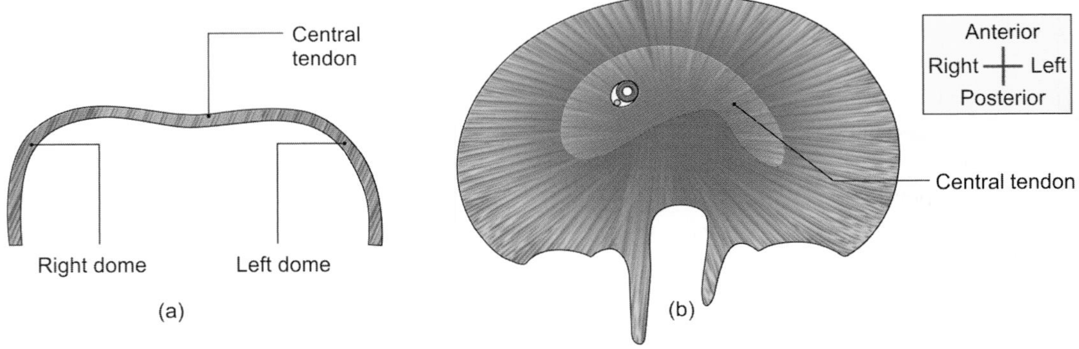

Figs 26.2a to c: Shape of the diaphragm: (a) Anteroposterior view shows the right and left domes, and (b) in superior view, it is kidney-shaped

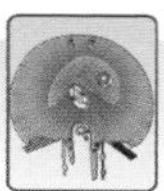

OPENINGS IN THE DIAPHRAGM

Large or Main Openings in the Diaphragm

The *aortic opening* is osseoaponeurotic. It lies at lower border of the 12th thoracic vertebra. It transmits:

a. Aorta
b. Thoracic duct
c. Azygos vein (Fig. 26.3).

The *oesophageal opening* lies in the muscular part of the diaphragm, at the level of the 10th thoracic vertebra. It transmits:

a. Oesophagus (Table 26.1)
b. Gastric or vagus nerves
c. Oesophageal branches of the left gastric artery, with some oesophageal veins that accompany the arteries.

The *vena caval opening* lies in the central tendon of the diaphragm at the level of the 8th thoracic vertebra. It transmits:

a. The inferior vena cava
b. Branches of the right phrenic nerve.
c. Lymphatics of liver.

Small Openings in the Diaphragm

1 Each crus of the diaphragm is pierced by the greater and lesser splanchnic nerves. The left crus is pierced in addition by the hemiazygos vein.

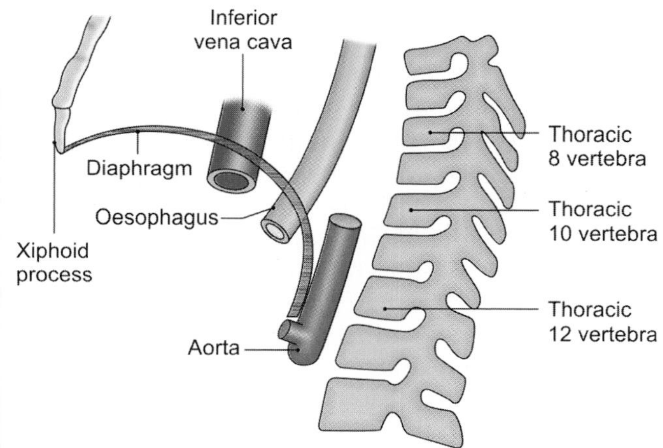

Fig. 26.3: Main openings in the diaphragm

2 The sympathetic chain passes from the thorax to the abdomen behind the medial arcuate ligament or medial lumbocostal arch.
3 The subcostal nerve and vessels pass behind the lateral arcuate ligament or lateral lumbocostal arch (Fig. 26.1).
4 The superior epigastric vessels and some lymphatics pass between the origins of the diaphragm from the xiphoid process and the 7th costal cartilage. This gap is known as Larry's space or foramen of Morgagni.
5 The musculophrenic vessels pierce the diaphragm at the level of 9th costal cartilage.

Relations

Superiorly

1 Pleurae, and
2 Pericardium.

Inferiorly

1 Peritoneum,
2 Liver,
3 Fundus of the stomach,
4 Spleen,
5 Kidneys, and
6 Suprarenals.

Nerve Supply

Motor

The phrenic nerves are the sole motor nerves to the diaphragm (ventral rami C3, **C4**, C5).

Sensory

The phrenic nerves are sensory to the central part, and the lower six thoracic nerves are sensory to the peripheral part of the diaphragm.

In addition to the diaphragm, the phrenic nerves also supply sensory fibres to the mediastinal and diaphragmatic pleurae, the fibrous pericardium, the parietal layer of serous pericardium, and the part of the parietal peritoneum lying below the central part of the diaphragm. Through its communications with the phrenic branches of the coeliac plexus, the phrenic

Table 26.1: Major openings

	Situation	*Shape*	*Structures passing*	*Effect of contraction*
Vena caval	T8, junction of right and median leaflet of central tendon	Quadrilateral	IVC, right phrenic nerve, lymphatics of liver	Dilatation
Oesophageal	T10, splitting of right crus	Elliptical	Oesophagus, gastric nerves oesophageal vessels	Constriction
Aortic	T12, behind median arcuate ligament	Rounded	Aorta, thoracic duct azygos vein	No change

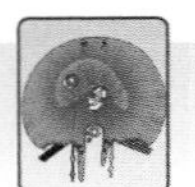

nerve is also distributed to the falciform and coronary ligaments of the liver, the inferior vena cava, the suprarenal glands, and the *gallbladder*.

Actions

1 The diaphragm is the *principal muscle of inspiration*. On contraction, the diaphragm descends increasing the vertical diameter of the thorax. The excursion of the diaphragm is about 1.5 cm during quiet breathing. In deep inspiration, it may be from 6 to 10 cm.
2 The diaphragm acts in all *expulsive acts* to give additional power to each effort. Thus before sneezing, coughing, laughing, crying, vomiting, micturition, defaecation, or parturition, a deep inspiration takes place. This is followed by closure of the glottis and powerful contraction of the trunk muscles.
3 The sphincteric action in lower end of oesophagus is due to the contraction of the intrinsic muscle in the lower 2 cm of the oesophagus.

The position of the diaphragm in the thorax depends upon three main factors. These are as follows.

a. The elastic recoil of lung tissue tends to pull the diaphragm upwards.
b. On lying down, the pressure exerted by the abdominal viscera pushes the diaphragm upwards. On standing or sitting, the viscera tend to pull the diaphragm downwards.
c. While standing, the muscles in the abdominal wall contract, increasing the intra-abdominal pressure. This pressure tends to push the diaphragm upwards. In sitting or lying down, the muscles are relaxed (*see* Chapter 13, Volume 1).

Because of these factors the level of the diaphragm is highest in the supine position, lowest while sitting, and intermediate while standing. The higher is the position of the diaphragm, the greater respiratory excursion.

DEVELOPMENT

Diaphragm develops from the following sources.

1 Septum transversum forms the central tendon.
2 Pleuroperitoneal membranes form the dorsal paired portion.
3 Lateral thoracic wall contributes to the circumferential portion of the diaphragm.
4 Dorsal mesentery of oesophagus forms the dorsal unpaired portion.

CLINICAL ANATOMY

- *Hiccough* or *hiccup* is the result of spasmodic contraction of the diaphragm. It may be:
  a. Peripheral, due to local irritation of the diaphragm or its nerve.
  b. Central, due to irritation of the hiccough centre in the medulla. Uraemia is an important cause of hiccough.
- *Shoulder tip pain:* Irritation of the diaphragm may cause referred pain in the shoulder because the phrenic and supraclavicular nerves have the same root values (C3, C4, C5) (*see* Figs 22.9 and 23.9).
- *Unilateral paralysis of the diaphragm*, due to a lesion of the phrenic nerve anywhere in its long course, is a common occurrence. The paralysed side moves opposite to the normal side, i.e. paradoxical movements. This can be seen both clinically and fluoroscopically.
- *Eventration* is a condition in which diaphragm is pushed upwards due to a congenital defect in the musculature of its left half which is represented only by a fibrous membrane containing a few scattered muscle fibres.
- *Diaphragmatic hernia* may be congenital or acquired:

  Congenital hernia

  a. *Retrosternal hernia:* It occurs through the space between the xiphoid and costal origins of the diaphragm, or foramen of Morgagni, or space of Larrey. It is more common on the right side and lies between the pericardium and the right pleura. Usually it causes no symptoms (Fig. 26.4).
  b. *Posterolateral hernia:* This is by far the commonest type of congenital diaphragmatic hernia. It occurs through the pleuro-peritoneal hiatus or *foramen of Bochdalek* situated at the periphery of the diaphragm in the region of attachments to the 10th and 11th ribs. It is more common on the left side. There is a free communication between the pleural and peritoneal cavities. Such a hernia may cause death of the infant within a few hours of birth due to acute respiratory distress caused by abdominal viscera filling the left chest. This hernia requires operation in the first few hours of life.
  c. *Posterior hernia:* This is due to failure of development of the posterior part of the diaphragm. One or both crus may be absent. The aorta and oesophagus lie in the gap, but there is no hernial sac.
  d. *Central hernia:* It is rare, left-sided, and is supposed to be the result of rupture of the foetal membranous diaphragm in the region of the left dome.

  Acquired hernia

  a. *Traumatic hernia:* It is due to bullet injuries of the diaphragm.

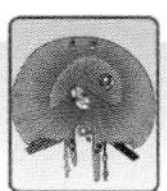

b. *Hiatal hernia:* It may be congenital or acquired.
   - A *congenital hiatal hernia* is due to persistence of an embryonic peritoneal process in the posterior mediastinum in front of the cardiac end of the stomach. The stomach can 'roll' upwards until it lies upside down in the posterior mediastinum. It is, therefore, called a rolling type of hernia. It is a rare type of hernia where the normal relationship of the cardio-oesophageal junction to the diaphragm is undisturbed, and, therefore, the mechanics of the cardio-oesophageal junction usually remains unaltered (Fig. 26.5a).
   - An *acquired hiatal hernia* or sliding type (Fig. 26.5b) is the commonest of all internal hernia. It is due to weakness of the phrenico-oesophageal membrane which is formed by the reflection of diaphragmatic fascia to the lower end of the oesophagus. It is often caused by obesity, or by operation in this area. The cardiac end can slide up through the hiatus. In this way the valvular mechanism at the cardio-oesophageal junction is disturbed causing reflux of gastric contents into the oesophagus.

- Summary of diaphragmatic hernia:
  a. *Congenital*
     i. Retrosternal,
     ii. Posterolateral,
     iii. Posterior, and
     iv. Central.
  b. *Acquired:*
     i. Traumatic
     ii. Hiatal
        - Congenital hiatal rolling hernia
        - Acquired hiatal sliding hernia (commonest).

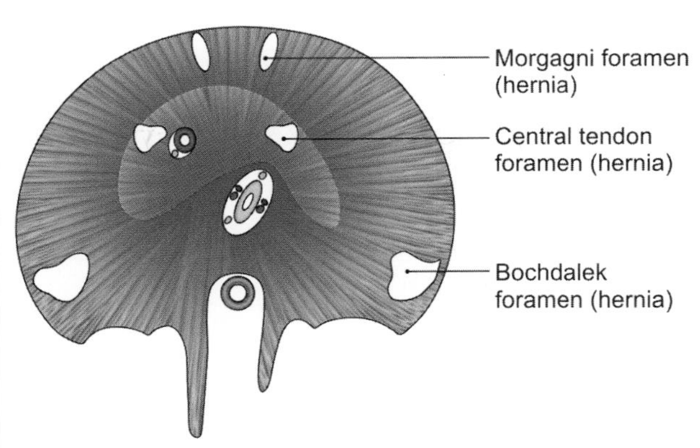

Fig. 26.4: Sites of diaphragmatic hernia

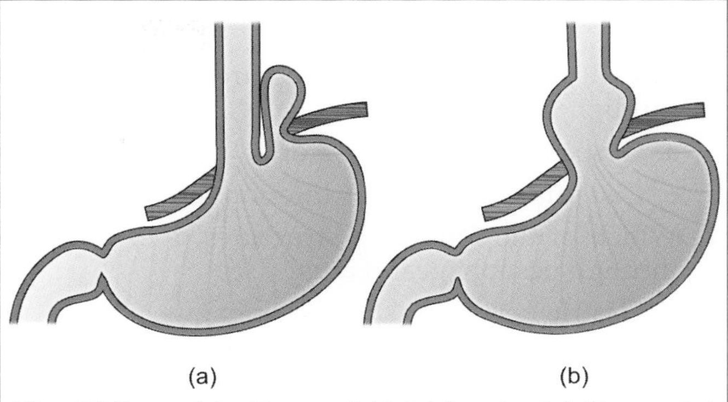

Figs 26.5a and b: Types of hiatal hernia: (a) Congenital rolling, and (b) acquired sliding

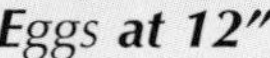

Mnemonics

Diaphragm apertures: spinal levels "I 8 10 Eggs at 12"

Inferior vena cava **(8)**
Oesophagus **(10)**
Aorta **(12)**

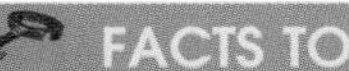

FACTS TO REMEMBER

- The sole motor nerve supply of the diaphragm is phrenic nerve (C4). It develops in the neck, but is carried downwards due to developmental factors.
- Inferior vena caval opening is in the central tendon. During inspiration the opening gets dilated allowing increased venous return.
- Right crus of diaphragm acts as a sphincter at the gastro-oesophageal junction.
- Hiatal hernia may be of rolling or sliding type. The rolling type is usually congenital while the sliding type is usually acquired.

CLINICOANATOMICAL PROBLEM

A busy obese businessman complains of acidity. He has been diagnosed as having sliding diaphragmatic hernia

- Why does this hernia occur?
- What is the relation of cardiac end of stomach to cardio-oesophageal junction?

Ans: This type of hernia occurs in busy executives or businessmen. It occurs due to weakness of phrenico-oesophageal membrane, which is formed by the reflection of diaphragmatic fascia to the lower end of oesophagus. The cardiac end may slide up through the hiatus. In this way the valvular mechanism at the cardio-oesophageal junction is disturbed, causing reflux of gastric contents up to the oesophagus.

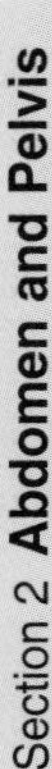

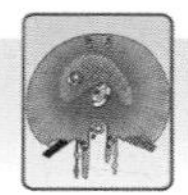

MULTIPLE CHOICE QUESTIONS

1. Which of the following structures does not pass through the diaphragm?
   a. Oesophagus b. Aorta
   c. Cisterna chyli d. Inferior vena cava
2. Which of the following structures does not pass through oesophageal hiatus?
   a. Gastric nerve b Oesophagus
   c. Left gastric artery d. Thoracic duct
3. Which of the following apertures lies in the central tendon of diaphragm?
   a. Oesophagus b. Inferior vena cava
   c. Thoracic duct d. Abdominal aorta
4. Which of the following structures form proper sphincter at the lower end of oesophagus?
   a. Left crus of diaphragm
   b. Intrinsic muscle of oesophagus
   c. Right crus of diaphragm
   d. Phrenico-oesophageal ligament
5. Patients with difficulty in breathing are comfortable in:
   a. Sitting up
   b. Lying down prone
   c. Lying down supine
   d. Standing up

ANSWERS

1. c **2.** d **3.** b **4.** c **5.** a

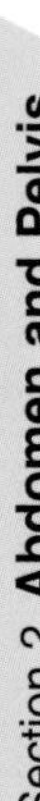

27

Posterior Abdominal Wall

Inferior vena cava is the largest vein of the body

INTRODUCTION

Posterior abdominal wall includes the study of the following structures.

1 Abdominal aorta.
2 Inferior vena cava.
3 Abdominal parts of the azygos and hemiazygos veins.
4 Lymph nodes of posterior abdominal wall and cisterna chyli.
5 Muscles of the posterior abdominal wall and thoracolumbar fascia.
6 Nerves of the posterior abdominal wall including lumbar plexus and the abdominal part of autonomic nervous system.

BLOOD VESSELS, MUSCLES AND NERVES

DISSECTION

Expose the centrally placed abdominal aorta and inferior vena cava to the right of aorta. Trace the ventral, lateral, posterior and terminal branches of abdominal aorta and the respective tributaries of inferior vena cava. Remove the big lymph nodes present in the posterior abdominal wall.

Identify the muscles of the posterior abdominal wall by removing their fascial coverings. These are psoas major, quadratus lumborum, and iliacus. Avoid injury to the vessels and nerves related to the muscles.

Detach psoas major from the intervertebral discs and vertebral bodies and trace the lumbar vessels and the rami communicans posteriorly deep to the tendinous arches from which psoas major arises. Dissect the genitofemoral nerve seen on the anterior surface of psoas major.

Trace the various branches of lumbar plexus, e.g. iliohypogastric, ilioinguinal, lateral cutaneous nerve of thigh and femoral nerve. These exit from the lateral border of psoas major. Identify obturator and lumbosacral trunk seen on the medial aspect of the muscle.

Locate the lumbar part of the right and left sympathetic chains. Trace their branches into the coeliac and superior mesenteric plexuses of nerves in addition to giving rami communicans to the lumbar spinal nerves.

ABDOMINAL AORTA

Beginning Course and Termination

The abdominal aorta begins in the midline at the aortic opening of the diaphragm, opposite the lower border of vertebra T12. It runs downwards and slightly to the left in front of the lumbar vertebrae, and ends in front of the lower part of the body of vertebra L4, about 1.25 cm to the left of the median plane, by dividing into the right and left common iliac arteries (Fig. 27.1). Due to the forward convexity of the lumbar vertebral column, aortic pulsations can be felt in the region of the umbilicus, particularly in slim persons.

Relations

Anteriorly

From above downwards, the aorta is related to:

1 Coeliac and aortic plexuses.
2 Body of the pancreas, with the splenic vein embedded in its posterior surface (*see* Fig. 23.15).
3 Third part of the duodenum (*see* Fig. 21.2).

Posteriorly

The aorta is related to:

1 The bodies of upper four lumbar vertebrae and the corresponding intervertebral discs (*see* Fig. 21.1).
2 Anterior longitudinal ligament.

To the right side of the aorta there are:

1 Inferior vena cava.
2 Right crus of the diaphragm.
3 Cisterna chyli and the azygos vein in the upper part.

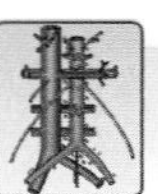

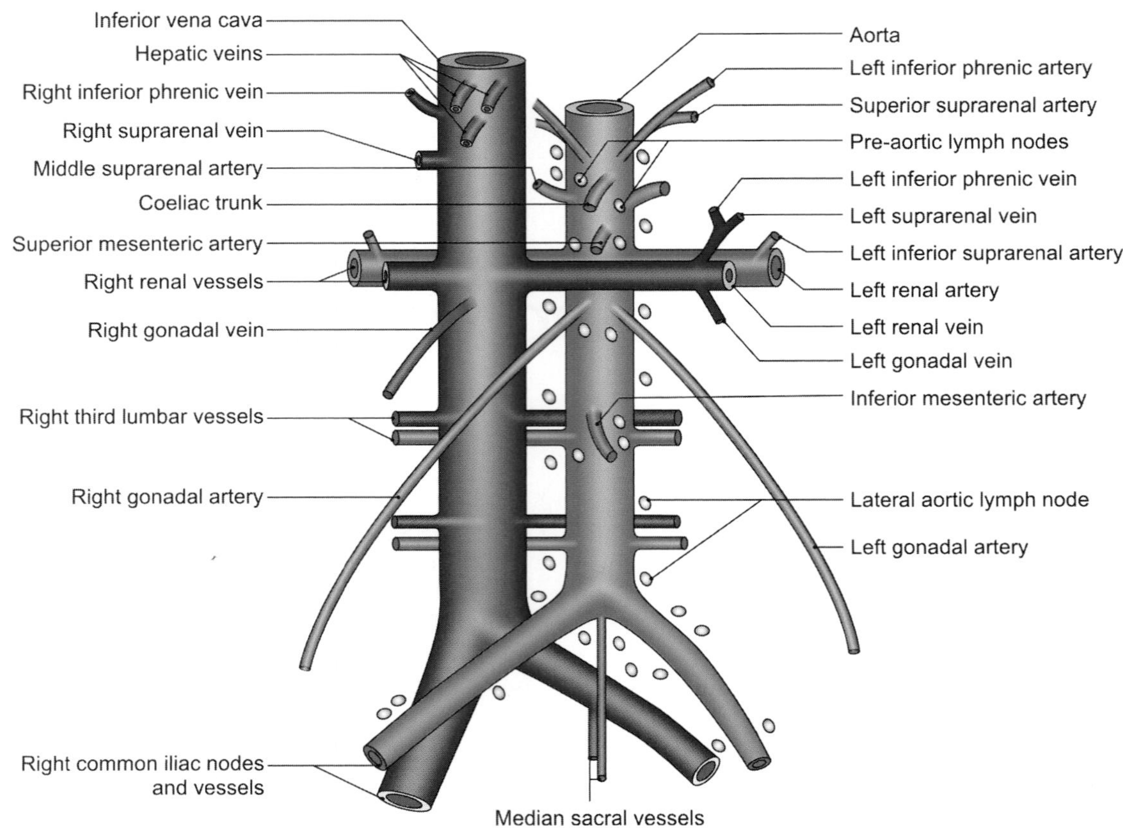

Fig. 27.1: The abdominal aorta, inferior vena cava and associated lymph nodes

To the left side of the aorta there are from above downwards:

a. Left crus of the diaphragm.
b. Pancreas.
c. Fourth part of the duodenum.

Branches

The branches of the abdominal aorta are classified as given below (Fig. 27.1).

Ventral branches, which develop from *ventral splanchnic* or *vitelline arteries* and supply the gut. These are as follows.

a. Coeliac trunk (*see* Chapter 21) gives left gastric, common hepatic and splenic branches.
b. Superior mesenteric artery (*see* Chapter 21) gives inferior pancreaticoduodenal, middle colic, right colic, ileocolic and 12–15 jejunal and ileal branches.
c. Inferior mesenteric artery (*see* Chapter 21) gives left colic, sigmoid arteries and continues as superior rectal.

Lateral branches, which develop from the *lateral splanchnic* or mesonephric arteries and supply the viscera derived from the intermediate mesoderm. These are right and left:

a. Inferior phrenic arteries.
b. Middle suprarenal arteries.
c. Renal arteries.
d. Testicular or ovarian arteries.

Dorsal branches represent the *somatic intersegmental* arteries and are distributed to the body wall. These are:

a. Lumbar arteries—four pairs.
b. Median sacral artery—unpaired.

Terminal branches are a pair of common iliac arteries. They supply the pelvis and lower limbs.

Inferior Phrenic Arteries

Inferior phrenic arteries arise from the aorta just above the coeliac trunk. Each artery runs upwards and laterally on the corresponding crus of the diaphragm, medial to the suprarenal gland. Each artery gives off two to three superior suprarenal arteries, and is then distributed to the diaphragm.

Middle Suprarenal Arteries

Middle suprarenal arteries arise at the level of the superior mesenteric artery. Each passes laterally and slightly upwards over the corresponding crus of the diaphragm, to reach the gland (*see* Fig. 25.4).

Renal Arteries

Renal arteries are large arteries which arise from the abdominal aorta just below the level of origin of the superior mesenteric artery. The *right renal artery* passes laterally behind the inferior vena cava to reach the hilum of the right kidney. The *left renal artery* runs behind the left renal vein, and the splenic vein. Each artery gives off the inferior suprarenal and ureteral branches, and is then distributed to the kidney (Fig. 27.1).

Gonadal: Testicular or Ovarian Arteries

Gonadal arteries are small and arise from the front of the aorta a little below the origin of the renal arteries. Each artery runs downwards and slightly laterally on the psoas major. On the right side the artery crosses in front of the inferior vena cava, the ureter and the genitofemoral nerve. It passes deep to the ileum. On the left side the artery crosses in front of the ureter and the genitofemoral nerve; and passes deep to the colon (*see* Figs 24.24 and 24.25).

The *testicular artery* joins the spermatic cord at the deep inguinal ring, and traverses the inguinal canal. Within the cord, it lies anterior to the ductus deferens. At the upper pole of the testis, it breaks up into branches which supply the testis and the epididymis.

The *ovarian artery* crosses the external iliac vessels at the pelvic brim to enter the suspensory or infundibulopelvic ligament of the ovary. It thus enters the broad ligament and runs below the uterine tube to reach the ovary through the mesovarium. The artery gives a branch which continues medially to anastomose with the uterine artery, and supplies twigs to the uterine tube and to the pelvic part of the ureter (*see* Fig. 31.4).

Lumbar Arteries

Four pairs of lumbar arteries arise from the aorta opposite the bodies of the upper four lumbar vertebrae. The small, fifth pair is usually represented by the lumbar branches of the iliolumbar arteries.

The upper four lumbar arteries run across the sides of the bodies of the upper four lumbar vertebrae, passing deep to the crura (upper arteries only), deep to the psoas major and the quadratus lumborum to end in small branches between the transversus and internal oblique muscles. Each artery gives off a dorsal branch, which arises at the root of the transverse process. The dorsal branch gives off a spinal branch to the vertebral canal, and then runs backwards to supply the muscles and skin of the back.

Median Sacral Artery

Median sacral artery represents the continuation of the primitive dorsal aorta. It arises from the back of the aorta just above the bifurcation of the latter, and runs downwards to end in front of the coccyx. It supplies the rectum and anastomoses with the iliolumbar and lateral sacral arteries.

COMMON ILIAC ARTERIES

Course

These are the terminal branches of the abdominal aorta, beginning in front of vertebra L4, 1.25 cm to the left of the median plane. On each side it passes downwards and laterally and ends in front of the sacroiliac joint, at the level of the lumbosacral intervertebral disc, by dividing into the external and internal iliac arteries.

The *right common iliac artery* passes in front of the commencement of the inferior vena cava. The right common iliac vein is posterior to the vena cava above, and medial to it below (Fig. 27.1).

The *left common iliac artery* is shorter than the right artery. It is crossed at its middle by the inferior mesenteric vessels. The left common iliac vein is medial to it. The structures lying on the left ala of the sacrum, i.e. sympathetic trunk, lumbosacral trunk, into lumbar artery and obturator nerve are deep to it.

INFERIOR VENA CAVA

The inferior vena cava is formed by the union of the right and left common iliac veins on the right side of the body of vertebra L5. It ascends in front of the vertebral column, on the right side of the aorta, grooves the posterior surface of the liver, pierces the central tendon of the diaphragm at the level of vertebra T8, and opens into the lower and posterior part of the right atrium (*see* Fig. 26.1).

Relations

Anteriorly

From above downwards, inferior vena cava is related to:

1 Posterior surface of the liver.
2 Epiploic foramen (*see* Fig. 18.22).
3 First part of the duodenum and the portal vein.
4 Head of the pancreas along with the bile duct.
5 Third part of duodenum (*see* Fig. 20.10a).

Posteriorly

Above, the right crus of the diaphragm is separated from the inferior vena cava by the right renal artery, the right coeliac ganglion, and the medial part of the right suprarenal gland. Below, it is related to the right sympathetic chain and to the medial border of the right psoas.

Tributaries

1 The *common iliac veins* formed by the union of the external and internal iliac veins unite to form the inferior vena cava. Each vein receives an iliolumbar vein. The median sacral vein joins the left common iliac vein (Fig. 27.1).
2 The *third* and *fourth lumbar veins* run along with the corresponding arteries and open into the posterior

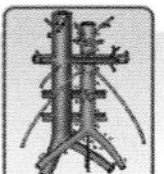

aspect of the inferior vena cava. The veins of the left side cross behind the aorta to reach the vena cava. The first and second lumbar veins end in the ascending lumbar vein, on the right and the left sides.

The ascending lumbar vein is an anastomotic channel which connects the lateral sacral, iliolumbar, and the subcostal veins. It lies within the psoas muscle, in front of the roots of the transverse processes of the lumbar vertebrae. On joining the subcostal vein it forms the azygos vein on the right side, and the hemiazygos vein on the left side.

3 The *right testicular* or *ovarian vein* opens into the inferior vena cava just below the entrance of the renal veins. *The left gonadal vein drains into the left renal vein* (Fig. 27.1).
4 The *renal veins* join the inferior vena cava just below the transpyloric plane. Each renal vein lies in front of the corresponding artery. The right vein is shorter than the left and lies behind the second part of the duodenum. The left vein crosses in front of the aorta, and lies behind the pancreas and the splenic vein. It receives the left suprarenal and gonadal veins (Fig. 27.1).
5 The *right suprarenal vein* is extremely short. It emerges from the hilum of the gland and soon opens into the inferior vena cava. The left suprarenal vein opens into the left renal vein.
6 The *hepatic veins* are three large and many small veins which open directly into the anterior surface of the inferior vena cava just before it pierces the diaphragm. These act as important support of liver (*see* Fig. 23.27).

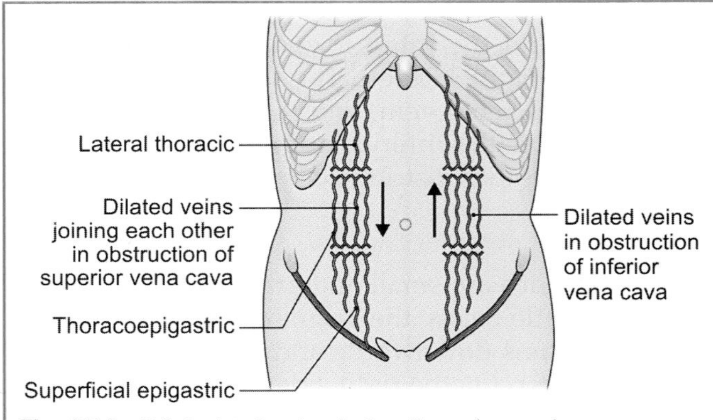

Fig. 27.2: Dilated veins in obstruction of superior vena cava and inferior vena cava

CLINICAL ANATOMY

Thrombosis in the inferior vena cava causes oedema of the legs and back. The collateral venous circulation between the superior and inferior venae cavae is established through the superficial or deep veins, or both. The participating main superficial veins include the (i) superficial epigastric, (ii) lateral thoracic, (iii) thoracoepigastric. Other veins are internal thoracic, posterior intercostal, external pudendal and lumbo-vertebral veins (Fig. 27.2). The deep veins are the azygos, hemiazygos and lumbar veins. The vertebral venous plexus may also provide an effective collateral circulation between the two venae cavae.

Abdominal aneurysm's (dilatation of the vessel) most common site is between the renal arteries and bifurcation of the abdominal aorta).

ABDOMINAL PARTS OF AZYGOS AND HEMIAZYGOS VEINS

These veins usually begin in the abdomen. The *azygos vein* arise from the posterior surface of the inferior vena cava near the renal veins; may be formed by the union of the right ascending lumbar vein and the right subcostal vein. It enters the thorax by passing through the aortic opening of the diaphragm.

The *hemiazygos vein* is the mirror image of the lower part of the azygos vein. It arise from the posterior surface of the left renal vein, or may be formed by the union of the left ascending lumbar vein and the left subcostal vein. It enters the thorax by piercing the left crus of the diaphragm.

LYMPH NODES OF POSTERIOR ABDOMINAL WALL

These are the external iliac, common iliac and lumbar or aortic nodes.

The *external iliac nodes* 8 to 10 lie along the external iliac vessels, being lateral, medial and anterior to them. They receive afferents from:

1 Inguinal lymph nodes
2 Deeper layers of the infraumbilical part of the anterior abdominal wall
3 Adductor region of the thigh
4 Glans penis or clitoris
5 Membranous urethra
6 Prostate
7 Fundus of the urinary bladder
8 Cervix uteri
9 Part of the vagina.

Their efferents pass to common iliac nodes. The inferior epigastric and circumflex iliac nodes are outlying members of the external iliac group.

The *common iliac nodes*, 4 to 6 in number lie along the common iliac artery below the bifurcation of the aorta in front of vertebra L5 or in front of the sacral promontory. They receive afferents from the external and internal iliac nodes, and send their efferents to the lateral aortic nodes (Fig. 27.1).

The *lumbar* or *aortic nodes* are divided into preaortic and lateral aortic groups. The *preaortic nodes* lie directly anterior to the abdominal aorta, and are divisible into coeliac, superior mesenteric and inferior mesenteric groups. They receive afferents from intermediate nodes associated with the subdiaphragmatic part of the gastrointestinal tract, the liver, the pancreas and the spleen (Fig. 27.1). Their efferents form the *intestinal trunks* which enter the cisterna chyli.

The *lateral aortic nodes* lie on each side of the abdominal aorta. They receive afferents from the structures supplied by the lateral and dorsal branches of the aorta and form the common iliac nodes. Their efferents from a *lumbar trunk* on each side, both of which terminate in the cisterna chyli (Fig. 27.1).

CISTERNA CHYLI

This is an elongated lymphatic sac, about 5 to 7 cm long. It is situated in front of the first and second lumbar vertebrae, immediately to the right of the abdominal aorta. It is overlapped by the right crus of the diaphragm. Its upper end is continuous with the thoracic duct. It is joined by the right and left lumbar and intestinal lymph trunks.

The lumbar trunks arise from the lateral aortic nodes, and bring lymph from the lower limbs, the pelvic wall and viscera, the kidneys, the suprarenal glands, the testes or ovaries, and the deeper parts of the abdominal wall. The intestinal trunks bring lymph from the stomach, the intestine, the pancreas, the spleen, and the anteroinferior part of the liver.

MUSCLES OF THE POSTERIOR ABDOMINAL WALL

These are the psoas major, the psoas minor, the iliacus and the quadratus lumborum. Their attachments are given in Table 27.1 and their nerve supply and actions are given in Table 27.2. Some additional facts about the psoas major (Fig. 27.3) are given below.

Relations of the Psoas Major

In the Posterior Mediastinum

The uppermost part of the psoas major lies in the posterior mediastinum, and is related anteriorly to the diaphragm and pleura.

In the Abdomen

Its *anterolateral surface* is related to:

1 Medial lumbocostal arch or medial arcuate ligament and psoas fascia (*see* Fig. 24.4).
2 Peritoneum and extraperitoneal connective tissue.

Table 27.1: Attachments of muscles of the posterior abdominal wall

Muscle	*Origin*	*Insertion*
1. **Psoas major** This is a fusiform muscle placed on the side of the lumbar spine and along the brim of the pelvis. The psoas and the iliacus are together known as the iliopsoas, due to their common insertion and actions (Fig. 27.3)	a. From anterior surfaces and lower borders of transverse process of all lumbar vertebrae (*see* Fig. 15.3) b. By 5 slips, one each from the bodies of two adjacent vertebrae and their intervertebral discs, from vertebrae, T12 to L5 c. From 4 tendinous arches extending across the constricted parts of the bodies of lumbar vertebrae, between the preceding slips. The origin is a continuous one from the lower border of T12 to upper border of L5	The muscle passes behind the inguinal ligament and in front of the hip joint to enter the thigh. It ends in a tendon which receives the fibres of the iliacus on its lateral side. It is then inserted into the tip and medial part of the anterior surface of the lesser trochanter of the femur
2. **Psoas minor** This is a small muscle which lies in front of the psoas major. It is frequently absent	Sides of the bodies of vertebrae T12 and L1 and the disc between them	The muscle ends in a long, flat tendon which is inserted into the pecten pubis and the iliopubic eminence
3. **Iliacus** This is a triangular muscle (Fig. 27.3)	a. Upper 2/3rd of iliac fossa (*see* Fig. 2.5) b. Inner lip of the iliac crest and the ventral sacroiliac and iliolumbar ligaments c. Upper surface of the lateral part of the sacrum	Lateral part of anterior surface of the lesser trochanter. The insertion extends for 2.5 cm below the trochanter
4. **Quadratus lumborum** This is a quadrate muscle lying in the lumbar region. Its origin lies below and the insertion is above (*see* Fig. 24.4)	a. Transverse process of vertebra L5 b. Iliolumbar ligament c. Adjoining 5 cm of the inner lip of the iliac crest (*see* Fig. 2.3)	a. Transverse processes of upper 4 lumbar vertebrae b. Medial half of the lower border of anterior surface of the 12th rib

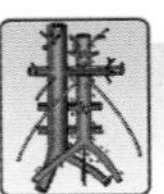

Table 27.2: Nerve supply and actions of muscles of the posterior abdominal wall

Muscle	*Nerve supply*	*Actions*
1. **Psoas major**	Branches from the roots of spinal nerve L2, L3 and sometimes L4.	1. With the iliacus, it acts as a powerful flexor of the hip, joint as in raising the trunk from recumbent to sitting posture 2. Helps in maintaining stability at the hip. Balances the trunk while sitting 3. When the muscle of one side acts alone, it brings about lateral flexion of the trunk on that side 4. It is a weak medial rotator of the hip. After fracture of the neck of the femur, the limb rotates laterally
2. **Psoas minor**	Branches from spinal nerve L1	Weak flexor of the trunk
3. **Iliacus**	Branches from femoral nerve (L2, 3)	With the psoas, it flexes the hip joint
4. **Quadratus lumborum**	Ventral rami of spinal nerves T12 to L4	1. Fixes the last rib during inspiration so that the contraction of the diaphragm takes place more effectively 2. When the pelvis is fixed, it may cause lateral flexion of the vertebral column 3. The muscles of both sides acting together can extend the lumbar vertebral column

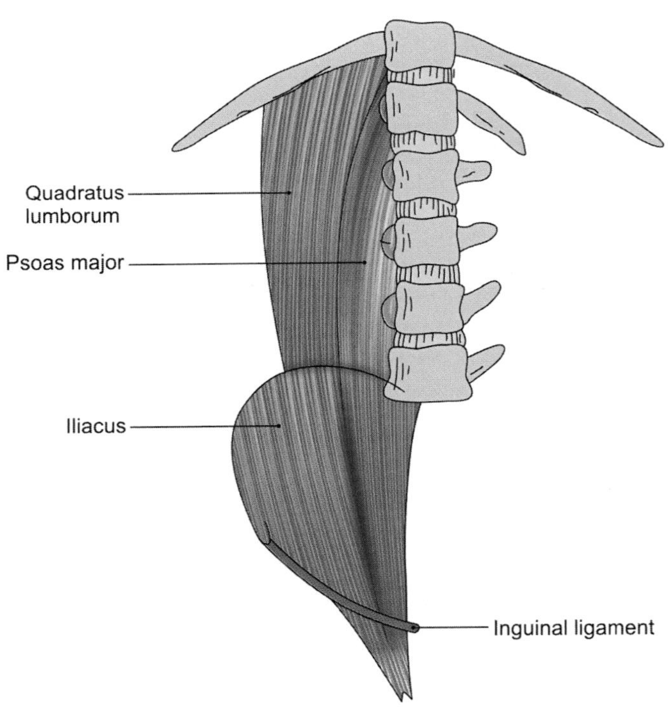

Fig. 27.3: Muscles of the posterior abdominal wall

3 Kidney and ureter (*see* Fig. 24.6).
4 Renal and gonadal vessels.
5 Genitofemoral nerve.
6 Psoas minor.
7 Inferior vena cava and the terminal ileum on the right side.
8 Colon on the left side.

The *posterior surface* is related to:
1 Transverse processes of lumbar vertebrae.
2 Lumbar plexus lies in substance of the muscle.

The *medial surface* is related to:
1 Bodies of the lumbar vertebrae (*see* Fig. 24.6).
2 Lumbar vessels.

The *medial (anterior) margin* is related to:
1 Sympathetic chain (Fig. 27.5).
2 Aortic lymph nodes.
3 Inferior vena cava on the right side.
4 Aorta on the left side.
5 External iliac vessels along the pelvic brim.

In the Thigh

Anteriorly: Femoral artery and fascia lata.

Posteriorly: Capsule of hip joint separated by a bursa.

Medially: Pectineus and femoral vein.

Laterally: Femoral nerve and iliacus (*see* Fig. 3.10b).

CLINICAL ANATOMY

Psoas abscess: The psoas is enclosed in the psoas sheath, a part of the lumbar fascia. Pus from tubercular infection of the thoracic and lumbar vertebrae may track down through the sheath into the thigh, producing a soft swelling in the femoral triangle (Fig. 27.4).

The typical posture of a laterally rotated lower limb following fracture of the neck of the femur is produced by contraction of the psoas muscle.

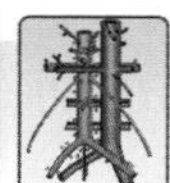

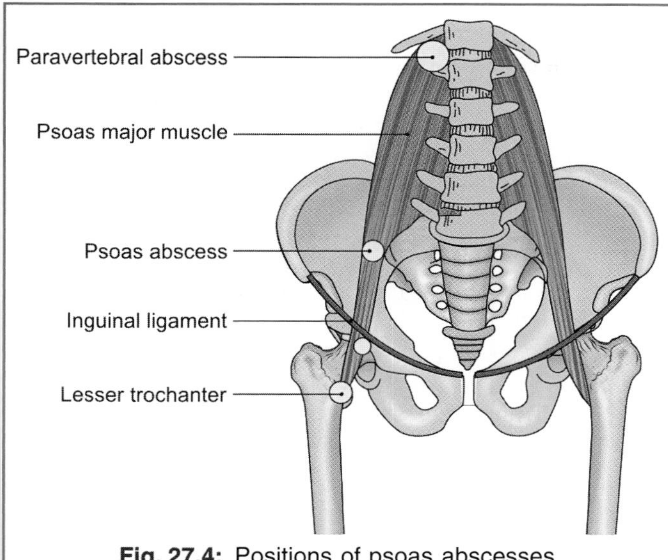

Fig. 27.4: Positions of psoas abscesses

THORACOLUMBAR FASCIA (LUMBAR FASCIA)

Lumbar fascia is the fascia enclosing the deep muscles of the back (*see* Fig. 24.11). It is made up of three layers—posterior, middle and anterior. The posterior layer is thickest and the anterior layer thinnest.

Extent

The posterior layer covers the loin and is continued upwards on the back of the thorax and neck. The middle and anterior layers are confined to the lumbar region.

Attachments

Posterior Layer

- *Medially,* the posterior layer is attached to the tips of the lumbar and sacral spines and the interspinous ligaments.
- *Laterally,* it blends with the middle layer at the lateral border of the erector spinae.
- *Superiorly,* it continues on to the back of the thorax where it is attached to the vertebral spines and the angles of the ribs.
- *Inferiorly,* it is attached to the posterior one-fourth of the outer lip of the iliac crest.

Middle Layer

- *Medially,* the middle layer is attached to the tips of the lumbar transverse processes and the intertransverse ligaments.
- *Laterally,* it blends with the anterior layer at the lateral border of the quadratus lumborum.
- *Superiorly,* it is attached to the lower border of the 12th rib and to the lumbocostal ligament.
- *Inferiorly,* it is attached to the posterior part of the intermediate area of the iliac crest.

Anterior Layer

- *Medially,* the anterior layer is attached to the vertical ridges on the anterior surface of the lumbar transverse processes.
- *Laterally,* it blends with the middle layer at the lateral border of the quadratus lumborum.
- *Superiorly,* it forms the lateral arcuate ligament, extending from the tip of the first lumbar transverse process to the 12th rib.
- *Inferiorly,* it is attached to the inner lip of the iliac crest and the iliolumbar ligament (*see* Fig. 24.11).

NERVES OF THE POSTERIOR ABDOMINAL WALL

Lumbar Plexus

The lumbar plexus lies in the posterior part of the substance of the psoas major muscle. It is formed by the ventral rami of the upper four lumbar nerves (*see* Fig. 3.3). The first lumbar nerve receives a contribution from the subcostal nerve, and the fourth lumbar nerve gives a contribution to the lumbosacral trunk; which takes part in the formation of the sacral plexus. The branches of the lumbar plexus are summarized.

Iliohypogastric Nerve (L1)

The *iliohypogastric nerve* (L1) emerges at the lateral border of the psoas, runs downwards and laterally in front of the quadratus lumborum, and behind the kidney and colon, pierces the transversus abdominis a little above the iliac crest, and runs in the abdominal wall supplying the anterolateral muscles.

Ilioinguinal Nerve (L1)

The *ilioinguinal nerve* (L1) has the same course as the iliohypogastric nerve, but on a slightly lower level. It exits through superficial inguinal ring.

Genitofemoral Nerve

The *genitofemoral nerve* (L1, L2 ventral divisions) emerges on the anterior surface of the psoas muscle near its medial border and runs downwards in front of the muscle. Near the deep inguinal ring it divides into femoral and genital branches. The *femoral branch* passes through the arterial compartment of the femoral sheath and is distributed to the skin of the upper part of the front of the thigh. The *genital branch* pierces the psoas sheath and enters the inguinal canal through the deep inguinal ring. In the male, it supplies the cremaster muscle, and in the female, it gives sensory branches to the round ligament of the uterus and to the skin of the labium majus (*see* Fig. 16.18).

Lateral Cutaneous Nerve of the Thigh

The *lateral cutaneous nerve of the thigh* (L2, L3; dorsal divisions) emerges at the lateral border of the psoas,

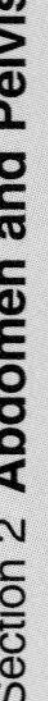

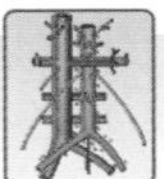

runs downwards and laterally across the right iliac fossa, over the iliacus and reaches the anterior superior iliac spine. Here it enters the thigh by passing behind the lateral end of the inguinal ligament (*see* Fig. 3.3).

Femoral Nerve

The *femoral nerve* (L2, L3, L4; dorsal divisions) emerges at the lateral border of the psoas below the iliac crest, and runs downwards and slightly laterally in the furrow between the psoas and iliacus. It lies under cover of the fascia iliaca. It passes deep to the inguinal ligament to enter the thigh lying on the lateral side of the femoral sheath. Before entering the thigh it supplies the iliacus and pectineus. In thigh it supplies quadriceps femoris and sartorius (*see* Fig. 3.26).

Obturator Nerve

The *obturator nerve* (L2, L3, L4; ventral divisions) emerges on the medial side of the psoas muscle and runs forwards and downwards on the pelvic wall, below the pelvic brim. Near its commencement it is crossed by the internal iliac vessels and the ureter. It enters the thigh by passing through the obturator canal. It supplies 3 adductor muscles, obturator externus and gracilis (*see* Fig. 4.4).

Lumbosacral Trunk

The *lumbosacral trunk* (L4, L5; ventral rami) is formed by union of the descending branch of nerve L4 with nerve L5. It enters the lesser pelvis by passing over and grooving the lateral part of the ala of the sacrum, posterior to the common iliac vessels and the medial part of the psoas. It is related medially to the sympathetic chain; and laterally to the iliolumbar artery and the obturator nerve (*see* Fig. 15.11). In the pelvis, it takes part in the formation of the sacral plexus.

ABDOMINAL PART OF THE AUTONOMIC NERVOUS SYSTEM

The abdomen is supplied by both sympathetic and parasympathetic nerves. The *sympathetic nerves* are derived from two sources.

1 The lumbar sympathetic trunk supplies somatic branches to the lower abdominal wall and the lower limb; and visceral branches for the pelvic organs (Fig. 27.5).
2 The coeliac plexus, formed by splanchnic nerves from the thorax, supplies all the abdominal organs, including the gonads.

The *parasympathetic nerves* are also derived from two sources.

a. The vagus joins the coeliac plexus.
b. The pelvic splanchnic nerves join the inferior hypogastric plexus.

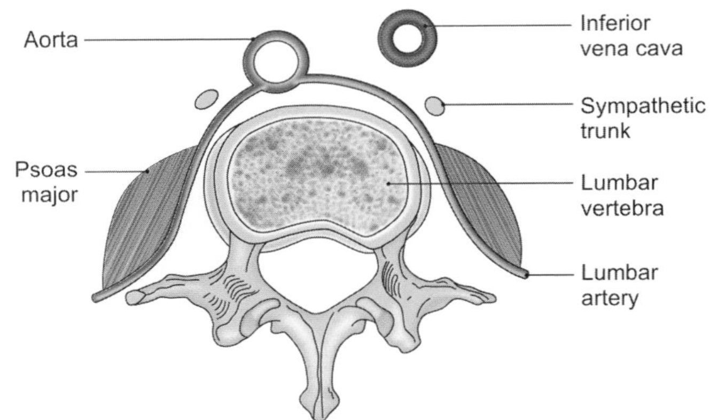

Fig. 27.5: Transverse section through the lumbar region showing location of the lumbar sympathetic chain

Lumbar Sympathetic Chain

This is ganglionated chain situated on either side of the bodies of the lumbar vertebrae containing five ganglia.

The lumbar sympathetic chain is continuous with the thoracic part deep to the medial arcuate ligament. It runs vertically downwards along the medial margin of the psoas major, and across the lumbar vessels. On the right side, it is overlapped by the inferior vena cava, and on the left by the lateral aortic lymph nodes.

The lumbar chain ends by becoming continuous with the sacral part of the sympathetic chain behind the common iliac vessels.

The anterior primary rami of the first and second lumbar nerves send white rami communicans to the corresponding ganglia.

Branches

Lateral

All the five lumbar nerves receive grey rami communicans from the corresponding lumbar ganglia. The grey rami carry fibres which are distributed to the lower abdominal wall and to the lower limb (Fig. 27.6).

Medial

The lumbar splanchnic nerves are generally four in number. The upper two join the coeliac and aortic plexuses, and the lower two join the superior hypogastric plexus.

Coeliac Ganglia and Coeliac Plexus

The *coeliac ganglion* (Fig. 27.7) is the largest ganglion in the body, situated one on each side of the coeliac trunk. Each ganglion is irregular in shape and is usually divided into a larger upper part which receives the greater splanchnic nerve, and a smaller lower part; aorticorenal ganglion which receives the lesser splanchnic nerve.

The *coeliac plexus* or solar plexus (Fig. 27.7) is closely related to the coeliac ganglion. The plexus is situated on

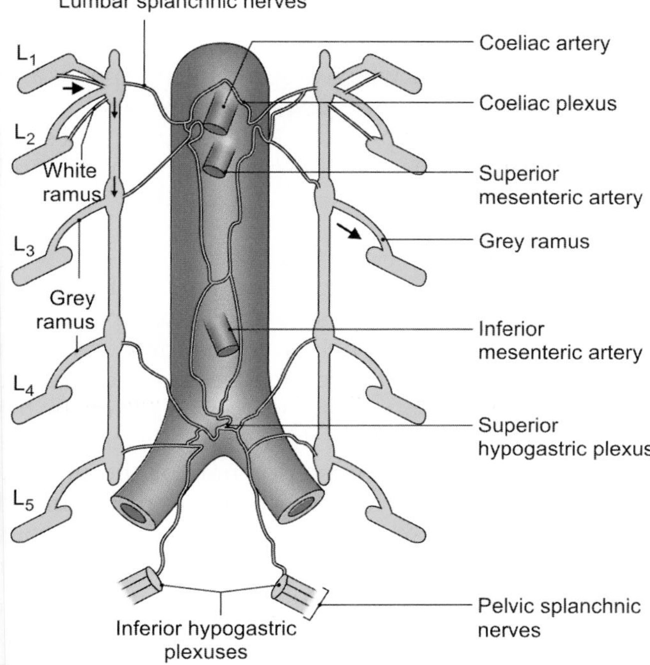

Fig. 27.6: The lumbar sympathetic chain and its branches. L1–L5 = lumbar spinal nerves; and G = lumbar sympathetic ganglion

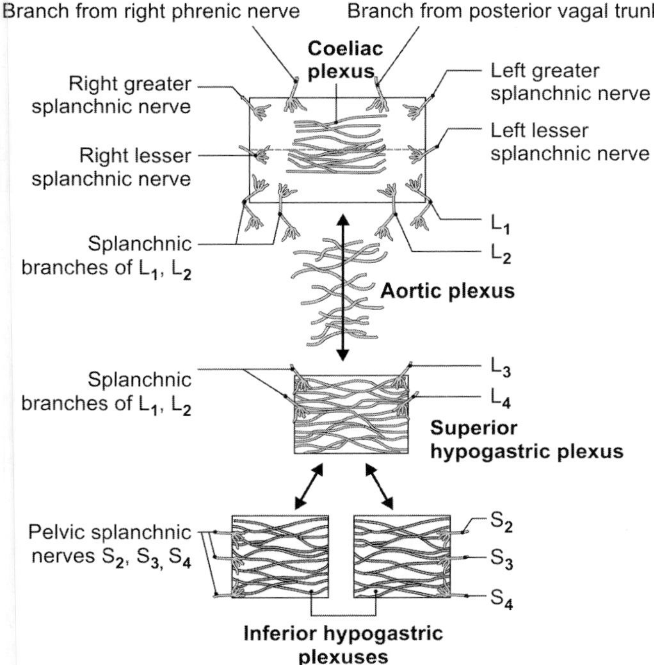

Fig. 27.7: Scheme to show the connections of the coeliac, superior hypogastric and inferior hypogastric plexuses

the aorta around the coeliac trunk and around the root of the superior mesenteric artery. The plexus extends on to the crura of the diaphragm. It is overlapped by the inferior vena cava and by the pancreas. The fibres making up the plexus are as follows:

a. Preganglionic sympathetic fibres reach it through the greater and lesser splanchnic nerves.
b. Postganglionic sympathetic fibres arising in the coeliac ganglion.
c. Preganglionic vagal fibres are derived from the posterior vagal trunk containing fibres from both the right and left vagal nerves. The fibres from the right vagus predominate.
d. Sensory fibres from the diaphragm reach the coeliac plexus along the inferior phrenic arteries.

Branches

The coeliac plexus forms a number of secondary plexuses which surround branches of the aorta.

1 The *phrenic plexus* passes along the inferior phrenic artery to diaphragm and to the suprarenal gland. The right phrenic plexus contains a right phrenic ganglion.
2 The *hepatic plexus* is distributed to the liver, the gallbladder and the bile ducts.
3 The *left gastric plexus* passes to the stomach.
4 The *splenic plexus* supplies the vessels and smooth muscle of the spleen.
5 The *suprarenal plexus* contains *preganglionic fibres*, that end in relation to the chromaffin cells of the suprarenal gland. These cells are homologous with postganglionic sympathetic neurons.
6 The *renal plexus* is formed by filaments from the coeliac plexus, the aorticorenal ganglion, the lowest thoracic splanchnic nerve, the first lumbar splanchnic nerve and the aortic plexus. It supplies the kidney and the upper part of the ureter.
7 The *testicular plexus* supplies the testis, the epididymis and the vas deferens.
8 The *ovarian plexus* supplies the ovary and the uterine tube.
9 The *superior mesenteric plexus* contains a superior mesenteric ganglion, and supplies the territory of the superior mesenteric artery.
10 The *abdominal aortic plexus* or intermesenteric plexus is formed by the coeliac plexus and filaments from the first and second lumbar splanchnic nerves (Fig. 27.8). It is situated on the sides and the front of the aorta, between the origins of the superior and inferior mesenteric arteries. Actually it is made up of four to twelve intermesenteric nerves connected by oblique filaments. It is continuous above with the coeliac plexus and below with the superior hypogastric plexus. Its branches form parts of the testicular, inferior mesenteric, iliac and superior hypogastric plexuses, and supply the inferior vena cava.

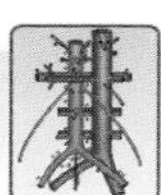

MULTIPLE CHOICE QUESTIONS

1. Ovarian artery is a branch of:
   a. Abdominal aorta b. Common iliac artery
   c. Internal iliac d. External iliac

2. Left gonadal vein drains into:
   a. Internal iliac vein b. Inferior vena cava
   c. Left renal vein d. Vena azygos

3. Following are ventral branches of aorta *except*:
   a. Coeliac axis
   b. Superior mesenteric artery
   c. Inferior mesenteric artery
   d. Gonadal artery

4. Following are lymph nodes of posterior abdominal wall *except*:
   a. Deep inguinal b. External iliac
   c. Common iliac d. Aortic group

5. Layers of thoracolumbar fascia are following *except*:
   a. Anterior layer b. Middle layer
   c. Medial layer d. Posterior layer

ANSWERS

1. a **2.** c **3.** d **4.** a **5.** c

28 Perineum

Women must not depend upon the protection of men, but must be taught to protect themselves
—S Anthony

INTRODUCTION

Perineum is the region at the lower end of the trunk, in the interval between the two thighs. The external genitalia are located, in the perineum. The perineum forms the lower division of the pelvis that lies below the pelvic diaphragm, formed by the levator ani and coccygeus, and fills in the pelvic outlet or inferior aperture of the pelvis.

In males there are two openings, one of the gastrointestinal system and the other being the common opening of urinary and genital system. In females there are three separate openings, one each of the gastrointestinal, genital and urinary systems. The perineal body supports the reproductive system. Its injury without repair, may lead to prolapse of the uterus. Pudendal nerve supplies muscles, skin, mucous membrane of both anal and urogenital triangles comprising the perineum. Pudendum means "to be ashamed of".

SUPERFICIAL BOUNDARIES

Anteriorly: The scrotum in males, and the mons pubis in females (Figs 28.1 and 28.2).

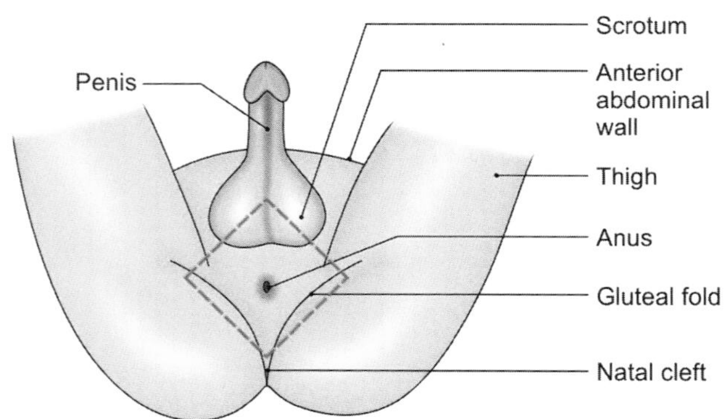

Fig. 28.1: The male perineum. Dotted lines indicate the outlines of pelvic outlet

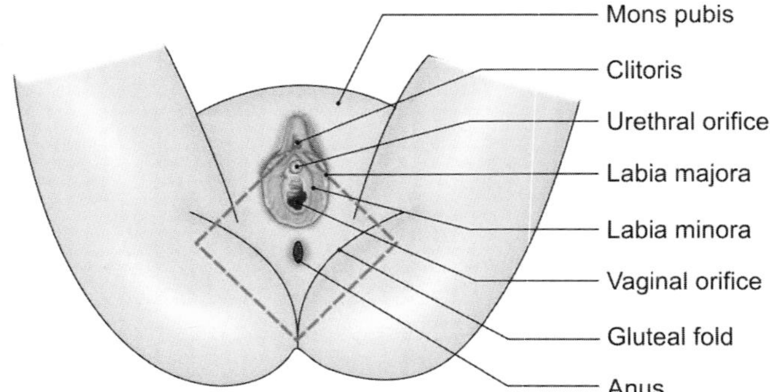

Fig. 28.2: The female perineum. Dotted lines indicate the position of pelvic outlet

Posteriorly: The buttocks.

On each side: The upper part of the medial side of the thigh.

DEEP BOUNDARIES OF THE PERINEUM

The deep boundaries of the perineum are the same as those of the pelvic outlet.

Anteriorly: Upper part of the pubic arch and the arcuate or inferior pubic ligament (Fig. 28.3).

Posteriorly: Tip of the coccyx.

On each side

- Conjoined ischiopubic rami.
- Ischial tuberosity.
- Sacrotuberous ligament.

Divisions of the Perineum

A transverse line joining the anterior parts of the ischial tuberosities, and passing immediately anterior to the anus, divides the perineum into two triangular areas, a posterior, *anal region* or triangle, and an anterior, *urogenital region* or triangle (Fig. 28.3).

The *anal region* contains the termination of the anal canal in the median plane and an ischioanal fossa on each side.

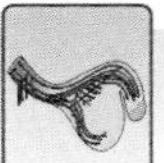

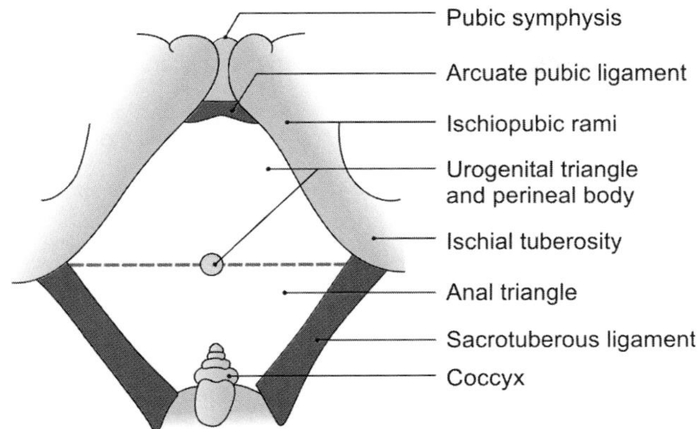

Fig. 28.3: Boundaries of perineum. Interrupted line shows the division of perineum into urogenital and anal regions

Urogenital region contains the external urogenital organs. In males, the urethra enclosed in the root of penis, partly hidden anteriorly by the scrotum; and in females, the female external genital organs.

In the urogenital region, there are the superficial perineal space or pouch and the deep perineal space or pouch.

The chief neurovascular bundle of the perineum occupies a fascial tunnel, the *pudendal canal*, and contains the pudendal nerve and the internal pudendal vessels. The pudendal canal lies in the lateral wall of the ischioanal fossa.

ANAL REGION

DISSECTION

Clean the sacrotuberous and sacrospinous ligaments. Identify coccyx in the midline posteriorly and locate the ischial tuberosity. Define the ischiopubic rami till the lower margins of pubic symphysis anteriorly.

Identify the openings of urethra, anal canal and vagina if it is a female cadaver. Define perineal body in the centre of perineum. Dissect the parts of external anal sphincter.

Pass a forceps downwards and backwards deep to the membranous layer of the superficial fascia of the anterior abdominal wall.

In the male, expose the membranous layer in the perineum. Make an incision in the membranous layer on one side and dissect the ischiocavernosus, bulbospongiosus and superficial transverse perinei muscles, nerves, blood vessels present in the superficial perineal space. The posterior scrotal/labial vessels and nerves pierce the posterolateral corner of perineal membrane to enter the superficial perineal space (Fig. 28.4).

In the female, remove the fat from the labium majus and expose the membranous layer. Incise it and expose the posterior part of this space and all its contents both in the male and female cadavers. Note the posterior limit where the membranous layer passes superiorly to fuse with the perineal membrane. Identify the various female external genital organs.

Identify the structures piercing the perineal membrane in both male and female. Note the ill-defined nature of the perineal membrane in female as it is pierced by vagina in addition to urethra.

Dissect the inferior rectal vessels and nerve and follow them to the lateral wall of the ischioanal fossa. Remove the fat from the ischioanal fossa. Identify and trace the pudendal nerve and vessels in the fascial pudendal canal on the lateral wall of the ischioanal fossa.

Cutaneous Innervation

The *inferior rectal nerve* (S2, S3, S4) supplies the skin around the anus and over the ischioanal fossa. The *perineal branch of the fourth sacral nerve* supplies the skin posterior to the anus.

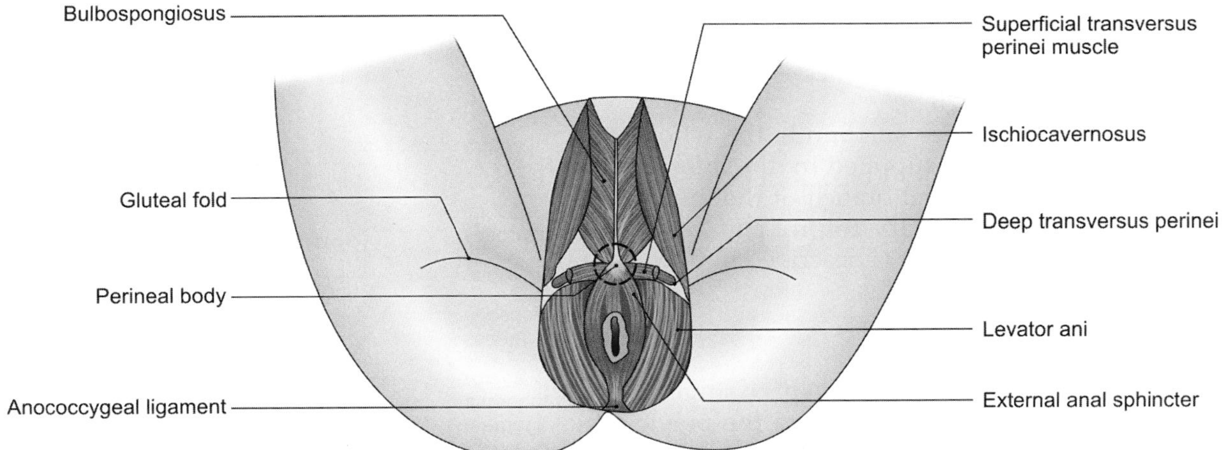

Fig. 28.4: Perineal body and the anococcygeal ligament in male

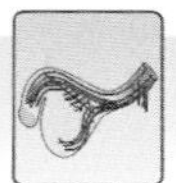

Superficial Fascia

It contains a large amount of fat which fills the ischioanal fossa.

Deep Fascia

It is formed by the inferior fascia of the pelvic diaphragm and the fascia covering the obturator internus below the attachment of the levator ani.

Anococcygeal Ligament

It is a fibrofatty mass permeated with muscle fibres derived from the levator ani and the external anal sphincter. It extends from the anus to the tip of the coccyx, and supports the rectum (Fig. 28.4).

PERINEAL BODY

The perineal body, or the central point of the perineum, is a fibromuscular node situated in the median plane, about 1.25 cm in front of the anal margin and close to the bulb of the penis. Ten muscles of the perineum converge and interlace in the perineal body.

Two unpaired:

- External anal sphincter.
- Fibres of longitudinal muscle coat of anal canal.

Paired:

- Bulbospongiosus.
- Superficial and deep transversus perenei.
- Levator ani.

All these converge and interlace in the perineal body. Nine are visible in Fig. 28.4. Last one is unstriped fibres of longitudinal muscle coat of the anal canal.

The perineal body is very important in the female for support of the pelvic organs. Sphincter urethrovaginalis in female is also attached here. It may be damaged during parturition or childbirth. This may result in prolapse of the urinary bladder, the uterus, the ovaries and even of the rectum.

EXTERNAL ANAL SPHINCTER

Anal canal is surrounded in its upper three-fourths by the internal anal sphincter which ends below at the level of white line of Hilton (Fig. 28.5).

The external anal sphincter surrounds the whole length of the anal canal. It is supplied by the inferior rectal nerve and by the perineal branch of the fourth sacral nerve. It is under voluntary control and keeps the anus and anal canal closed. It is described in detail in Chapter 33.

ISCHIOANAL FOSSA

The ischioanal fossa is a wedge-shaped space situated one on each side of the anal canal below the pelvic diaphragm. Its base is directed downwards, towards the surface. The apex is directed upwards.

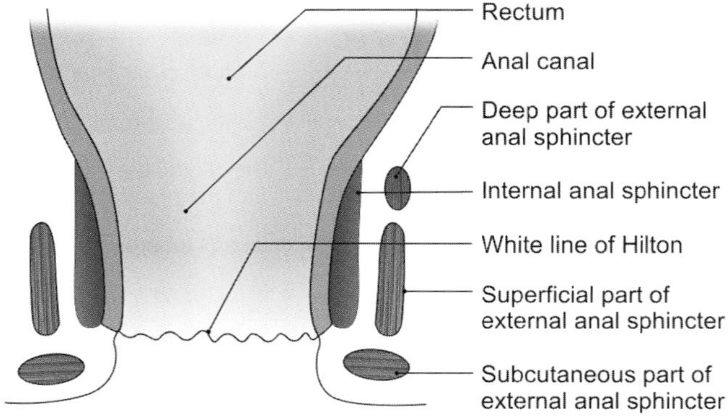

Fig. 28.5: The external and internal anal sphincters

Dimensions

Length (anteroposteriorly), 5 cm; width (side to side), 2.5 cm; and depth (vertically), 5 to 6.2 cm.

Boundaries

The *base* is formed by the skin.

The *apex* is formed by the line where the obturator fascia meets the inferior fascia of the pelvic diaphragm or anal fascia. The line corresponds to the origin of the levator ani from the lateral pelvic wall.

Anteriorly, the fossa is limited by the posterior border of the perineal membrane (but for the anterior recess of the fossa) (Fig. 28.6).

Posteriorly, the fossa reaches.

a. Lower border of the gluteus maximus.
b. Sacrotuberous ligament.

The *lateral wall* is vertical, and is formed by:

a. Obturator internus with the obturator fascia.
b. Medial surface of the ischial tuberosity, below the attachment of obturator fascia (Fig. 28.7).

The *medial wall* slopes upwards and laterally, and is formed by:

a. The external anal sphincter, with the fascia covering it in the lower part.
b. The levator ani with the anal fascia in the upper part (Fig. 28.7).

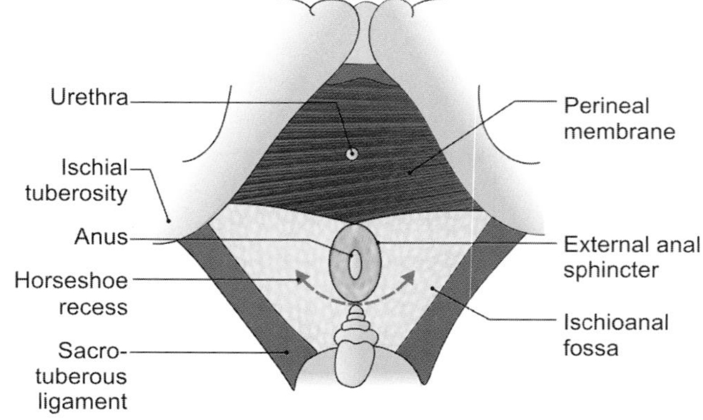

Fig. 28.6: Surface view of the ischioanal fossa, and perineal membrane

Section 2 **Abdomen and Pelvis**

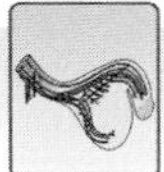

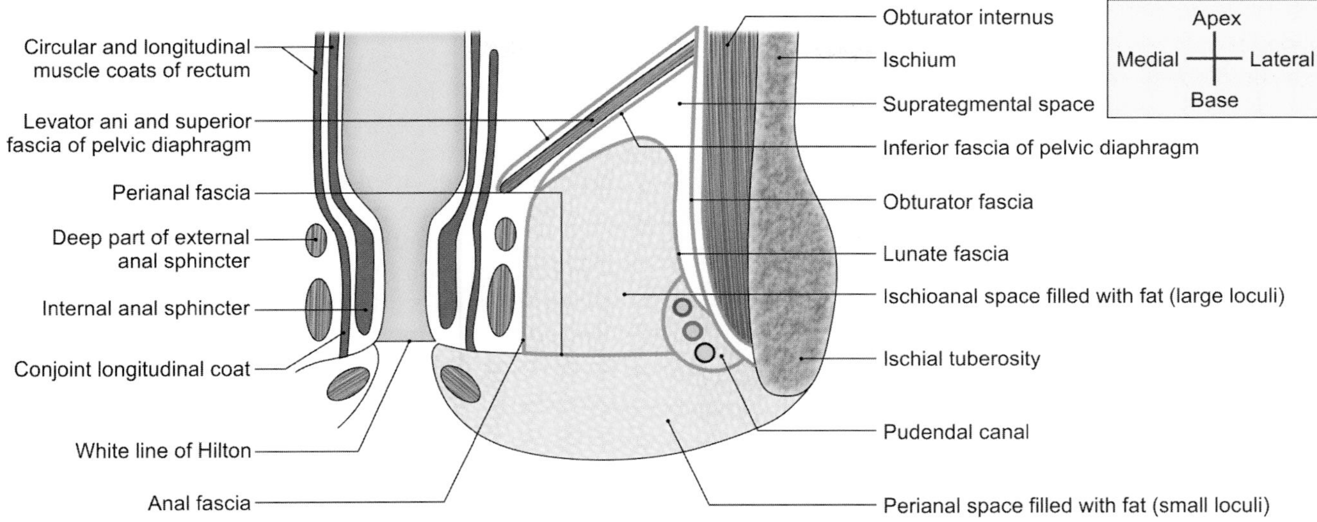

Fig. 28.7: Coronal section through the ischioanal fossa

Recesses

These are narrow extensions of the fossa beyond its boundaries.

1 The *anterior recess* extends forwards above the perineal membrane, reaching almost up to the posterior surface of the body of the pubis. It is closely related to the prostate or the vagina (Fig. 28.8).
2 The *posterior recess* is smaller than the anterior. It extends deep to sacrotuberous ligament.
3 The horseshoe recess connects the two ischioanal fossae behind the anal canal (Fig. 28.6).

Spaces and Canals of the Fossa

The arrangement of the fascia in this region forms the following spaces.

Perianal Space

The perianal fascia is in the form of a septum that passes laterally from the lower end of the longitudinal coat of the anal canal. It extends medially from the white line of Hilton to the pudendal canal laterally. It separates a shallow subcutaneous *perianal space* from the deep *ischioanal space*. The fat in the perianal space is tightly arranged in small loculi formed by complete septa. The infections of this space are, therefore, very painful due to the tension caused by swelling.

Ischioanal Space

This is large and deep. The fat in this space is loosely arranged in large loculi formed by incomplete delicate septa. The infections of this space are, therefore, least

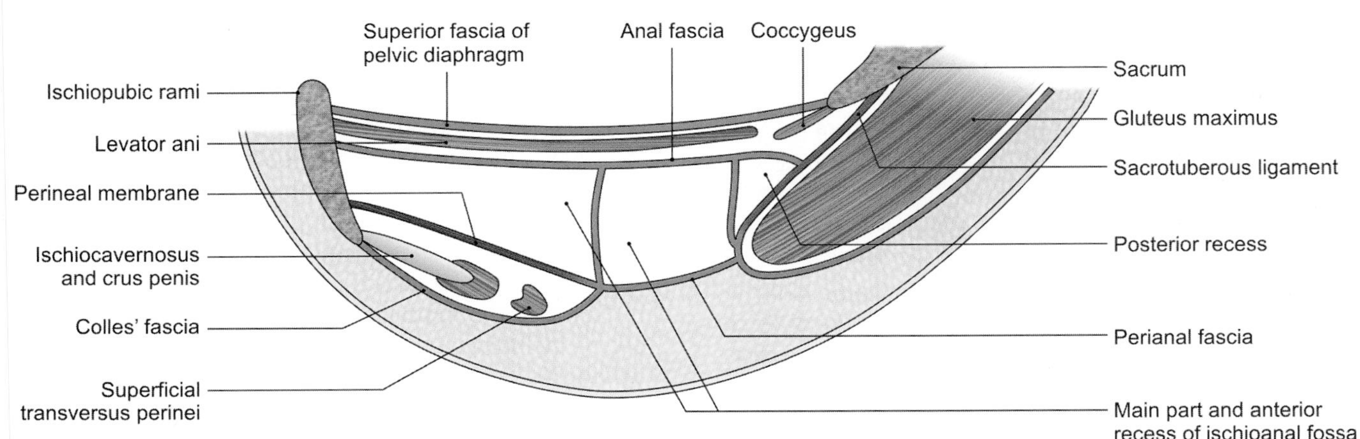

Fig. 28.8: Parasagittal section through the ischioanal fossa, showing its recesses

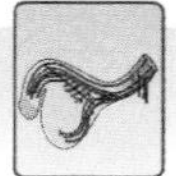

painful because swelling can occur without tension (Fig. 28.7).

The *lunate fascia* arches over the ischioanal fat. It begins laterally at the pudendal canal and merges medially with the fascia covering the deep part of the external anal sphincter. The fascia divides the ischioanal space into:

a. *Suprategmental space*, above the fascia.
b. *Tegmental space*, below the fascia.

Pudendal Canal

This is a fascial canal in the lateral wall of the ischioanal fossa, enclosing the pudendal nerve and internal pudendal vessels. The fascia of the canal is fused with the lower part of the obturator fascia laterally, with the lunate fascia above, with the perianal fascia medially, and with the falciform process of the sacrotuberous ligament below.

Contents of Ischioanal Fossa

1. Ischioanal pad of fat.
2. Inferior rectal nerve and vessels. They pass through the fossa from lateral to medial side. They arch upwards above the fat (Fig. 28.9) to supply mucous membrane, external sphincter and the skin around the anus.
3. Pudendal canal with its contents. This canal lies along the lateral wall of the fossa (Fig. 28.7).
4. Posterior scrotal or posterior labial (in females) nerves and vessels. They cross the anterolateral part of the fossa and enter the urogenital triangle.
5. Perineal branch of the fourth sacral (S4) nerve. It enters the posterior angle of the fossa and runs over the levator ani to the external anal sphincter.
6. Perforating cutaneous branches of nerves S2, S3. They appear at the lower border of the gluteus maximus, in the posterior part of the fossa.

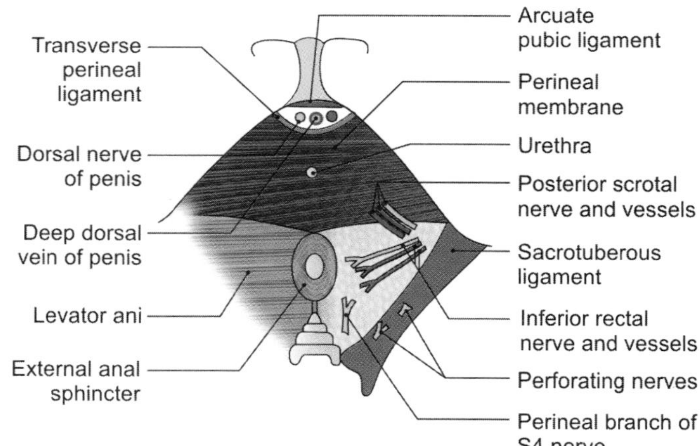

Fig. 28.9: Surface view of the ischiorectal fossa, showing some of its contents

CLINICAL ANATOMY

- The two ischioanal fossae allow distention of the rectum and anal canal during passage of faeces.
- Both the perianal and ischioanal spaces are common sites of abscesses (Fig. 28.10).

  Sometimes an abscess may burst into the anal canal or rectum internally, and on to the surface of the perineum externally. In this way an ischioanal type of *anorectal fistula* or *fistula in ano* may be produced. The most common site of the internal opening is in the floor of one of the anal crypts. If the abscess bursts only externally, and healing does not follow, an *external sinus* is produced. Through the horseshoe recess a unilateral abscess may become bilateral.
- The ischioanal fat acts as a cushion-like support to the rectum and anal canal. Loss of this fat in debilitating diseases like diarrhoea in children may result in *prolapse of the rectum.*
- The occasional gap between the tendinous origin of levator ani and the obturator fascia is known as *hiatus of Schwalbe*. Rarely pelvic organs may herniate through this gap into the ischioanal fossa, resulting in an *ischioanal hernia*.

MALE PERINEUM

DISSECTION

Place a finger in the ischioanal fossa and push it gently forwards. It will pass easily above the urogenital diaphragm, lateral to levator ani. Strip the ischiocavernosus muscles from the crus of the penis or clitoris. Trace them to their termination.

Detach the superficial perineal muscles, including right crus of the penis from the ischiopubic rami. Turn it forwards to expose the deep artery and vein on the superior surface of perineal membrane also called inferior fascia of urogenital diaphragm.

In the male detach the bulb of the penis from the central perineal tendon. Turn it forwards to expose the urethra and the artery of the bulb.

In the female raise the posterior end of the bulb of the vestibule to expose the greater vestibular gland.

Detach the perineal membrane from the pubic arch on the right side. Carefully, reflect the membrane medially to visualise the urethra and a pair of posteriorly placed deep transversus perinei muscles.

Remove the exposed muscles of the deep perineal space including the endopelvic fascia. Clean the area to see the perineal surface of the levator ani.

Male External Genital Organs

These have been described in Chapter 17.

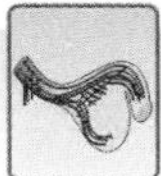

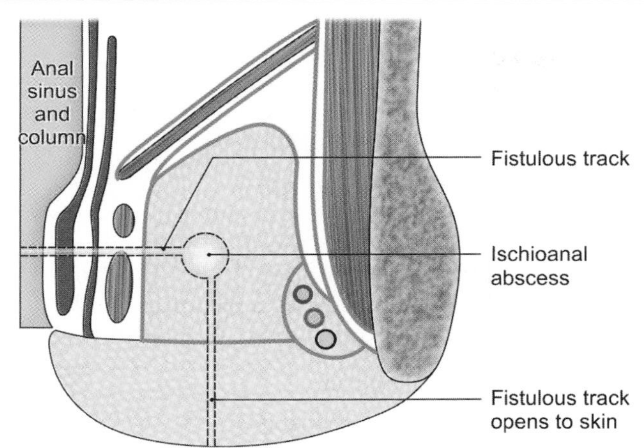

Fig. 28.10: Ischiorectal type of fistula in ano. Internally it usually opens into one of anal crypts. The track traverses the superficial parts of external anal sphincter and lower part of internal anal sphincter. A blind sinus lies high up in the ischiorectal fossa

Male Urogenital Region

The anterior division of the perineum is the urogenital region. It contains the superficial and deep perineal spaces or pouches.

Cutaneous Innervation

1 *Dorsal nerve of penis*: It supplies the skin of the penis, except at its root (Fig. 28.11).
2 *Ilioinguinal nerve* and *genital branch of the genitofemoral nerve*: These supply the skin of the *anterior one-third* of the scrotum and the root of the penis.
3 *Perineal branch of posterior cutaneous nerve of thigh:* It supplies the skin of the lateral part of the urogenital region and the lateral part of the *posterior two-thirds* of the scrotum.

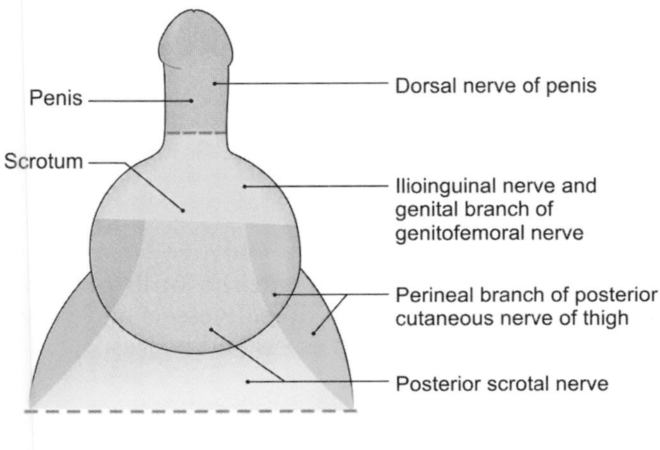

Fig. 28.11: Cutaneous innervation of the male perineum

4 *Posterior scrotal:* These supply the skin of the medial part of the urogenital region and the medial part of the posterior two-thirds of the scrotum.
5 The mucous membrane of urethra is supplied by the *perineal branch of the pudendal nerve.*

CLINICAL ANATOMY

The cutaneous nerves of perineum are derived from the sacral nerves (S2, S3, S4). These segments also supply parasympathetic fibres to the pelvic organs. Diseases of these organs may, therefore, cause *referred pain* in the perineum.

Superficial Fascia

It is made up of two layers as in the lower part of the anterior abdominal wall. The superficial *fatty layer* is continuous with the superficial fascia of the surrounding regions. The deep *membranous layer* or Colles' fascia is attached posteriorly to the posterior border of perineal membrane, and on each side to pubic arch below the crus penis. Anteriorly, it is continuous with the fascia of the scrotum containing the dartos, fascia of the penis, and with the membranous layer of the superficial fascia of the anterior abdominal wall or fascia of Scarpa.

Deep Fascia

It is also made up of one layer that lines the deep perineal space inferiorly.

This fascia of the urogenital diaphragm is thick. It is also called the perineal membrane.

Boundaries

The urogenital region is bounded posteriorly by the interischial line which usually overlies the posterior border of the transverse perinei muscles. Anteriorly and laterally, it is bounded by symphysis pubis and ischiopubic rami.

Urogenital region extends superficially to encompass the scrotum and root of penis.

Urogenital region is divided into two parts by strong perineal membrane.

Above it: Deep perineal space.

Below it: Superficial perineal space.

DEEP PERINEAL SPACE

Previous view: Space between superior fascia of urogenital diaphragm and perineal membrane that contained urethra and urethral sphincter.

Present view: Now the urethral sphincter is known to be contained inside the urethra itself (within). The urogenital diaphragm does not exist. The deep perineal space is thin and open above (Fig. 28.12 and Table 28.1).

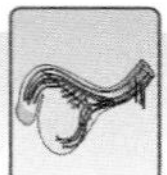

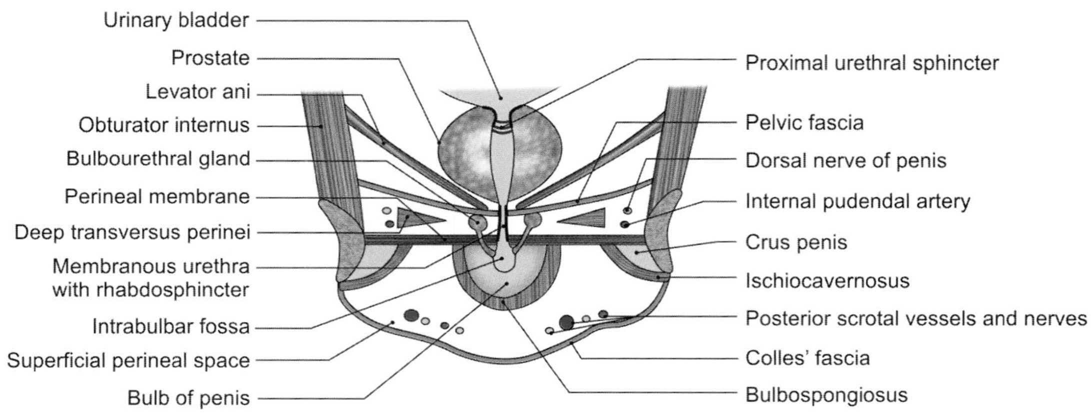

Fig. 28.12: Coronal section through the urogenital region of the male perineum

Table 28.1: Deep perineal space

Features	*Male*	*Female*
Definition	This is the thin space of the urogenital region situated deep to the perineal membrane Contributes to pelvic floor	Same
Boundaries		
a. Superficial	Perineal membrane (Fig. 28.12)	Same (Fig 28.19)
b. Deep	Open above	Same
c. On each side	Ischiopubic rami	Same
d. Anteriorly	Gap between perineal membrane and inferior pubic ligament	Same
Contents		
1. Tubes	Part of urethra	Parts of urethra and vagina
2. Muscles	a. Sphincter urethrae or distal urethral sphincter within the wall of urethra b. Deep transversus perinei. Mainly skeletal muscle	a. Sphincter urethrae within the wall of urethra b. Same attachment. Mainly smooth muscle c. Compressor urethrae d. Sphincter urethrovaginalis (Fig. 28.20)
3. Nerves on each side	a. Dorsal nerve of penis b. Muscular branches from perineal nerve	a. Dorsal nerve of clitoris b. Muscular branches from perineal nerve
4. Vessels	a. Artery of penis b. Stems of origin of four branches namely, artery to the bulb of penis, urethral artery, deep and dorsal arteries of penis	a. Artery of clitoris b. Stems of origin of four branches namely artery to bulb of vestibule, urethral artery, deep and dorsal arteries of clitoris
5. Glands	Bulbourethral glands	No glands

Boundaries

Deep aspect: Endopelvic fascia of pelvic floor.

Superficial aspect: Perineal membrane. Between these two fascial layers lie deep transverse perinei; superficial to the proximal urethral sphincter mechanism and pubourethralis (Fig. 28.12).

The previous view was that sphincter urethrae extended between the two ischiopubic rami and was pierced by urethra but as of now the sphincter urethrae lies within wall of urethra as distal urethral sphincter.

These muscles do not form a true diaphragmatic sheet as such because fibres from the several parts extend through the visceral outlet in the pelvic floor into the lower reaches of the pelvic cavity. (There is no sphincter urethrae outside urethra. So, no urogenital diaphragm exists).

Contents

Urethra, vessels and nerve to the bulb of penis, bulbourethral glands, deep dorsal vessels and nerves of penis, posterior scrotal vessels and nerves.

Deep Transverse Perinei

It forms an incomplete sheet of skeletal muscle extending across the urogenital triangle from the medial aspects of the ischiopubic rami. Posteriorly, the sheet is attached to perineal body where its fibres decussate with those of opposite side.

Anteriorly, the muscles are deficient and the visceral structures pass across the endopelvic fascia and the perineal membrane. Some fibres pass to the deep part of external anal sphincter posteriorly and sphincter urethrae (contained within the urethra).

Together with superficial transverse perinei the muscles act to tether (hold) the perineal body in median plane. The muscle gives dynamic support for pelvic viscera.

Supplied by perineal branches of pudendal nerve and vessels.

Distal Urethral Sphincter Mechanism

Consists of intrinsic striated and smooth muscles of urethra and the pubourethralis component of levator ani which surrounds the urethra at the point of maximum concentration of those muscles. It surrounds the membranous urethra in the male.

Smooth muscle fibres also reach up to the lowest part of the neck of the bladder and between the two, fibres lie on the surface of prostate.

Bulk of fibres surround the membranous urethra. There are circularly disposed striated muscle fibres called *rhabdosphincter* which forms main part of distal urethral sphincter mechanism (Fig. 28.12). Some fibres are attached to inner surface of the ischiopubic ramus, *forming compressor urethrae.*

PERINEAL MEMBRANE

Perineal membrane is almost triangular membrane:

- Laterally attached to periosteum of ischiopubic rami.
- Apex attached to arcuate ligament of pubis, where the membrane is attached to this arcuate ligament of pubis, it is particularly thick and is called *transverse perineal ligament.*
- Posterior border is fused to deep parts of perineal body and is continuous with the fascia over deep transversus perinei.

Perineal membrane (Fig. 28.13) is crossed by or pierced by:

- Urethra 2–3 cm behind the inferior border of pubic symphysis.
- Artery to the bulb of penis.
- Duct of bulbourethral gland.
- Muscular branches to muscles of Fig. 28.14.
- Deep artery of the penis, urethral artery.
- Dorsal artery and dorsal nerves of penis.
- Posterior scrotal vessels and nerves, anterior to transverse perinei.

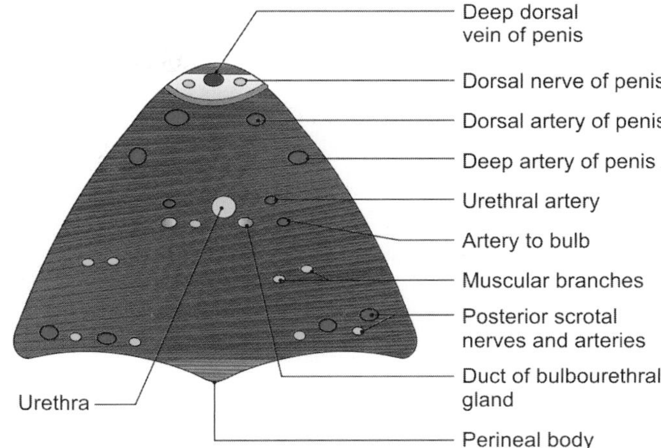

Fig. 28.13: Structures piercing the perineal membrane (male)

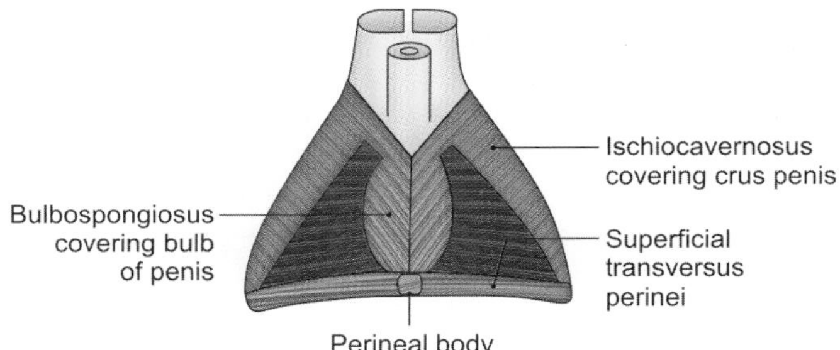

Fig. 28.14: Superficial muscles of the male perineum

Superficial perineal space is given in Tables 28.2 and 28.3.

CLINICAL ANATOMY

- *The membranous part of the male urethra* is the narrowest and least dilatable part of the urethra. In inexperienced hands, it is likely to be ruptured during instrumentation. The urethra can also rupture in accidental injuries.
- Rupture of the urethra leads to extravasation of urine, which may be superficial or deep. In *superficial extravasation*, the urine spreads downwards deep to the membranous layer of the superficial fascia. It first fills the superficial perineal space; and then the scrotum, the penis and the lower part of the anterior abdominal wall. It is prevented from going to the ischioanal fossa or the thigh by the firm attachment of the membranous layer of superficial fascia to their boundaries (Fig. 28.15).

  In *deep extravasation*, the urine spreads upwards into the extraperitoneal space of the pelvis around bladder and prostate into the anterior abdominal wall (Fig. 28.16).

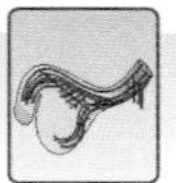

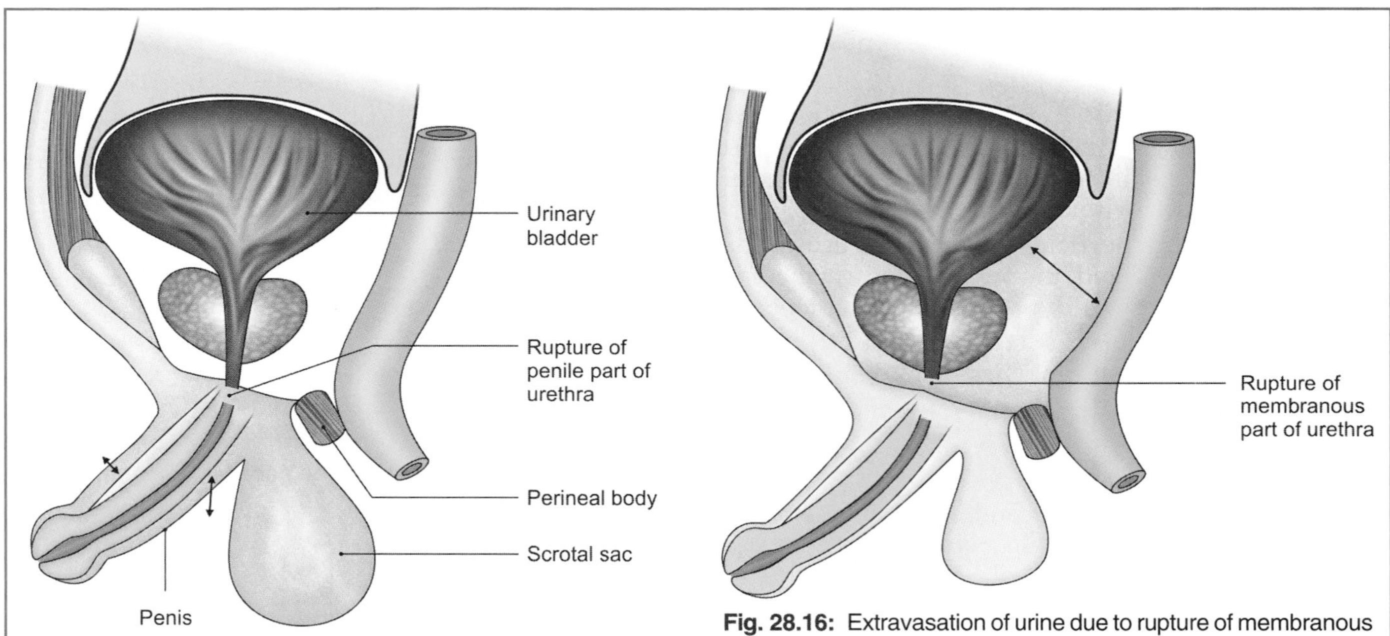

Fig. 28.15: Extravasation of urine due to rupture of penile urethra

Fig. 28.16: Extravasation of urine due to rupture of membranous urethra

FEMALE PERINEUM

It comprises of female external genital organs and female urogenital region.

FEMALE EXTERNAL GENITAL ORGANS/ PUDENDUM/VULVA

Pudendum includes:

- Mons pubis (Fig. 28.17)
- Labia majora
- Labia minora.
- Clitoris.
- Vestibule of the vagina.
- Bulbs of the vestibule.
- Greater vestibular glands.

Mons Pubis

Mons pubis is a rounded eminence present in front of the pubic symphysis. It is formed by accumulation of subcutaneous fat. It is covered with pubic hair. The hair bearing area has a nearly horizontal upper limit.

Labia Majora

Labia majora are two thick folds of skin enclosing fat. They form the lateral boundaries of the *pudendal cleft*. Their outer surfaces are covered with hair, and the inner surfaces are studded with large sebaceous glands. The larger anterior ends are connected to each other below the mons pubis to form the *anterior commissure*. The skin connecting the less prominent posterior ends of the labia is known as the *posterior*

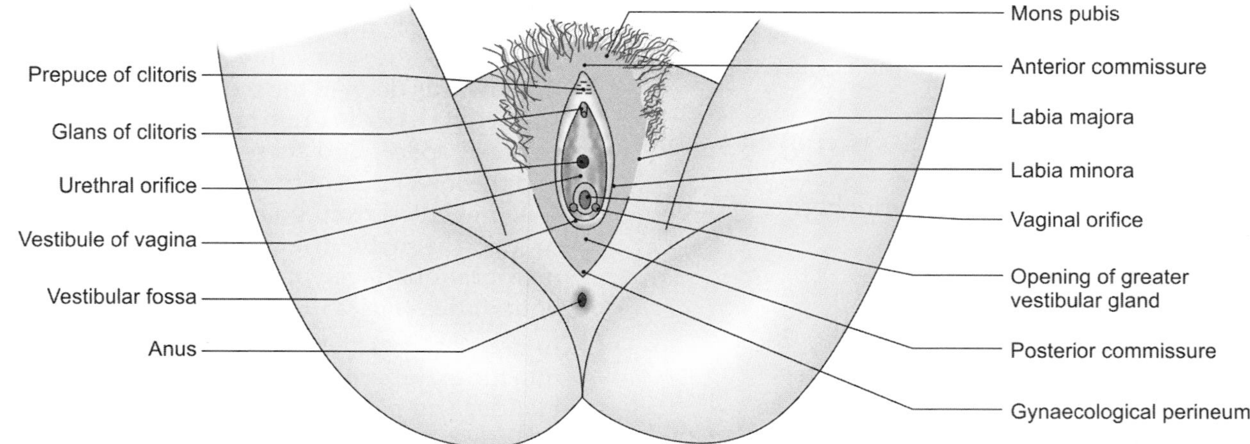

Fig. 28.17: The female external genital organs

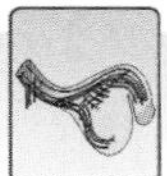

commissure. The area between the posterior commissure and the anus which is about 2.5 cm long constitutes the *gynaecological perineum*.

Labia Minora

Labia minora are two thin folds of skin, which lie within the pudendal cleft. Anteriorly, each labium minus splits into two layers; the upper layer joins the corresponding layer of the opposite side to form the *prepuce of the clitoris*. Similarly the lower layers of the two sides join to form the *frenulum of the clitoris*. Posteriorly, the two labia minora meet to form the *frenulum of the labia minora*. The inner surface of the labia minora contains numerous sebaceous glands.

Clitoris

The clitoris is an erectile organ, homologous with the penis. However, *it is not traversed by urethra*. It lies in the anterior part of pudendal cleft. The body of clitoris is made up of two *corpora cavernosa* enclosed in a fibrous sheath and partly separated by an incomplete *pectiniform septum*. *The corpus spongiosum is absent*. Each corpus cavernosum is attached to the ischiopubic rami. The down-turned free end of clitoris is formed by a rounded tubercle, *glans clitoridis*, which caps the free ends of corpora. The glans is made up of erectile tissue continuous posteriorly with the commissural venous plexus uniting right and left bulbs of vestibule called *bulbar commissure*. The surface of glans is highly sensitive and plays an important role in sexual responses.

Vestibule of the Vagina

Vestibule of the vagina is space between two labia minora. It presents the following features.

1 The *urethral orifice* lies about 2.5 cm behind the clitoris and just in front of the vaginal orifice.
2 *Vaginal orifice* or *introitus* lies in the posterior part of the vestibule, and is partly closed, in the virgin, by a thin membrane called the *hymen*. In married women, the hymen is represented by rounded tags of tissue called the carunculae hymenales.
3 *Orifices of the ducts of greater vestibular glands* lie one on each side of vaginal orifice, between the hymen and labium minus (Fig. 28.19).
4 Numerous *lesser vestibular* or *mucous glands* open on the surface of vestibule.
5 The posterior part of vestibule between vaginal orifice and frenulum of labia minora forms a shallow depression known as *vestibular fossa*.

Bulbs of the Vestibule

Bulbs of the vestibule are two oval bodies of erectile tissue that correspond to the two halves of the bulb of the penis. The bulbs lie on either side of the vaginal and urethral orifices, superficial to the perineal membrane. The tapering anterior ends of the bulbs are united in front of the urethra by a venous plexus, called the *bulbar commissure*. The expanded posterior ends of the bulbs partly overlap the greater vestibular glands.

Greater Vestibular Glands of Bartholin

Greater vestibular glands are homologous with the bulbourethral glands of Cowper in the male. These lie in the superficial perineal space. Each gland has a long duct about 2 cm long which opens at the side of the hymen, between the hymen and the labium minus.

FEMALE UROGENITAL REGION

Cutaneous Innervation

1 *Dorsal nerve* of clitoris. It supplies the skin of the clitoris (Fig. 28.18).
2 *Ilioinguinal nerve* and *genital branch of the genitofemoral nerve*. These supply the skin of the *anterior one-third* of the labium majus.
3 *Perineal branch of posterior cutaneous nerve of thigh:* It supplies the skin of the lateral part of the urogenital region and the lateral part of the *posterior two-thirds* of the labium majus.
4 *Posterior scrotal or labial nerves:* These supply the skin of the medial part of the urogenital region including the labium minus in females and the medial part of the posterior two-thirds of the labium majus.
5 The mucous membrane of urethra is supplied by the *perineal branch of the pudendal nerve*.

CLINICAL ANATOMY

The cutaneous nerves of perineum are derived from the sacral nerves (S2, S3, S4). These segments also supply parasympathetic fibres to the pelvic organs. Diseases of these organs may, therefore, cause *referred pain* in the perineum.

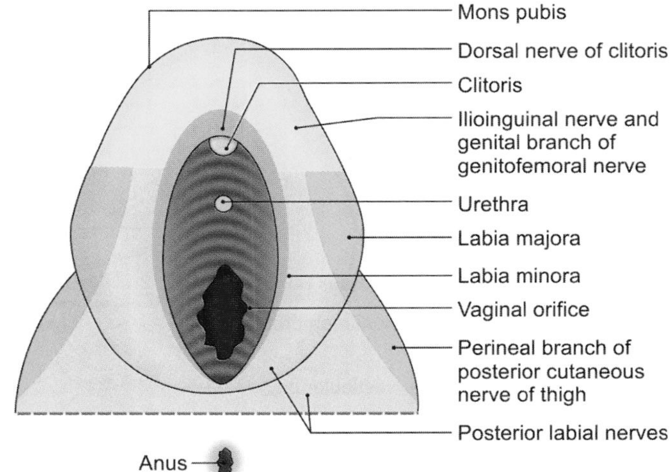

Fig. 28.18: Cutaneous innervation of the female perineum

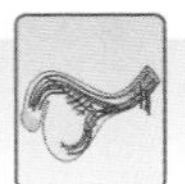

Superficial Fascia

It is made up of two layers as in the lower part of the anterior abdominal wall. The superficial *fatty layer* is continuous with the superficial fascia of the surrounding regions. The deep *membranous layer* or Colles' fascia is attached posteriorly to the posterior border of perineal membrane, and on each side to pubic arch below the crus penis. Anteriorly, it is continuous with the fascia of the scrotum containing the dartos, fascia of the penis, and with the membranous layer of the superficial fascia of the anterior abdominal wall or fascia of Scarpa.

Deep Fascia

It is also made up of one layer that lines the deep perineal space inferiorly.

This fascia of the urogenital diaphragm is thick. It is also called the perineal membrane.

Boundaries

The urogenital region is bounded by the interischial line which usually overlies the posterior border of the transverse perinei muscles.

Anteriorly and laterally, it is bounded by symphysis pubis and ischiopubic rami.

In the female, urogenital region extends to the labia majora and mons pubis.

Urogenital region is divided into two parts by perineal membrane.

Above it: Deep perineal space.

Below it: Superficial perineal space.

DEEP PERINEAL SPACE

Previous view: Space between urogenital diaphragm and perineal membrane that contained urethra and urethral sphincter.

Present view: Now the urethral sphincter is known to be contained inside the urethra itself (within). The urogenital diaphragm does not exist. It is thin space, open above (Fig. 28.19).

Boundaries

Superficial aspect: Perineal membrane. On the deep aspect of perineal membrane lie deep transverse perenei; superficial to compressor urethrae and sphincter urethrovaginalis.

Previous view was that sphincter urethrae extended between the two ischiopubic rami and was pierced by urethra and vagina but as of now the sphincter urethrae lies within urethra.

These muscles do not form a true diaphragmatic sheet as such because fibres from the several parts extend through the visceral outlet in the pelvic floor into the lower reaches of the pelvic cavity. There is no sphincter urethrae outside urethra. So no urogenital diaphragm exists.

Deep transverse perinei is mainly *smooth* muscle in female.

In female perineal membrane is less well defined and divided into two halves by urethra and vagina so that it forms triangle on two sides.

The pubourethral ligament links the two sides anteriorly behind pubic arch.

Contents

Urethra, vagina, deep dorsal vessels and nerves of clitoris, posterior labial vessels and nerves.

Urethral Sphincter Mechanism

Consists of intrinsic smooth muscle, intrinsic skeletal muscle. This is anatomically separate from the pubourethralis component of levator ani.

The sphincter mechanism surrounds more than the middle third of urethra. It blends above with the smooth muscle of bladder neck and below with the smooth muscle of lower urethra and vagina. Skeletal muscle fibres are circularly disposed, called *rhabdosphincter*.

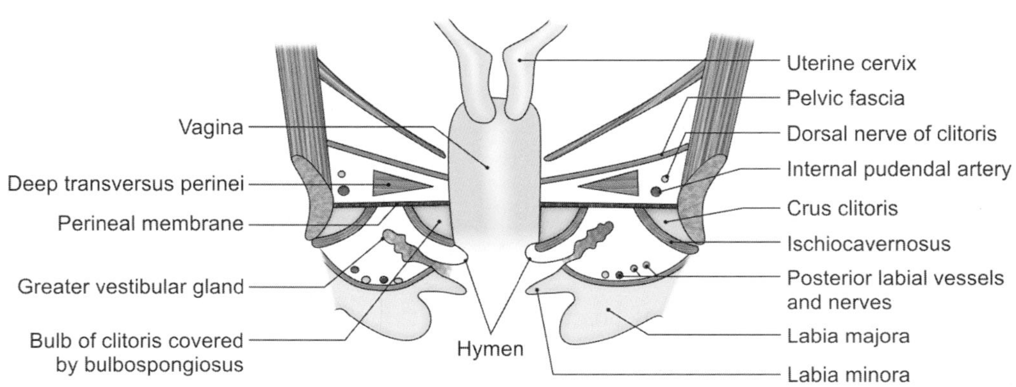

Fig. 28.19: Coronal section through the urogenital region of the female perineum

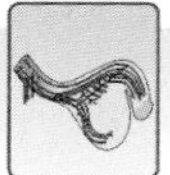

This forms main part of external urethral sphincter. This in reality is not distal but just urethral sphincter mechanism, since there is no proximal urethral sphincter in female (Fig. 28.20).

Actions

Compresses the urethra, particularly when bladder contains fluid. It contracts to expel the final drops of urine.

Nerve Supply

Perineal branch of pudendal nerve and pelvic splanchnic nerves.

Extensions of the muscles are:

Compressor Urethrae

Compressor urethrae arises from ischiopubic rami of each side by a small tendon. Fibres pass anteriorly to meet their counterparts in a flat band which lies anterior to urethra. A variable number of these fibres pass medially to reach the lower wall of vagina. Sphincter urethrae is within the wall of urethra (Fig. 28.21).

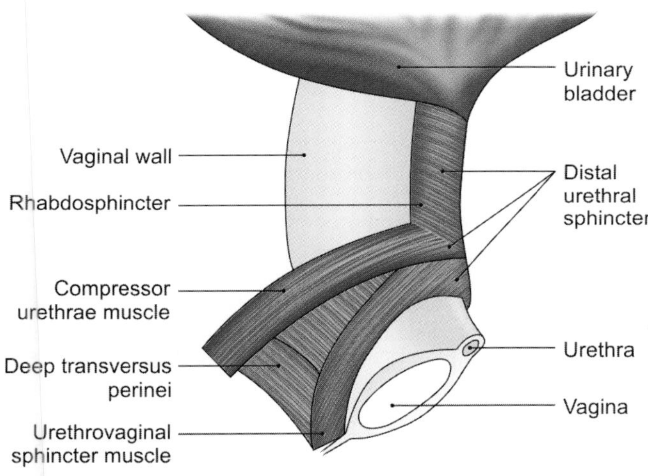

Fig. 28.20: Muscles in the deep perineal pouch in female

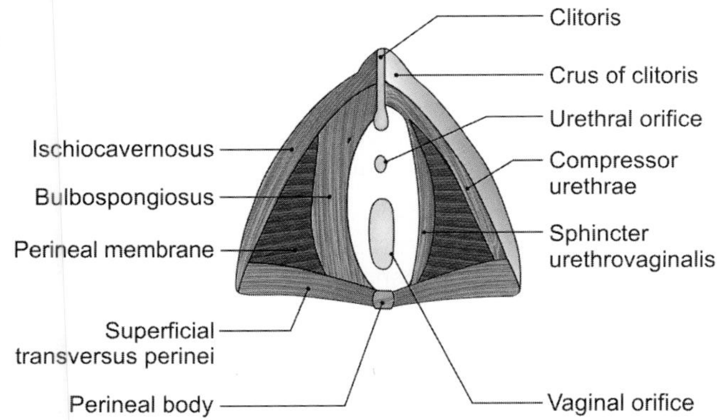

Fig. 28.21: Female perineum showing superficial muscles on right half and deep perineal muscles on left half

Sphincter Urethrovaginalis

Sphincter urethrovaginalis arises from perineal body. Its fibres pass forwards on either side of urethra and vagina to meet their counterparts in a flat band, anterior to urethra below compressor urethrae.

Actions

Direction of the fibres of compressor urethrae and sphincter urethrovaginalis suggest that these produce elongation as well as compression of the membranous urethra and thus aid continence in females. Both are supplied by perineal nerve.

PERINEAL MEMBRANE

Perineal membrane (Fig. 28.22) is pierced by:

- Urethra, 2–3 cm behind the inferior border of pubic symphysis.
- Vagina (centrally), behind urethra.
- Deep artery of clitoris.
- Dorsal vessels and nerves of clitoris.
- Artery to bulb of vestibule.

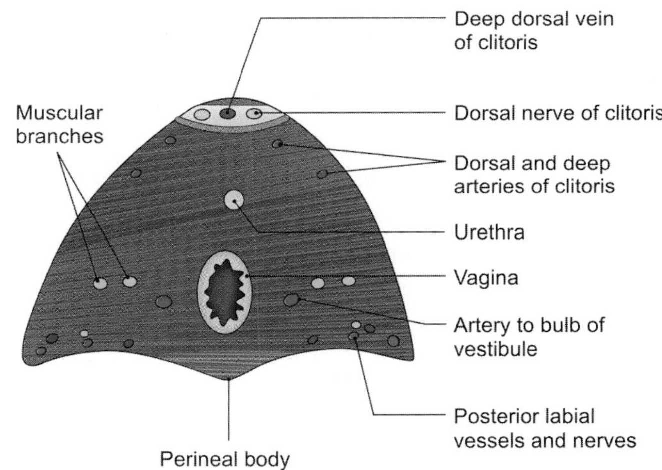

Fig. 28.22: Structures piercing the perineal membrane (female)

- Muscular branches to muscles of Fig. 28.21.
- Posterior labial vessels and nerves, anterior to transverse perinei.

PERINEAL SPACES/POUCHES

The arrangement of the superficial and deep fasciae in the urogenital region results in the formation of two triangular spaces, the superficial and deep perineal spaces or pouches (Fig. 28.18).

The boundaries and contents of the deep space are summarised in Table 28.1.

Table 28.2 summarises the boundaries and contents of superficial perineal space.

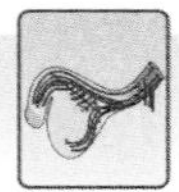

Muscles of the Urogenital Region

These muscles are arranged in superficial and deep, groups. The superficial muscles are the ischiocavernosus, the bulbospongiosus and the superficial transversus perinei, described in Table 28.3. The deep muscles are the distal urethral sphincter mechanism, sphincter urethrae with extensions and the deep transversus perinei (described earlier).

PUDENDAL CANAL

This is a fascial tunnel present in the lateral wall of the ischioanal fossa, just above the sacrotuberous ligament. It transmits the pudendal nerve and the internal pudendal vessels.

The canal extends from the lesser sciatic notch to the posterior border of the perineal membrane (Fig. 28.23).

Formation

The pudendal canal is a space between obturator fascia and the lunate fascia. Others believe that it is formed by splitting of the obturator fascia (Fig. 28.7).

Contents

1 *Pudendal nerve* (S2, S3, S4): In the posterior part of the canal, pudendal nerve gives off the inferior rectal nerve and then soon divides into a larger perineal nerve and a smaller dorsal nerve of penis.

Table 28.2: The superficial perineal space

Features	*Male*	*Female*
Definition	This is the superficial space of the urogenital region situated superficial to the perineal membrane	Same
Boundaries		
a. Superficial	Colles' fascia	Same
b. Deep	Perineal membrane	Same
c. On each side	Ischiopubic rami	Same
d. Posteriorly	Closed by the fusion of perineal membrane with Colles' fascia.	Same
e. Anteriorly	Open and continuous with the spaces of the scrotum, penis and the anterior abdominal wall	Open and continuous with the spaces of the clitoris and the anterior abdominal wall
Contents	Root of penis, made up of two corpora cavernosa and one corpus spongiosum traversed by the urethra (Fig. 28.12)	Body of clitoris, made up only of two corpora cavernosa *separated by an incomplete septum. The corpus* spongiosum *is absent.* Urethral orifice lies 2 cm behind the clitoris. Vaginal orifice just behind urethral orifice. Two bulbs of vestibule are there, one on each side of these two orifices. These unite and get attached to the glans clitoridis.
Muscles on each side	a. Ischiocavernosus covering the corpora cavernosa of penis (Fig. 28.14) b. Bulbospongiosus covering corpus spongiosum; both are united by a median raphe c. Superficial transversus perinei	a. Ischiocavernosus covering the corpora cavernosa of clitoris (Fig. 28.21) b. Bulbospongiosus covering bulb of vestibule. These remain separated to give passage to urethra and vagina (Fig. 28.19) c. Superficial transversus perinei
Nerves	a. Three sets of branches from perineal nerve namely posterior scrotal nerve, branch to bulb and muscular branches b. Long perineal nerve from posterior cutaneous nerve of thigh	a. Three sets of branches from perineal nerve namely posterior labial nerve, branch to bulb of vestibule and muscular branches b. Same
Vessels	a. Two branches of perineal artery namely, the posterior scrotal and transverse perineal b. Four branches from the artery of penis namely, artery to the bulb of penis, urethral artery, deep and dorsal arteries of penis	a. Two branches of perineal artery namely posterior labial and transverse perineal b. Four branches from the artery of clitoris, namely artery to bulb of vestibule, urethral artery, deep and dorsal arteries of clitoris
Glands and ducts	Only the ducts of bulbourethral glands	Greater vestibular glands and their ducts

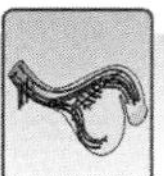

Table 28.3: The superficial perineal muscles in male/female

Muscle	*Origin*	*Fibres*	*Insertion*	*Nerve supply*	*Actions*
1. **Ischiocavernosus** It covers the crus penis or crus clitoridis; smaller in females	a. Medial surface of ischial ramus behind the crus b. Posterior part of perineal membrane	Fibres run forwards and spiral over the crus	Inserted by an aponeurosis into the sides and undersurface of the anterior part of the crus	Perineal branch of pudendal nerve	It helps in maintaining erection of the penis by compressing the crus Causes erection of clitoris in female
2. **Bulbospongiosus** It covers the bulb of penis and the two muscles are united by a median raphe	a. Perineal body b. Median raphe over the bulb of penis	a. Posterior fibres embrace the posterior end of the bulb b. Middle fibres embrace the corpus spongiosum c. Anterior fibres embrace the entire body of penis	a. Posterior *fibres,* into the perineal membrane b. Middle fibres embrace the bulb and corpus spongiosum, and the raphe on their upper surface c. Anterior fibres are inserted into the raphe on the dorsal surface of the penis	Perineal branch of pudendal nerve	1. Helps in ejaculation of semen and ejecting the last drops of urine 2. Middle fibres assist in the erection of the corpus spongiosum penis by compressing the bulb 3. Anterior fibres also help in the erection of penis by compressing the deep dorsal vein of penis
In females, it covers the bulb of vestibule and the two muscles are separated by the vagina and urethra	Perineal body	Fibres pass anteriorly	a. Perineal membrane b. Bulb of vestibule c. Body of clitoris and corpus spongiosum		In females it acts as sphincter of vagina and assists in erection of clitoris
3. **Superficial transversus perinei** Narrow slip running transversely in front of anus on either side	Medial surface of the root of ischial ramus	Fibres run medially	Inserted into the perineal body where it interlaces with other converging muscles	Perineal branch of pudendal nerve	Steadies the perineal body

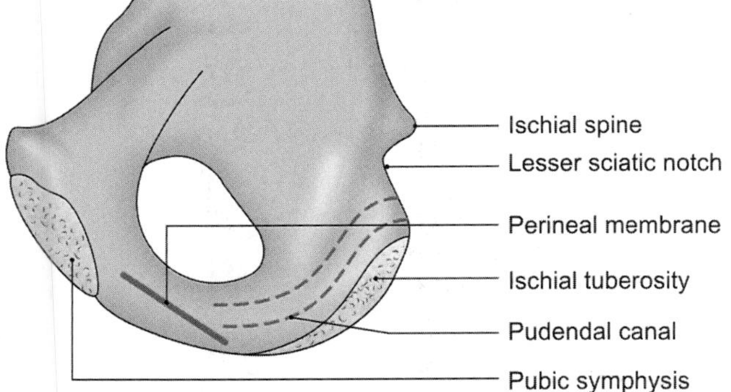

Fig. 28.23: Inner surface of the right hip bone showing the position of pudendal canal

2 *Internal pudendal artery*: This artery gives off the inferior rectal artery in the posterior part of the canal. In the anterior part of the canal, the artery divides into the perineal artery and the artery of penis. Vein accompanies the artery.

PUDENDAL NERVE

Pudendal nerve is the chief nerve of the perineum and of the external genitalia. It is accompanied by the internal pudendal vessels.

Origin

Pudendal nerve arises from the sacral plexus in the pelvis. It is derived from spinal nerves S2, S3, S4.

Course

It originates in the pelvis, enters gluteal region through greater sciatic notch, leaves it through lesser sciatic notch to enter the pudendal canal in the lateral wall of ischioanal fossa. It terminates by dividing into branches.

Relations

1 *In the pelvis*, the pudendal nerve descends in front of the piriformis deep to its fascia. It leaves the pelvis, to enter the gluteal region, by passing through the

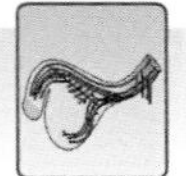

lower part of the greater sciatic foramen, between the piriformis and the coccygeus, medial to internal pudendal vessels.

2 *In the gluteal region*, the pudendal nerve crosses the apex of the sacrospinous ligament, under cover of gluteus maximus. Here it lies medial to the internal pudendal vessels which cross the ischial spine. Accompanying these vessels, the nerve leaves the gluteal region by passing through the lesser sciatic foramen, and enters the pudendal canal.

3 *In the pudendal canal*, the neurovascular bundle lies in the lateral wall of the ischioanal fossa (Fig. 28.7).

Branches

In the posterior part of the pudendal canal the pudendal nerve gives off the inferior rectal nerve, and then divides into two terminal branches, the perineal nerve and the dorsal nerve of the penis or clitoris (Figs 28.24 and 28.25).

The *inferior rectal nerve* pierces the medial wall of the pudendal canal, crosses the ischioanal fossa from lateral to medial side, and supplies the external anal sphincter, the skin around the anus, and the lining of the anal canal below the pectinate line (Fig. 28.9).

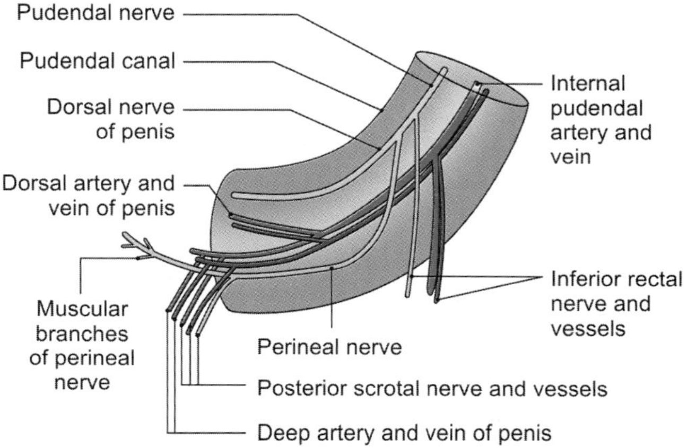

Fig. 28.24: Contents of pudendal canal

The *perineal nerve* is the larger terminal branch of the pudendal nerve. It runs forwards below the internal pudendal vessels, and terminates by dividing into:

a. Medial and lateral *posterior scrotal* or labial nerves.
b. *Muscular branches* to the urogenital muscles, and to anterior parts of external anal sphincter and the levator ani. The nerve to the bulbospongiosus also gives off the nerve to bulb which supplies corpus spongiosum, penis and the urethra.

The *dorsal nerve of the penis* or *clitoris* is the smaller terminal branch of the pudendal nerve. It runs forwards first in the pudendal canal above the internal pudendal vessels; and then in the deep perineal space between these vessels and the pubic arch. Next it passes through the lateral part of the oval gap between the apex of the perineal membrane and the arcuate pubic ligament, runs on the dorsum of the penis or clitoris, and ends in the glans penis or glans clitoridis. It supplies the skin of the body of the penis or clitoris and of the glans.

CLINICAL ANATOMY

The pudendal nerve supplies sensory branches to the lower of the vagina, through the inferior rectal and posterior labial branches. Therefore, in vaginal operations, general anaesthesia can be replaced by a *pudendal nerve block*. The nerve is infiltrated near the ischial spine by a needle passed through the vaginal wall and then guided by a finger (Fig. 28.26).

INTERNAL PUDENDAL ARTERY

This is the chief artery of the perineum and of the external genital organs. It is smaller in females than in males.

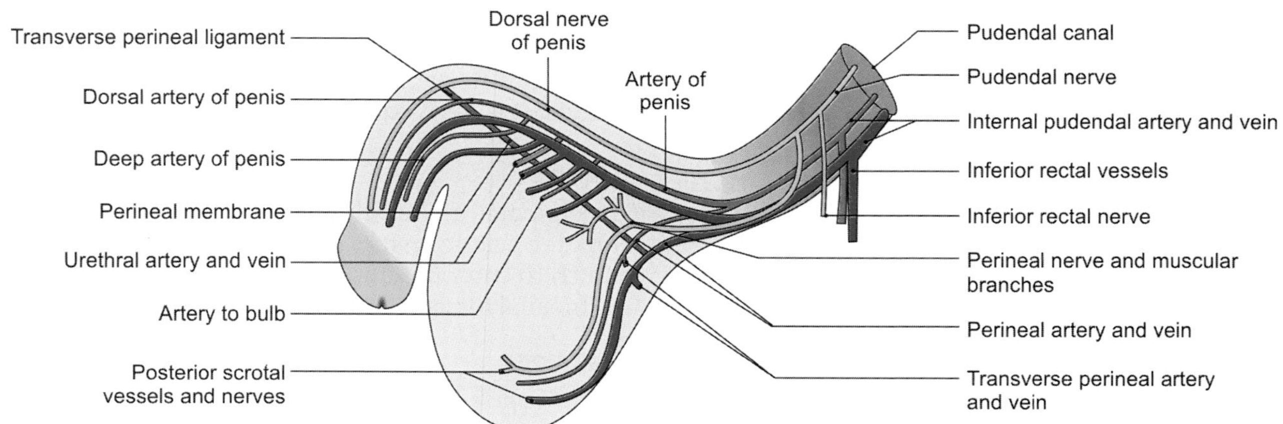

Fig. 28.25: Course and distribution of the pudendal nerve, and of the internal pudendal artery

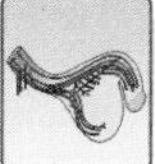

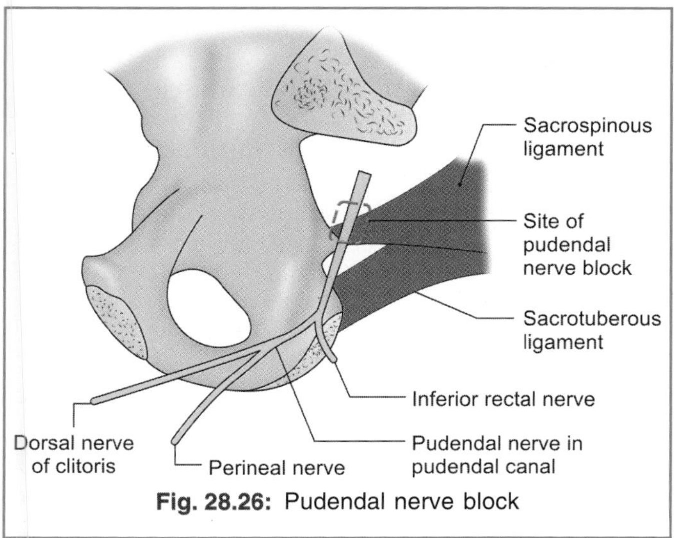

Fig. 28.26: Pudendal nerve block

Origin

The artery is the smaller terminal branch of the anterior division of the internal iliac artery, given off in the pelvis; the larger branch is the inferior gluteal.

Course

The course of internal pudendal artery is similar to the course of pudendal nerve.

Relations

In the pelvis, the artery runs downwards in front of the piriformis, the sacral plexus and the inferior gluteal artery. It leaves the pelvis by piercing the parietal pelvic fascia and passing through the greater sciatic foramen, below the piriformis, thus entering the gluteal region.

In the gluteal region, the artery crosses the dorsal aspect of the tip of the ischial spine, under cover of the gluteus maximus. Here it lies between the pudendal nerve medially and the nerve to the obturator internus laterally. It leaves the gluteal region by passing through the lesser sciatic foramen, and thus enters the pudendal canal.

In the pudendal canal, the artery runs downwards and forwards in the lateral wall of the ischioanal fossa, about 4 cm above the lower margin of the ischial tuberosity. Here it is related to the dorsal nerve above and the perineal nerve below. The artery gives off the inferior rectal artery in the posterior part of the canal, and the perineal artery in the anterior part. The internal pudendal artery continues into the deep perineal space as the artery of the penis or of the clitoris (Fig. 28.24).

In the deep perineal space, the artery of the penis or clitoris which is continuation of internal pudendal artery, runs forwards close to the side of pubic arch, medial to the dorsal nerve of penis or of clitoris. The artery ends a little behind the arcuate pubic ligament by dividing into the deep and dorsal arteries of penis or of the clitoris (Fig. 28.25).

Branches

1 The *inferior rectal artery* arises near the posterior end of the pudendal canal, and accompanies the nerve of the same name. The artery supplies the skin, muscles and mucous membrane of the anal region, and anastomoses with the superior and middle rectal arteries (Fig. 28.24).
2 The *perineal artery* arises near the anterior end of the pudendal canal, and pierces the base of the perineal membrane to reach the superficial perineal space. Here it divides into the *transverse perineal* and the *posterior scrotal* or *posterior labial* branches.
3 The *artery of the penis* or *the clitoris* runs in the deep perineal space and gives off:
   a. Artery to the bulb.
   b. Urethral artery.
   c. Deep artery of the penis or the clitoris.
   d. Dorsal artery of the penis or the clitoris.

   All of them pierce the perineal membrane and reach the superficial perineal space. The *artery to the bulb* supplies the bulb of the penis or bulb of vestibule and the posterior part of the urethra or only the urethra. The *urethral artery* supplies the corpus spongiosum and the anterior part of the urethra. The *deep artery of the penis* or *the clitoris* traverses and supplies the crus and the corpus cavernosum. The *dorsal artery of the penis* or *the clitoris* supplies the skin and fasciae of the body of the penis and of the glans or the glans clitoridis.

INTERNAL PUDENDAL VEIN

The tributaries of internal pudendal vein follow the branches of the internal pudendal artery. The vein drains into internal iliac vein.

HISTOLOGY OF BODY OF PENIS/CLITORIS

Penis consists of two corpora cavernosa containing the deep artery of the penis and a single corpora spongiosum with the urethra. All three erectile masses contain spaces or caverns. The spaces are larger in corpora cavernosa and smaller in corpus spongiosum. These three corpora are covered by fasciae and skin. In the deep fascia lie deep dorsal vein of penis, two dorsal arteries and two dorsal nerves of penis. The superficial dorsal vein of the penis lies in the superficial fascia.

Clitoris comprises two corpora cavernosa only. *Corpus spongiosum is absent*. The two erectile masses contain caverns or spaces.

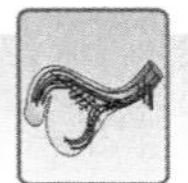

FACTS TO REMEMBER

- Perineum is divided into anterior by placed urogenital triangle and posteriorly placed anal triangle.
- Anal triangle comprises terminal part of anal canal in the centre with right and left ischioanal fossae on each side. Ischioanal fossa contains internal pudendal vessels and pudendal nerve.
- Fat in ischioanal fossa keeps the anal canal closed except at the time of defaecation.
- Sphincter urethrae is within the wall of urethra. So there is hardly any deep perineal space.
- Perineal membrane is the key structure in urogenital triangle. Main difference in male and female perineum about the structures piercing the perineal membrane is the additional vaginal opening in female and two ducts of bulbourethral glands in the male only.
- Key structure and central tendon of perineum is perineal body.
- Body of clitoris in female is made up of only two corpora cavernosa and *no* corpus spongiosum
- There is corpus spongiosum with urethra in the penis of male in addition to two corpora cavernosa (*see* Fig. 17.2).
- Clitoris is much smaller than the penis and is *not traversed by the urethra*. Urethral orifice lies 2 cm behind clitoris.
- Bulbspongiosus of two sides are separate in female and overlie the bulb of vestibule. In male the two are united by a median septum and overlie the bulb of penis.
- Pudendal nerve supplies all the muscles and skin of perineum.
- Inferior rectal nerve supplies mucous membrane of the lower part of the anal canal, external anal sphincter and the skin around anal opening.
- The labium majora contains sebaceous glands, sweat glands and hair follicles.
- There are four openings in the vestibule one each, of urethra, and vagina and two of ducts of Bartholin's glands.

CLINICOANATOMICAL PROBLEM

A woman few days after childbirth complained of a painful swelling in her perianal region.

- Name is the fossa related to anal canal.
- What vessel passes through the fossa?
- Disruption of which vessel causes collection of blood after the childbirth?

Ans: The fossa related to the anal region is the ischioanal fossa. There is one fossa on each side of the anal canal. The internal pudendal artery and pudendal nerve course through the pudendal canal, lying in the lateral wall of the fossa.

The swelling occurred due to disruption of a small branch of internal pudendal artery, probably as a result of infection during childbirth or infection the episiotomy area.

MULTIPLE CHOICE QUESTIONS

1. Deep boundaries of the perineum are all *except*:
 a. Inferior pubic ligament
 b. Tip of the coccyx
 c. Sacrotuberous ligament
 d. Sacrospinous ligament

2. Following are the paired muscles attached to the perineal body *except*:
 a. Bulbospongiosus
 b. Deep transverses perenei
 c. Levator ani
 d. Part of sphincter ani externus

3. Following are the contents of ischioanal fossa *except*:
 a. Inferior rectal nerve and vessels
 b. Pudendal nerve and internal pudendal vessels
 c. Middle rectal vessels
 d. Ischioanal pad of fat

4. Main bulk of distal urethral sphincter mechanism is formed by:
 a. Compressor urethrae
 b. Smooth muscle of urethra
 c. Rhabdosphincter
 d. Pubourethralis part of levator ani

5. Following structures pierce the perineal membrane in male *except*:
 a. Vagina
 b. Urethra
 c. Deep artery of penis
 d. Dorsal artery of penis

6. Which part of urethra is the least dilatable?
 a. External opening b. Prostatic part
 c. Membranous part d. Penile part

ANSWERS

1. d **2.** d **3.** c **4.** c **5.** a **6.** c

29

Preliminary Consideration of Boundaries and Contents of Pelvis

It is a basin for housing lower parts of digestive and excretory systems.
It chiefly lodges the genital system, the only system different in the male and female

INTRODUCTION

Pelvis is formed by articulation of each of the two hip bones with the sacrum behind and with each other in front. The greater pelvis is comfortably occupied by the abdominal viscera, leaving only the lesser pelvis for the pelvic viscera. Urinary bladder lies behind pubic symphysis; rectum and anal canal are close to the sacrum and coccyx. The middle space left is for the genital organs. Many structures cross the brim of the pelvis, i.e. curved line extending around the pelvis at the junction of greater and lesser pelves (linea terminalis).

The bony pelvis is formed by *four bones* united at *four joints*. The bones are the two hip bones in front and on the sides, and the sacrum and coccyx behind. The joints are the two sacroiliac joints, the pubic symphysis and the sacrococcygeal joint.

The pelvis is divided by the plane of the *pelvic inlet* or pelvic brim, or superior aperture of the pelvis into two parts.

a. Upper part is known as greater or *false pelvis.*
b. Lower part is known as the *lesser* or *true pelvis.* The plane of the pelvic inlet passes from the sacral promontory to the upper margin of the pubic symphysis. The *greater* or *false pelvis* includes the two iliac fossae, and forms a part of the posterior abdominal wall. The *lesser* or *true pelvis* contains the pelvic viscera.

LESSER PELVIS

Pelvic Walls

The pelvic walls are made up of bones, ligaments and muscles.

Bony Walls

These are formed:

1 *Anteriorly* by the pubic symphysis and bodies of the pubic bones.
2 *Posteriorly* by the sacrum and coccyx.
3 *On each side* by the two rami of the pubis, the ischium with its ramus, and the lower part of the ilium (Fig. 29.1).

Ligaments and Membranes

1 *Obturator membrane* closes the greater part of the obturator foramen, and completes the lower part of the lateral wall of the pelvis (Fig. 29.2).
2 *Sacrotuberous* ligament and *sacrospinous* ligaments bridge the gap between the hip bone and the sacrum, and convert the greater and lesser sciatic notches into the foramina of the same name (Fig. 29.3).

Muscles

1 The *obturator internus* with its fascia reinforces the lateral wall of the pelvis from the inside.
2 The *piriformis* with its fascia forms the posterior wall of the pelvis. It also helps in filling the gap of the greater sciatic foramen (Figs 29.4 and 29.5).

Pelvic Inlet: Superior Aperture of Pelvis

The pelvic inlet is an oblique plane, making an angle of 50 to 60 degrees with the horizontal. It is *bounded*

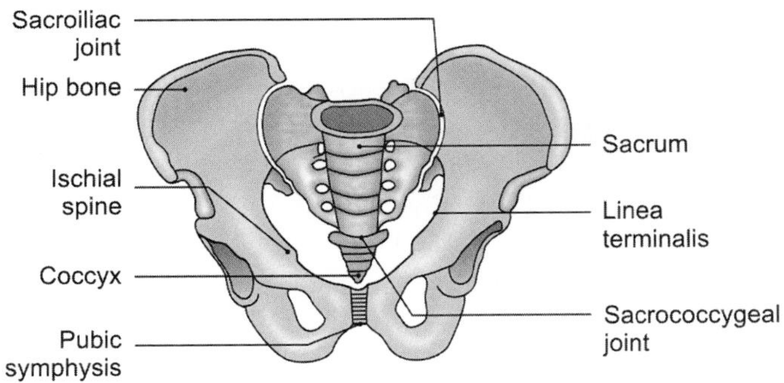

Fig. 29.1: Anterior view of the male pelvis

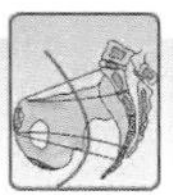

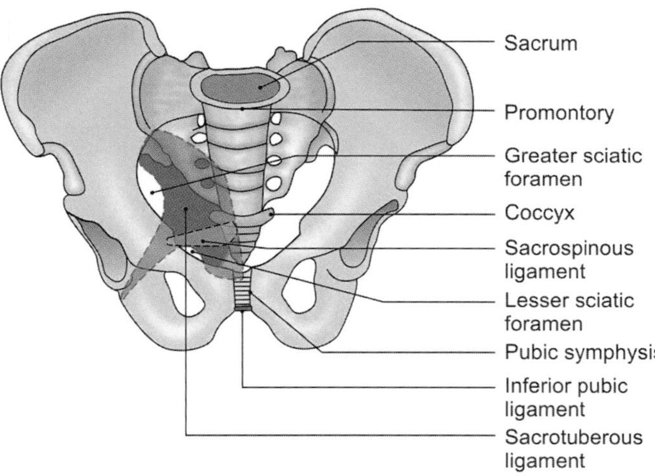

Fig. 29.2: Bones and ligaments of pelvis seen from the front

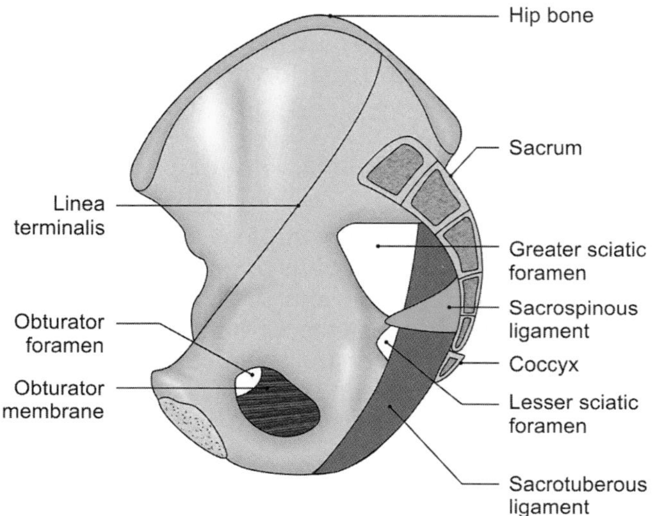

Fig. 29.3: Pelvic bones and ligaments seen from the medial side

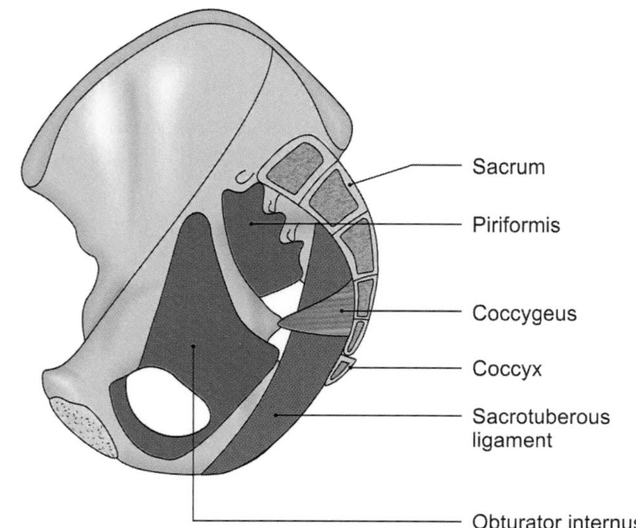

Fig. 29.4: Muscles of the pelvic wall seen from the medial side

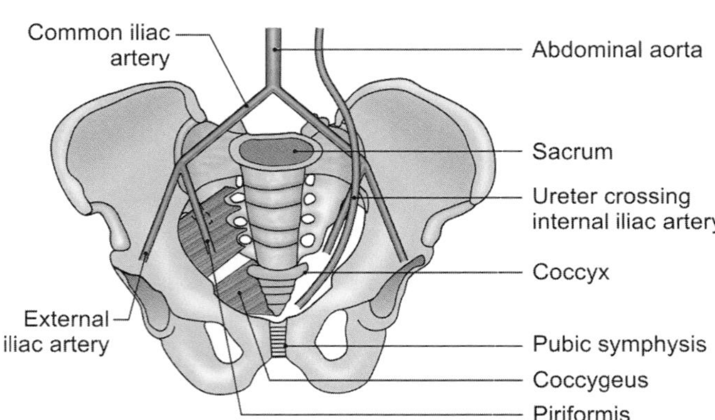

Fig. 29.5: Muscles of the posterior part of the pelvic wall seen from the front

posteriorly by the sacral promontory, *anteriorly* by the upper margin of the pubic symphysis, and on *each side* by the linea terminalis. The linea terminalis includes the anterior margin of the ala of the sacrum, the arcuate line or lower part of the medial border of the ilium, the pectineal line of the pubis or pecten pubis, and the pubic crest (Fig. 29.6).

The pelvic inlet is heart-shaped *in the male*, and is widest in its posterior part. *In the female*, it is oval, and is widest more anteriorly than in the male. Posteriorly, the inlet is indented by the sacral promontory, more so in the male than in the female (Fig. 29.7).

Pelvic Outlet: Inferior Aperture of Pelvis

The pelvic outlet is *bounded anteriorly* by the arcuate or inferior pubic ligament; *posteriorly* by the coccyx; and *on each side* by the ischiopubic rami or side of the pubic arch, the ischial tuberosities and the sacrotuberous

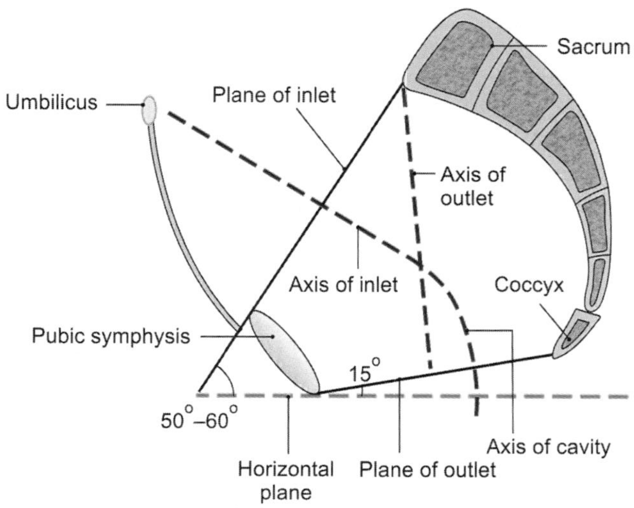

Fig. 29.6: Sagittal section of the pelvis showing the planes of its inlet and outlet and their axes. The axis of the pelvic cavity is J-shaped

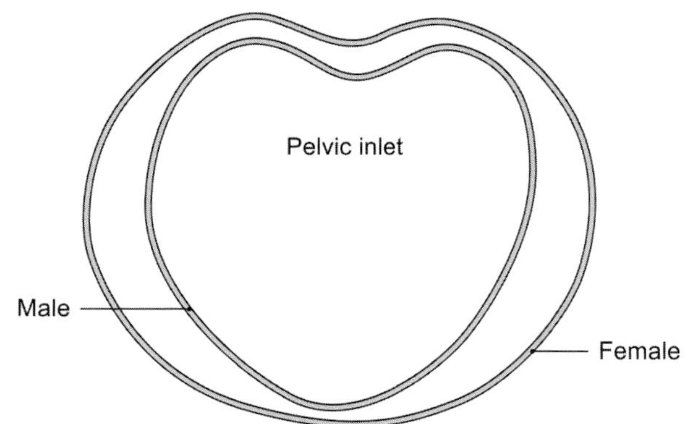

Fig. 29.7: Shape of pelvic inlet in the male, and in the female

ligaments. The posterior part of the outlet is formed by the coccyx and the sacrotuberous ligaments. It is mobile on the sacrum, and the sacrum itself is slightly mobile at the sacroiliac joints (Fig. 29.6).

The pubic arch is formed by the ischiopubic rami of the two sides and by the lower margin of the pubic symphysis which is rounded off by the arcuate pubic ligament (Fig. 29.2).

CLINICAL ANATOMY

- The pelvis is a basin with its various walls and many openings. The posterior wall contains 5 pairs of anterior sacral foramina. The greater and lesser sciatic notches are converted into foramina of the same name with the help of sacrotuberous and sacrospinous ligaments. Greater sciatic foramen is the "doorway" of the gluteal region. Pudendal nerve enters the region through the greater sciatic notch and quickly leaves it through lesser sciatic notch to enter the perineum. The lateral wall contains obturator foramen for the passage of obturator nerve which supplies adductors of the hip joint.
- Fracture may occur in the true (ring-like) pelvis. If fracture is at one point, the fracture will be stable.
- In athletes, anterior superior iliac spine may be pulled off by forcible contraction of sartorius. Similarly anterior inferior iliac spine or ischial tuberosity may get **avulsed** by the contraction of their attached muscles.

Pelvic Floor

The pelvic floor is formed by the pelvic diaphragm which consists of the levator ani and the coccygeus (*see* Chapter 34). It resembles a hammock, or a gutter because it slopes from either side towards the median plane where it is traversed by the urethra and the anal canal, and also by the vagina in the female. The pelvic diaphragm separates the perineum below from the pelvis above.

The muscles of the true pelvis, its blood vessels and nerves are considered in Chapter 34.

CLINICAL ANATOMY

- Pelvic floor formed by two gutter-shaped levator ani muscles supports the pelvic viscera, especially during raised intra-abdominal pressure. The foetal head travels in the axis of pelvic cavity (Fig. 29.8). During second stage of labor, the head of the baby on reaching the pelvic floor rotates from earlier transverse position to the anteroposterior position. The occiput moves downwards and forwards and reaches below the 80°–85° angled pubic arch. Then the head passes through the anterior hiatus of the levator ani to reach the perineum and then deliver. Sometimes episiotomy is given to enlarge the perineum (Fig. 29.9).
- Injury to pelvic floor which mostly occurs during vaginal delivery, may cause uterine, vaginal or even rectal prolapse.
- Appendicitis occurring due to pelvic position of the appendix may irritate the obturator nerve leading to referred pain in the medial side of thigh (*see* Fig. 20.23).
- Inflammation of ovaries may cause referred pain in the medial side of thigh due to irritation of the obturator nerve (*see* Fig. 31.1).
- The 2nd to 4th sacral nerves and coccygeal nerve can be anaesthetised by the anaesthetic agent put into the sacral canal. It is called *caudal anaesthesia* and is used in obstetrics practice.
- Pain in the sacroiliac joint is felt on pressing the posterior superior iliac spine present in a dimple on the lower back (*see* Fig. 5.1).

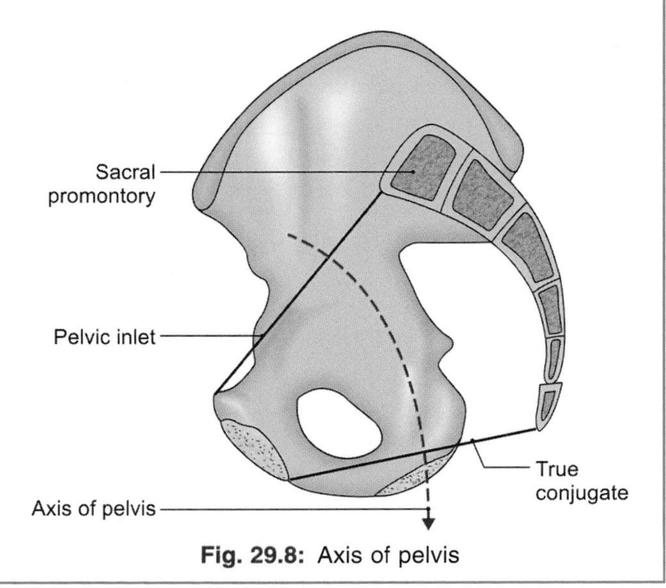

Fig. 29.8: Axis of pelvis

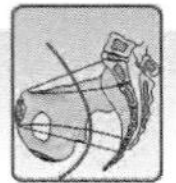

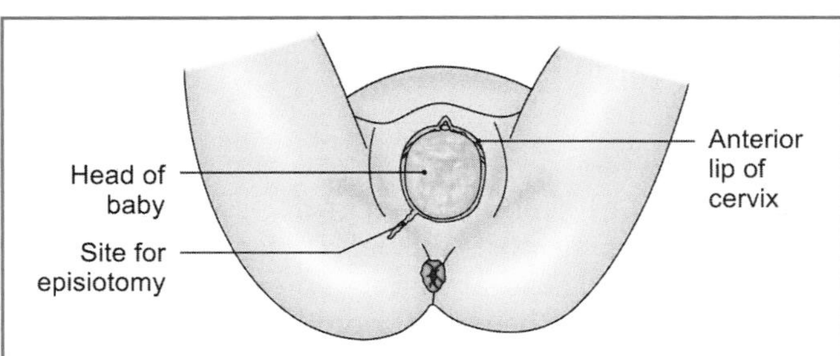

Fig. 29.9: Head of the delivering baby seen at the perineum. Site of episiotomy is also seen

Pelvic Cavity

The pelvic cavity is continuous above with the abdominal cavity at the pelvic brim, and is limited below by the pelvic diaphragm. The cavity is curved in such a way that it is first directed downwards and backwards, and then downwards and forwards (J-shaped) as shown in (Fig. 29.10). It has unequal walls, measuring only about 5 cm anteriorly and 15 cm posteriorly. The cavity is more roomy or larger in the female than in the male.

Contents

1 Sigmoid colon and rectum occupy the posterior part of the pelvis.
2 Urinary bladder lies anteriorly. The prostate lies below the neck of urinary bladder.
3 In between the bladder and rectum, there is a transverse septum or *genital septum* made up of connective tissue. In the male, the septum is small. It contains the ductus deferens, the seminal vesicle and the ureter on each side.

In the female, the septum is large, and contains the uterus, the uterine tubes, the round ligament of the uterus, the ligaments of the ovary, ovaries, the vagina and the ureters.

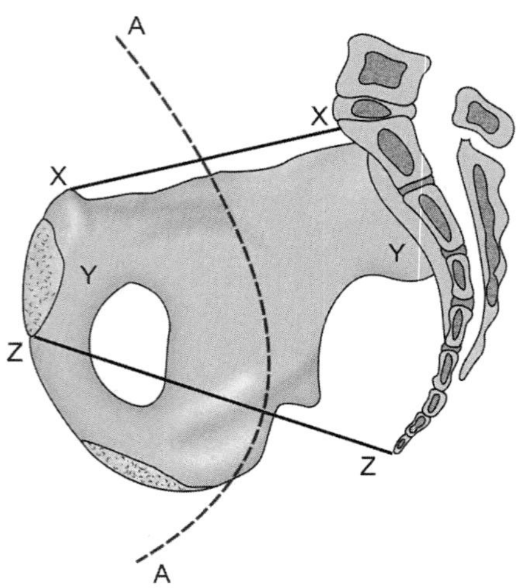

Fig. 29.10: Side view of bony female pelvis. AA—Axis of pelvic cavity (X–X—Plane of inlet, Y–Y—Zone of cavity, Z–Z—Plane of outlet)

These contents are considered in detail in the chapters that follow.

Structures Crossing the Pelvic Inlet/Brim of the Pelvis

From posterior median plane sweeping laterally and anteriorly:

1 Median sacral vessels (Fig. 29.11).
2 Sympathetic trunk.
3 Lumbosacral trunk (Fig. 29.11).
4 Iliolumbar artery.
5 Obturator nerve.
6 Internal iliac vessels (Fig. 29.5)
7 Medial limb of sigmoid mesocolon with superior rectal vessels—left side only (Fig. 29.11).

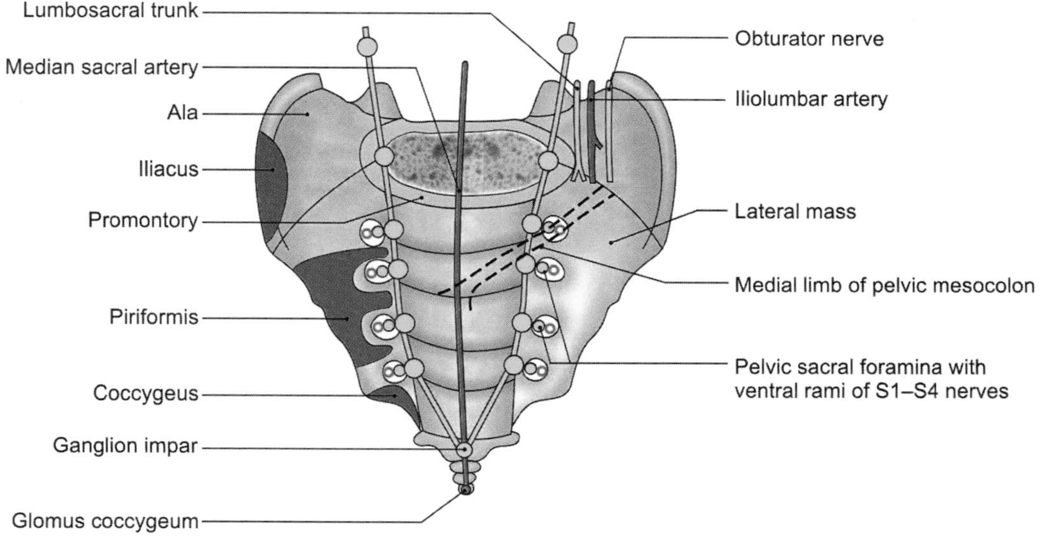

Fig. 29.11: Anterior (pelvic) view of the sacrum and attachment of sigmoid mesocolon

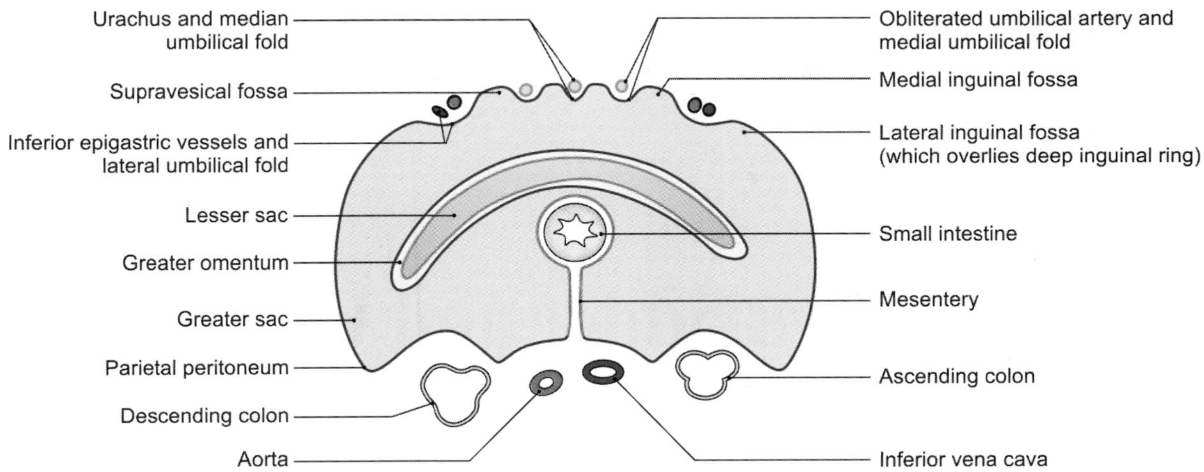

Fig. 29.12: Urachus and obliterated umbilical artery will cross the pelvic brim

8 Ureter (*see* Figs 24.22, 29.5 and 30.3).
9 Sigmoid colon—on left side only.
10 Ovarian vessels in female (*see* Fig. 31.5).
11 Ductus deferens in male/round ligament of uterus in female (*see* Fig. 31.11 and 32.2).
12 Lateral umbilical ligament (Fig. 29.12).
13 Median umbilical ligament or urachus (Fig. 29.12).
14 Autonomic nerve plexuses.
15 Coils of intestine and pregnant uterus.
16 Full urinary bladder.

FACTS TO REMEMBER

- Axis of pelvic cavity is "J" shaped. Plane of outlet of pelvis makes an angle of 15° with the horizontal plane. Plane of inlet of pelvis makes an angle of 50°–60° with the horizontal plane.
- Shallowest wall of pelvis is its anterior wall. Distance between two ischial spines is the least.

CLINICOANATOMICAL PROBLEM

During childbirth, a woman was given pudendal nerve block. She still complained of some pain during her labour

- What is pudendal nerve block?
- Which other nerves have to be anaesthetized to get painless childbirth?

Ans: Pudendal nerve arises from ventral rami of S2, S3, S4 segments of spinal cord. It is the nerve of the perineum. It supplies three muscles of superficial perineal space including most of the skin and mucous membrane of perineum. So it is blocked by an anaesthetic agent given above the ischial tuberosity.

Since sensations from perineum are also carried by ilioinguinal (L1), genitofemoral (L1, L2), and posterior cutaneous nerve of thigh, these nerves also need to be blocked by making an injection of the same agent along the lateral margin of labia majora.

MULTIPLE CHOICE QUESTIONS

1. All the following are the characteristic features of the female bony pelvis *except*:
   a. Pelvic inlet is oval or round
   b. Subpubic angle is 50–60 degrees
   c. Obturator foramen is small and triangular
   d. Sciatic notches are wider
2. Axis of pelvic inlet is:
   a. Vertical
   b. Downwards and backwards
   c. Transverse
   d. Downwards and forwards
3. Angle of horizontal plane with plane of inlet is:
   a. 70°–80° b. 50°–60°
   c. 40°–50° d. 45°–65°
4. Angle of horizontal plane with plane of outlet is:
   a. 10° b. 15°
   c. 20° d. 25°
5. All the following structures cross the brim of pelvis in male *except*:
   a. Internal iliac vessels b. Ovarian vessels
   c. Iliolumbar artery d. Sympathetic trunks

ANSWERS

1. b **2.** b **3.** b **4.** b **5.** b

30

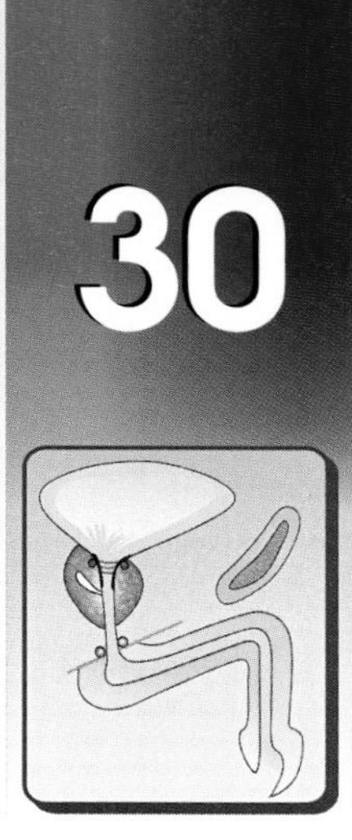

Urinary Bladder and Urethra

Poisons and medicines are often times the same substance given with different doses and different intents
— S Anthony

INTRODUCTION

Urinary bladder is the temporary store house of urine which gets emptied through the urethra. The external urethral sphincter is the sphincter urethrae which is placed proximally in the wall of urethra, and not at the terminal part of the urethra. In the case of pylorus and anal canal, the sphincters are placed at their terminal ends.

The male urethra subserving the functions of urination and ejaculation, i.e. expulsion of semen is 18–20 cm long with curvatures and comprises preprostatic, prostatic, membranous and longest anterior bulbar and penile parts.

The female urethra is for urination only and is 4 cm long. The cathetarisation if required is much easier in the female than in the male.

DISSECTION

Clean and define the muscles, membranes and ligaments in the pelvic cavity. These are the levator ani obturator internus muscles; medial and lateral pubo prostatic ligaments and median, medial umbilical folds.

Identify the peritoneum on the superior surface of the bladder situated just behind the pubic symphysis. Identify and follow the median umbilical ligament from the apex of bladder. Define the surfaces, blunt borders and the openings in the urinary bladder.

In the male, trace the ductus deferens and ureter to the base of the bladder on both sides. Pull the bladder medially and identify the structures on its lateral surface, e.g. the levator ani, obturator vessels and nerve, superior vesical branch of umbilical artery and the obliterated umbilical artery.

In female, the cervix and vagina lie behind the urinary bladder.

Make the incision through the bladder wall along the junction of the superior and inferolateral surface on both sides. Extend these incisions till the lateral extremities of the base. Incise the superior wall of the bladder to be able to visualise its interior.

In the male, make a median section through the penis, opening the entire length of the spongy part of the urethra. Examine the internal structure of the urethra.

URINARY BLADDER

Features

The urinary bladder is a muscular reservoir of urine, which lies in the anterior part of the pelvic cavity. The detrusor muscle of urinary bladder is arranged in whorls and spirals and is adapted for mass contraction rather than peristalsis.

Size, Shape and Position

The bladder varies in its size, shape and position according to the amount of urine it contains.

When empty, it lies entirely within the pelvis; but as it fills it expands and extends upwards into the abdominal cavity, reaching up to the umbilicus or even higher.

External Features

An *empty bladder is tetrahedral* in shape and has:

1 *Apex*, directed forwards.
2 *Base* or fundus, directed backwards.
3 *Neck*, which is the lowest and most fixed part of the bladder.
4 *Three surfaces*, superior, right and left inferolateral.
5 *Four borders*, two lateral, one anterior and one posterior (Figs 30.1 and 30.2).

A *full bladder is ovoid* in shape and has:

1 *An apex*, directed upwards towards the umbilicus.
2 *A neck*, directed downwards.
3 *Two surfaces*, anterior and posterior.

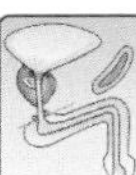

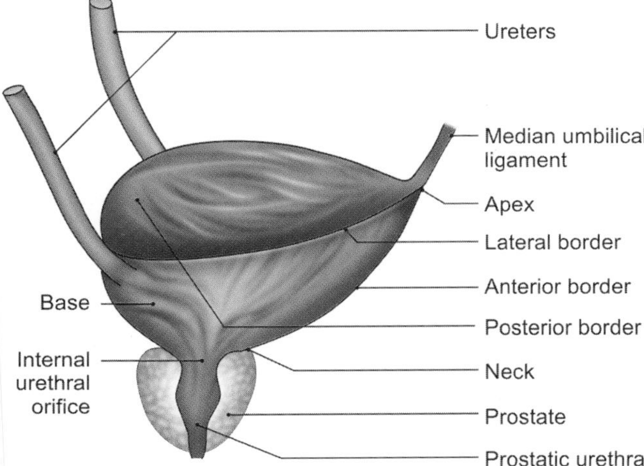

Fig. 30.1: The shape of the urinary bladder

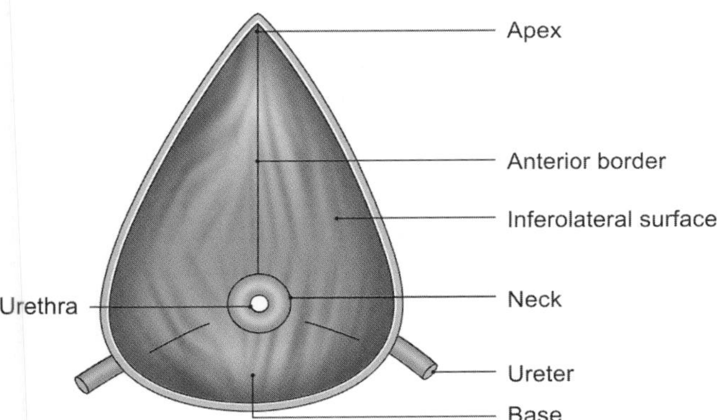

Fig. 30.2: Urinary bladder seen from below

Relations

1 The *apex* is connected to the umbilicus by the median umbilical ligament which represents the obliterated embryonic urachus (Fig. 30.1).

2 *Base:*

a. *In the female,* it is related to the uterine cervix and to the vagina (*see* Fig. 31.21).

b. *In the male,* the upper part of the base is separated from the rectum by the rectovesical pouch (*see* Fig. 18.17a) and the contained coils of intestine; and the lower part is related to the seminal vesicles and the terminations of the vas deferens (Fig. 30.3). The triangular area between the two deferent ducts is separated from the rectum by the rectovesical fascia of Denonvilliers.

3 The *neck* is the lowest and most fixed part of the bladder. It lies 3 to 4 cm behind the lower part of the pubic symphysis, a little above the plane of the pelvic outlet. It is pierced by the internal urethral orifice.

a. *In males,* smooth muscle bundles surround the bladder neck and preprostatic urethra. These are arranged as distinct circular collar with its own

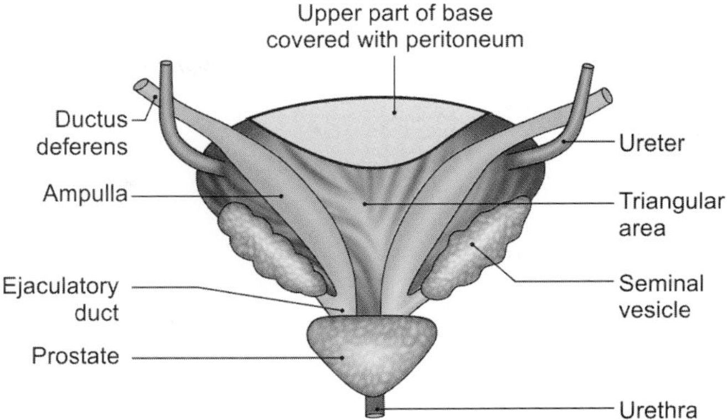

Fig. 30.3: Posterior view of a male urinary bladder and its relations to the genital ducts and glands

distinct adrenergic innervations. This is the preprostatic sphincter and is devoid of parasympathetic cholinergic nerves. It is part of proximal urethral sphincter mechanism.

b. *In females,* neck is related to the pelvic fascia which surrounds the upper part of the urethra.

In infants, the bladder lies at a higher level. The internal urethral orifice lies at the level of the superior border of the pubic symphysis. It gradually descends to reach the adult position after puberty.

4 *Superior surface:*

a. *In males,* it is completely covered by peritoneum, and is in contact with the sigmoid colon and coils of the terminal ileum (*see* Fig. 18.17a).

b. *In females,* peritoneum covers the greater part of the superior surface, except for a small area near the posterior border, which is related to the supravaginal part of the uterine cervix. The peritoneum from the superior surface is reflected to the isthmus of the uterus to form the vesicouterine pouch (*see* Fig. 18.17b).

5 *Inferolateral surfaces:* These are devoid of peritoneum, and are separated from each other anteriorly by the anterior border, and from the superior surface by the lateral borders.

a. *In the male,* each surface is related to the pubis, the puboprostatic ligaments, the retropubic fat, the levator ani and the obturator internus (Fig. 30.4).

b. *In the female,* the relations are same, except that the puboprostatic ligaments are replaced by the pubovesical ligaments.

As the bladder fills, the inferolateral surfaces form the anterior surface of the distended bladder, which is covered by peritoneum only in its upper part. The lower part comes into direct contact with the anterior abdominal wall, there being no intervening peritoneum. This part can be approached surgically without entering the peritoneal cavity.

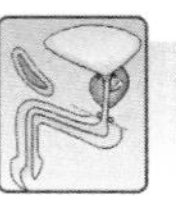

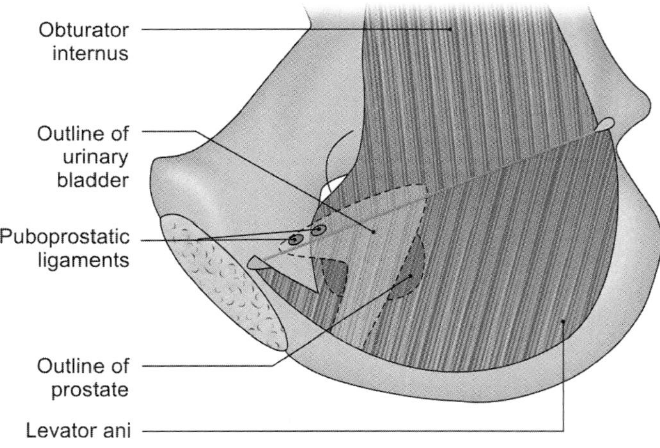

Fig. 30.4: Medial view of the lower part of the pelvic wall and the pelvic diaphragm. The urinary bladder has been superimposed to show relations of its inferolateral surface

Ligaments of the Bladder

True Ligaments

These are condensations of pelvic fascia around the neck and base of the bladder. They are continuous with the fascia on the superior surface of the levator ani.

1 The *lateral true ligament* of the bladder extends from the side of the bladder to the tendinous arch of the pelvic fascia (Fig. 30.5).
2 The *lateral puboprostatic ligament* is directed medially and backwards. It extends from the anterior end of the tendinous arch of the pelvic fascia to the upper part of the prostatic sheath (*see* Fig. 32.8).
3 The *medial puboprostatic ligament* is directed downwards and backwards. It extends from the back of the pubic bone (near the pubic symphysis) to the prostatic sheath. The ligaments of the two sides form the floor of the retropubic space (*see* Fig. 32.8).

In females, bands similar to the puboprostatic ligaments are known as the *pubovesical ligaments*. They end around the neck of the bladder (Fig. 30.5).

4 The *median umbilical ligament* is the remnant of the urachus (Fig. 30.1).
5 The *posterior ligament* of the bladder is directed backwards and upwards along the vesical plexus of veins. It extends on each side from the base of bladder to the wall of pelvis (Fig. 30.5).

False Ligaments

These are peritoneal folds, which do not form any support to the bladder. They include:

1 Median umbilical fold.
2 Medial umbilical fold.
3 Lateral false ligament, formed by peritoneum of the paravesical fossa.
4 Posterior false ligament formed by peritoneum of the sacrogenital folds (*see* Fig. 18.20).

Interior of the Bladder

It can be examined by cystoscopy, at operation or at autopsy.

In an empty bladder, the greater part of the mucosa shows irregular folds due to its loose attachment to the muscular coat.

In a small triangular area over the lower part of the base of the bladder, the mucosa is smooth due to its firm attachment to the muscular coat. This area is known as the *trigone* of the bladder. The apex of the trigone is directed downwards and forwards. The internal urethral orifice, opening into the urethra is located here. The ureters open at the posterolateral angles of the trigone. Their openings are 2.5 cm apart in the empty bladder, and 5 cm apart in a distended bladder (Fig. 30.6).

A slight elevation on the trigone immediately posterior to the urethral orifice produced by the median lobe of the prostate, is called the *uvula vesicae*. The base of the trigone is formed by the *interureteric ridge* or *bar of Mercier* produced by the continuation of the inner longitudinal muscle coats of the two ureters. The ridge

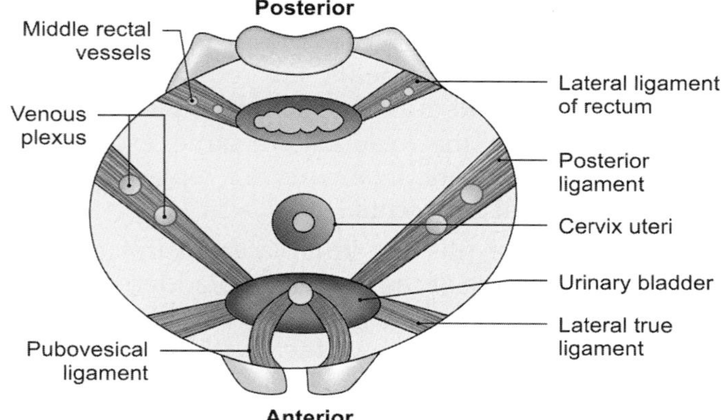

Fig. 30.5: True ligaments of the bladder in female

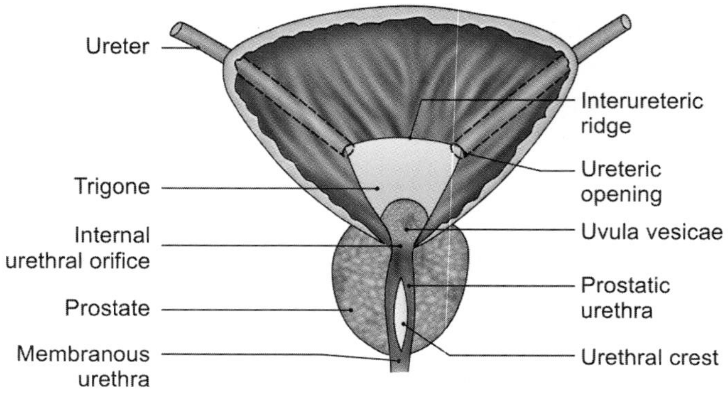

Fig. 30.6: Coronal section through the bladder and prostate to show the interior of the bladder

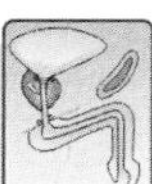

extends beyond the ureteric openings as the *ureteric folds* over the interstitial part of the ureters.

CLINICAL ANATOMY

- The interior of the bladder can be examined in the living by *cystoscope* (Fig. 30.7).
- A distended bladder may be *ruptured* by injuries of the lower abdominal wall. The peritoneum may or may not be involved.
- Chronic obstruction to the outflow of urine by an enlarged prostate causes hypertrophy of bladder leading to trabeculated bladder.
- In the operation of *suprapubic cystotomy*, the bladder is distended with about 300 ml of fluid. As a result the anterior aspect of the bladder comes into direct contact with the anterior abdominal wall, and can be approached without entering the peritoneal cavity.

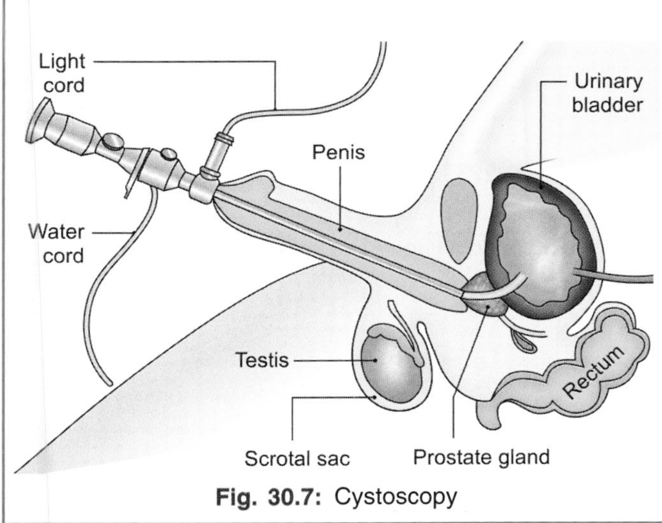

Fig. 30.7: Cystoscopy

Capacity of the Bladder

The mean capacity of the bladder in an adult male is 220 ml, varying from 120 to 320 ml. Filling beyond 220 ml causes a desire to micturate, and the bladder is usually emptied when filled to about 250 to 300 ml. Filling up to 500 ml may be tolerated, but beyond this it becomes painful. Referred pain is felt in the lower part of the anterior abdominal wall, perineum and penis (T11 to L2; S2 to S4).

Arterial Supply

1. The main supply comes from the superior and inferior vesical arteries, branches of anterior trunk of the internal iliac artery (*see* Fig. 34.1).
2. Additional supply is derived from the obturator, and inferior gluteal arteries; and in females from the uterine and vaginal arteries instead of inferior vesical.

Venous Drainage

Lying on the inferolateral surfaces of the bladder there is a vesical venous plexus. Veins from this plexus pass backwards in the posterior ligaments of the bladder, and drain into the internal iliac veins.

Lymphatic Drainage

Most of the lymphatics from the urinary bladder terminate in the external iliac nodes. A few vessels may pass to the internal iliac nodes or to the lateral aortic nodes.

Nerve Supply

The urinary bladder is supplied by the vesical plexus of nerves which is made up of fibres derived from the inferior hypogastric plexus. The vesical plexus contains both sympathetic and parasympathetic components, each of which contains motor or efferent and sensory or afferent fibres.

1. *Parasympathetic efferent* fibres or nervi erigentes, S2, S3, S4 are motor to the detrusor muscle. These nerves do not supply the preprostatic sphincter. If these are destroyed, normal micturition is not possible.
2. *Sympathetic efferent* fibres (T11 to L2) are said to be inhibitory to the detrusor and motor to the preprostatic sphincter mechanism.
3. The somatic, *pudendal nerve* (S2, S3, S4) supplies the sphincter urethrae which is voluntary and is situated within the wall of urethra.
4. *Sensory nerves:* Pain sensations, caused by distension or spasm of the bladder wall, are carried mainly by parasympathetic nerves and partly by sympathetic nerves. In the spinal cord, pain arising in bladder passes through the *lateral spinothalamic tract*, and awareness of bladder distension is mediated through the *posterior columns. Bilateral anterolateral cordotomy*, therefore, selectively abolishes pain without affecting the awareness of bladder distension and the desire to micturate.

CLINICAL ANATOMY

- *Emptying of bladder:* Emptying of the bladder is essentially a reflex function, involving the motor and sensory pathways. Voluntary control over this reflex is exerted through upper motor neurons, and as long as one pyramidal tract is functioning normally, control of the bladder remains normal. Acute injury to the cervical/thoracic segments of spinal cord leads to a state of spinal shock. The muscle of the bladder is relaxed, the sphincter vesicae contracted, but sphincter urethrae relaxed. The bladder distends and urine dribbles.

After a few days, the bladder starts contracting reflexly. When it is full, it contracts every 2–4 hours. This is "automatic reflex bladder" (Fig. 30.8).

Damage to the sacral segments of spinal cord situated in lower thoracic and lumbar one vertebra results in "autonomous bladder". The bladder wall is flaccid and its capacity is greatly increased. It just fills to capacity and overflows. So there is continuous dribbling (Fig. 30.9).

- Urinary bladder is one of sites for stone formation as concentrated urine lies here.

MALE URETHRA

Male urethra is 18–20 cm long that extends from the internal urethral orifice in the urinary bladder to the external opening (meatus) at the end of the penis.

Considered in two parts:

1 Relatively short posterior urethra which is 4 cm long, lies in the pelvis proximal to corpus spongiosum and is acted upon by urogenital sphincter mechanisms and also acts as a conduit.

Posterior urethra

a. Preprostatic segment (Fig. 30.10).
b. Prostatic segment.
c. Membranous segment.

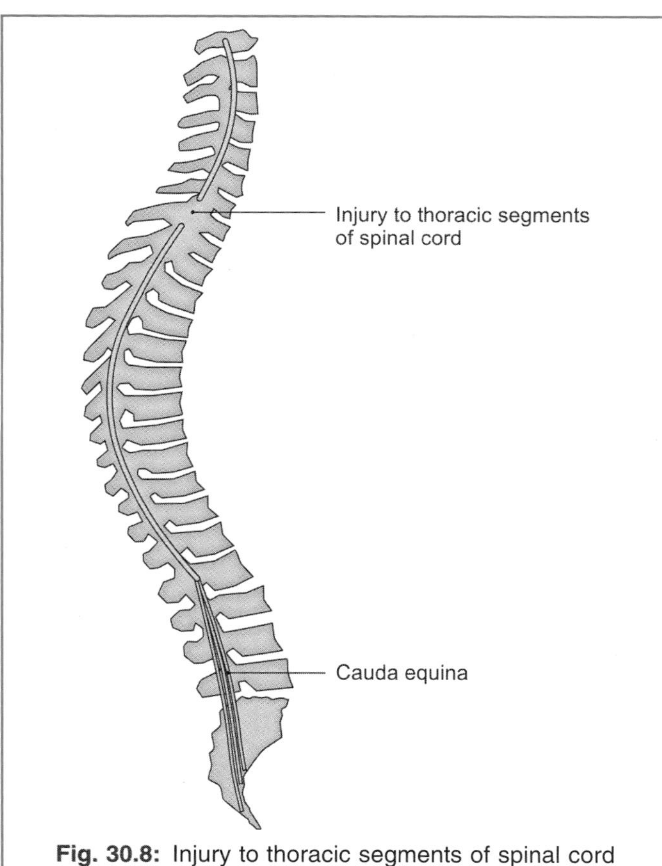

Fig. 30.8: Injury to thoracic segments of spinal cord

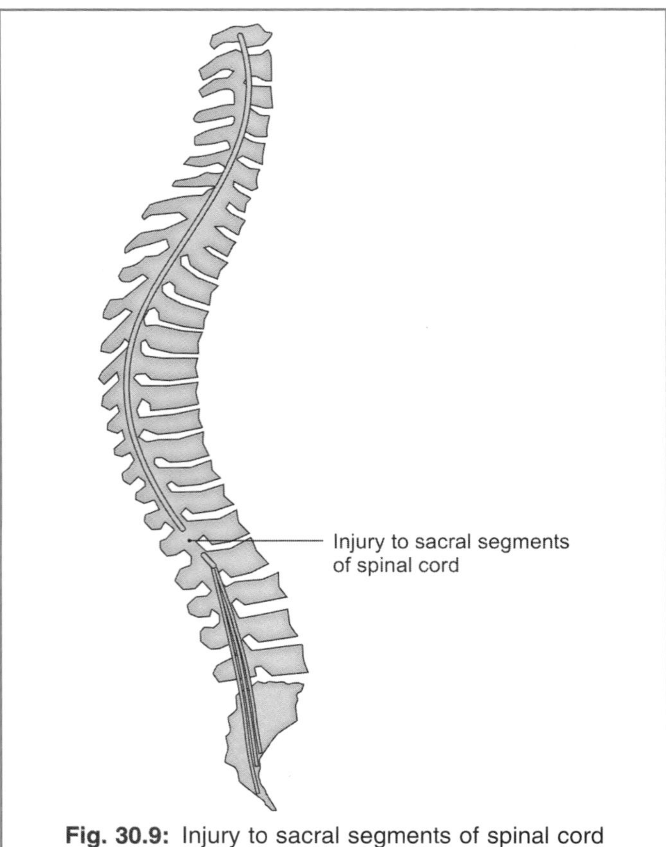

Fig. 30.9: Injury to sacral segments of spinal cord

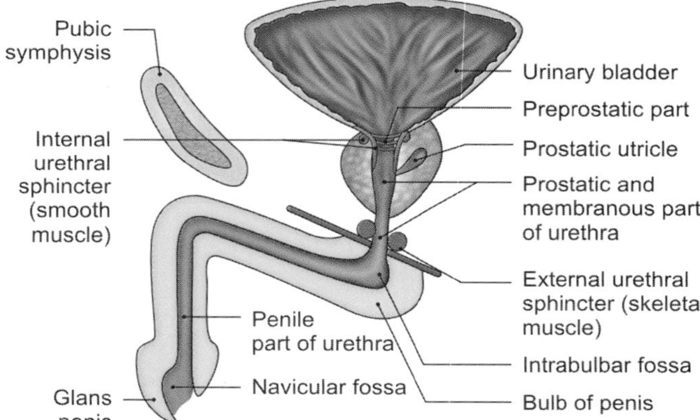

Fig. 30.10: Left view of a sagittal section through the male urethra showing its subdivisions

2 Relatively long anterior urethra which is 16 cm long within the perineum (proximally) and penis (distally). It is surrounded by corpus spongiosum and is functionally a conduit.

Anterior urethra

a. Bulbar urethral (proximal) component surrounded by bulbospongiosus. Entirely within perineum (Fig. 30.11).

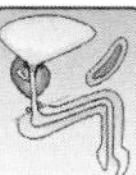

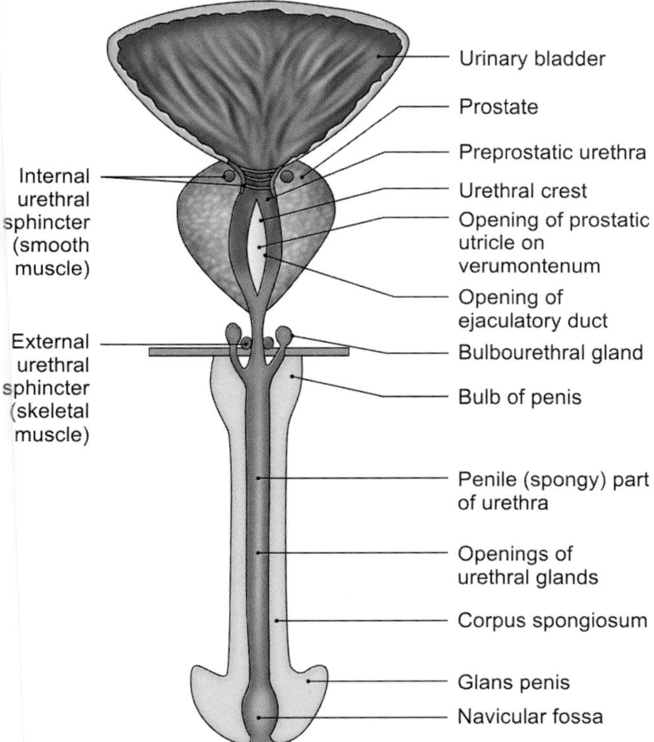

Fig. 30.11: Anterior view of the male urethra straightened and cut open

b. Pendulous/penile component that continues to the tip of penis.

In flaccid penis, urethra as a whole represents double curve except during the passage of fluid along it. The urethral canal is a mere slit.

In transverse section:

- The urethral slit is crescentic or transversely arched in prostatic part (Fig. 30.12).
- In the preprostatic and membranous part it is stellate.

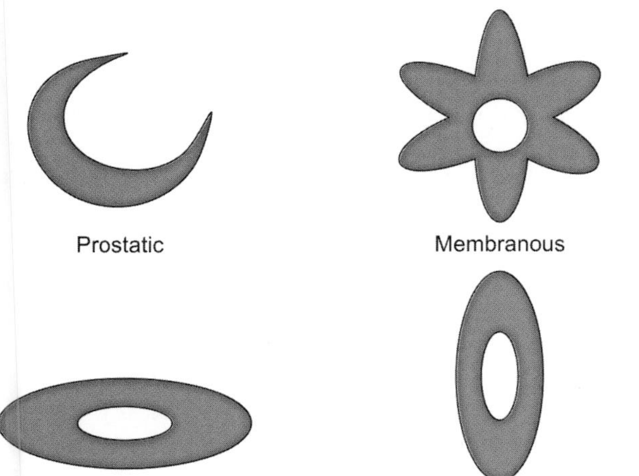

Fig. 30.12: Shape of different parts of the male urethra

- In bulbar and penile portions it is transverse.
- In external urethral orifice it is sagittal.

Passage of urine through different shapes of urethra causes it to flow in a continuous stream. Since it is passing under pressure, stream falls a little away from the body. Males can urinate standing without wetting themselves.

Posterior Part

Preprostatic Part

1–1.5 cm in length. It extends almost vertically from bladder neck to verumontanum (superior aspect) in prostatic urethra.

The preprostatic part is surrounded by proximal urethral sphincter mechanism (Fig. 30.10).

Proximal urethral sphincter mechanism

In addition to the smooth muscle bundles which run in continuity from the bladder neck down to the prostatic urethra and distinct from the smooth muscle within the prostate, smooth muscle bundles, surround the bladder neck and preprostatic urethra. They are arranged as distinct circular collar which has its own distinct adrenergic innervations.

The bundles which form this preprostatic sphincter are small in size compared with the muscle bundles of detrusor and are separated by a relatively larger connective tissue component rich in elastic fibres.

It is also different in that unlike detrusor and rest of urethral smooth muscle (common to both sexes), the preprostatic sphincter is almost totally devoid of parasympathetic cholinergic nerves.

Contraction of preprostatic urethra serves to prevent retrograde flow of ejaculate through proximal urethra into bladder.

It may maintain continence when external sphincter has been damaged. It is extensively disrupted in vast majority of men with:

a. Bladder neck surgery.

b. Transurethral resection of prostate.

So retrograde ejaculation occurs in such patients.

It is absent in female.

Simple mucus-secreting glands lie in the tissue around the preprostatic urethra and surrounded by the preprostatic sphincter. These simple glands are similar to those in the female urethra and are unlike the glands of prostate.

Prostatic Part

3–4 cm in length. It tunnels through the substance of prostate closer to anterior than the posterior surface of gland. Emerging from the prostate slightly anterior to the apex (most inferior part), urethra turns inferiorly as it passes through the prostate making an angle of 35°.

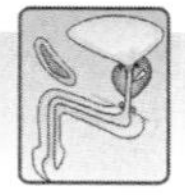

Throughout its length, the posterior wall has a midline ridge called as *urethral crest*. This crest projects into the lumen causing the lumen to appear crescentic in transverse section.

On each side of crest are shallow depression called *prostatic sinus*, the floor of which is perforated by orifices of 15–20 ducts prostatic ducts.

There is an elevation called *verumontanum* (colliculus seminalis) at about middle of urethral crest. It contains slit-like orifice of prostatic utricle.

On both side of or just within this orifice are the two small openings of the ejaculatory ducts (Fig. 30.11).

Prostatic utricle

It is a cul-de-sac 6 mm long, which runs upwards and backwards in the substance of prostate behind its median lobe. The walls are composed of fibrous tissue, muscle fibres and mucous membrane. The mucous membrane is pitted by the openings of numerous small glands. It develops from paramesonephric ducts or urogenital sinus and is thought to be homologous with the vagina of female.

So vagina masculine is also a name for this prostatic utricle.

Lowermost part of prostatic urethra is fixed by puboprostatic ligaments and is, therefore, immobile.

Membranous Part

It is 1.5 cm, shortest, least dilatable and with the exception of external orifice is the narrowest section of urethra. Descends with a slight ventral concavity from the prostate to bulb of penis, passing through the perineal membrane. 2.5 cm posteroinferior to pubic symphysis.

Wall of membranous urethra, i.e. part of external or distal urethral sphincter mechanism

Its muscle coat is separated from epithelium by narrow layer of fibroelastic connective tissue. Muscle coat consists of relatively thin layer of bundles of smooth muscle, which are continuous proximally with those of prostatic urethra and a prominent outer layer of the circularly oriented striated muscle fibres (rhabdosphincter) which form external urethral sphincter.

External sphincter represents points of highest intransurethral pressure in the normal, contracted state.

Intrinsic striated muscle is made of fibres of very small diameter, devoid of muscle spindles, physiologically being slow twitch type, unlike pelvic floor with heterogenous mixture of slow and fast twitch type of larger diameter. So slow twitch fibres of sphincter are capable of sustained contraction over long period of time and contribute to tone that closes the urethra and maintains urinary continence.

So several components of distal urethral sphincter mechanism are:

a. Urethral smooth muscle.
b. Urethral striated muscle (of rhabdosphincter). It is most important component as it is capable of sustained contractions.
c. Pubourethral part of levator ani, important to resist surges of intra-abdominal pressure (on coughing or exercise).

Anterior Part

Anterior or spongiosus part lies in corpus spongiosum and is 16 cm long when penis is flaccid. It extends from membranous urethra to external urethral orifice on glans penis. It starts below the perineal membrane at a point anterior to the lowest part of pubic symphysis (Fig. 30.11).

Part of anterior urethra which is surrounded by bulbospongiosus is called *bulbar urethra* and is wide part of urethra. Bulbourethral glands open in this section 2.5 cm below the perineal membrane.

From here, when penis is flaccid, urethra curves downwards as *penile urethra*. It is narrow and slit-like when empty and has diameter of 6 mm when passing urine. It is dilated at its termination within the glans penis and dilatation is called "navicular fossa".

External urethral orifice is the narrowest part of urethra and is a sagittal slit, 6 mm long, bounded on each side by a small labium.

Epithelium of urethra, particularly in bulbar and distal penile segment presents orifice of numerous small glands and follicles situated in the submucous tissue called *urethral glands*. It contains a number of small pit-like recesses, or lacunae of varying size whose orifice are directed forwards.

One lacuna larger than the rest is *lacuna magna* which is situated on the roof of navicular fossa.

CLINICAL ANATOMY

Traumatic to urethra injured by a fall-astride (or straddle) results in injury to penile urethra in the perineum (*see* Fig. 28.15).

Extravasation of urine occurs but is prevented from going:

a. Posteriorly as the perineal membrane and the membranous layer of superficial fascia are continuous with the fascia around superficial transverse perinei.
b. Laterally by ischial and pubic rami.
c. Above to lesser pelvis by intact perineal membrane. So, extravasated urine goes anteriorly into the loose connective tissue of scrotum and penis and then to anterior abdominal wall.

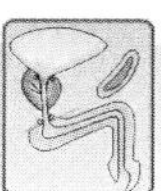

Arteries

1. Urethral artery arises from internal pudendal artery just below perineal membrane and travels through corpus spongiosum to reach glans penis.
2. Dorsal penile artery via circumflex branches on each side.

Veins

Anterior urethra → dorsal vein of penis → internal pudendal vein which drains into prostatic venous plexus → internal iliac veins.

Posterior urethra → prostatic and vesical venous plexus → internal iliac veins.

Lymphatic

1. Prostatic urethra → internal iliac.
2. Membranous urethra → internal iliac.
3. Anterior urethra → accompany that of glans → deep inguinal.

Innervation

Prostatic plexus supplies the smooth muscle of prostate and prostatic urethra. Greater cavernous nerves are sympathetic to preprostatic sphincter during ejaculation. Parasympathetic nerves are from 2nd–4th sacral segments.

Nerve supply of rhabdosphincter is controversial but is said to be by neurons in Onuf's nucleus situated in sacral 2 segment of spinal cord; fibres pass via perineal branch of pudendal nerve.

FEMALE URETHRA

Female urethra is only 4 cm long and 6 mm in diameter. It begins at the internal urethral orifice of bladder, approximately opposite middle of the pubic symphysis and runs anteroinferiorly behind the symphysis pubis, embedded in anterior wall of vagina. It crosses the perineal membrane and ends at external urethral orifice as an anteroposterior slit with rather prominent margins situated directly anterior to the opening of vagina and 2.5 cm behind glans clitoridis.

Except during passage of urine anterior and posterior wall of canal possesses a ridge which is termed urethral crest. Many small mucous urethral glands and minute pit-like recess or lacunae open into urethra. On each side, near the lower end of urethra, a number of these glands are grouped and open into a duct, named *paraurethral duct*.

Each paraurethral duct runs down in the submucous tissue and ends in a small aperture on the lateral margins of external urethral orifice.

Arteries

Superior vesical and vaginal arteries.

Veins

Venous plexus around urethra → vesical venous plexus → internal pudendal vein → internal iliac vein.

Lymphatic

Internal and external iliac nodes.

Innervation

Parasympathetic preganglionic fibres from 2nd–4th sacral segments of spinal cord. These run through pelvic splanchnic nerves and synapse in vesical venous plexus. Postganglionic fibres reach smooth muscles.

Somatic fibres from same segments (S2–S4) reach the striated muscles through pelvic splanchnic nerves that do not synapse in vesical plexus.

Sensory fibres in pelvic splanchnic nerves reach to 2nd–4th sacral segments of spinal cord. Postganglionic sympathetic fibres arise from plexus around the vaginal arteries.

WALLS OF URETHRA

Wall has outer muscle coat and inner mucosa that lines the lumen and is continuous with that of bladder.

Muscle coat: Outer sheath of striated muscle/external urethral sphincter or distal sphincter mechanism together with smooth muscle.

Female external urethral sphincter is anatomically separate from the adjacent periurethral striated muscle of the anterior pelvic floor, i.e. pubourethralis part of levator ani.

The sphincter form a sleeve which is thickest anteriorly in the middle one-third of urethra, and is relatively deficient posteriorly. The striated muscle extends into the anterior wall of both proximal and distal thirds of urethra, but is deficient posteriorly. Muscle cells forming external urethral sphincter are all small diameter slow twitch fibres.

Smooth muscle coat (inner) extends throughout the length of urethra. A few circularly arranged muscle fibres occur in the outer aspect of nonstriated muscle layer which are oblique or longitudinally oriented and these intermingle with striated muscle fibres forming inner parts of external urethral sphincter.

Proximally, the urethral smooth muscle extends as far as the neck of bladder where it is replaced by detrusor smooth muscle. But this region in the females ***lacks*** well-defined circular smooth muscle components comparable to the ***preprostatic sphincter*** of male. Women do not possess an internal urethral sphincter.

Distally, urethral smooth muscle terminate in subcutaneous adipose tissue around external urethral meatus.

Smooth muscle of female urethra receives an extensive presumptive cholinergic nerve supply, but few noradrenergic fibres.

In the absence of an anatomical sphincter, competence of female bladder neck and proximal urethra is unlikely to be totally dependent on smooth muscle activity and is probably related to support provided by ligamentous structures which surround them.

Longitudinal orientation and the innervation of muscles suggests that urethral smooth muscle in female is active during micturition and serves to shorten and widen urethral lumen.

MICTURITION

1 Initially the bladder fills without much rise in the intravesical pressure. This is due to adjustment of bladder tone.
2 When the quantity of urine exceeds 220 cc, the intravesical pressure rises. This stimulates sensory nerves and produces a desire to micturate. If this is neglected, rhythmic reflex contractions of the detrusor muscle start, which become more and more powerful as the quantity of urine increases. This gives a feeling of fullness of the bladder, which later on becomes painful. The voluntary holding of urine is due to contraction of the sphincter urethrae and of the perineal muscles, with coincident inhibition of the detrusor muscle.
3 Micturition is initiated by the following successive events.
   a. First there is relaxation of perineal muscles, except the distal urethral sphincter and contraction of the abdominal muscles.
   b. This is followed by firm contraction of the detrusor and relaxation of the proximal urethral sphincter mechanism.
   c. Lastly, distal urethral sphincter mechanism relaxes, and the flow of urine begins.
4 The bladder is emptied by the contraction of the detrusor muscle. Emptying is assisted by the contraction of abdominal muscles.
5 When urination is complete, the detrusor muscle relaxes, the proximal urethral sphincter mechanism contracts, and finally the distal urethral sphincter mechanism contracts. In the male, the last drops of urine are expelled from the bulbar portion of the urethra by contraction of the bulbospongiosus.

HISTOLOGY OF URINARY BLADDER

The epithelium of urinary bladder is of transitional variety. The luminal cells are well-defined dome shaped squamous cells with prominent nuclei. The middle layers are pear-shaped cells and the basal layer is of short columnar cells (Fig. 24.30). The muscle coat is admixture of longitudinal, circular and oblique layers. Outermost layer is the serous or adventitial coat.

DEVELOPMENT OF URINARY BLADDER AND URETHRA

Cloaca (Latin *sewer)* is divided by the *urorectal septum* into posterior *anorectal canal* and anterior *primitive urogenital sinus*. The cranial and largest part of primitive urogenital sinus called the *vesicourethral canal* forms most of the urinary bladder. It is connected with the *allantois*. The lumen of allantois gets obliterated to form *urachus* connecting the apex of the bladder to the umbilicus. This ligament is the *median umbilical ligament*. *Trigone* of bladder is formed by the absorption of *mesonephric ducts* and is mesodermal in origin. With time, the mesodermal lining is replaced by endodermal epithelium. So the epithelium is wholly endodermal, while muscles are of splanchnic origin.

1 Vesicourethral canal formed by endoderm forms the anterior wall of prostatic urethra above the opening of prostatic utricle.
2 Absorbed portions of the mesonephric ducts, i.e. mesoderm forms posterior wall of prostatic urethra above the opening of prostatic utricle.
3 Definitive urogenital sinus formed by endoderm forms the lower part of prostatic urethra and the membranous urethra.
4 Urethral plate or endoderm forms most of the anterior part of urethra.
5 Surface epithelium of glans penis or ectoderm forms the terminal portion of penile urethra.

CLINICAL ANATOMY

- *Catheterization of bladder:* In some cases, the patient is unable to pass urine leading to retention of urine. In such cases a rubber tube called a *catheter* is passed into the bladder through the urethra. While passing a catheter one has to remember the normal curvatures of the urethra. It has also to be remembered that the lacunae are directed forwards, and may intercept the point of the catheter (Fig. 30.13). Forceful insertion of instruments may create false passages in the urethra.
- *Rupture of urethra:* The urethra is commonly ruptured beneath the pubis by a fall astride a sharp object. This causes extravasation of urine (*see* Figs 28.15 and 28.16).
- Infection of the urethra is called *urethritis*.
- A constriction of the urethra is called *stricture* of the urethra. It is usually a result of infection.

- *Hypospadias* is a common anomaly in which the urethra opens on the undersurface of the penis or in the perineum.
- *Epispadias* is a rare condition in which the urethra opens on the dorsum of the penis. The condition is associated with ectopia vesicae and absence of infraumbilical part of anterior abdominal wall.

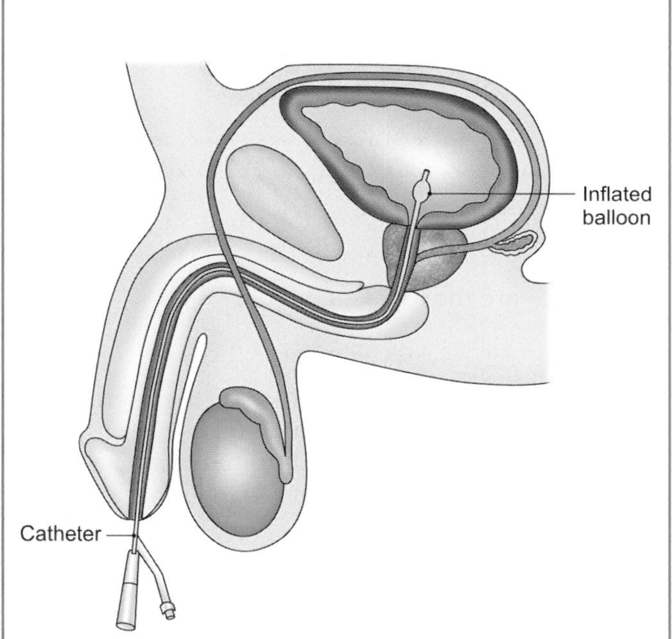

Fig. 30.13: Catheterisation of urinary bladder in male

FACTS TO REMEMBER

- Most fixed part of urinary bladder is the neck of bladder.
- Widest part of male urethra is prostatic part
- Least dilatable part of male urethra is the membranous part. Narrowest part of urethra is external urethral orifice.
- Prostatic utricle represents the vagina of female.
- Proximal urethral sphincter is lacking in the female.

CLINICOANATOMICAL PROBLEM

A female patient about 50 years suffered injuries in her pelvic region. X-ray showed fracture of pubic bones and catheterized urine specimen showed the presence of blood.

- What organ is most likely to be injured?
- Why is there blood in the urine specimen?
- Where would the extravasated urine go from the ruptured urinary bladder?

Ans: The organ ruptured is the urinary bladder. The pubic bones have also got fractured. As the bladder has ruptured few blood vessels are injured, making the urine red.

Urine would pass in the pelvic cavity and behind ascending and descending colons into the paracolic gutters. On percussion over descending colon, the note would be dull, When the patient is rolled to right side, urine escapes to right side and the note over the descending colon gets resonant.

MULTIPLE CHOICE QUESTIONS

1. Which of the following is true regarding the innervations of urinary bladder?
   a. Parasympathetic efferent fibres are motor to detrusor muscle
   b. Sympathetic nerves are sensory to sphincter urethrae
   c. Pudendal nerve innervates sphincter vesicae
   d. Awareness of distension of urinary bladder is mediated by lateral spinothalamic tract

2. Which of the following is the shortest part of urethra?
   a. Prostatic
   b. Membranous
   c. Perineal
   d. Penile

3. Capacity of urinary bladder is adult is about:
   a. 300 ml   b. 200 ml
   c. 500 ml   d. 1500 ml

4. Which of the following sphincters is missing in female?
   a. Rhabdosphincter
   b. Preprostatic sphincter
   c. Urethral smooth muscle
   d. Pubourethral part of levator ani

5. Urinary bladder develops from the following *except*:
   a. Vesico-urethral canal
   b. Absorption of mesonephric ducts
   c. Urachus
   d. Urethral plate

ANSWERS

1. a **2.** b **3.** a **4.** b **5.** d

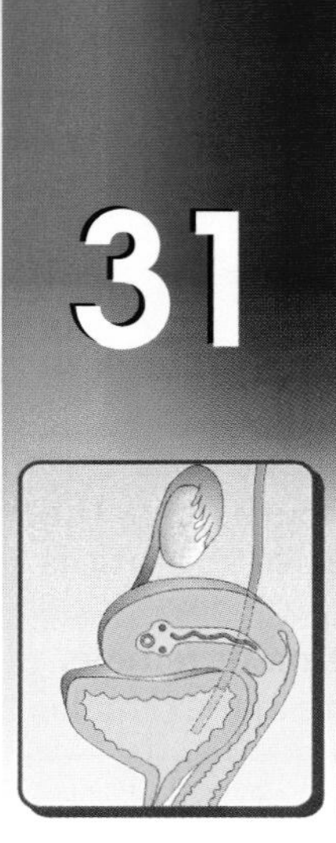

31 Female Reproductive Organs

No woman can call herself free who does not own and control her body.
No woman can call herself free until she can choose consciously whether she will or will not be a mother
—Margaret Sanger

INTRODUCTION

Female reproductive organs include external and internal genital organs. The external genital organs have been described in Chapter 28.

The internal genital organs comprise a pair of ovaries, a pair of uterine/fallopian tubes, single uterus and vagina. The ovaries are homologous to the testes of males but lie within the pelvis. The ovaries are much smaller than the testes.

INTERNAL GENITAL ORGANS

DISSECTION

Cut through the pubic symphysis with a knife in the median plane and extend the incision into the urethra. Make a median dorsal cut with a saw through the fourth and fifth lumbar vertebrae, the sacrum and coccyx to meet the knife. Cut through the soft tissues.

Separate the two halves of the pelvis and examine the cut surface of all the tissues.

Locate the ovary on the lateral wall of pelvis in the female cadaver. Identify the ovarian vessels in the infundibulopelvic ligament and trace these to the ovary and uterine tube. Follow, the ovarian artery till its anastomosis with the uterine artery.

Identify the uterus and follow the peritoneum on its superior and inferior surfaces which is thus free to move. Trace the uterus downwards till the supravaginal part of cervix which is attached to the lateral pelvic wall by transverse cervical ligaments and to the sacrum by uterosacral ligaments.

The vaginal part of cervix is surrounded on all sides by fornices of the vagina. The posterior fornix is the deepest. These can be felt by putting index and middle fingers through the vagina.

Identify the broad ligament attaching uterus to the lateral pelvic wall and note various structures present in its borders and surfaces.

OVARIES

The ovaries are the female gonads.

Situation

Each ovary lies in the ovarian fossa on the lateral pelvic wall. The ovarian fossa is bounded:

1 *Anteriorly* by the obliterated umbilical artery.
2 *Posteriorly* by the ureter and the internal iliac artery (Fig. 31.1).

Position

The position of the ovary is variable. In nulliparous women, its long axis is nearly vertical, so that the ovary is usually described as having an upper pole and a lower pole. However, in multiparous women, the long axis becomes horizontal; so that the upper pole points laterally and the lower pole medially (Figs 31.2a and b).

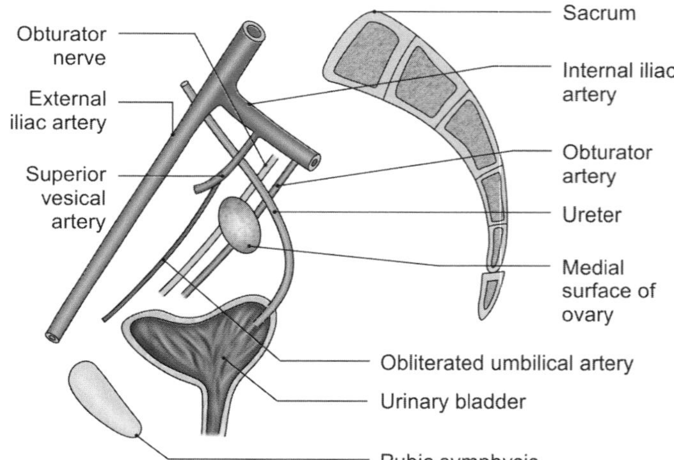

Fig. 31.1: Medial view of the boundaries of the ovarian fossa as seen in a sagittal section

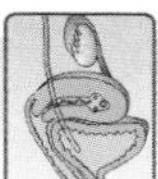

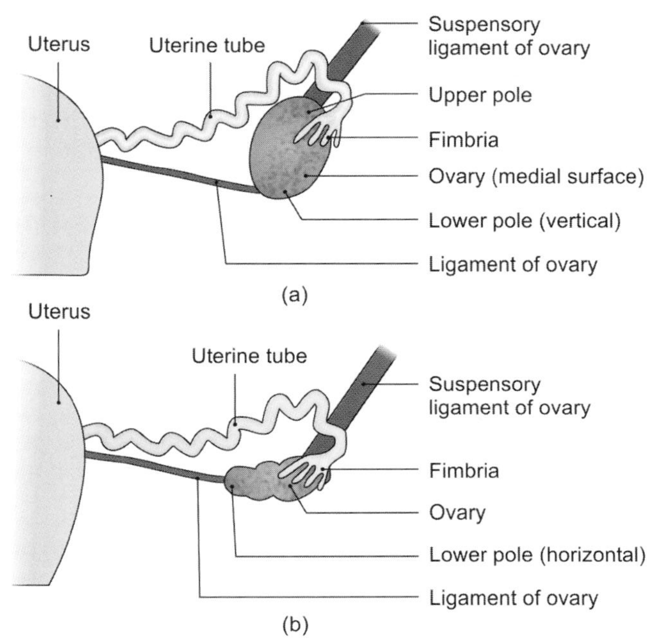

Figs 31.2a and b: Positions of the ovary. (a) It is vertical in nullipara, and (b) horizontal in multipara (after one or more deliveries) due to the pull by the pregnant uterus

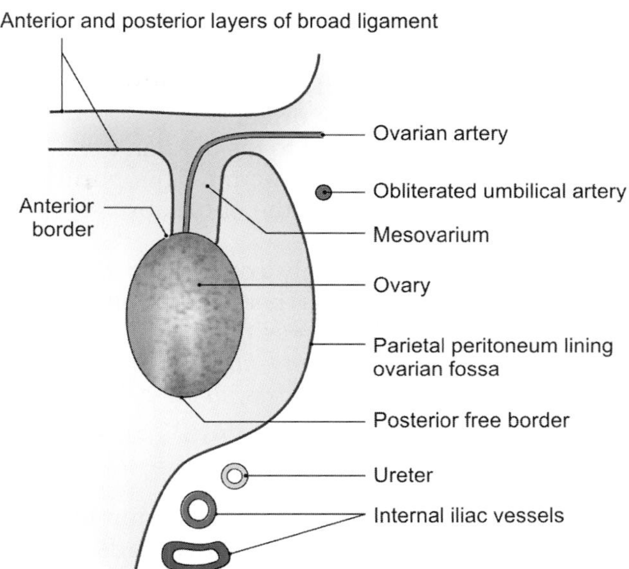

Fig. 31.3: Superior view of a horizontal section through the right ovarian fossa and the lateral part of the broad ligament

EXTERNAL FEATURES

In young girls, *before the onset of ovulation,* the ovaries have smooth surfaces which are greyish pink in colour. *After puberty,* the surface becomes uneven and the colour changes from pink to grey.

Each ovary has *two poles or extremities,* the upper or tubal pole, and the lower or uterine pole; *two borders,* the anterior or mesovarian border, and the posterior or free border; and *two surfaces,* lateral and medial.

Relations

Peritoneal Relations

The ovary is almost entirely covered with peritoneum, except along the mesovarian or anterior border where the two layers of the covering peritoneum are reflected on to the posterior layer of the broad ligament of the uterus. The ovary is connected to the posterior layer of the broad ligament by a short fold of peritoneum, called the *mesovarium* (Fig. 31.3). The squamous epithelium of the *mesovarium* is continuous with the cubical epithelium of the ovary. The mesovarium transmits the vessels and nerves to and from the ovary (*see* Fig. 18.21).

The lateral part of the broad ligament of uterus, extending from the infundibulum of the uterine tube and the upper pole of the ovary, to the external iliac vessels, forms a distinct fold known as *suspensory ligament of the ovary* or *infundibulopelvic ligament.* It contains the ovarian vessels and nerves (Fig. 31.4).

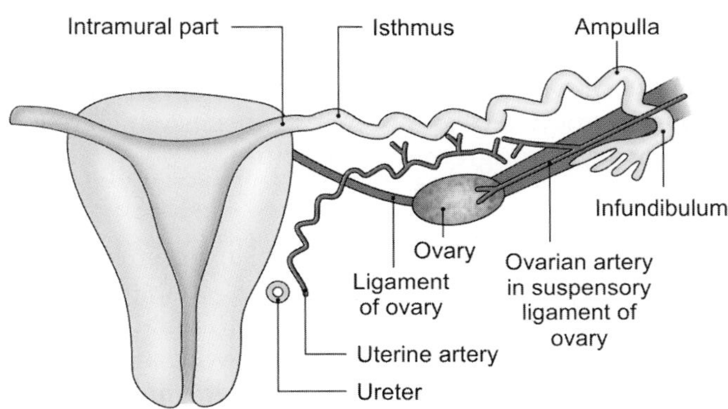

Fig. 31.4: The subdivisions, relations and blood supply of the uterine tube

Visceral Relations

1 *Upper or tubal pole:* It is broader than the lower pole, and is related to the uterine tube and the external iliac vein. The right ovary may be related to the appendix if the latter is pelvic in position. The ovarian fimbria and the suspensory ligament of the ovary are attached to the upper pole of the ovary (Fig. 31.2).
2 *Lower or uterine pole:* It is narrower than the upper pole and is related to the pelvic floor. It is connected, by the ligament of the ovary, to the lateral angle of the uterus, posteroinferior to the attachment of the uterine tube. The ligament lies between the two layers of the broad ligament of the uterus and contains some smooth muscle fibres (Fig. 31.2).
3 *Anterior or mesovarian border:* It is straight and is related to the uterine tube and the obliterated umbilical artery. It is attached to the back of the broad

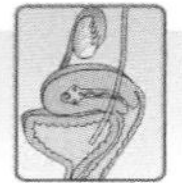

ligament of the uterus by the mesovarium, and forms the *hilus* of the ovary (Fig. 31.3).

4 *Posterior or free border:* It is convex and is related to the uterine tube and the ureter.
5 *Lateral surface:* It is related to the ovarian fossa which is lined by parietal peritoneum. This peritoneum separates the ovary from the obturator vessels and nerve (Fig. 31.1).
6 *Medial surface:* It is largely covered by the uterine tube. The peritoneal recess between the mesosalpinx and this surface is known as the *ovarian bursa*.

Only the lower pole and lateral surfaces are not related to utrine tube, remaining two borders, upper pole and medial surface are related to the tube.

Arterial Supply

1 The *ovarian artery* arises from the abdominal aorta just below the renal artery. It descends over the posterior abdominal wall and enters the suspensory ligament of the ovary. It sends branches to the ovary through the mesovarium, and continues medially through the broad ligament of the uterus to anastomose with the uterine artery (Fig. 31.4). In addition to ovary, the ovarian artery also supplies the uterine tube, the side of uterus and the ureter.
2 The uterine artery gives some branches which reach the ovary through the mesovarium.

Venous Drainage

The veins emerge at the hilus and form a pampiniform plexus around the artery. The plexus condenses into a single ovarian vein near the pelvic inlet. This vein ascends on the posterior abdominal wall and drains into the *inferior vena cava* on the right side and into the *left renal vein* on the left side.

Lymphatic Drainage

The lymphatics from the ovary communicate with the lymphatics from the uterine tube and fundus of the uterus. They ascend along the ovarian vessels to drain into the lateral aortic and preaortic nodes.

Nerve Supply

The ovarian plexus, derived from the renal, aortic and hypogastric plexuses, accompanies the ovarian artery. It contains both sympathetic and parasympathetic nerves. Sympathetic nerves (T10, T11) are afferent for pain as well as efferent or vasomotor. Parasympathetic nerves (S2, S3, S4) are vasodilator.

Functions

1 *Production of oocytes:* During reproductive life of about 30 years (from puberty to menopause), the ovaries produce alternately one secondary oocyte per month (per ovarian cycle of 28 days).

Liberation of oocyte from the ovary is called *ovulation*. It occurs on or about the 14th day of the 28-day menstrual cycle. Variations in the length of menstrual cycle are due to variations in the preovulatory phase; the postovulatory phase is constant.

An oocyte is viable (capable of being fertilized) for about 12–24 hours.

2 *Production of hormones:*
   a. *Oestrogen* is secreted by the follicular and paraluteal cells.
   b. *Progesterone* is secreted by the luteal cells.

HISTOLOGY

Histologically, the ovary is made up of the following parts from without inwards.

1 *Germinal epithelium* of cubical cells, derived from peritoneum.
2 *Tunica albuginea* is a thin layer of connective tissue.
3 The *cortex* contains *ovarian follicles* at various stages of development. Each follicle contains one oocyte. One follicle matures every month and sheds an oocyte. Total of 400 oocytes are ovulated in the reproductive life. After the oocyte is liberated the Graafian follicle is converted into a structure called the *corpus luteum*.
4 The hormone oestrogen is secreted by follicular cells of ovarian follicles. Another hormone, progesterone, is produced by the corpus luteum.
5 Medulla has rich vascular connective tissue, containing vessels, nerves and lymphatics.

CLINICAL ANATOMY

- *Determination of ovulation:* In cases of sterility, the ovulation can be determined by repeated ultrasonography.
- *Prolapse of ovaries:* Ovaries are frequently displaced to the pouch of Douglas where they can be palpated by a PV or per vaginal examination.
- *Ovarian cysts:* The developmental arrest of the ovarian follicles may result in the formation of one or more small ovarian cysts.

  Multiple small theca lutein cysts involve both the ovaries in cases with *Stein-Leventhal syndrome*. The syndrome is characterized by mild hirsutism, deep voice, secondary amenorrhoea, and cystic enlargement of both the ovaries.
- *Carcinoma of ovary* is common, and accounts for 15% of all cancers and 20% of gynaecological cancers.
- Ovaries are the commonest site in the abdomen for endometriosis. The endometrial cysts in the ovary are called the *chocolate cysts*.

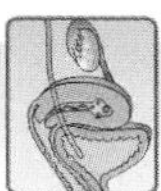

UTERINE TUBES

Synonym

The uterine tubes are also called *fallopian tubes/salpinx*.

Definition

They are tortuous ducts which convey oocyte from the ovary to the uterus. Spermatozoa introduced into the vagina pass up into the uterus, and from there into the uterine tubes. Fertilization usually takes place in the lateral part of the tube.

Situation

These are situated in the free upper margin of the broad ligament of uterus.

Dimensions

Each uterine tube is about 10 cm long. At the lateral end, the uterine tube opens into the peritoneal cavity through its *abdominal ostium*. This ostium is about 3 mm in diameter.

Subdivisions

1 The lateral end of the uterine tube is shaped like a funnel and is, therefore, called the *infundibulum*. It bears a number of finger-like processes called *fimbriae* and is, therefore, called the *fimbriated end*. One of the fimbriae is longer than the others and is attached to the tubal pole of the ovary. It is known as the *ovarian fimbria* (Fig. 31.2).
2 The part of the uterine tube medial to the infundibulum is called the *ampulla*. It is thin-walled, dilated and tortuous, and forms approximately the lateral two-thirds or 6 to 7 cm of the tube. It arches over the upper pole of the ovary. The ampulla is about 4 mm in diameter (Fig. 31.4). This is the site for fertilisation.
3 The *isthmus* succeeds the ampulla. It is narrow, rounded and cord-like. It forms approximately the medial one-third or 2 to 3 cm of the tube.
4 The *uterine* or *intramural* or *interstitial* part of the tube is about 1 cm long and lies within the wall of the uterus. It opens at the superior angle of the uterine cavity by a narrow *uterine ostium*. This ostium is about 1 mm in diameter.

Course and Relations

1 The isthmus and the adjoining part of the ampulla are directed posterolaterally in a horizontal plane. Near the lateral pelvic wall, the ampulla arches over the ovary and is related to its anterior and posterior borders, its upper pole and its medial surface. The infundibulum projects beyond the free margin of the broad ligament.
2 The uterine tube lies in the upper free margin of the broad ligament of the uterus. The part of the broad ligament between the attachment of the mesovarium and the uterine tube is known as the *mesosalpinx* (Fig. 31.5). It contains the termination of the uterine and ovarian vessels and the epoophoron.

Blood Supply

The *uterine artery* supplies approximately the medial two-thirds, and the ovarian artery supplies the lateral one-third, of the tube. The *veins* run parallel with the arteries and drain into the pampiniform plexus of the ovary and into the uterine veins (Fig. 31.4).

Lymphatic Drainage

Most of the tubal lymphatics join the lymphatics from the ovary and drain with them into the *lateral aortic* and *preaortic nodes*. The lymphatics from the isthmus accompany the round ligament of the uterus and drain into the *superficial inguinal nodes*.

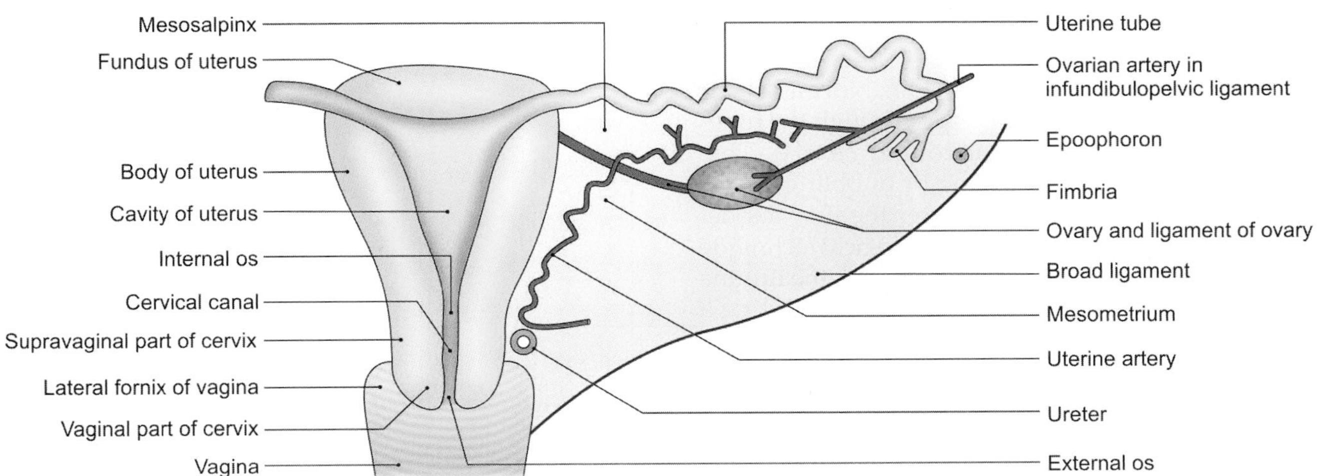

Fig. 31.5: Posterosuperior view of the uterus and the right broad ligament

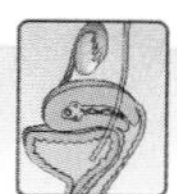

Nerve Supply

The uterine tubes are supplied by both the sympathetic and parasympathetic nerves running along the uterine and ovarian arteries.

1 The *sympathetic nerves* from T10 to L2 segments are derived from the hypogastric plexuses. They contain both visceral afferent and efferent fibres. The latter are vasomotor and perhaps stimulate tubal peristalsis. However, peristalsis is mainly under hormonal control.
2 *Parasympathetic nerves* are derived from the vagus for the lateral half of the tube and from the pelvic splanchnic nerves from S2, S3, S4 segments of spinal cord for the medial half. They inhibit peristalsis and produce vasodilatation.

HISTOLOGY

Uterine tube is made up of the following coats.

1 An outer *serous coat,* derived from peritoneum.
2 The middle *muscular coat,* which is thick in the isthmus and thin in the ampulla. The circular muscle coat is thickest in the isthmus and acts as a sphincter which delays the progress of the zygote towards the uterus until it is sufficiently mature for implantation.
3 The inner *mucous membrane,* which is lined by the ciliated columnar epithelium mixed with the non-ciliated secretory cells or peg cells. The mucous membrane is thrown into *complicated folds* which fill up the lumen of the tube. In the isthmus, there are only 3–6 primary folds and the cilia tend to disappear. But in the ampulla, the folds are more complex and exhibit the secondary and even tertiary folds.

CLINICAL ANATOMY

- *Salpingitis:* Inflammation of the uterine tube is called salpingitis (Salpinx=trumpet or tube).
- *Sterility:* Inability to have a child is called sterility. The most common cause of sterility in the female is tubal blockage which may be congenital, or caused by infection. Patency of the tube can be investigated by:
  a. *Insufflation test* or *Rubin's test*. Normally, air pushed into the uterus passes through the tubes and leaks into the peritoneal cavity. This leakage produces a hissing or bubbling sound which can be auscultated over the iliac fossae.
  b. *Hysterosalpingography* is a radiological technique by which the cavity of the uterus and the lumina of the tubes can be visualized, after injecting a radiopaque oily dye into the uterus (Fig. 31.6).
- *Tubal pregnancy*: Sometimes the fertilized ovum instead of reaching the uterus adheres to the walls of the uterine tube and starts developing there. This is known as *tubal pregnancy*. The enlarging embryo may lead to rupture of tube.
- *Tubectomy:* For purposes of family planning a woman can be sterilized by removing a segment of the uterine tube on both sides. This can be done by laparoscopy (Fig. 31.7) or through an incision in abdominal wall (Fig. 31.8).
- *Transport of ovum:* The transport of ovum is chiefly due to muscular contractions. The ciliary movements create an effective stream of lymph towards the uterus which assists in the nourishment of ovum in the lumen of the tube over the mucosal ridges.

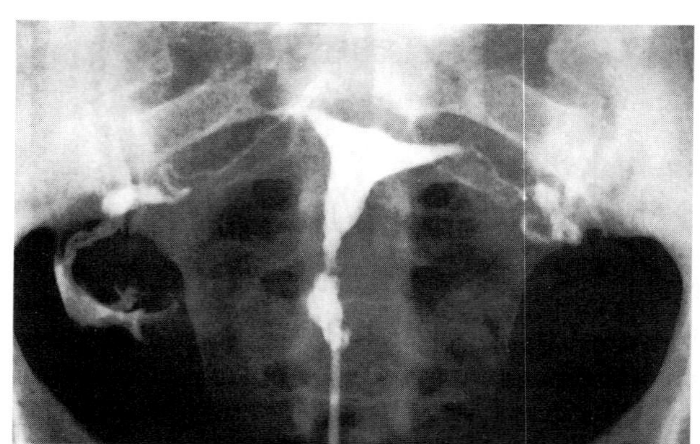

Fig. 31.6: Hysterosalpingogram

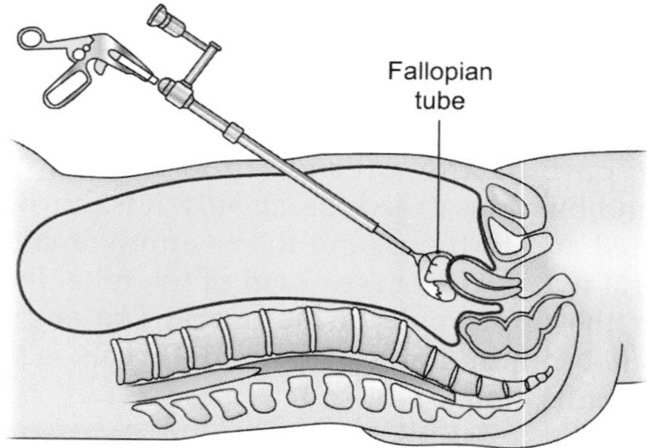

Fig. 31.7: Laparoscopic sterilisation

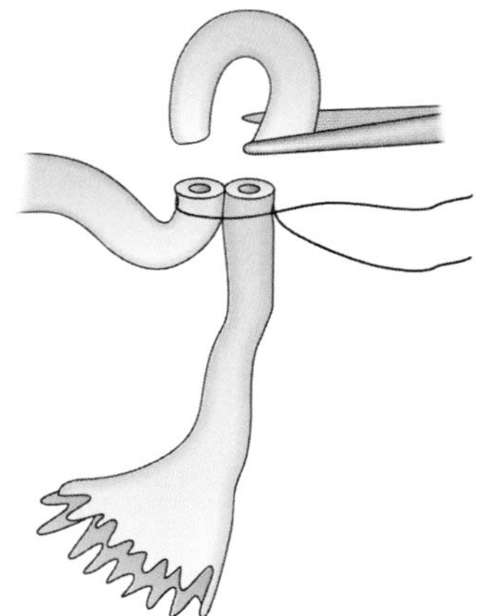

Fig. 31.8: Abdominal sterilisation

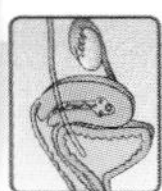

UTERUS

Synonym

In layman's language, the uterus is called the womb. It is also called *hystera*, on which word hysterectomy is based.

Definition

Uterus is a child-bearing organ in females, situated in the pelvis between bladder and rectum. Though hollow, it is thick walled and firm, and can be palpated bimanually during a PV (per vaginal) examination.

It is the organ which protects and provides nutrition to a fertilized ovum, enabling it to grow into a fully formed foetus. At the time of childbirth or parturition contractions of muscle in the wall of the organ result in expulsion of the foetus from the uterus.

Size and Shape

The uterus is pyriform in shape. It is about 7.5 cm long, 5 cm broad, and 2.5 cm thick. It weighs 30 to 40 grams. It is divisible into an upper expanded part called the *body* and a lower cylindrical part called the *cervix*. The junction of these two parts is marked by a circular constriction called the isthmus. Part of uterus above the opening of fallopian tube is called the fundus. The body forms the upper two-thirds of the organ, and the cervix forms the lower one-third.

The superolateral angle of the body project outwards at the junction of body and fundus and is called cornua of uterus. The uterine tube, ligament of ovary and round ligament are attached to it on each side.

Normal Position and Angulation

Normally, the long axis of the uterus forms an angle of about 90 degrees with the long axis of the vagina. The angle is open forwards. The forward tilting of the uterus relative to the vagina is called *anteversion*. The backward tilting of the uterus relative to vagina is known as *retroversion*. The uterus is also slightly flexed at the level of internal os of cervix; this is referred to as *anteflexion*. The angle of anteflexion is 125 degrees (Figs 31.9a to c).

Roughly, the long axis of the uterus corresponds to the axis of the pelvic inlet, and the axis of the vagina to the axis of the pelvic cavity and of the pelvic outlet (*see* Fig. 29.6).

It is normally deviated to right side and is called dextrorotation.

Communications

Superiorly, the uterus communicates on each side with the uterine tube, and inferiorly, with the vagina (Fig. 31.5).

Parts of Uterus

The uterus comprises:

1 A fundus,
2 Body with two surfaces, anterior or vesical and posterior or intestinal.
3 Two lateral borders.

The *fundus* is formed by the free upper end of the uterus. Fundus lies above the openings of the uterine tubes. It is convex like a dome. It is covered with peritoneum and is directed forward when the bladder is empty. The fertilized oocyte is usually implanted in the posterior wall of the fundus (Fig. 31.5).

The *anterior* or *vesical surface* of the body is flat and related to the urinary bladder. It is covered with peritoneum and forms the posterior or superior wall of the uterovesical pouch.

The *posterior* or *intestinal surface* is convex and is related to coils of the terminal ileum and to the sigmoid colon. It is covered with peritoneum and forms the anterior wall of the rectouterine pouch (*see* Figs 18.17b and 18.21).

Each *lateral border* is rounded and convex. It provides attachment to the broad ligament of the uterus which connects it to the lateral pelvic wall. The uterine tube opens into the uterus at the upper end of this border. This end of the border gives attachment to the round ligament of the uterus, anteroinferior to the tube; and to the ligament of the ovary posteroinferior to the tube. The uterine artery ascends along the lateral border of the uterus between the two layers of the broad ligament (Figs 31.10 and 31.11).

In sagittal section, the cavity of the body of the uterus is seen as a mere slit because the uterus is compressed anteroposteriorly. In coronal section, the cavity is seen to be triangular in shape, the apex being directed downwards. At the apex, the cavity becomes continuous with the canal of the cervix. The junction is called the *internal os*. The superolateral angles of the cavity receive the openings of the right and left uterine tubes (Fig. 31.5).

Cervix of Uterus

The cervix is the lower, cylindrical part of the uterus. It is less mobile than the body. It is about 2.5 cm long, and is slightly wider in the middle than at either end. The lower part of the cervix projects into the anterior wall of the vagina which divides it into supravaginal and vaginal parts.

The *supravaginal part of the cervix* is related:

a. Anteriorly to the bladder.
b. Posteriorly to the rectouterine pouch, containing coils of intestine and to the rectum (*see* Fig. 18.17b).
c. On each side, to the ureter and to the uterine artery, embedded in parametrium. The fibrofatty

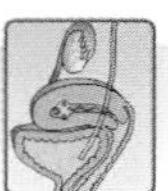

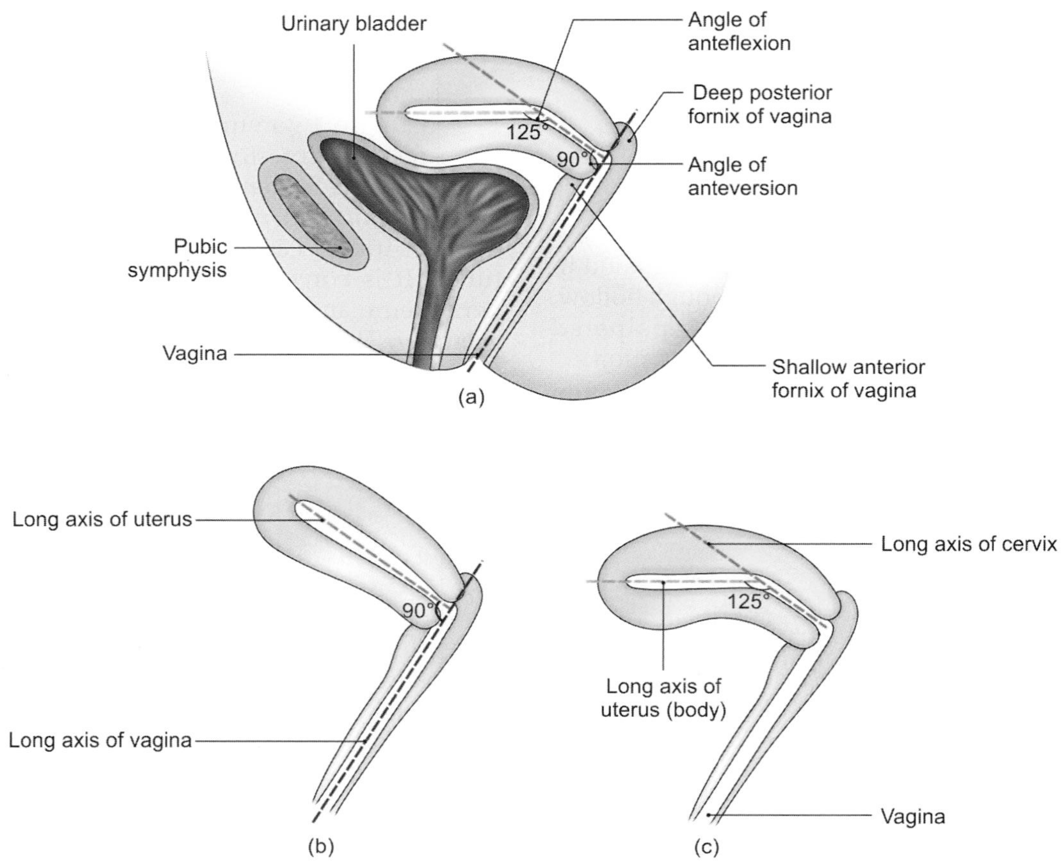

Figs 31.9a to c: (a) Angulations of the uterus and vagina, and their axes, (b) angle of anteversion, and (c) angle of anteflexion

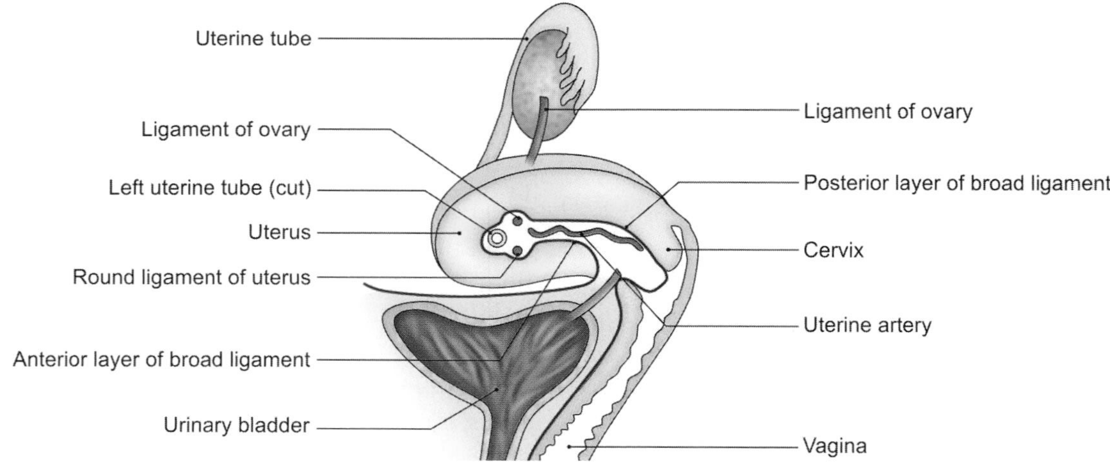

Fig. 31.10: Uterus, vagina and urinary bladder seen from the left side after removing the left broad ligament

tissue between the two layers of the broad ligament and below it, is called the *parametrium*. It is most abundant near the cervix and vagina (Fig. 31.10).

The *vaginal part* of the cervix projects into the anterior wall of the vagina. The spaces between it and the vaginal wall are called the *vaginal fornices*. The cervical canal opens into the vagina by an opening called the *external os*. In a nulliparous woman, i.e. a woman who has not borne children, the external os is small and circular (Fig. 31.5). However, in multiparous women, the external os is bounded by anterior and posterior lips, both of which are in contact with the posterior wall of the vagina.

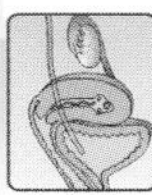

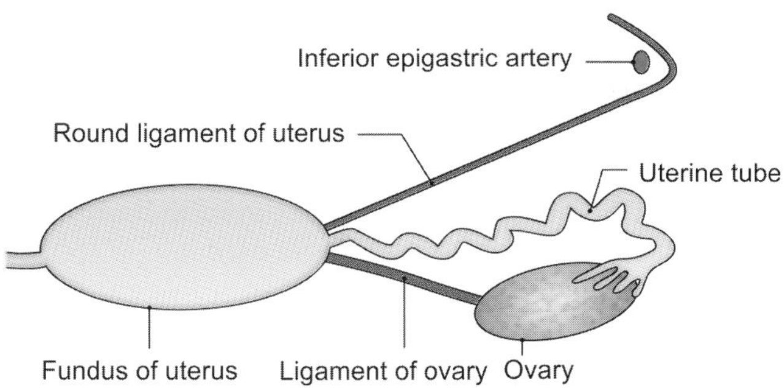

Fig. 31.11: Fundus of the uterus seen from above

The *cervical canal,* i.e. the cavity of the cervix is fusiform in shape. It communicates above with the cavity of the body of the uterus, through the *internal os,* and below with the vaginal cavity through the *external os.* The canal is flattened from before backwards so that it comes to have anterior and posterior walls. These walls show mucosal folds which resemble the branches of a tree called the *arbor vitae uteri.* The folds in the anterior and posterior walls interlock with each other and close the canal.

Ligaments of Uterus

Peritoneal Ligaments

These are mere peritoneal folds which do not provide any support to the uterus.

1 The *anterior ligament* consists of the uterovesical fold of peritoneum.
2 The *posterior ligament* consists of the rectovaginal fold of peritoneum (*see* Fig. 18.17).
3 The right and left *broad ligaments* are folds of peritoneum which attach the uterus to the lateral pelvic wall. When the bladder is full, the ligament has anterior and posterior surfaces, and upper, lower, medial and lateral borders. The upper border is free. The anterior and posterior layers of peritoneum forming the ligament become continuous here. The lateral and inferior borders of the ligament are attached to the corresponding parts of the pelvic wall. The medial border is attached to the lateral margin of the uterus (*see* Fig. 18.21).

The ovary is attached to the posterior layer of the broad ligament through the *mesovarium* (Fig. 31.3). The ligament of the ovary passes from the lower pole of the ovary to the lateral angle of the uterus. The part of the broad ligament lying between the uterine tube and the ligament of ovary is called the *mesosalpinx,* while the part below the ligament of ovary is called the *mesometrium.* The part of the broad ligament that stretches from the upper pole of the ovary and the infundibulum of the uterine tube to the lateral pelvic wall is called the *suspensory ligament of the ovary* or the *infundibulopelvic ligament* (Fig. 31.5).

The broad ligament contains the following structures.

1 The uterine tube (Figs 31.5 and 31.11).
2 The round ligament of the uterus.
3 The ligament of the ovary.
4 Uterine vessels near its attachment to the uterus (Fig. 31.4).
5 Ovarian vessels in the infundibulopelvic ligament.
6 The uterovaginal and ovarian nerve plexuses.
7 Epoophoron (Fig. 31.5).
8 Paroophoron.
9 Some lymph nodes and lymph vessels.
10 Dense connective tissue or parametrium present on the sides of the uterus.

Fibromuscular Ligaments

The fibromuscular ligaments are:

1 Round ligaments of the uterus.
2 Transverse cervical ligaments
3 Uterosacral ligaments.

These are described separately under the heading of "supports" of uterus.

Arterial Supply

The uterus is supplied:

1 Chiefly by the two uterine arteries which are markedly enlarged during pregnancy.
2 Partly by the ovarian arteries.

The *uterine artery* is a branch of the anterior division of the internal iliac artery. It first runs medially towards the cervix, crossing the ureter above the lateral fornix of the vagina and 2 cm lateral to the cervix. Then the artery ascends along the side of the uterus, with a tortuous course. Finally, it runs laterally towards the hilus of the ovary, and ends by anastomosing with the ovarian artery. The tortuosity of the artery without stretching the artery permits expansion of the uterus during pregnancy (Fig. 31.12). Apart from the uterus, the artery also gives branches to without stretching the artery.

a. Vagina.
b. Medial two-thirds of the uterine tube.
c. Ovary.
d. Ureter.
e. Structures present in the broad ligament (Fig. 31.5).

Venous Drainage

The veins form a plexus along the lateral border of the uterus. The plexus drains through the uterine, ovarian and vaginal veins into the internal iliac veins.

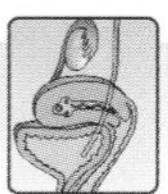

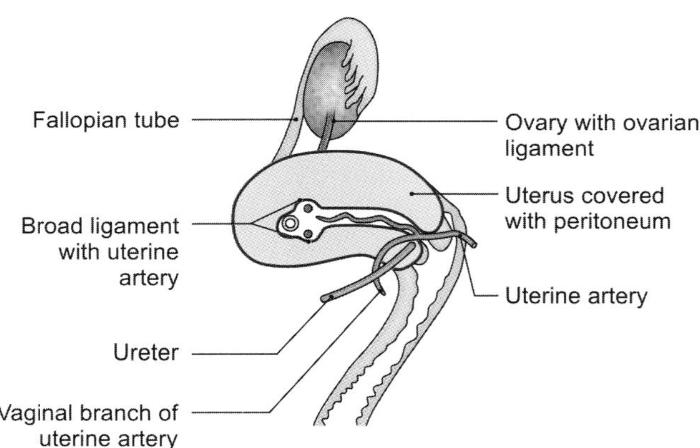

Fig. 31.12: Arterial supply of the uterus

Lymphatic Drainage

Lymphatics of the uterus begin at three intercommunicating networks, endometrial, myometrial and subperitoneal. These plexuses drain into lymphatics on the side of the uterus. Of these, the *upper lymphatics* from the fundus and upper part of the body drain mainly into the aortic nodes, and only partly to the superficial inguinal nodes along the round ligament of the uterus. The *lower lymphatics* from the cervix drain into the external iliac, internal iliac and sacral nodes. The *middle lymphatics* from the lower part of body drain into the external iliac nodes (Fig. 31.13).

Nerve Supply

The uterus is richly supplied by both sympathetic and parasympathetic nerves, through the inferior hypogastric and ovarian plexuses. Sympathetic nerves from T12, L1 segments of spinal cord produce uterine contraction and vasoconstriction. The parasympathetic nerves (S2, S3, S4) produce uterine inhibition and vasodilatation. However, these effects are complicated by the pronounced effects of hormones on the genital tract.

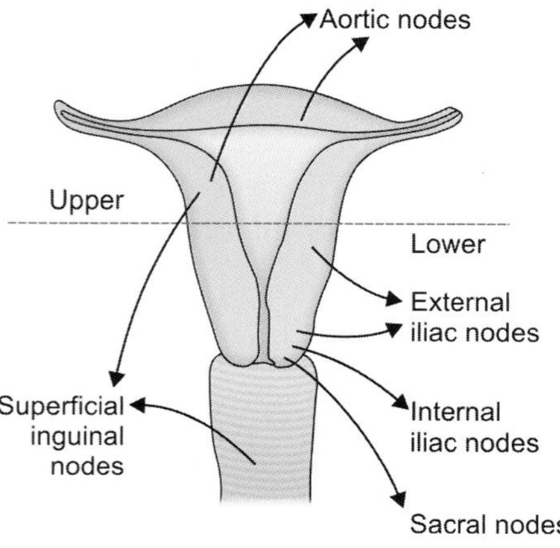

Fig. 31.13: Lymphatic drainage of uterus and vagina

Pain sensation from the body of the uterus pass along the sympathetic nerves, and from the cervix, along the parasympathetic nerves.

Age and Reproductive Changes

1 *In foetal life:* The cervix is larger than the body which projects a little above the pelvic brim.
2 *At puberty:* The uterus enlarges and descends to the adult position. The arbor vitae uteri also appear.
3 *During menstruation:* The uterus is slightly enlarged and becomes more vascular. The lips of the *external os* are swollen.
4 *During pregnancy:* The uterus is enormously enlarged, mainly due to hypertrophy of the smooth muscle fibres and partly due to hyperplasia. As pregnancy advances the uterine wall becomes progressively thinner. After parturition the uterus gradually involutes and returns almost to the nonpregnant size.
5 *In old age:* The uterus becomes atrophic and smaller in size and more dense in texture. The *internal os* is frequently obliterated. The lips of the *external os* disappear, and the *os* itself may be obliterated.

Supports of the Uterus

The uterus is a mobile organ which undergoes extensive changes in size and shape during the reproductive period of life. It is supported and prevented from sagging down by a number of factors which are chiefly muscular and fibromuscular.

Primary Supports

Muscular or active supports

1 Pelvic diaphragm.
2 Perineal body.
3 Distal urethral sphincter mechanism.

Fibromuscular or mechanical supports

1 Uterine axis.
2 Pubocervical ligaments.
3 Transverse cervical ligaments of Mackenrodt.
4 Uterosacral ligaments.
5 Round ligaments of uterus.

Secondary Supports

These are of doubtful value and are formed by peritoneal ligaments.

1 Broad ligaments (Fig. 31.5).
2 Vesicouterine pouch and fold of peritoneum.
3 Rectovaginal or rectouterine pouch and fold of peritoneum (*see* Fig. 18.17b).

Role of Individual Supports

Pelvic Diaphragm

The pelvic diaphragm (Fig. 31.14) supports the pelvic viscera and resists any rise in the intra-abdominal

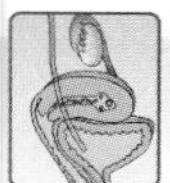

pressure. The pubococcygeus part of the levator ani is partly inserted into the perineal body between the vagina and the rectum. Some of these fibres also form a supporting sling and a sphincter for the vagina, and so indirectly for the uterus and the urinary bladder. If the pubococcygeus is torn during parturition, the support to the vagina is lost, and the latter tends to sink into the vestibule along with the uterus, thus causing *prolapse* of the uterus. The efficacy of the levator ani as a support is also lost when the perineal muscles are torn. They normally fix the perineal body, and make it an anchor for the levator ani (Fig. 31.14).

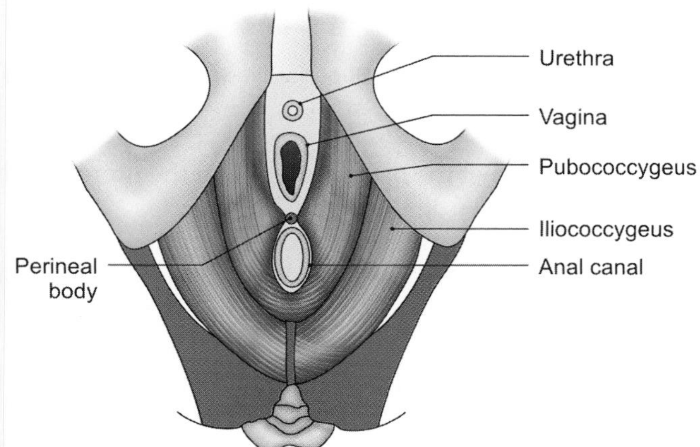

Fig. 31.14: Superior view of the pelvic diaphragm (the levator ani and coccygeus)

Perineal Body

It is a fibromuscular node to which ten muscles are attached. It acts as an anchor for the pelvic diaphragm, and thus maintains the integrity of the pelvic floor. The muscles are two superficial transversus perinei two deep transversus perinei, two pubococcygeus part of levator ani, two bulbospongiosus and single sphincter ani externus and unstriped fibres of longitudinal muscle coat of the anal canal (*see* Fig. 28.4).

Urethral Sphincter Mechanism

The urogenital diaphragm does not exist as sphincter urethrae is within the wall of the urethra. The urethral sphincter mechanism exists. In addition there is compressor urethrae and sphincter urethrae vaginalis. Since these are inserted into vagina, they support the uterus indirectly (*see* Fig. 28.20).

Uterine Axis

The anteverted position of the uterus itself prevents the organ from sagging down through the vagina. Any rise in intra-abdominal pressure tends to push the uterus against the bladder and pubic symphysis, which further accentuates anteversion. The angle of anteversion is

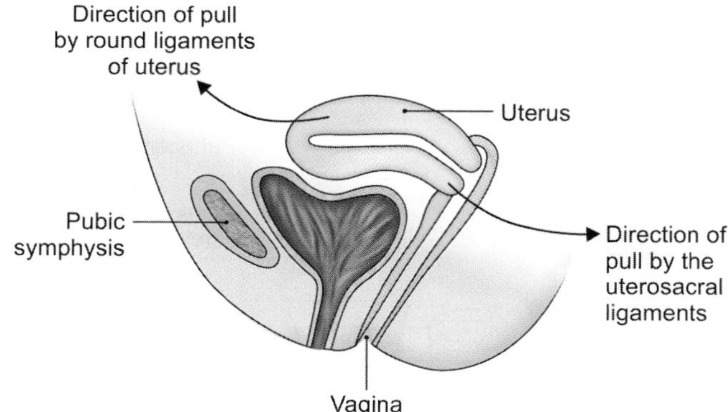

Fig. 31.15: Anteversion of the uterus is maintained by the couple of forces provided by the pull of the uterosacral ligament and the round ligament of the uterus

maintained by the uterosacral and round ligaments (Figs 31.9 and 31.15).

Pubocervical Ligaments

These ligaments connect the cervix to the posterior surface of pubis. They are derived from the endopelvic fascia, and correspond to the medial and lateral puboprostatic ligaments in the male (Fig. 31.16a).

Transverse Cervical Ligaments of Mackenrodt

These are also known by various other names like lateral cervical ligaments; cardinal ligaments; paracervical ligaments; retinacula uterine sustentaculum of Bonny (Figs 31.16b and 31.17).

These are fan shaped condensations of the endopelvic fascia on each side of the cervix above the levator ani and around the uterine vessels. They connect the lateral aspects of the cervix and of the upper vaginal wall to the lateral pelvic wall, about 2.5 cm ventral to the ischial spine. They form a 'hammock' that supports the uterus.

Uterosacral Ligaments

These are also condensations of the endopelvic fascia. They connect the cervix to the periosteum of the sacrum (S2, S3) and are enclosed within rectouterine folds of peritoneum (which form the lateral boundaries of the rectouterine pouch). The *uterosacral ligaments* keep the cervix braced backwards against the forward pull of the round *ligaments*. The two ligaments form a couple that maintains the uterine axis (Figs 31.16a and 31.18).

Round Ligaments of Uterus

The round ligaments are two fibromuscular flat bands, 10 to 12 cm long, which lie between the two layers of the broad ligament, anteroinferior to the uterine tube. Each ligament begins at the lateral angle of the uterus, runs forwards and laterally, passes through the deep

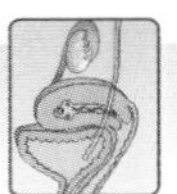

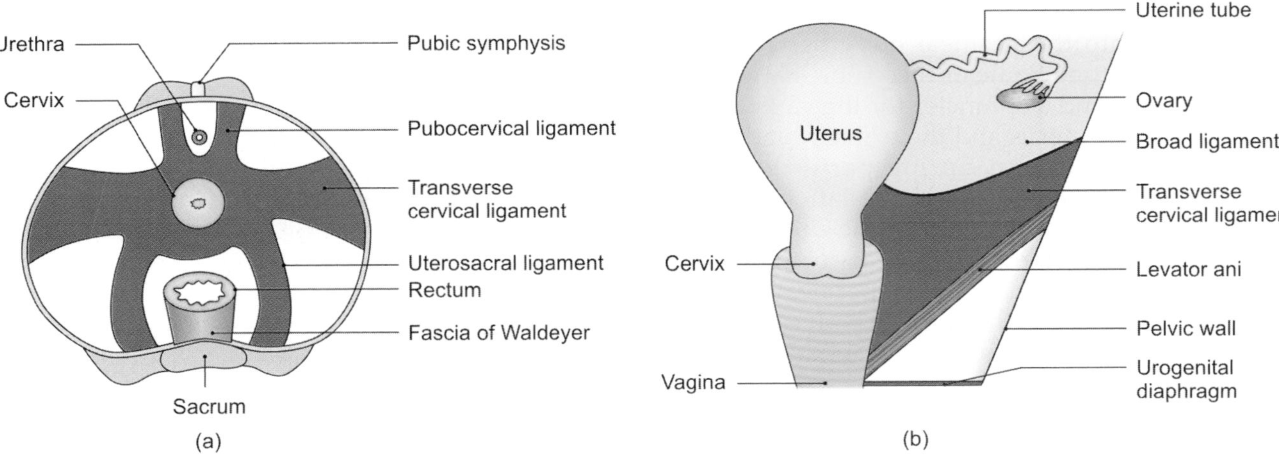

Figs 31.16a and b: Condensation of pelvic fascia forming the supports of the pelvic organs. (a) Superior view of the ligamentous supports of the uterus and rectum, (b) coronal view of the right cardinal ligament

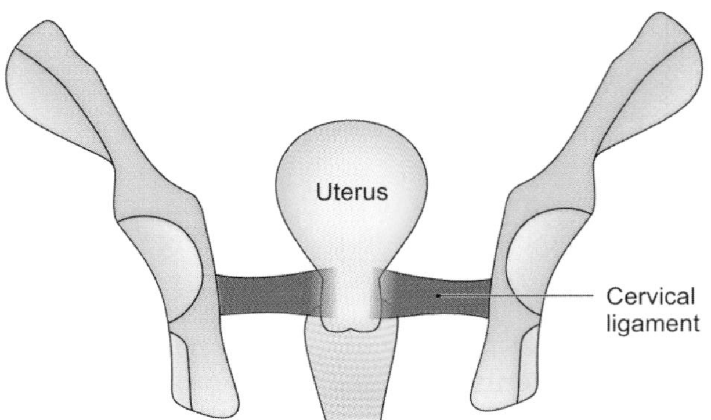

Fig. 31.17: Cervical ligaments supporting the uterus

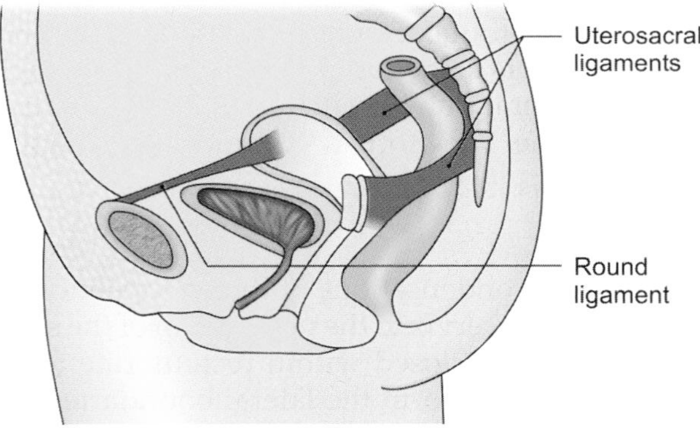

Fig. 31.18: Uterosacral and round ligaments supporting the uterus

inguinal ring, traverses the inguinal canal and merges with the areolar tissue of the labium majus after breaking up into thin filaments. In the inguinal canal, it is accompanied by a process of peritoneum during foetal life. If it persists after birth, it is known in females as the *canal of Nuck*. The round ligament keeps the fundus pulled forwards and maintains the angle of anteversion against the backward pull of the uterosacral ligaments (Figs 31.10, 31.11 and 31.15).

HISTOLOGY

The mucous membrane is called the endometrium, which undergoes cyclic changes in three phases in one menstrual cycle. There is no submucous coat.

Myometrium is thickest layer made of an outer and an inner longitudinal coats and middle thick circular coat with lots of arterioles.

The serous lining of peritoneum forms the outer covering.

Following are the three phases of endometrium.

1 *Proliferative phase:* The lining comprises simple columnar epithelium. Stroma contains simple tubular glands. Its deeper part contains sections of coiled arteries.
2 *Progestational phase:* The glands get sacculated and tortuous. The sections of coiled arteries are seen in the superficial part of thick endometrium.
3 *Menstrual phase:* This phase occurs due to decline of both the hormones. The endometrium becomes ischaemic and starts being shed. The vessel wall gets necrosed and blood enters the stroma and menstrual flow starts.

CLINICAL ANATOMY

- *Colpotomy and colporrhaphy:* Posterior colpotomy is done to drain the pus from the pouch of Douglas.
- Intrauterine contraceptive device is used to prevent implantation of fertilised oocyte (Fig. 31.19).
- Uterus is common site of formation of fibroids (Fig. 31.20).
- Perineal body is one of the chief supports of pelvic organs. Damage to the perineal body often leads to prolapse of the uterus and of other pelvic organs.

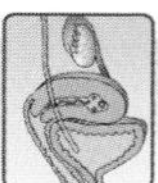

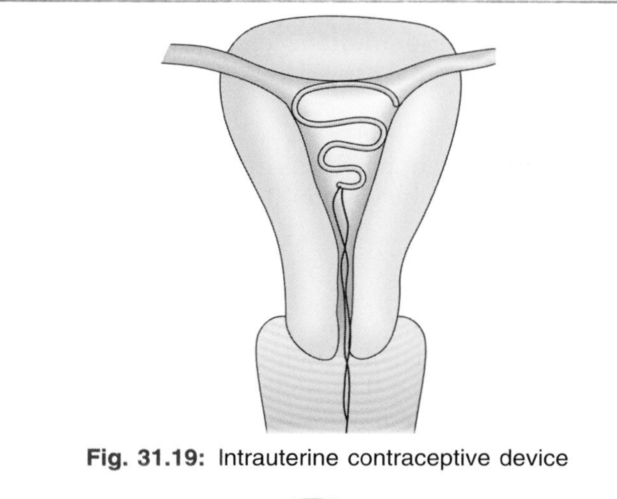

Fig. 31.19: Intrauterine contraceptive device

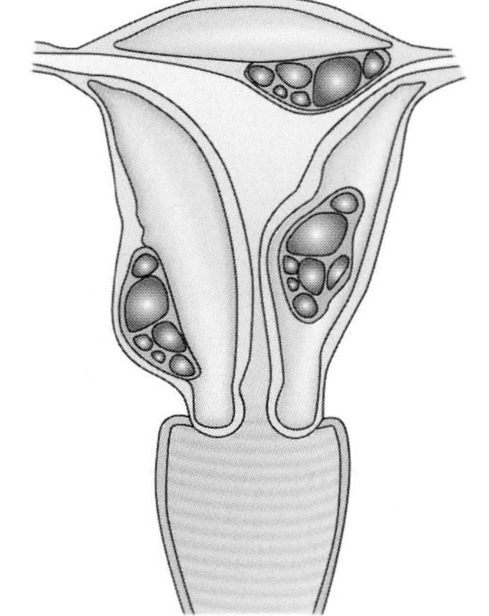

Fig. 31.20: Common sites of formation of fibroids

VAGINA

Synonym

Kolpos=Vagina (use of the terms colposcopy, colpotomy and colporrhaphy).

Definitions

The vagina is a fibromuscular canal, forming the female copulatory organ. The term 'vagina' means a sheath.

Extent and Situation

The vagina extends from the vulva to the uterus, and is situated behind the bladder and the urethra, and in front of the rectum and anal canal.

Direction

In the erect posture, the vagina is directed upwards and backwards. Long axis of uterus and cervix forms an angle of 90° with long axis of vagina (Figs 31.9b and 31.21).

Size and Shape

The anterior wall of the vagina is about 8 cm long and the posterior wall about 10 cm long.

The *diameter* of the vagina gradually increases from below upwards. The upper end or vault is roughly 5 cm twice the size of the lower end (2.5 cm). However, it is quite distensible and allows passage of the head of the foetus during delivery (Figs 31.5 and 31.10).

The *lumen* is circular at the upper end because of the protrusion of the cervix into it. Below the cervix, the anterior and posterior walls are in contact with each other, so that the lumen is a transverse slit in the middle part, and is H-shaped in the lower part.

In the virgin, the lower end of the vagina is partially closed by a thin annular fold of mucous membrane called the *hymen*. In married women the hymen is represented by rounded elevations around the vaginal orifice, the *caruncular hymenales*.

Fornices of Vagina

The interior of the upper end of the vagina or vaginal vault is in the form of a circular groove that surrounds the protruding cervix. The groove becomes progressively deeper from before backwards and is arbitrarily divided into four parts called the vaginal fornices. The *anterior fornix* lies in front of the cervix and is shallowest. The *posterior fornix* lies behind the cervix and is deepest. The *lateral fornices* lie one on each side of the cervix (Figs 31.5 and 31.9).

Relations

Anterior Wall

1 Upper half is related to the base of the bladder.
2 Lower half to the urethra (Fig. 31.21).

Posterior Wall

1 Upper one-fourth is separated from the rectum by the rectouterine pouch.
2 Middle two-fourths are separated from the rectum by loose connective tissue.
3 Lower one-fourth is separated from the anal canal by the perineal body and the muscles attached to it.

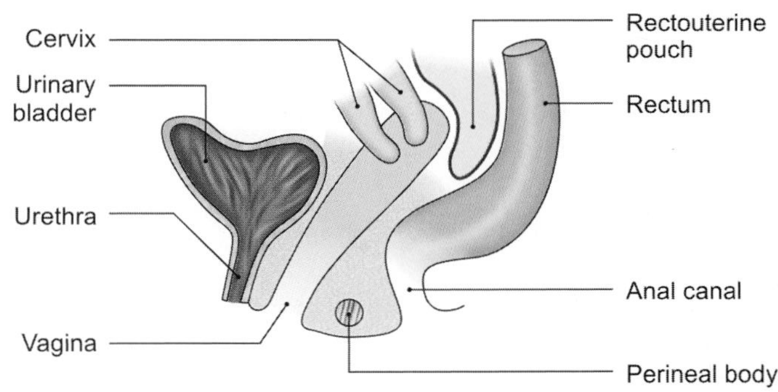

Fig. 31.21: Vagina and some related structures as seen in sagittal section

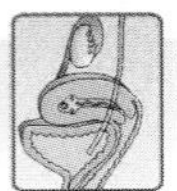

Lateral Walls

On each side:

1 Upper one-third is related to the transverse cervical ligament of pelvic fascia in which are embedded a network of vaginal veins, and the *ureter gets crossed by the uterine artery* (Fig. 31.22).
2 Middle one-third is related to the pubococcygeus part of the levator ani.
3 Lower one-third pierces the perineal membrane, below which it is related to the bulb of the vestibule, the bulbospongiosus and the duct of greater vestibular gland of Bartholin (*see* Figs 28.19, 31.22 and 31.23).

Arterial Supply

The vagina is a very vascular organ, and is supplied by the following arteries.

1 The main artery supplying it is the vaginal branch of the internal iliac artery.
2 In addition, the upper part is supplied by the cervicovaginal branch of the uterine artery (Fig. 31.23). The lower part is by the middle rectal and internal pudendal arteries.

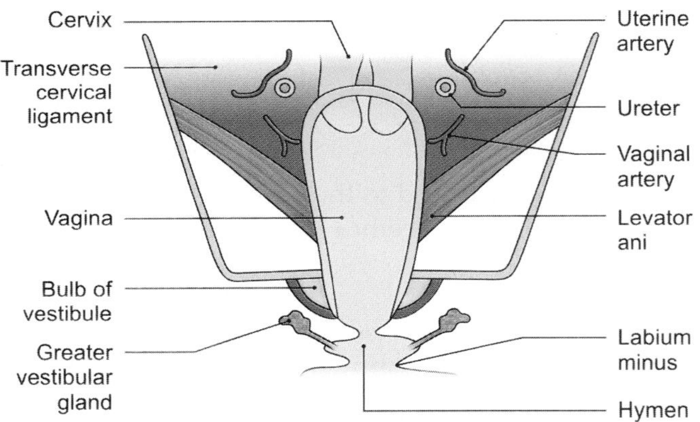

Fig. 31.22: Vagina and some related structures as seen in coronal section

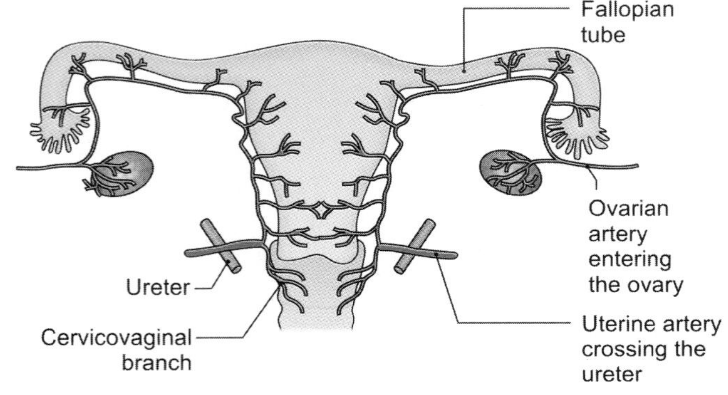

Fig. 31.23: Arterial supply of vagina and uterus by the uterine artery

Branches of these arteries anastomose to form anterior and posterior midline vessels called the *vaginal azygos arteries*.

Venous Drainage

The rich vaginal venous plexus drains into the internal iliac veins through the vaginal veins which accompany the vaginal arteries.

Lymphatic Drainage

Lymphatics from the upper one-third of the vagina drain into the external iliac nodes; from the middle one-third into the internal iliac nodes; and from the lower one-third into the medial group of superficial inguinal nodes.

Nerve Supply

1 The lower one-third of the vagina is pain sensitive and is supplied by the pudendal nerve through the inferior rectal and posterior labial branches of the perineal nerve.
2 The upper two-thirds of the vagina are pain insensitive and are supplied by sympathetic L1, L2 and parasympathetic segments S2 to S4. Nerves are derived from the inferior hypogastric and uterovaginal plexuses. Sympathetic nerves are vasoconstrictor and parasympathetic nerves vasodilator. The fibres which accompany the vaginal arteries form the vaginal nerves.

Ureter in Female Pelvis

As ureter lies anterior to internal iliac artery and immediately behind ovary it forms the posterior boundary of the ovarian fossa. It descends down till ischial spine. Then it courses anteromedially towards urinary bladder (Figs 31.1, 31.10, 31.12 and 31.23).

In its anteromedial part, ureter is related to the uterine artery, cervix and vaginal fornices. Ureter lies in endopelvic fascia in inferomedial part of broad ligament of uterus, where it may be damaged.

In the broad ligament, uterine artery is antero-superior to ureter by 2.5 cm and then crosses the ureter to ascend along lateral side of the uterus (Fig. 31.5).

Ureter runs forwards slightly above the lateral fornix of vagina and is 2 cm lateral to supravaginal part of cervix. It then turns medially towards urinary bladder and is apposed to vagina.

Left ureter to often more close to vagina, as uterus is slightly on the right side and vagina is on the left side of median plane.

One has to be careful of ureter, especially during ligation of the uterine artery. Ureter exhibits peristaltic movements with longitudinal plexus of blood vessels. It is pale glistening and is palpated as firm cord.

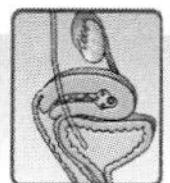

HISTOLOGY

1 Mucous membrane is lined by nonkeratinised stratified squamous epithelium.
2 Lamina propria is made up of loose connective tissue.
3 Muscle coat consists of an outer longitudinal and an inner circular layer.
4 The outer fibrous coat is the usual connective tissue.

There are no glands in the vaginal mucosa. It is kept moist by the cervical glands from above and the greater vestibular glands from below. The vaginal fluid is acidic in nature because of the fermentation of glycogen (in vaginal cells) by the Doderlein's bacilli.

CLINICAL ANATOMY

- *Vaginal Examination*
  a. *Inspection:* Vagina is first inspected at the introitus by separating the labia minora with the left hand. Next the speculum examination is done to inspect the cervix and vaginal vault, and to take the vaginal swab.
  b. *Palpation* of the pelvic organs can be done by a per vaginal (PV) digital examination (Fig. 31.24). With the examining fingers one can feel:
    - *Anteriorly,* the urethra, bladder and pubic symphysis;
    - *Posteriorly,* the rectum and pouch of Douglas;
    - *Laterally,* the ovary, tube, lateral pelvic wall, thickened ligaments, and ureters; and
    - *Superiorly,* the cervix.

  Bimanual (abdominovaginal) examination helps in the assessment of the size and position of the uterus, enlargements of the ovaries and tubes, and the other pelvic masses.
- *Vaginal lacerations:* Traumatic lacerations of vagina are common, and may be caused by forcible coitus (rape), during childbirth, or by accidents. This may give rise to profuse bleeding.
- Hymen is examined in medicolegal cases to confirm virginity.
- *Vaginitis:* It is common before puberty and after menopause because of the thin delicate epithelium. In adults, the resistant squamous epithelium prevents the infection. Vaginitis is commonly caused by the trichomonas, monilial and gonococcal infections. It causes leucorrhoea or white discharge.
- *Prolapse:* Prolapse of the anterior wall of vagina drags the bladder (cystocoele) and urethra (urethrocoele); the posterior wall drags the rectum (rectocoele).

  Weakness of supports of uterus can give rise to different degrees of prolapse.

  Similarly, trauma to the anterior and posterior walls of vagina can cause the vesicovaginal, urethrovaginal and rectovaginal fistulae.
- *Neoplasms:* Primary new growths of vagina, like the infections, are uncommon. However, secondary involvement of vagina by the cancer cervix is very common.
- Episiotomy is an incision given in posterolateral side of vagina to increase the size of outlet for the baby during delivery. The position of episiotomy incision during 2nd stage of labor is shown (*see* Fig. 29.9). Some muscles of superficial perineal space are incised.

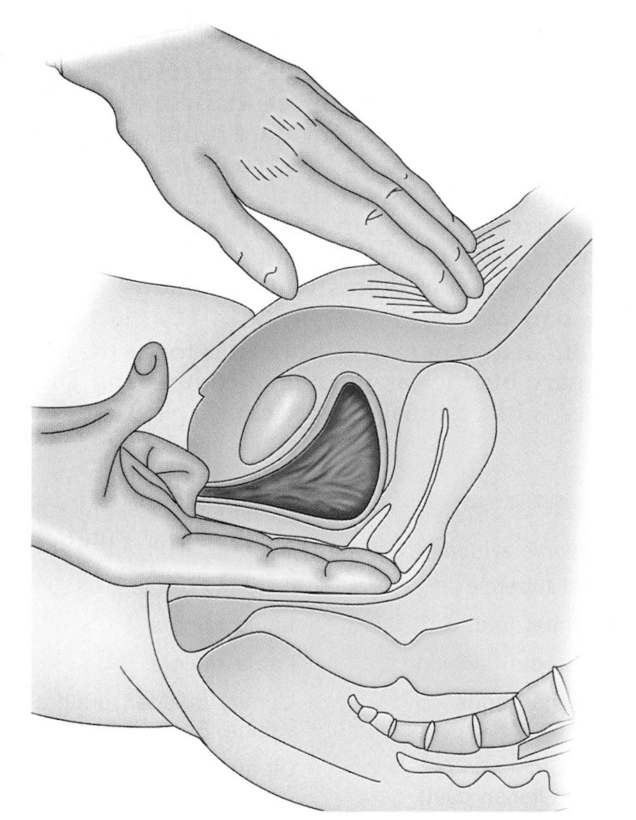

Fig. 31.24: Bimanual examination of the female internal genital organs

DEVELOPMENT

Female reproductive system comprises two ovaries and

1 Genital ducts
2 External genitalia

Ovary

Sex of the embryo is determined at the time of fertilization.

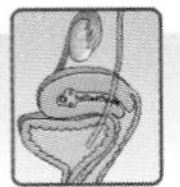

The chromosomal complement in female is 'XX'. Various components of ovary are germs cells, follicular cells and the stromal cells.

Germ cells get migrated from the dorsocaudal end of the yolk sac. Follicular cells are derived from the epithelial cells of the coelomic epithelium, while stromal cells are derived from mesoderm.

There is no tunica albuginea in the ovary and the *cortical part* of the gonad predominates.

Ovary descends down till the pelvis. Its descent is interrupted due to the presence of the single uterus, which divides the gubernaculum into ligament of ovary and round ligament of uterus.

Ducts

In female, müllerian or paramesonephric duct predominates. This duct is situated lateral to mesonephric duct. It opens caudally into definitive urogenital sinus. Müllerian duct proliferates due to presence of oestrogens and absence of testosterone and of mullerian inhibiting substance. Müllerian duct forms all four parts of fallopian tube. The distal part of the two ducts fuse to form the single uterovaginal canal which gives rise to uterus with its fundus, body and cervix parts.

Wolffian duct or mesonephric duct forms the trigone of urinary bladder as functional component. Duct of Gartner is its vestigial component (Table 31.1).

Mesonephric Tubules

These only form vestigial elements in female. These are epoophoron, paroophoron and aberrant ductules.

Epoophoron

It consists of 10 to 15 parallel tubules situated in the lateral part of the mesosalpinx between the ovary and the uterine tube. The tubules end in a longitudinal duct. These tubules represent cranial mesonephric tubules while the duct is a remnant of the mesonephric duct (Fig. 31.5).

Paroophoron

It consists of a few very short rudimentary tubules situated in the broad ligament between the ovary and uterus. These represent caudal mesonephric tubules which are not attached to the mesonephric duct.

Duct of Gartner

Occasionally, the duct of the epoophoron is much larger than usual and is called the *duct of Gartner*. It can be traced first along the uterine tube, and then along the lateral margin of the uterus up to the level of the *internal os*. Further down it runs through the cervix and the lateral wall of the vagina, and ends near the free margin of the hymen. It represents the mesonephric duct. It may form a cyst in the anterior or lateral wall of the vagina.

Table 31.1: Comparison between the derivatives of female and male urogenital structures

Embryonic structure	*Female*	*Male*
Genital tubercle	Clitoris	Penis
Urogenital folds	Labia minora	Ventral aspect of penis
Labioscrotal swelling	Labia majora	Scrotum
Urogenital sinus	Urinary bladder, urethral glands vagina, Bartholin's glands	Urinary bladder urethra its glands and prostate Bulbourethral glands
Paramesonephric duct (müllerian duct)	Uterus, cervix, fallopian tubes, upper part of vagina	Appendix of testis
Mesonephric duct (Wolfian duct)	Duct of Gartner Duct of epoophoron Trigone of urinary bladder	Epididymis, vas deferens Seminal vesicle Trigone of urinary bladder
Mesonephric tubules	Epoophoron Paroophoron	Efferent ductules Paradidymis
Gonad	Ovary secretes oestrogen and progesterone hormones	Testis secretes testosterone hormone
	Ovary is a pelvic organ	Testis descends outside the abdominal cavity as spermatogenesis requires 3 degree lower temperature
Gubernaculum	Ligament of ovary	Gubernaculum
	Round ligament of uterus	Testis
Mullerian tubercle	Hymen	Seminal colliculus

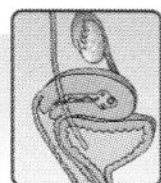

Vesicular Appendix

Occasionally, one or two pedunculated cysts are found attached to the fimbriated end of the uterine tube. These are called the *vesicular appendices* or *paramesonephric appendices*. These are believed to develop from the cranial end of the paramesonephric duct.

VAGINA

As the fused müllerian or paramesonephric ducts which form the uterovaginal canal open into the definitive urogenital sinus, the endoderm bulges to form the müllerian tubercle. Uterovaginal canal forms upper 1/3rd of vagina.

Endoderm on either side of müllerian tubercle proliferates to form two sinovaginal bulbs which fuse to form vaginal plate. The vaginal plate surrounds the caudal end of the uterovaginal canal.

Soon there is canalisation of the vaginal plate to form lower 2/3rd of vagina and vaginal fornices. It opens through an endodermal partial septum—the hymen in the definitive urogenital sinus.

EXTERNAL GENITALIA

Mesenchymal cells migrate around cloacal membrane to form cloacal folds. These folds fuse ventrally to form genital tubercle.

Cloacal folds get divided into urethral folds anteriorly and anal folds posteriorly. This occurs at the same time that the cloacal membrane gets divided into urogenital membrane and anal membrane.

Lateral to urethral folds another pair of folds, the genital swellings, make their appearance.

Genital tubercle forms clitoris; urethral folds form labia minora, genital swellings form labia majora, urogenital membrane gets ruptured to form the vestibule.

Mnemonics

Female pelvic organs "3 organs, each gets 2 blood supplies"

Vagina: Uterine, vaginal

Rectum: Middle rectal, inferior rectal (inferior rectal is the branch of pudendal)

Bladder in female: Superior vesical, vaginal

FACTS TO REMEMBER

- Cervix is the least movable part of uterus.
- Main ligamentous support of uterus is the transverse cervical ligament.
- Site of implantation of the blastocyst is posterior wall of fundus of uterus, close to its body.
- Uterine artery crosses ureter from lateral to medial side anteriorly to run tortuously along lateral surface of uterus.
- The epithelium of uterus is simple columnar type. The glands are simple, tubular. The submucous layer is absent. Tall columnar cells line the cervical canal.
- The cortex of the ovary is full of follicles. The medulla contains hilus cells, homologous to the interstitial cells of the testis.
- Pelvic part of the ureter about 13 cm long, lies close to the supravaginal part of the cervix. It is narrow at (i) where ureter crosses the brim of pelvis, (ii) where it is crossed by the uterine artery and (iii) in the intravesical part.
- Broad ligament has four parts: (i) infundibulo-pelvic ligament, (ii) mesovarium, (iii) mesosalpinx and (iv) mesometrium.
- Round ligament is 10–12 cm long with one end attached to uterine cornua and other to anterior third of labia majora.
- Before PV examination, the urinary bladder must be emptied.
- Forced penetration of penis into vagina is known as "rape". It is a punishable crime.
- Caesarean section is the delivery of the baby by cutting open the anterior abdominal wall and the uterus.

CLINICOANATOMICAL PROBLEM

Due to repeated child births, a female felt something out at the perineum, especially while standing.

- What organ descends down?
- Name the supports of the organ?

Ans: The organ which descends down is the uterus. It occurs due to repeated childbirths. Normally the organ is supported by number of muscles and ligaments. These may get weakened and stretched and thus are unable to support uterus. So uterus descends down through vagina. Its supports are:

Muscular: All parts of levator ani, perineal body with its attached muscles and distal urethral sphincter mechanism.

Ligaments: Transverse cervical ligament, uterosacral ligament, these are true supports

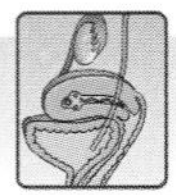

MULTIPLE CHOICE QUESTIONS

1. Normal position of uterus is:
   a. Anteverted and anteflexed
   b. Retroverted and retroflexed
   c. Anteverted and retroflexed
   d. Retroverted and anteflexed
2. Cervix is supplied by which of the following nerves?
   a. Pudendal
   b. Pelvic splanchnic nerve
   c. Sacral
   d. Lumbar 5, Sacral 1
3. Which of the following is not a content of broad ligament?
   a. Cervix
   b. Uterine tube
   c. Ligament of the ovary
   d. Round ligament
4. Uterine artery is a branch of which artery?
   a. External iliac
   b. Internal iliac
   c. Abdominal aorta
   d. Common iliac
5. Following are the muscular supports of uterus *except*:
   a. Pelvic diaphragm
   b. Perineal body
   c. Proximal urethral sphincter mechanism
   d. Distal urethral sphincter mechanism

ANSWERS

1. a **2.** b **3.** a **4.** b **5.** c

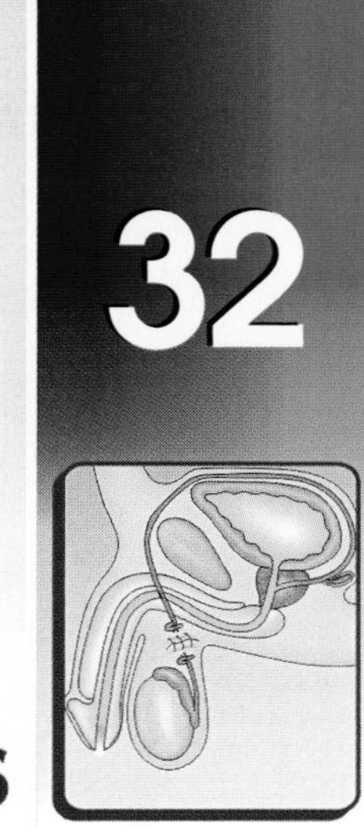

32 Male Reproductive Organs

There is no medicine like hope, no incentive so great, and no tonic so powerful as expectation of something tomorrow
—O S Mardern

INTRODUCTION

The male reproductive organs include the external and internal genitalia. The external genitalia are the penis and the scrotum containing testis, epididymis and part of ductus deferens. The internal genitalia on each side are, the part of ductus deferens, the seminal vesicle, the ejaculatory ducts, and the prostate.

The external genitalia have been described in Chapter 17, and the male urethra in Chapter 30. The remaining structures are considered below.

MALE REPRODUCTIVE ORGANS

DISSECTION

The ductus deferens has been seen till the deep inguinal ring in the anterior abdominal wall. Follow it from there as it hooks round the lateral side of inferior epigastric artery to pass backwards and medially across the external iliac vessels to enter into the lesser pelvis. There it crosses the ureter and lies on the posterior surface of urinary bladder medial to the seminal vesicle (Fig. 32.2). Separate the ductus from the adjacent seminal vesicle and trace these till the base of the prostate gland (*refer* to).

Follow the deep dorsal vein of the penis and its two divisions into the prostatic venous plexus situated in the angle between the bladder and the prostate.

Feel the thickened puboprostatic ligaments. Feel the firm prostate lying just at the neck of the urinary bladder.

Identify the levator prostatae muscle lying inferolateral to the prostate. This is identifiable by pulling both the bladder and prostate medially. The first part of urethra traverses the prostate. Cut through the anterior one-third of the gland to expose the prostatic urethra.

DUCTUS DEFERENS

Synonyms

The *ductus deferens* is also called the *vas deferens* or the *deferent duct*.

Definition

The ductus deferens is a thick-walled, muscular tube which transmits spermatozoa from the epididymis to the ejaculatory duct (Fig. 32.1). It feels cord-like at the upper lateral part of scrotum. Ductus deferens has a narrow lumen except at the terminal dilated part called the ampulla (Fig. 32.2).

Length

The ductus deferens is about 45 cm long when straightened.

Location and Course

In its course, the vas lies successively:

1 Within the scrotum along the posterior border of the testis.
2 In the inguinal canal as part of the spermatic cord (Fig. 32.1).
3 In the greater pelvis.
4 In the lesser pelvis.

Course and Relations

1 The ductus deferens begins as a continuation of the tail of the epididymis (Fig. 32.1).
2 *Along the posterior border of the testis:* At first it is very tortuous, but gradually straightens as it ascends along the posterior border of the testis, medial to the epididymis.
3 *In the spermatic cord:* The ductus deferens lies vertically in posterior part of spermatic cord. It runs upwards to the superficial inguinal ring, and then traverses the

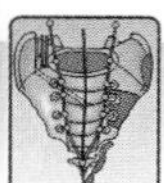

2 *Middle rectal vein:* The tributaries of this vein drain, chiefly, the muscular walls of the rectal ampulla, and open into the internal iliac veins (Fig. 33.6).
3 *Median sacral vein:* It joins left common iliac vein.

Lymphatic Drainage

1 Lymphatics from more than the *upper half* of the rectum pass along the superior rectal vessels to the inferior mesenteric nodes after passing through the pararectal and sigmoid nodes (Fig. 33.7).
2 Lymphatics from the *lower half* of the rectum pass along the middle rectal vessels to the internal iliac nodes.
3 Lymphatics from the lower part of anal canal drain into superficial inguinal nodes.

Nerve Supply

The rectum is supplied by both sympathetic (L1, L2) and parasympathetic (S2, S3, S4) nerves through the superior rectal or inferior mesenteric and inferior hypogastric plexuses.

Sympathetic nerves are vasoconstrictor, inhibitory to the rectal musculature and motor to the internal sphincter. Parasympathetic nerves are motor to the musculature of the rectum and inhibitory to the internal sphincter.

Sensations of distension of the rectum pass through the parasympathetic nerves, while pain sensations are carried by both the sympathetic and parasympathetic nerves.

Supports of Rectum

1 Pelvic floor formed by levator ani muscles (*see* Fig. 31.14).
2 *Fascia of Waldeyer:* It attaches the lower part of the rectal ampulla to the sacrum. It is formed by condensation of the pelvic fascia behind the rectum. It encloses the superior rectal vessels and lymphatics.
3 *Lateral ligaments of the rectum:* They are formed by condensation of the pelvic fascia on each side of the rectum. They enclose the middle rectal vessels, and branches of the pelvic plexuses, and attach the rectum to the posterolateral walls of the lesser pelvis.
4 *Rectovesical fascia of Denonvilliers:* It extends from the rectum behind to the seminal vesicles and prostate in front (*see* Fig. 32.3).
5 The *pelvic peritoneum* and the related *vascular pedicles* also help in keeping the rectum in position (Fig. 33.3).
6 Perineal body with its muscles (*see* Fig. 28.4).

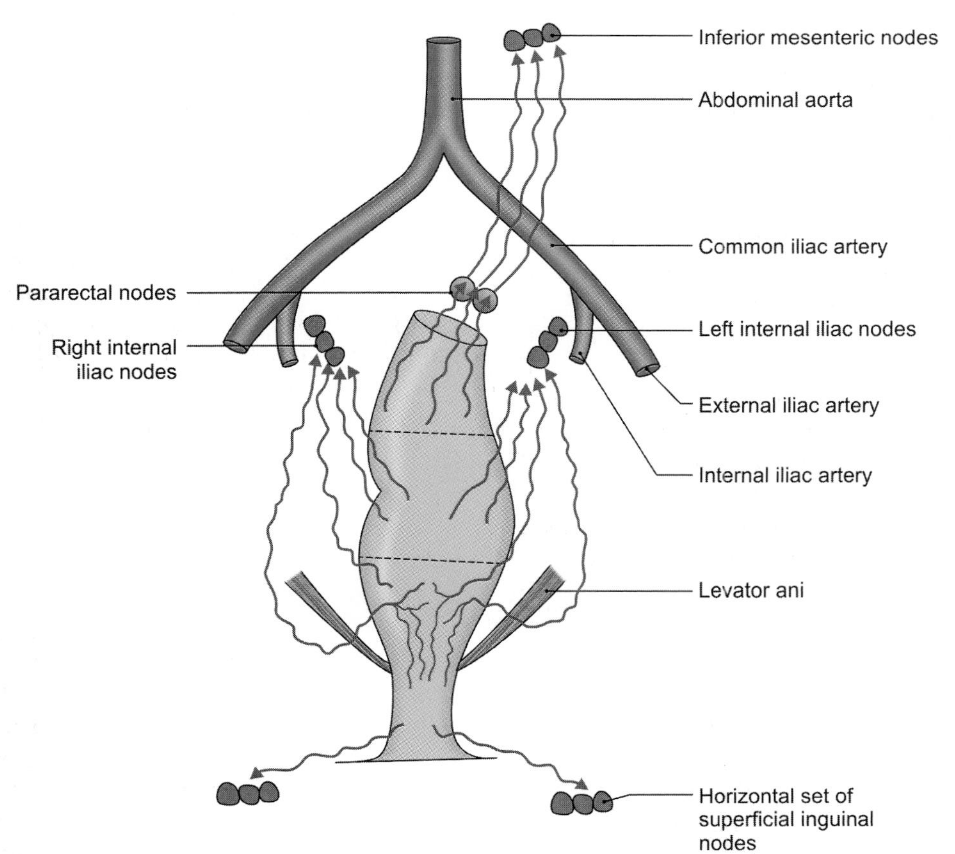

Fig. 33.7: Lymph drainage of rectum and anal canal

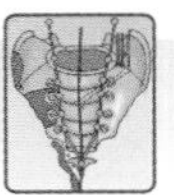

CLINICAL ANATOMY

- Digital per rectum (PR) examination: In PR examination the finger enters anal canal before reaching lower end of rectum.
  In a normal person, the following structures can be palpated by a finger passed per rectum.
  In males (Fig. 33.8):
  1. Posterior surface of prostate.
  2. Seminal vesicles.
  3. Vas deferens.

  In females (Fig. 33.9):
  1. Perineal body.
  2. Cervix.
  3. Presenting part of the foetus during delivery.

  In both sexes:
  1. Anorectal ring.
  2. Coccyx and sacrum.
  3. Ischioanal fossae and ischial spines.

  In patients, a PR examination can help in the palpation of following abnormalities.
  a. Within the lumen: Faecal impaction and foreign bodies, bleeding piles or haemorrhoids.
  b. In the rectal wall: Rectal growths and strictures, and thrombosed piles.
  c. Outside the rectal wall: In males, the enlargements of prostate, seminal vesicles and bulbourethral glands, and stone in membranous urethra; in females, enlargements of uterus, tubes and ovaries, and abnormalities in the pouch of Douglas; and in both sexes, the distended bladder, lower ureteric stones, and tumours of the bony pelvis.

  During parturition the dilatation of cervix is commonly assessed through the rectal wall to avoid infection by repeated vaginal examinations (Fig. 33.9).
- *Proctoscopy and sigmoidoscopy:* The interior of the rectum and anal canal can be examined under direct vision with special instruments, like a proctoscope or a sigmoidoscope. Proctoscopy shows internal piles and growths in lower part of rectum. Sigmoidoscopy helps in revealing the ulcers, growths and diverticula, and in taking a rectal biopsy.
- *Prolapse of rectum: Incomplete* or *mucosal prolapse* of the rectum through the anus may occur following violent straining. This is due to imperfect support of the rectal mucosa by the submucosa which is made up of loose areolar tissue.
  Complete prolapse or *procidentia* is the condition in which the whole thickness of the rectal wall protrudes through the anus. The contributory factors in its causation are:
  a. Laxity of the pelvic floor.
  b. Excessively deep rectovesical or rectouterine pouch.
  c. Inadequate fixation of the rectum in its presacral bed.
- *Neurological disturbances of the rectum:* In spite of the identical innervation of the rectum and bladder, the rectal involvement in nervous lesions is less severe than that of the bladder.
  After sacral denervation of the rectum the peripheral nervous plexus controls the automatic evacuation of the rectum. This reflex activity is more massive and complete when sacral innervation is intact, e.g. complete cord lesion above the sacral region. However, due to weak musculature of the rectum and sparing of the tone of the external sphincter by transverse lesions of the cord, rectal disturbances tend to cause constipation, although complete lesions may cause reflex defaecation.
- *Carcinoma of rectum:* It is quite common, and is generally situated at the rectosigmoid junction (constricting type), or in the ampulla (proliferating type). It causes bleeding per rectum from an indurated raised ulcer. The condition is surgically treated by an abdominoperineal excision in which the anus, anal canal and rectum with their fascial sheaths, and a varying amount of distal colon along with its mesocolon containing the lymph nodes are removed en bloc, and a permanent colostomy in the left iliac fossa is done with the proximal cut end of the colon.
- *Rectal continence:* Rectal continence depends solely on the anorectal ring. Damage to the ring results in rectal incontinence. The surgeon has to carefully protect the anorectal ring in operating on the region.

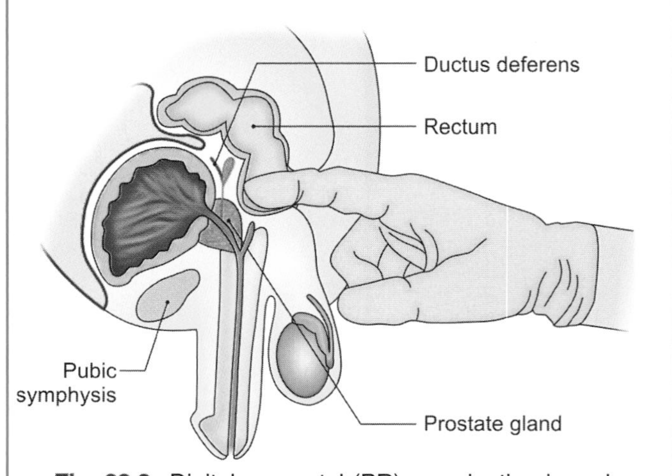

Fig. 33.8: Digital per rectal (PR) examination in male

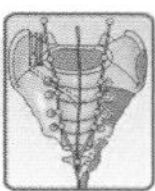

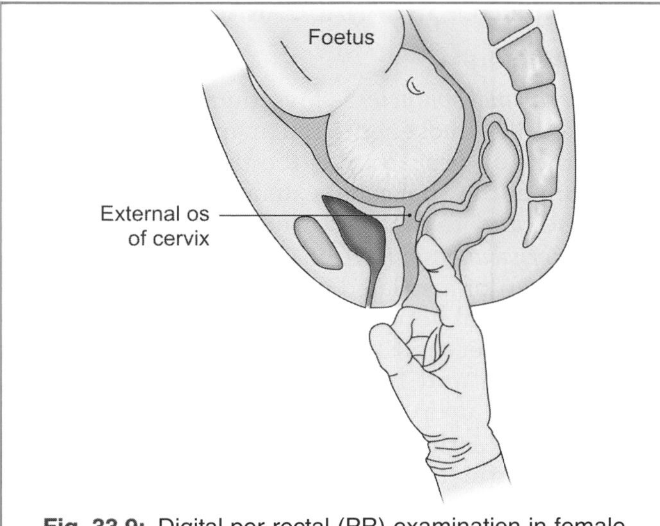

Fig. 33.9: Digital per rectal (PR) examination in female

ANAL CANAL

DISSECTION

Identify the relations of the anal canal in both male and female. Examine the lining of the anal canal. Strip the mucous membrane and skin from a sector of the anal canal. Identify the thickened part of the circular muscle layer forming the internal sphincter of the anus. Locate the external anal sphincter with its parts, partly overlapping the internal sphincter. The anal canal is the terminal part of the large intestine.

Introduction

Anal canal is the terminal part of gastrointestinal tract and is situated below the level of the pelvic diaphragm. It lies in the anal triangle of perineum in between the right and left ischioanal fossae, which allows its expansion during passage of the faeces. The sacculations and taeniae are absent here also.

Length, Extent and Direction

The anal canal is 3.8 cm long. It extends from the anorectal junction to the anus. It is directed downwards and backwards. The anal canal is surrounded by inner involuntary and outer voluntary sphincters which keep the lumen closed in the form of an anteroposterior slit.

The *anorectal junction* is marked by the forward convexity of the perineal flexure of the rectum (Fig. 33.2) and lies 2–3 cm in front of and slightly below the tip of the coccyx. Here the ampulla of the rectum suddenly narrows and pierces the pelvic diaphragm. In males it corresponds to the level of the apex of the prostate.

The *anus* is the surface opening of the anal canal, situated about 4 cm below and in front of the tip of the coccyx in the cleft between the two buttocks. The surrounding skin is pigmented and thrown into radiating folds, and contains a ring of large apocrine glands.

RELATIONS OF THE ANAL CANAL

Anteriorly

1 *In both sexes:* Perineal body.
2 *In males:* Membranous urethra and bulb of penis.
3 *In females:* Lower end of the vagina (*see* Fig. 31.21).

Posteriorly

1 Anococcygeal ligament.
2 Tip of the coccyx (*see* Fig. 28.6).

Laterally: Ischioanal fossae (*see* Fig. 28.6).

All-round: Anal canal is surrounded by the sphincter muscles, the tone of which keeps the canal closed.

INTERIOR OF THE ANAL CANAL

The interior of the anal canal shows many important features and can be divided into three parts: the upper part about 15 mm long; the middle part about 15 mm long; and the lower part about 8 mm long. Each part is lined by a characteristic epithelium and reacts differently to various diseases of this region (Fig. 33.10).

Upper Mucous Part

1 This part is about 15 mm long. It is lined by mucous membrane, and is of endodermal origin.
2 The mucous membrane shows:
   a. 6 to 10 vertical folds; these folds are called the *anal columns* of Morgagni.
   b. The lower ends of the anal columns are united to each other by short transverse folds of mucous membrane; these folds are called the *anal valves*.
   c. Above each valve there is a depression in the mucosa which is called the *anal sinus*.
   d. The anal valves together form a transverse line that runs all-round the anal canal. This is the

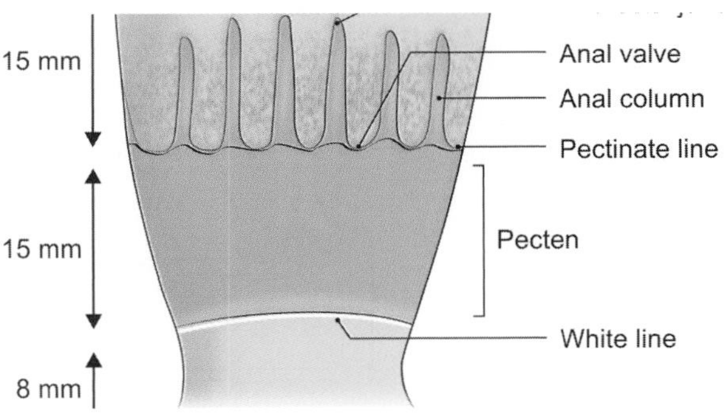

Fig. 33.10: Interior of the anal canal

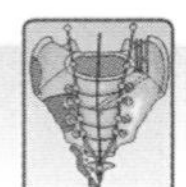

pectinate line. It is situated opposite the middle of internal anal sphincter, the junction of ectodermal and endodermal parts. Occasionally the anal valves show epithelial projections called *anal papillae*. These papillae are remnants of the embryonic anal membrane (Fig. 33.11).

e. The anal sinus contains anal glands. The secretion of these glands produce peculiar small which is important in lower animals to attract.

Middle Part or Transitional Zone or Pecten

1 The next 15 mm or so of the anal canal is also lined by mucous membrane, but anal columns are not present here. The mucosa has a bluish appearance because of a dense venous plexus that lies between it and the muscle coat. The mucosa is less mobile than in the upper part of the anal canal. This region is referred to as the *pecten* or *transitional zone*. The lower limit of the pecten often has a whitish appearance because of which it is referred to as the *white line of Hilton*. Hilton's line is situated at the level of the interval between the subcutaneous part of external anal sphincter and the lower border of internal anal sphincter.

2 It marks the lower limit of pecten or stratified squamous epithelium which is thin, pale and glossy and is devoid of sweat glands.

Lower Cutaneous Part

It is about 8 mm long and is lined by true skin containing sebaceous glands. The epithelium of the lowest part resembles that of pigmented skin in which sebaceous glands, sweat glands and hair are present.

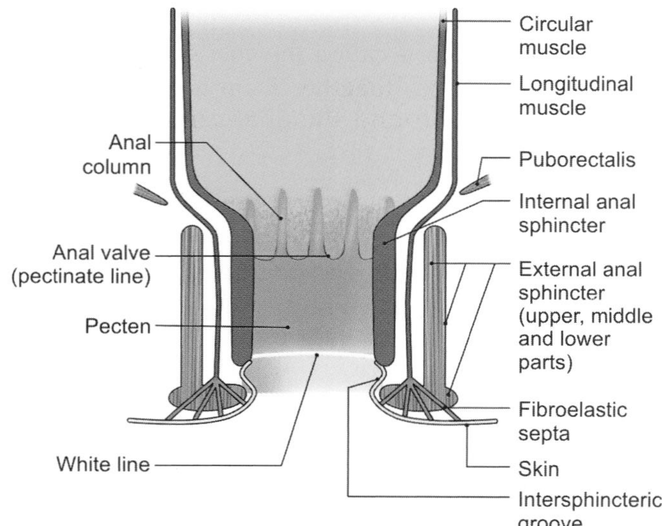

Fig. 33.11: Coronal section through the wall of the anal canal

MUSCULATURE OF THE ANAL CANAL

Anal Sphincters

The *internal anal sphincter* is involuntary in nature. It is formed by the thickened circular muscle coat of this part of the gut. It surrounds the upper three-fourths, i.e. 30 mm of the anal canal extending from the upper end of the canal to the white line of Hilton.

The *external anal sphincter* is under voluntary control. It is made up of a striated muscle and is supplied by the inferior rectal nerve and the perineal branch of the fourth sacral nerve. It surrounds the whole length of the anal canal and has three parts, subcutaneous, superficial and deep.

Contrary to earlier view, the external anal sphincter forms a single functional and anatomic entity. Uppermost fibres blend with fibres of puborectalis. Anteriorly some fibres decussate with superficial transverse perinei muscle and posterior fibres get attached to anococcygeal raphe (Fig. 33.12a).

Middle fibres surround lower part of internal anal sphincter. These are attached to perineal body anteriorly and to coccyx via anococcygeal ligament posteriorly. Some fibres of each side decussate to form a commissure in the midline.

Lower fibres lie below the level of internal anal sphincter and are separated from anal epithelium by submucosa.

In males transverse perinei and bulbospongiosus end in central point of perineum, so that there is a surgical plane of cleavage between urogenital triangle and anal canal.

In females, the puborectalis is separate from external anal sphincter. Its anterior portion is thinner and shorter (Fig. 33.12b).

In addition, in females, transverse perinei and bulbospongiosus fuse with external anal sphincter in lower part of perineum.

Conjoint Longitudinal Coat

It is formed by fusion of the puborectalis with the longitudinal muscle coat of the rectum at the anorectal junction. It lies between the external and internal sphincters. When traced downwards it becomes fibroelastic and at the level of the white line it breaks up into a number of fibroelastic septa which spread out fan wise, pierce the subcutaneous part of the external sphincter, and are attached to the skin around the anus called as corrugator cutis ani. The most lateral of these septa forms the perianal fascia. The most medial septum forms, the *anal intermuscular septum*, which is attached to the white line. In addition, some strands pass obliquely through the internal sphincter and end in the submucosa below the anal valves (Fig. 33.11).

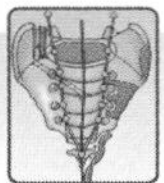

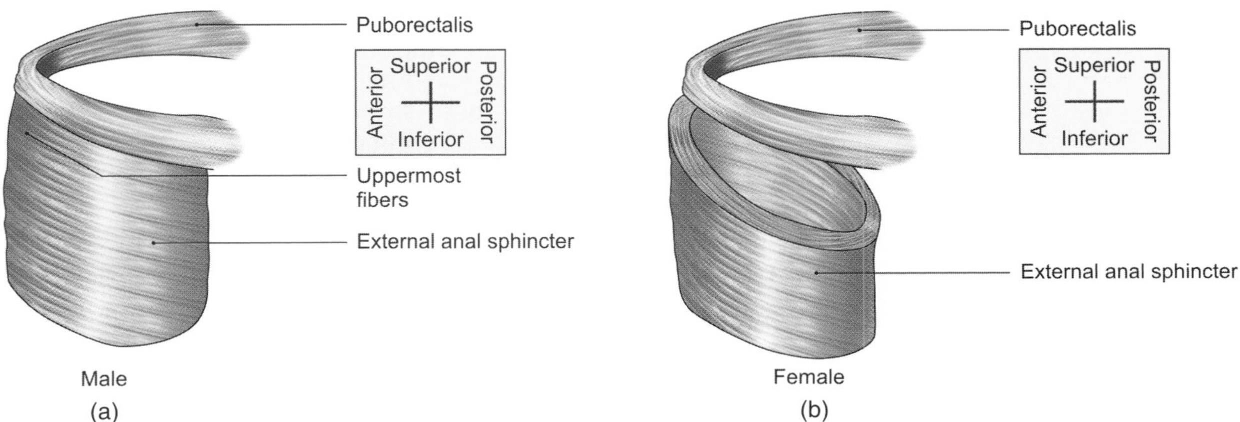

Figs 33.12a and b: Relation of puborectalis and external anal sphincter (a) in male, and (b) in female

Anorectal Ring

This is a muscular ring present at the anorectal junction. It is formed by the fusion of the puborectalis, uppermost fibres of external sphincter and the internal sphincter. It is easily felt by a finger in the anal canal. Surgical division of this ring results in rectal incontinence. The ring is less marked anteriorly where the fibres of the puborectalis are absent (Figs 33.12a and b).

Surgical Spaces Related to the Anal Canal

1. The *ischioanal space* or fossa lies on each side of the anal canal. It is described in Chapter 28.
2. The *perianal space* surrounds the anal canal below the white line. It contains the lower fibres of external sphincter, the external rectal venous plexus, and the terminal branches of the inferior rectal vessels and nerves. Pus in this space tends to spread to the anal canal at the white line or to the surface of the perineal skin rather than to the ischioanal space.
3. The *submucous space* of the canal lies above the white line between the mucous membrane and the internal sphincter. It contains the internal rectal venous plexus and lymphatics (Fig. 33.13).

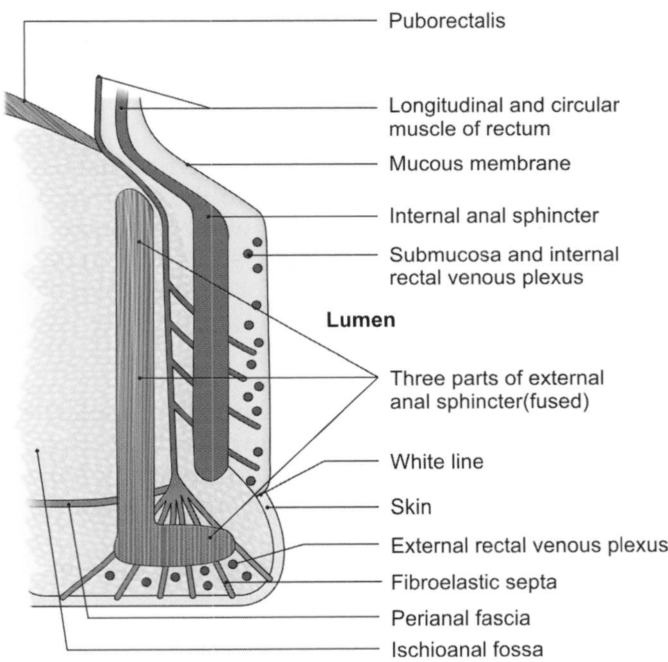

Fig. 33.13: Coronal section through the anal canal (magnified)

Arterial Supply

1. The part of the anal canal above the pectinate line is supplied by the superior rectal artery.
2. The part below the pectinate line is supplied by the inferior rectal arteries (Fig. 33.6).

Venous Drainage

1. The *internal rectal venous plexus* or haemorrhoidal plexus lies in the submucosa of the anal canal. It drains mainly into the superior rectal vein, but communicates freely with the external plexus and thus with the middle and inferior rectal veins. The internal plexus is, therefore, an important site of communication between the portal and systemic veins. The internal plexus is in the form of a series of dilated pouches connected by transverse branches around the anal canal (Fig. 33.6).

   Veins present in the three anal columns situated at 3, 7 and 11 o'clock positions as seen in the lithotomy position are large and constitute potential sites for the formation of primary internal piles (Fig. 33.14).
2. The *external rectal venous plexus* lies outside the muscular coat of the rectum and anal canal, and communicates freely with the internal plexus. The lower part of the external plexus is drained by the inferior rectal vein into internal pudendal vein; the middle part by middle rectal vein into internal iliac vein; and the upper part by superior rectal vein which continues as the inferior mesenteric vein.
3. The *anal veins* are arranged radially around the anal margin. They communicate with the internal rectal

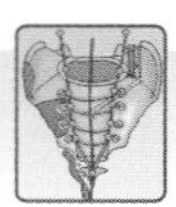

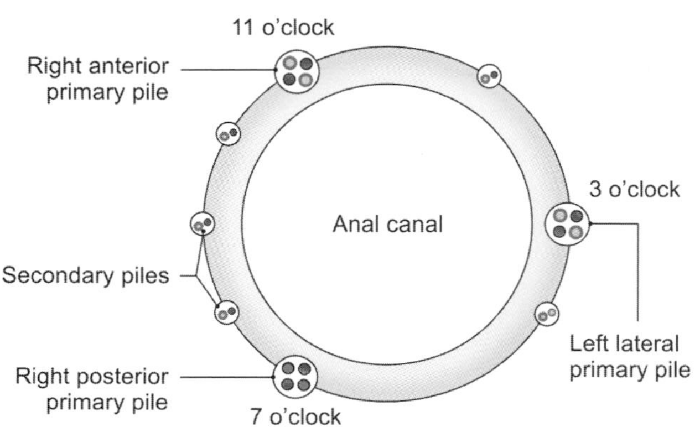

Fig. 33.14: Position of primary and secondary piles haemorrhoids

plexus and with the inferior rectal veins. Excessive straining during the defaecation may rupture one of these veins, forming a subcutaneous perianal haematoma known as external piles.

Lymphatic Drainage

Lymph vessels from the part above the pectinate line, drain with those of the rectum into the internal iliac nodes. Vessels from the part below the pectinate line drain into the medial group of the superficial inguinal nodes (Fig. 33.7). Pectinate line forms the water shed line of anal canal.

Nerve Supply

1 *Above the pectinate line*, the anal canal is supplied by autonomic nerves, both sympathetic (inferior hypogastric plexus; L1, L2) and parasympathetic (pelvic splanchnic, S2, S3, S4). Pain sensations are carried by both of them.
2 *Below the pectinate line*, it is supplied by somatic (inferior rectal, S2, S3, S4) nerves.
3 *Sphincters:* The internal sphincter is caused to contract by sympathetic nerves and is relaxed by parasympathetic nerves. The external sphincter is supplied by the inferior rectal nerve and by the perineal branch of the fourth sacral nerve.

HISTOLOGY

Rectum: The mucous membrane of rectum has many large folds. The epithelium and crypts contain abundant goblet cells. Submucosa contains plexus of nerves and capillaries. Muscularis externa is of uniform thickness. Serosa is seen in upper part and adventitia in lower part.

Anal canal: The epithelium lining of upper 15 mm is simple or stratified columnar, while that of middle 15 mm is stratified squamous without any sweat gland or sebaceous gland or hair follicle. The epithelium of lowest 8 mm resembles that of true skin with sweat and sebaceous glands and hair follicles.

The thick inner circular layer covers the upper three-fourths of anal canal to form the internal anal sphincter. The outer longitudinal layer is a thin layer. Outside these smooth muscle layers is the striated external anal sphincter.

DEVELOPMENT

Rectum

The distal part of hindgut known as cloaca is divided by urorectal septum into primitive anorectal canal posteriorly and vesicourethral canal anteriorly. Primitive anorectal canal forms the lower part of rectum and proximal part of anal canal. Its distal part of anal canal is formed by the proctodeum.

Upper part of rectum, i.e. part above the third transverse fold of rectum, develops from endoderm of hindgut. This part is related to peritoneum. Lower part, below the third transverse fold, is formed from the dorsal part of the cloaca. It is devoid of peritoneum.

Anal Canal

Upper 15 mm develops from the primitive anorectal canal. Lower part below the pectinate line (lower 15 + 8 mm) is formed from ectodermal invagination, i.e. proctodeum (Greek *on the way to*). Non-continuity of the two parts results in imperforate anus.

Table 33.1 shows comparison of upper and lower parts of anal canal.

CLINICAL ANATOMY

- *Piles/haemorrhoids: Internal piles* or true piles are saccular dilatations of the internal rectal venous plexus. They occur above the pectinate line and are, therefore, painless. They bleed profusely during straining at stool. The *primary piles* occur in 3, 7 and 11 o'clock positions of the anal wall when viewed in the lithotomy position. They are formed by enlargement of the three main radicles of the superior rectal vein which lie in the anal columns, which occupy the left lateral, right posterior, and right anterior positions (Fig. 33.14). Varicosities in other positions of the lumen are called *secondary piles*. The various *factors* responsible for causing internal piles are:
  a. Poor support to veins from the surrounding loose connective tissue, so that the veins are less capable of resisting increased blood pressure;
  b. Absence of valves in the superior rectal and portal veins;
  c. Compression of the veins at the sites where they pierce the muscular coat of the rectum; and
  d. Direct transmission of the increased portal pressure at the portosystemic communications.

  For these reasons the development of piles is

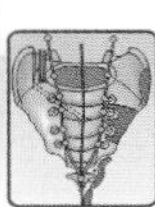

Table 33.1: Comparison of upper (15 mm) and lower (23 mm) parts of anal canal

	Upper part 15 mm	*Lower part 15 + 8 mm*
1. Development	Hindgut (endoderm)	Proctodaeum (ectoderm)
2. Lining	Simple columnar epithelium squamous.	Stratified columnar and stratified
3. Arterial supply of mucosa	Mainly superior rectal	Mainly inferior rectal
4. Venous drainage	Chiefly into portal vein.	Chiefly into systemic veins
5. Lymph drainage	Internal iliac lymph nodes.	Superficial inguinal lymph nodes.
6. Nerve supply	Autonomic nerves: Sympathetic L1, L2 Parasympathetic S2, S3, S4	Inferior rectal (somatic) nerve, S2, S3, S4
7. Sensory to	Ischaemia, distension and spasm	Pain, touch, temperature and pressure.
8. Type of piles	Internal painless piles	External painful piles

favoured by constipation, prolonged standing, excessive straining at stool, and portal hypertension.

- *External piles* or false piles occur below the pectinate line and are, therefore, very painful. They do not bleed on straining at stool.
- *Fissure in ano:* Anal fissure is caused by the rupture of one of the anal valves, usually by the passage of dry hard stool in a constipated person. Each valve is lined with mucous membrane above, and with skin below. Because of the involvement of skin the condition is extremely painful and is associated with marked spasm of the anal sphincters.
- *Fistula in ano:* A fistula is an abnormal epithelialised track connecting two cavities, or one cavity with the exterior (*see* Fig. 28.10).
- Fistula in ano is caused by spontaneous rupture of an abscess around the anus or may follow surgical drainage of the abscess. Most of these abscesses are formed by the small vestigial glands opening into the anal sinuses. Such an anorectal abscess tends to track in various directions and may open medially into the anal sinus, laterally into the ischioanal fossa, inferiorly at the surface, and superiorly into the rectum. A fistula can also be caused by an ischioanal or a pelvirectal abscess. The fistula is said to be complete when it opens both internally into the lumen of the gut and externally at the surface.
- More severe malformations of the anorectal region include the following.
  a. Anal stenosis.
  b. Anal agenesis with or without a fistula.
  c. Anorectal agenesis with or without a fistula. Most of the anorectal malformations are caused by abnormal partitioning of the cloaca by the urorectal septum.

FACTS TO REMEMBER

- Middle lateral curvature of rectum is most prominent. It is convex to the left side.
- Chief artery of rectum is superior rectal and chief vein is superior rectal vein.
- Perineal body and levator ani form the main supports of rectum.
- Most of the anal canal is surrounded by internal and external anal sphincters.
- Only middle fibres of external anal sphincter have a bony attachment.
- Proximal 15 mm of anal canal develops from anorectal canal (endoderm) and distal 23 mm develops from the proctodaeum (ectoderm)
- Primary piles appear at 3, 7, 11 o'clock positions.

CLINICOANATOMICAL PROBLEM

A female patient aged 40 years complained of a painless, bleeding with some structure coming out of anus at the time of defaecation

- What is the painless structure which bleeds during defaecation?
- Identify the reasons for this development

Ans: The patient has developed internal haemorrhoids or piles. These are due to prolapse of the mucous membrane containing the tributaries of internal rectal venous plexus draining blood from the anal canal. Since this part of mucous membrane is supplied by autonomic nerves, these piles are not painful. Since these contain varicose venous radicles, these rupture due to pressure, resulting in painless bleeding during defaecation.

These types of piles may result from irregular bowel habits, chronic constipation, too much straining during defaecation and also in case of portal hypertension resulting due to liver cirrhosis.

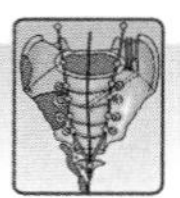

MULTIPLE CHOICE QUESTIONS

1. Inferior rectal artery is a branch of:
   a. Internal iliac
   b. Inferior mesenteric
   c. Internal pudendal
   d. Superior mesenteric

2. Superior rectal is a branch/continuation of:
   a. Superior mesenteric
   b. Inferior mesenteric
   c. Internal iliac
   d. External iliac

3. Which artery supplies the posterior part of anorectal junction and posterior part of anal canal?
   a. Inferior rectal
   b. Superior rectal
   c. Median sacral
   d. Middle rectal

4. Middle rectal artery chiefly supplies:
   a. Mucous membrane b. Muscle layers
   c. Connective tissue d. All of the above

5. Which vessel is present in the lateral rectal ligament?
   a. Superior rectal b. Middle rectal
   c. Inferior rectal d. All of the above

6. Following structures form the anorectal ring *except*:
   a. Deep external sphincter
   b. Internal sphincter
   c. Puborectalis
   d. Conjoint longitudinal coat

7. Which part of sphincter ani externus has a bony attachment?
   a. Superficial b. Subcutaneous
   c. Deep d. All of the above

ANSWERS

1. c **2.** b **3.** c **4.** b **5.** b **6.** d **7.** a

34

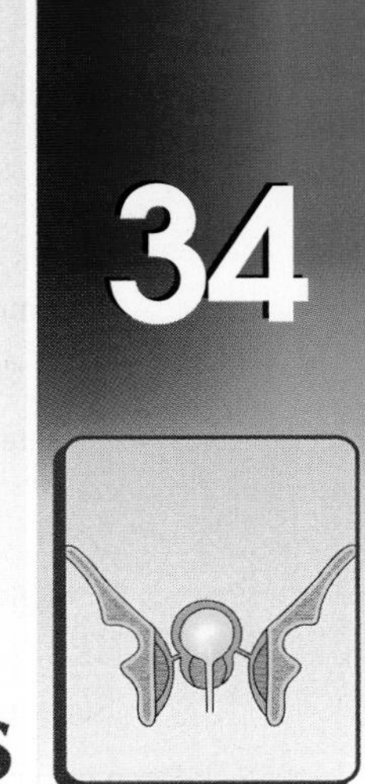

Walls of Pelvis

There is a great man who makes every one feel small. But the real great man is the man who makes every one feel great
—Charles Dickens

All the pelvic viscera, i.e. terminal parts of digestive and urinary system; and components of genital system are located in the pelvis. These organs are provided due protection and nutrition by the bones, muscles, fascia, blood vessels, lymphatics and nerves of the pelvis. The posterior superior iliac spine seen as a dimple (mostly covered) lies opposite the middle of the sacroiliac joint.

Contents: In this chapter the vessels, nerves, muscles, fascia, and joints of the pelvis will be considered.

VESSELS OF THE PELVIS

DISSECTION

Remove the viscera from the pelvic wall and the pelvic cavity. Trace the internal iliac artery and its two divisions. Follow the branches of each of its divisions to the position of the viscera and the parieties. Remove the veins and venous plexuses as these obstruct the view of the arteries. Clean the hypogastric plexus.

INTERNAL ILIAC ARTERY

The internal iliac artery is the smaller terminal branch of the common iliac artery. It is 3.75 cm long. It supplies:

1 Pelvic organs except those supplied by the superior rectal, ovarian and median sacral arteries.
2 Perineum.
3 Greater part of the gluteal region.
4 Iliac fossa.

In the foetus, internal iliac artery is double the size of the external iliac artery because it transmits blood to the placenta through the umbilical artery. The umbilical artery with the internal iliac then forms the direct continuation of the common iliac artery. After birth the proximal part of the umbilical artery persists to form superior vesical artery, and the rest of it degenerates into a fibrous cord, the medial umbilical ligament.

Course

The internal iliac artery begins in front of the sacroiliac joint, at the level of the intervertebral disc between the fifth lumbar vertebra and the sacrum. Here it lies medial to the psoas major muscle. The artery runs downwards and backwards, and ends near the upper margin of the greater sciatic notch, by dividing into anterior and posterior divisions or trunks (Fig. 34.1).

Relations

Anterior	:	Ureter. In female to the ovary and lateral end of the uterine tube (*see* Fig. 31.1)
Posterior	:	Internal iliac vein, lumbosacral trunk and the sacroiliac joint (*see* Figs 24.27 and 34.7)
Lateral	:	External iliac vessels and obturator nerve (Fig. 34.1)
Medial	:	Peritoneum and to a few tributaries of the internal iliac vein.

Branches

Branches of Anterior Division

In the male, it gives off six branches.

1 Superior vesical.
2 Obturator.
3 Middle rectal.
4 Inferior vesical.
5 Inferior gluteal.
6 Internal pudendal. The last two are the terminal branches.

In the female, it gives off seven branches. The inferior vesical artery is replaced by the vaginal artery. The uterine artery is the seventh branch.

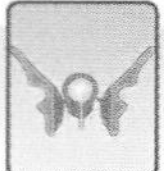

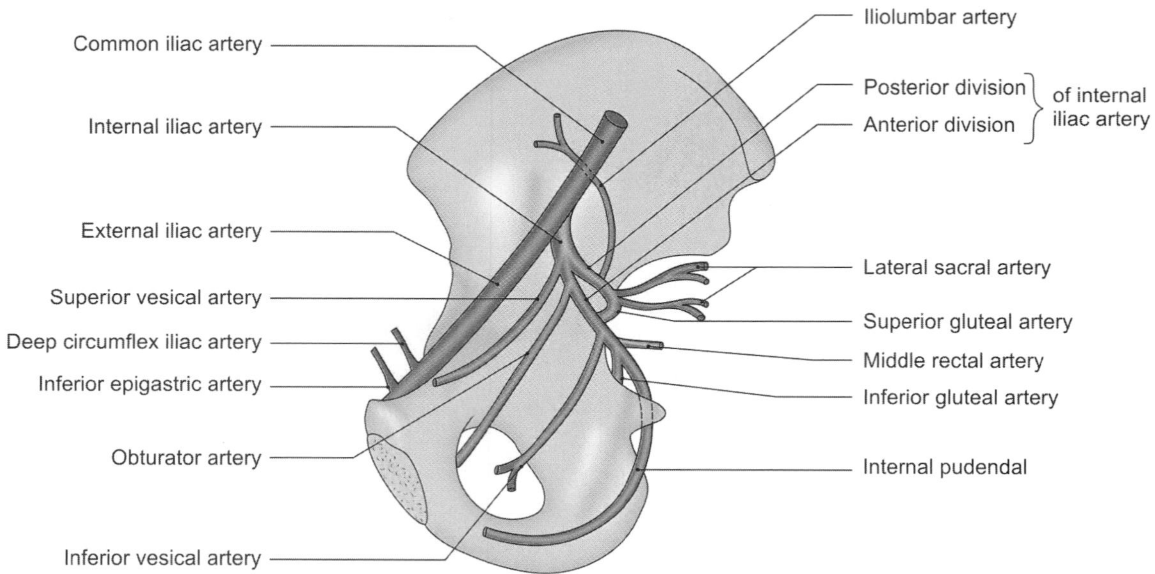

Fig. 34.1: Branches of the right internal iliac artery in a male

Branches of Posterior Division

It gives off:
1 Iliolumbar.
2 Two lateral sacral.
3 Superior gluteal arteries (Flow chart 34.1).

Parietal Branches of Anterior Division

1 *Inferior gluteal artery:* It is the largest branch of the anterior division of the internal iliac artery. It is the *axial artery* of the lower limb. It supplies chiefly the buttock and the back of the thigh. In the pelvis, it runs downwards in front of the sacral plexus and piriformis. Next, it pierces the parietal pelvic fascia, passes below the first sacral nerve and then between the piriformis and the coccygeus, and enters the gluteal region through the lower part of the greater sciatic foramen (Fig. 34.2). In the pelvis, it supplies:
   a. Muscular branches to nearby muscles.
   b. Vesical branches to the base of the bladder, the seminal vesicles and the prostate.
2 *Obturator artery:* It runs forwards and downwards on the obturator fascia below the obturator nerve and above the obturator vein (NAV). Medially, it is crossed by the ureter and the ductus deferens, and is covered with peritoneum. It passes through the obturator foramen to leave the pelvis and enter the thigh. In the pelvis it gives off:
   a. Iliac branches to the iliac fossa.
   b. A vesical branch to the urinary bladder.
   c. A pubic branch to the back of the pubis, which anastomoses with the pubic branch of the inferior epigastric artery and with its fellow of the opposite side.

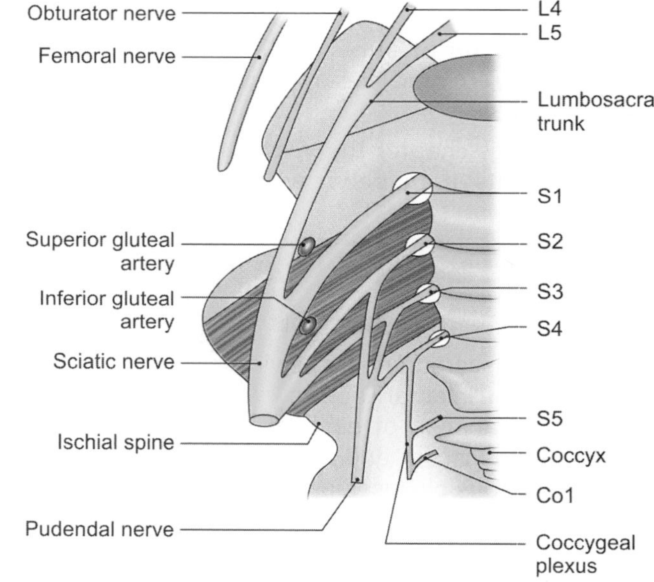

Fig. 34.2: Anterior view of the right sacral and coccygeal plexuses

Visceral Branches of Anterior Division

1 *Superior vesical artery:* The proximal 2.5 cm or so of the superior vesical artery represents the persistent part of the umbilical artery. It supplies many branches to the upper part of the urinary bladder. One of these branches gives off the artery to the ductus deferens.
2 *Middle rectal artery:* It is characterized by three features.
   a. It is often absent, especially in females.
   b. Very little of its blood goes to the rectum, and that too goes only to its muscle coats.
   c. Most of its blood goes to the prostate and seminal vesicles.

Flow chart 34.1: Branches of internal Iliac artery

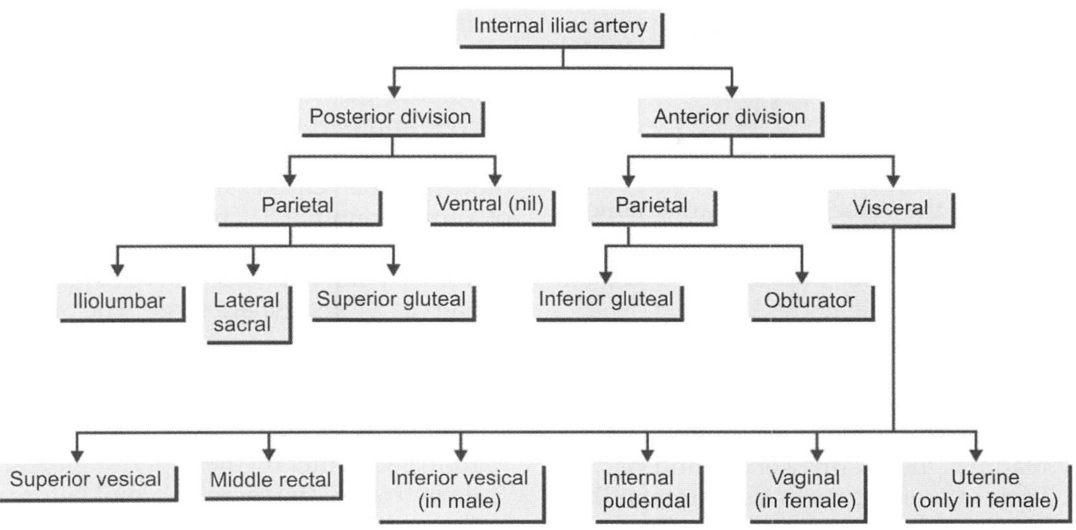

3 *Inferior vesical artery:* It supplies the trigone of the bladder, the prostate, the seminal vesicles, and the lower part of the ureter.

4 *Internal pudendal artery:* It is the smaller terminal branch of the anterior division of the internal iliac artery. It supplies the perineum and external genitalia. Its branches are inferior rectal, perineal, artery to bulb, urethral, deep and dorsal arteries. It is described in Chapter 28.

5 *Vaginal artery:* It corresponds to the inferior vesical artery of the male, and supplies the vagina, the bulb of the vestibule, the base of the urinary bladder, and the adjacent part of the rectum (*see* Chapter 31).

6 *Uterine artery:* It has a tortuous course. Crosses the ureter 2 cm lateral to cervix. Runs along side of uterus. Supplies vagina, cervix uterus, fallopian tube (*see* Chapter 31).

Branches of Posterior Division

1 *Iliolumbar artery:* It runs upwards in front of the sacroiliac joint and lumbosacral trunk, and behind the obturator nerve and external iliac vessels (Fig. 34.1). Behind the psoas major, it divides into the lumbar and iliac branches.

The *lumbar branch* represents the fifth lumbar artery, and supplies the psoas, the quadratus lumborum and the erector spinae. Its spinal branch supplies the cauda equina.

The *iliac branch* supplies the iliac fossa and the iliacus. It participates in the anastomoses around the anterior superior iliac spine.

2 *Lateral sacral arteries:* These are usually two in number, upper and lower. They run downwards and medially over the sacral nerves. Their branches enter the four anterior sacral foramina to supply the contents of the sacral canal. Their terminations pass out through the posterior sacral foramina and supply the muscles and skin on the back of the sacrum (*see* Fig. 33.4).

3 *Superior gluteal artery:* It runs backwards, pierces the pelvic fascia, passes above the first sacral nerve, and leaves the pelvis through the greater sciatic foramen above the piriformis (Fig. 34.2). It supplies gluteus maximus muscle. Also takes part in anastomoses around anterior superior iliac spine and in trochanteric anastomoses to supply nearby muscles and overlying skin. For further course *see* Chapter 5.

INTERNAL ILIAC VEIN

It ascends posteromedial to the internal iliac artery, and joins the external iliac vein to form the common iliac vein at the pelvic brim, in front of the lower part of the sacroiliac joint. Its tributaries correspond with the branches of the artery, except for the iliolumbar vein which joins the common iliac vein. The tributaries are as follows.

Veins arising in and outside the pelvic wall

1 Superior gluteal is the largest tributary,
2 Inferior gluteal,
3 Internal pudendal,
4 Obturator, and
5 Lateral sacral veins.

Veins arising from the plexuses of pelvic viscera

1 Rectal venous plexus is drained by the superior, middle and inferior rectal veins.
2 Prostatic venous plexus is drained by the vesical and internal iliac veins.
3 Vesical venous plexus is drained by the vesical veins.

4 Uterine venous plexus is drained by the uterine veins.
5 Vaginal venous plexus is drained by the vaginal veins.

LYMPH NODES OF THE PELVIS

The pelvic lymphatics drain into the following lymph nodes, which lie along the vessels of the same name.

1 4 to 6 *common iliac nodes* receive lymphatics from the external and internal iliac nodes, and send their efferents to the lateral aortic nodes.
2 8 to 10 *external iliac nodes* receive lymphatics from the inguinal nodes, the deeper layers of the infraumbilical part of the anterior abdominal wall, the membranous urethra, the prostate, the base of the urinary bladder, the uterine cervix, and part of the vagina. Their efferents pass to the common iliac nodes. The *inferior epigastric* and *circumflex iliac nodes* are outlying members of this group.
3 The *internal iliac nodes* receive lymphatics from all the pelvic viscera, the deeper parts of the perineum, and muscles of the buttocks and of the back of the thigh. Their efferents pass to the common iliac nodes. The sacral and obturator nodes are outlying members of this group.

NERVES OF THE PELVIS

DISSECTION

Expose the lumbosacral trunk and ventral rami of sacral one to sacral five nerves. Lift the sacral plexus forwards and expose its terminal branches, the sciatic and pudendal nerves.

Find the nerves arising from the dorsal surface of plexus, e.g. superior gluteal, inferior gluteal, perforating cutaneous and perineal branch of fourth sacral nerve.

Trace the two branches, e.g. nerve to quadratus femoris and nerve to obturator internus arising from the pelvic surface of the plexus.

Trace the sympathetic trunks in the pelvis till these terminate in the single *ganglion impar* on the coccyx. Trace the large grey rami communicans from the ganglia to the ventral rami of the sacral nerves.

Find the inferior hypogastric plexus around the internal iliac vessels. In addition, trace the pelvic splanchnic nerves reaching the inferior hypogastric plexus from the ventral rami of second, third and fourth sacral nerves.

The nerves of the pelvis include:

1 Lumbosacral plexus,
2 Coccygeal plexus, and
3 Pelvic splanchnic nerves.

LUMBOSACRAL PLEXUS

Formation

The lumbosacral plexus is formed by the lumbosacral trunk and the ventral rami of the first to third sacral nerves, and part of the fourth sacral nerve (Fig. 34.2).

The *lumbosacral trunk* is formed by the descending branch of the ventral ramus of nerve L4 and the whole of ventral ramus L5. The trunk descends over the ala of the sacrum, crosses the pelvic brim in front of the sacroiliac joint, and joins nerve S1 (*see* Fig. 33.4).

Nerves S1 and S2 are large. The other sacral nerves become progressively smaller in size.

Relations

1 The lumbosacral trunk and ramus S1 are separated from each other by the superior gluteal vessels. Both lie in front of the sacroiliac joint before passing on to the surface of the piriformis. Thus both may be involved in pathological conditions of the joint (Fig. 34.2).
2 Ramus S1 is separated from ramus S2 by the inferior gluteal vessels.
3 Rami S2, S3 and a part of S4 lie between the anterior surface of the piriformis and the pelvic fascia.
4 The main plexus lies in front of the piriformis deep to the pelvic fascia, and behind the internal iliac vessels and the ureter (Fig. 34.4).

Layout of Connections and Branches

1 Each ventral ramus receives a *grey ramus communicans* from the sympathetic chain at the anterior sacral foramen.
2 Before uniting to form the plexus, the ventral rami give off:
   a. Twigs to the piriformis (S1, S2).
   b. Twigs to the levator ani, the coccygeus and the sphincter ani externus (S4).
   c. Pelvic splanchnic nerves (S2, S3, S4).
3 The plexus gives rise to two main branches namely, the sciatic and pudendal nerves, concerned respectively with locomotion and reproduction.
4 As in other plexuses, the rami tend to divide into ventral and dorsal divisions which supply the corresponding aspects of the lower limb and trunk. In general, the *dorsal divisions* supply the extensors and the abductors, and the *ventral divisions* supply the flexors and the adductors, of the limb.

Branches

Branches derived from both dorsal and ventral divisions are as follows.

1 *Sciatic nerve:* The common peroneal nerve component arises from dorsal divisions of L4, L5, S1, S2. It supplies evertors of foot and dorsiflexors

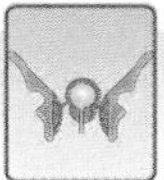

of ankle joint. The tibial nerve component arises from ventral divisions of L4, L5, S1, S2, S3. It supplies the hamstring muscles, all muscles of calf and intrinsic muscles of the sole. This nerve is described in Chapter 7.

2 *Posterior cutaneous nerve of thigh:* Dorsal divisions of S1, S2 and ventral divisions of S2, S3 (*see* Chapter 7).

Branches from Dorsal Divisions

1 Superior gluteal nerve: L4, L5, S1 (*see* Fig. 5.14).
2 Inferior gluteal nerve: L5, S1, S2 (*see* Fig. 5.14).
3 Nerve to piriformis: S1, S2.
4 Perforating cutaneous nerve: S2, S3.

Branches from Ventral Division

1 Nerve to quadratus femoris: L4, L5, S1.
2 Nerve to obturator internus: L5, S1, S2.
3 Pudendal nerve: S2, S3, S4: Supplies sphincter ani externus and all muscles in urogenital triangles.
4 Muscular branches to the levator ani, the coccygeus and the sphincter ani externus, including perineal branch of nerve S4.
5 Pelvic splanchnic nerves: S2, S3, S4.

Muscular Branches

Nerves to the levator ani or iliococcygeus part and the coccygeus or ischiococcygeus arise from nerve S4 and enter their pelvic surfaces.

The nerve to the middle part of the sphincter ani externus is called the *perineal branch of the fourth sacral nerve*. It runs forwards on the coccygeus and reaches the ischioanal fossa by passing between the coccygeus and the levator ani. In addition to the lower end of external sphincter, it supplies the skin between the anus and the coccyx.

COCCYGEAL PLEXUS

1 It is formed by the ventral rami of spinal nerves S4 (descending branch), S5 and the coccygeal nerve (Fig. 34.2).
2 The three nerves join on the pelvic surface of the coccygeus to form a small plexus known as the coccygeal plexus.
3 The plexus gives off the anococcygeal nerves, which pierce the sacrotuberous ligament and supply the skin in the region of the coccyx.

CLINICAL ANATOMY

The lumbosacral trunk (L4, L5) and the ventral ramus of nerve S1 cross the pelvic surface of the joint and may be involved in disease of the joint, causing pain in the area of their distribution below the knee. L4 supplies medial aspect of leg and sole. S1 supplies lateral aspect of sole refer (*see* Fig. 10.2).

PELVIC AUTONOMIC NERVES

Pelvic Sympathetic System

The pelvic part of the sympathetic chain runs downwards and slightly medially over the body of sacrum, and then along the medial margins of the anterior sacral foramina. The two chains unite in front of the coccyx to form a small *ganglion impar*. The chain bears four sacral ganglia on each side and the single ganglion impar in the central part.

The *branches* of the chain are:

a. Grey rami communicans to all sacral and coccygeal ventral rami.
b. Branches to the inferior hypogastric plexus from the upper ganglia.
c. Branches to the median sacral artery from the lower ganglia.
d. Branches to the rectum from the lower ganglia.
e. Branches to the glomus coccygeum (*see* Fig. 29.11) from the ganglion impar.

The *inferior hypogastric plexus* (*see* Chapter 27) one on each side of the rectum and other pelvic viscera is formed by the corresponding hypogastric nerve from the superior hypogastric plexus; branches from the upper ganglia of the sacral sympathetic chain; and the pelvic splanchnic nerves. Branches of the plexus accompany the visceral branches of the internal iliac artery; and are named:

a. Rectal plexus,
b. Vesical plexus,
c. Prostatic plexus, and
d. Uterovaginal plexus.

Pelvic Splanchnic Nerves

Nervi Erigentes

The nervi erigentes represent the sacral outflow of the parasympathetic nervous system. The nerves arise as fine filaments from the ventral rami of S2, S3 and S4. They join the inferior hypogastric plexus and are distributed to the pelvic organs. Some parasympathetic fibres ascend with the hypogastric nerve to the superior hypogastric plexus and thence to the inferior mesenteric plexus. Others ascend independently and directly to the part of the colon derived from the hindgut.

PELVIC FASCIA AND MUSCLES

PELVIC FASCIA

The pelvic fascia is distributed in the extraperitoneal space of the pelvis. It covers the lateral pelvic wall and the pelvic floor called *parietal pelvic fascia*; and also surrounds the pelvic viscera called *visceral pelvic fascia*.

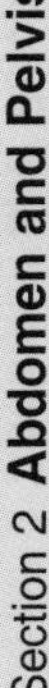

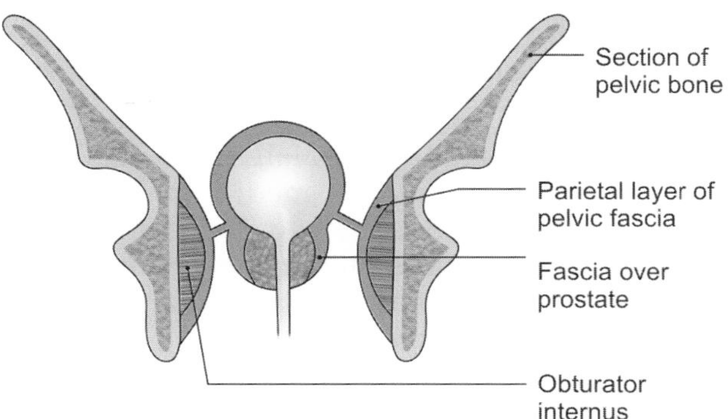

Fig. 34.3: Pelvic fascia

Principles Governing its Distribution

1. The fascia is dense and membranous over nonexpansile structures, e.g. lateral pelvic wall, but is only loosely arranged over expansile structures, e.g. viscera, and over mobile structures, e.g. the pelvic floor (Fig. 34.3).
2. As a rule the fascia does not extend over bare bones; at the margins of the muscles it fuses with the periosteum. In this respect, the fascia of Waldeyer is an exception, which extends from the sacrum to the ampulla of rectum.

Parietal Fascia of the Lateral Pelvic Wall

1. The fascia covering the muscles of the lateral pelvic wall is condensed to form thick and strong membranes. It is closely adherent to the walls of the pelvic cavity. It is attached along a line from iliopectineal line to the inferior border of pubic bone.
2. The fascia covering the obturator internus is called the *obturator fascia*. It shows a linear thickening or tendinous arch for the origin of the levator ani. Below this origin it is closely related to the lunate fascia and to the pudendal canal.
3. The *fascia covering the piriformis* is thin. The nerves over the piriformis, i.e. the sacral plexus lie external to the pelvic fascia and, therefore, do not pierce the fascia while passing out of the pelvis. The gluteal vessels, on the other hand, lie internal to the pelvic fascia and, therefore, have to pierce the fascia while passing out of the pelvis (Fig. 34.4).

Parietal Fascia of the Pelvic Floor

1. The pelvic fascia covers both the surfaces of the pelvic diaphragm, forming the superior and inferior layers. The inferior fascia is also known as the *anal fascia*.
2. In general, the fascia of the pelvic floor is loosely arranged between the peritoneum and the pelvic floor, forming a dead space for distension of the bladder, the rectum, the uterus and the vagina. Because of the loose nature of the fascia infections can spread rapidly within it.

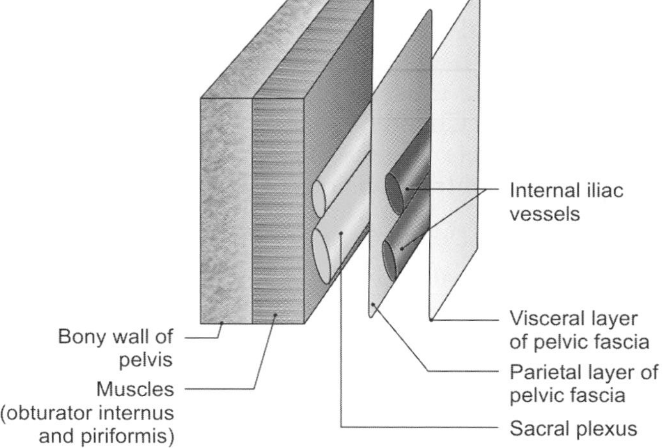

Fig. 34.4: Arrangement of structures on the walls of true pelvis

3. However, the fascia is condensed at places to form fibromuscular ligaments which support the pelvic viscera. The various ligaments are dealt with individual viscera including the prostate, bladder, uterus and the rectum.

Visceral Pelvic Fascia

This fascia surrounds the extraperitoneal parts of the pelvic viscera. It is loose and cellular around distensible organs like bladder, rectum and vagina, but is dense around non-distensible organs, like the prostate. The visceral layer is attached along a line extending from the middle of back of pubis to the ischial spine.

PELVIC MUSCLES

DISSECTION

Muscles of lesser pelvis

Identify the origin of piriformis from the ventral surface of the sacrum. Trace it through the greater sciatic foramen to its insertion into the upper border of greater trochanter of femur.

Feel the ischial spine and trace the fibres of coccygeus and levator ani that arise from it. Trace the origin of levator ani from thickened fascia, i.e. tendinous arch over the middle of obturator internus muscle till the back of body of the pubis. Note that the right and left sheet like levator ani muscles are united and the muscles are inserted into central perineal tendon or perineal body, anal canal, anococcygeal ligament.

Detach the origin of levator ani from obturator fascia. While removing obturator fascia identify pudendal canal with its contents in the lower part of the fascia.

Trace the tendon of obturator internus muscle. This tendon along with superior and inferior gemelli muscles leaves through the lesser sciatic foramen to be inserted into the medial surface of greater trochanter of femur.

Features

The pelvic muscles include two groups.

1 Piriformis and obturator internus, which are short lateral rotators of the hip joint and are described with the muscles of the lower limb.
2 Levator ani and coccygeus, which with the corresponding muscles of the opposite side, form the pelvic diaphragm. The diaphragm separates the pelvis from the perineum (Figs 34.5a and b).

The levator ani and coccygeus may be regarded as one morphological entity, divisible from before backwards into the pubococcygeus, the iliococcygeus and the ischiococcygeus or coccygeus. They have a continuous linear origin from the pelvic surface of the body of the pubis, the obturator fascia or white line or tendinous arch and the ischial spine. The muscle fibres slope downwards and backwards to the midline, making a gutter-shaped pelvic floor. These muscles are described below.

THE LEVATOR ANI

The muscle is divisible into a pubococcygeus part, an iliococcygeus part and a ischiococcygeus part (Fig. 34.6).

Pubococcygeus Part

1 The anterior fibres of this part arise from the medial part of the pelvic surface of the body of the pubis. In the male these fibres closely surround the prostate and constitute the *levator prostatae*. In the female these fibres surround the vagina and form the *sphincter vaginae*. In both cases the anterior fibres are inserted into the perineal body.
2 The middle fibres constitute the puborectalis. These arise from the lateral part of the pelvic surface of the body of the pubis. They partly form a loop or sling around the anorectal junction; and are partly continuous with the longitudinal muscle coat of the rectum. In female the anterior portion of puborectalis is thinner and shorter (*see* Fig. 33.12b).
3 The posterior fibres of the pubococcygeus arise from the anterior half of the white line on the obturator fascia. These get attached to anococcygeal ligament and tip of coccyx.

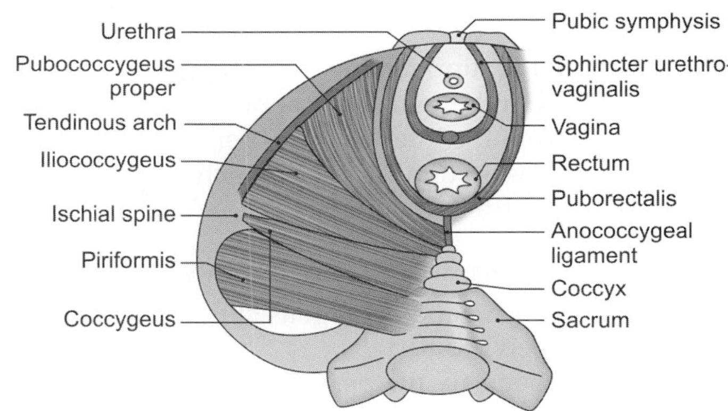

Fig. 34.6: The levator ani, the coccygeus and the piriformis in a female

Iliococcygeus Part

The fibres of this part arise from:

1 The posterior half of the white line on the obturator fascia.
2 The pelvic surface of the ischial spine. They are inserted into the anococcygeal ligament and into the side of the last two pieces of coccyx.

Coccygeus

This muscle represents the posterior or ischiococcygeus part of the pelvic diaphragm. It is triangular in shape. It is partly muscular and partly tendinous.

Its fibres arise from:

a. The pelvic surface of the ischial spine.
b. The sacrospinous ligament. It is inserted into the side of the coccyx, and into the fifth sacral vertebra.

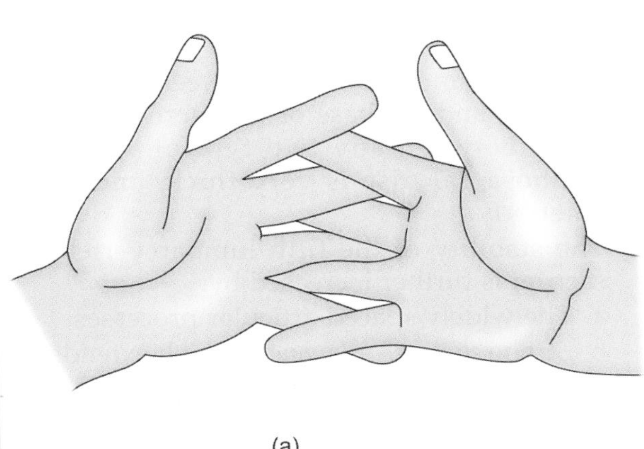

(a)

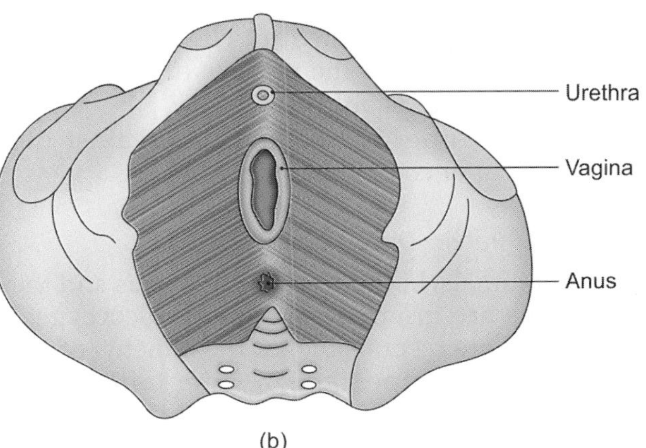

(b)

Figs 34.5a and b: (a) Interlocking hands represent the enterlocking fibres of two levator ani muscles, and (b) openings in the pelvic diaphragm in female

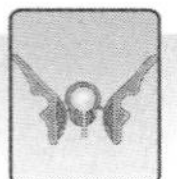

Nerve Supply

The levator ani is supplied by:

1 A branch from the fourth sacral nerve.
2 A branch from the inferior rectal nerve.

The coccygeus is supplied by a branch derived from the fourth and fifth sacral nerves.

Actions of Levators Ani and Coccygeus

1 The levatores ani and coccygeus close the posterior part of the pelvic outlet.
2 The levators ani fix the perineal body and support the pelvic viscera.
3 During coughing, sneezing, lifting and other muscular efforts, the levators ani and coccygei counteract or resist increased intra-abdominal pressure and help to maintain continence of the bladder and the rectum.

   In micturition, defaecation and parturition, a particular pelvic outlet is open, but contraction of fibres around other openings resists increased intra-abdominal pressure and prevents any prolapse through the pelvic floor. The increase in the intra-abdominal pressure is momentary in coughing and sneezing and is more prolonged in yawning, micturition, defaecation and lifting heavy weights. It is most prolonged and intense in second stage of labour.

4 The coccygeus pulls forwards and support the coccyx, after it has been pressed backwards during defaecation, parturition or childbirth.

Relations of the Levator Ani

1 The superior or pelvic surface is covered with pelvic fascia which separates it from the bladder, prostate, rectum and the peritoneum.
2 The inferior or perineal surface is covered with anal fascia and forms the medial boundary of the ischioanal fossa (*see* Fig. 28.7).
3 The anterior borders of the two muscles are separated by a triangular space for the passage of the urethra and the vagina (Fig. 34.5b).
4 The posterior border is free and lies against the anterior margin of coccygeus (Fig. 34.6).

Morphology of Pelvic Diaphragm

1 In lower mammals, both the pubococcygeus and the iliococcygeus are inserted only into the coccygeal vertebrae and are responsible for movements of the tail. With the disappearance of the tail during evolution, the muscles have been modified to form the pelvic diaphragm which supports the viscera. Such support became necessary with the adoption of the erect posture by man.
2 In lower mammals, the levator ani arises from the pelvic brim. In man, the origin has shifted down to the side wall of the pelvis.
3 The coccygeus muscle corresponds exactly with the sacrospinous ligament, which is a degenerated part of the aponeurosis of this muscle. The two are inversely proportional in their development.

CLINICAL ANATOMY

The muscles of the pelvic floor may be injured during parturition. When the perineal body is torn, and has not been repaired satisfactorily, the contraction of anterior fibres of the levator ani increases the normal gap in the pelvic floor, instead of decreasing it. This results in prolapse of the uterus.

JOINTS OF PELVIS

DISSECTION

Joints

Remove the remains of any muscle of the back or thoracolumbar fascia. Identify the iliolumbar and dorsal sacroiliac ligaments. Remove the dorsal sacroiliac ligament to identify the deeply placed interosseous sacroiliac ligament. Divide this interosseous ligament and open the joint from the posterior aspect.

Define the attachments of ventral sacroiliac ligament. Cut through this thin ligament to open the sacroiliac joint.

The following parts are considered.

1 Lumbosacral joints,
2 Sacrococcygeal and intercoccygeal joints,
3 Sacroiliac joints with vertebropelvic ligaments,
4 Pubic symphysis; followed by
5 The mechanism of pelvis.

LUMBOSACRAL JOINTS

1 The joints and ligaments between the fifth lumbar vertebra and the base of the sacrum are similar to those between any two typical vertebrae. The lumbosacral disc is very thick, and is thickest anteriorly.
2 The stability of the fifth lumbar vertebra on the sacrum is further increased by:
   a. The widely spaced articular processes.
   b. Strong *iliolumbar ligament* which extends from the stout transverse process of the fifth lumbar vertebra to the iliac crest. The ligament fans out inferiorly to be attached to the lateral part of the ala of the sacrum as the lumbosacral ligament (Figs 34.7a and b).

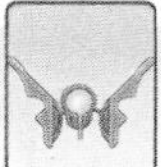

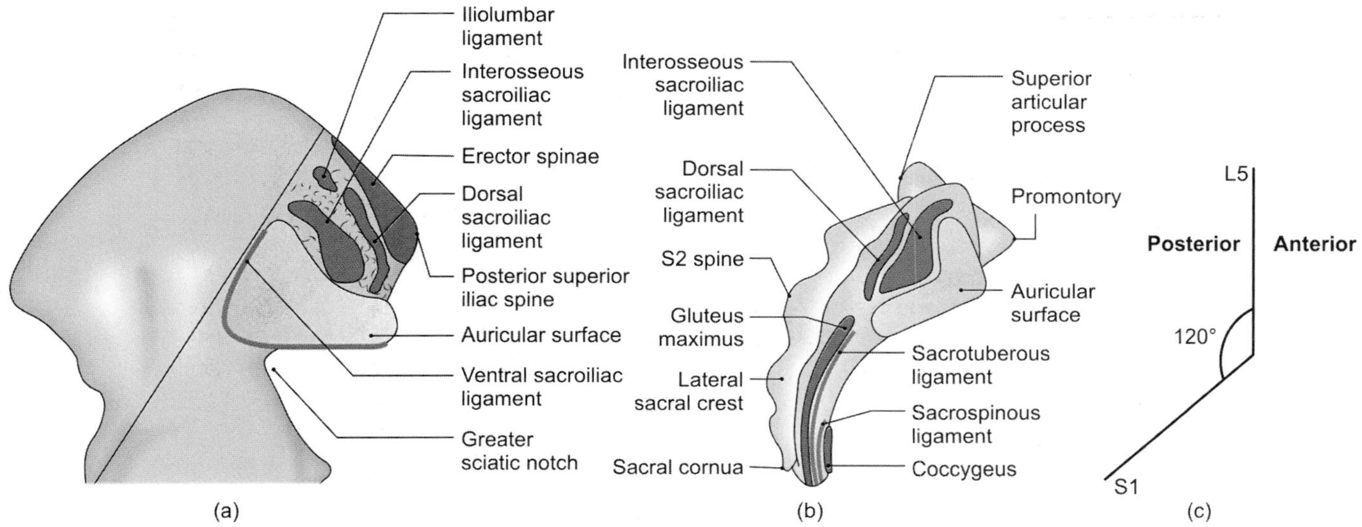

Figs 34.7a to c: Articular surfaces of the right sacroiliac joint. (a) Medial view of the upper part of the right hip bone, (b) right lateral view of the sacrum, and (c) lumbosacral angle is 120° opening backwards

3 The body of the fifth lumbar vertebra makes an angle of about 120 degrees opens backwards with the sacrum. This is the lumbosacral or sacrovertebral angle, and opens backwards (Fig. 34.7c).
4 This region is subject to a number of variations which give rise to symptoms of backache. These are:
   a. Sacralization of the fifth lumbar vertebra.
   b. Lumbralization of the first sacral vertebra.
   c. Spina bifida.
   d. Spondylolisthesis, etc.

SACROCOCCYGEAL AND INTERCOCCYGEAL JOINTS

The *sacrococcygeal joint* is a secondary cartilaginous joint between the apex of the sacrum and the base of the coccyx. The bones are united by:

1 A thin intervertebral disc.
2 Ventral sacrococcygeal ligament corresponding to the anterior longitudinal ligament.
3 Deep dorsal sacrococcygeal ligament corresponding to the posterior longitudinal ligament.
4 Superficial dorsal sacrococcygeal ligament, completing the lower part of the sacral canal.
5 Lateral sacrococcygeal ligament corresponding to the intertransverse ligament and completing the foramen for the fifth sacral nerve.
6 Intercornual ligament, connecting the cornua of the sacrum and the coccyx. In old age the joint is obliterated and the ligaments are ossified. Sometimes the joint is synovial, and the coccyx is freely mobile.

The *intercoccygeal joints* are present only in young subjects. Fusion of the segments begins at the age of 20 years and is complete by about 30 years.

SACROILIAC JOINT

Type

This is a synovial joint of the plane variety. The articular surfaces are flat in infants; but in adults show interlocking irregularities which discourage movements at this joint.

Articular Surface

The joint is formed between:

1 Auricular surface of the sacrum, which is covered with fibrocartilage.
2 Auricular surface of the ilium, which is covered with hyaline cartilage (Fig. 34.7).

Ligaments

1 The *fibrous capsule* is attached close to the margins of the articular surfaces. It is lined by synovial membrane (Fig. 34.8).
2 The *ventral sacroiliac ligament* is a thickening of the anterior and inferior parts of the fibrous capsule. Its lower part is attached to the preauricular sulcus.
3 The *interosseous sacroiliac ligament* is massive and very strong, forming the chief bond of union between the sacrum and the ilium. It connects the wide, rough areas adjoining the concave margins of the auricular surfaces, and is covered by the dorsal sacroiliac ligament.
4 The dorsal sacroiliac ligament covers the interosseous sacroiliac ligament, from which it is separated by the dorsal rami of the sacral spinal nerves and vessels.

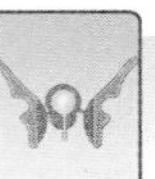

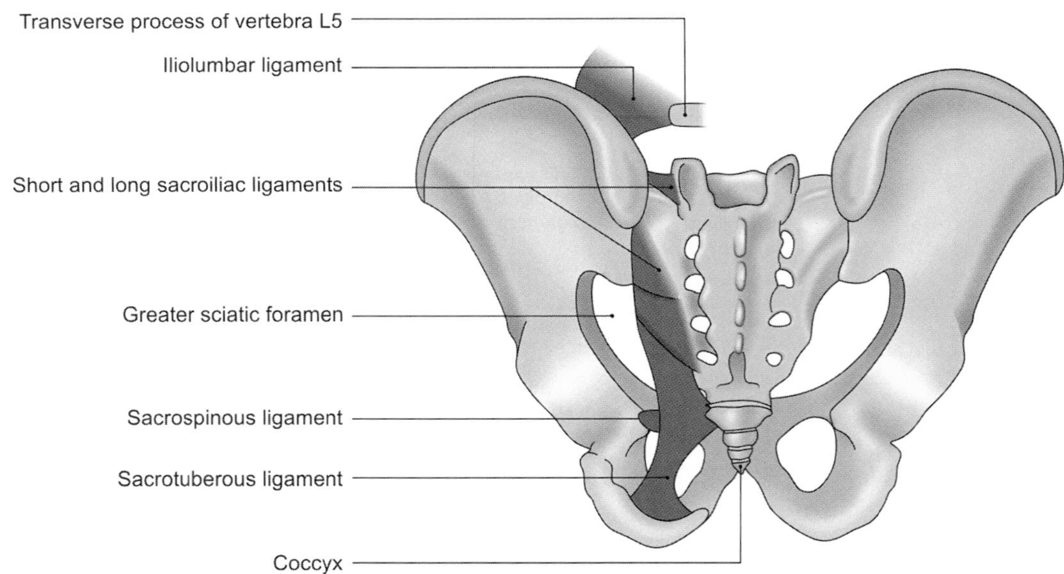

Fig. 34.8: Ligaments of the pelvis as seen from behind

Dorsal sacroiliac consists of:

a. Short transverse fibres or *short posterior sacroiliac ligament* passing from the ilium to the transverse tubercles of the first two sacral pieces.

b. A long, more vertical, band or *long posterior sacroiliac ligament* passing from the posterior superior iliac spine to the transverse tubercles of the third and fourth sacral pieces; it is continuous laterally with medial edge of the sacrotuberous ligament.

5 The *vertebropelvic ligaments* include the iliolumbar, sacrotuberous and sacrospinous ligaments. These are accessory ligaments to the sacroiliac joint and are important in maintaining its stability.

a. The *iliolumbar ligament* is a strong, triangular ligament, extending from the thick transverse process of the fifth lumbar vertebra to the posterior part of the inner lip of the iliac crest. It is continuous with the middle and anterior layers of the thoracolumbar fascia and gives partial origin to the quadratus lumborum. It is covered anteriorly by the psoas, and posteriorly by the erector spinae. It prevents anteroinferior slipping of the fifth lumbar vertebra under the influence of body weight, and also prevents forward movement at the sacroiliac joint (Fig. 34.8).

b. The *sacrotuberous ligament* is a long and strong band which forms parts of the boundaries of the pelvic outlet and of the sciatic foramina. Its superomedial end or base is wide. It is attached to the posterior superior and posterior inferior iliac spines, the lower transverse tubercles of the sacrum, the lateral margin of the lower part of the sacrum and the upper part of the coccyx. The inferolateral end is narrow. It is attached to the medial margin of the ischial tuberosity. A part of it that extends along the ramus of the ischium is called the falciform process. The ligament is covered by and also gives partial origin to gluteus maximus, and is pierced by the perforating cutaneous nerve, the fifth sacral and first coccygeal nerves, and branches of the coccygeal plexus (*see* Figs 5.14 and 34.8).

c. The *sacrospinous ligament* is a thin, triangular ligament, which lies deep to sacrotuberous ligament, and separates the greater and lesser sciatic foramina. Its base is attached to the lateral margins of the last piece of the sacrum and to the coccyx and its apex to the ischial spine. Its pelvic surface is covered by and also gives origin to the coccygeus. Morphologically, the ligament is a degenerated part of the coccygeus (Fig. 34.8).

The sacrotuberous and sacrospinous ligaments bind the sacrum to the ischium. They oppose upward tilting of the lower end of the sacrum and therefore, downward tilting of its upper end under body weight.

Relations

Posteriorly

1 Joint is covered by the erector spinae, the gluteus maximus and the sacrotuberous ligament (Fig. 34.7b).

2 Dimple overlying the posterior superior iliac spine lies opposite the middle of joint (*see* Fig. 5.1).

Abdominal Surface

1 It is covered by the psoas and iliacus (*see* Fig. 2.5).

2 Deep to the psoas, the joint is crossed by the iliolumbar vessels and the obturator nerve (*see* Fig. 15.11).

3 Femoral nerve is separated from the joint by the iliacus muscle.

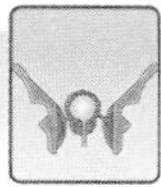

The *pelvic surface* is related to:

1 Lumbosacral trunk and the posterior division of the internal iliac artery.
2 Internal iliac vein and the anterior division of the internal iliac artery.
3 Superior gluteal vessels and the first sacral nerve (S1) (Fig. 34.2).
4 Upper part of the piriformis.

Factors Providing Stability

Stability is the primary requirement of the joint as it transmits body weight from the vertebral column to the lower limbs. Stability is maintained by a number of factors which are as follows.

1 Interlocking of the articular surfaces.
2 Thick and strong interosseous and dorsal sacroiliac ligaments play a very important role in maintaining stability (Fig. 34.7).
3 Vertebropelvic ligaments, i.e. iliolumbar, sacrotuberous and sacrospinous are equally important in this respect.
4 With advancing age, partial synostosis of the joint takes place which further reduces movements.

Blood Supply

Sacroiliac joint is supplied by twigs from all the three branches of posterior division of internal iliac artery, i.e. iliolumbar, lateral sacral and superior gluteal arteries.

Nerve Supply

The joint is supplied by the following nerves.

1 Superior gluteal.
2 Ventral rami and the lateral branches of dorsal rami of the first and second sacral nerves.

Movements

During flexion and extension of the trunk, stooping and straightening, i.e. the sacroiliac joint permits a small amount of *anteroposterior rotatory movement* around a transverse axis passing 5 to 10 cm vertically below the sacral promontory. This little movement serves the important function of *absorbing the shocks* of jumping and bearing of loads. The range of movement is increased temporarily in pregnancy in which all the ligaments of the pelvis become loose, under the influence of hormones, to facilitate delivery of the foetus.

PUBIC SYMPHYSIS

This is a secondary cartilaginous joint between the bodies of the right and left pubic bones. Each articular surface is covered with a thin layer of hyaline cartilage. The fibrocartilaginous disc is reinforced by surrounding ligamentous fibres. The fibres are thickest inferiorly where they form the *arcuate pubic ligament*. Anteriorly, the fibres form the *anterior pubic ligament* (*see* Fig. 15.14a).

The pubic symphysis permits slight movement between the hip bones, which helps in absorbing shocks. The range of movement is increased during pregnancy.

THE MECHANISM OF PELVIS

The most important mechanical function of the pelvis is to transmit the weight of trunk to the lower limb. The weight passes mainly through the alae of sacrum and through the thick part of hip bone lying between sacroiliac joint and acetabulum.

Theoretically, the weight falling on the lumbosacral joint is divided into two components.

a. *One component of the force* is expanded in trying to drive the sacrum downwards and backwards between the iliac bones. This is resisted by the ligaments of pubic symphysis.
b. *Second component of the force* tries to push the upper end of sacrum downwards and forwards towards the pelvic cavity. This is resisted by the middle segment of the sacroiliac joint, where the auricular surface of the sacrum is wider posteriorly, i.e. wedge-shaped and is concave for interlocking with the reciprocal surface of the ilium.

Because of the poor wedging and poor locking of the articular surfaces in the anterior and posterior segments of the sacroiliac joint, the sacrum is forced to rotate under the influence of body weight. In this rotation, the anterior segment is tilted downwards and the posterior segment upwards. The downward tilt of the anterior segment is prevented chiefly by the dorsal and interosseous sacroiliac ligaments; and the upward tilt of the posterior segment is prevented chiefly by the sacrotuberous and sacrospinous ligaments.

During all these movements the separation of iliac bones is resisted by sacroiliac and iliolumbar ligaments, and the ligaments of pubic symphysis.

CLINICAL ANATOMY

- During pregnancy the pelvic joints and ligaments are relaxed, so that the range of movement is increased and locking mechanism becomes less efficient. This naturally puts greater strain on the ligaments. The *sacroiliac strain* thus produced may persist even after pregnancy.

  After childbirth the ligaments are tightened up again, so that the locking mechanism returns to its original efficiency. Sometimes locking occurs in the rotated position of the hip bones adopted during pregnancy. This results in *subluxation* of the joint, causing low backache due to strain on ligaments.
- The *diseases of the lumbosacral and sacroiliac joints can be differentiated* by the following tests.
  a. In lumbosacral lesions, the tenderness is present over the spines and above the dimple of posterior

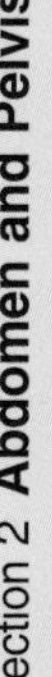

superior iliac spine (over the iliolumbar ligament); in sacroiliac lesions, the tenderness is located inferomedial to the dimple (over the posterior sacroiliac ligament) (Fig. 34.9).

b. In lumbosacral disease, the movements of vertebral column are restricted in all directions; in sacroiliac disease, the movements are free, except for extreme forward bending, when the tension on hamstrings causes backward rotation of the hip bones, opposite to that of sacrum, producing pain in a diseased joint.

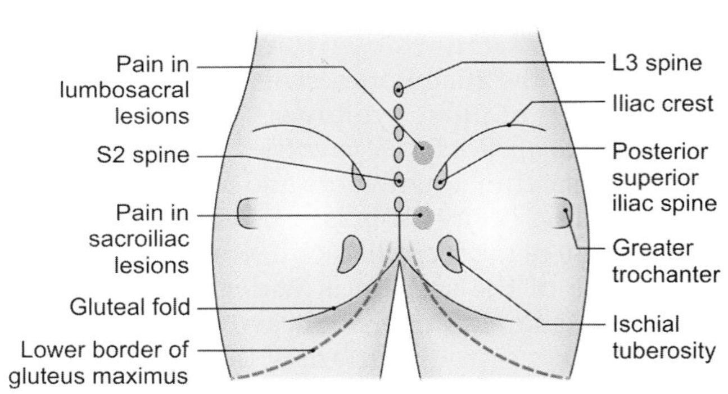

Fig. 34.9: Sites of tenderness in lumbosacral and sacroiliac lesions

FACTS TO REMEMBER

- Inferior gluteal artery is the largest branch of anterior division of internal iliac artery. It is also part of the axial artery of lower limb.
- Pelvic viscera are supported by pelvic diaphragm formed by levator ani and coccygeus muscles in the large posterior part of pelvic outlet. In its small anterior part, the muscles of urogenital region support the viscera.
- Inferior vesical is replaced by vaginal artery in female.
- Uterine artery is the additional artery exclusively in the female.
- Ventral ramus of L4 nerve takes part both in formation of lumbar plexus as well as sacral plexus and is called *nervi furcalis*.
- Nerves forming sacral plexus lie outside the parietal layer of pelvic fascia. Blood vessels of the pelvis lie inside the parietal layer.
- Interosseous sacroiliac ligament is the strongest ligament of the body.
- The free anastomoses between superior rectal vein of portal and the middle and inferior rectal veins of the caval system explain the metastases in the liver from cancers of the genital organs.
- The sensory nerve supply of the ovary and fallopian tube is from T10–T12 nerves.

CLINICOANATOMICAL PROBLEM

An elderly person was hit by a speeding car. As he fell down, he was run over by the vehicle. He was taken to the hospital.

- Which bones are likely to be fractured?
- What structures form the pelvic ring?
- Which viscera are likely to be injured?
- What type of joints are pubic symphysis and sacroiliac joints?

Ans:

- Pubic bone of one side is fractured and sacroiliac joint of the other side is dislocated.
- Pelvic ring comprises of pubic rami, acetabulum, ischium, ilium and sacrum.
- Urinary bladder is likely to be injured.
- Pubic symphysis is secondary cartilaginous joint and sacroiliac joint is plane synovial joint.

MULTIPLE CHOICE QUESTIONS

1. Following are the branches of anterior division of the internal iliac artery *except*:
   a. Superior vesical b. Inferior vesical
   c. External pudendal d. Internal pudendal
2. Following are the branches of posterior division of internal iliac artery *except*:
   a. Iliolumbar b. Two lateral sacral
   c. Superior gluteal d. Inferior gluteal
3. Branches of anterior division of internal iliac artery in female are as follows *except*:
   a. Obturator
   b. Uterine
   c. Vaginal
   d. Inferior vesical
4. Nervi erigentes arises from:
   a. Ventral rami of S2, S3, S4 segments
   b. Ventral rami of S2, S3, S4 and S5 segments
   c. Ventral rami of S1, S2, S3 segments
   d. Dorsal rami of S2, S3, S4 segments
5. Parts of levator ani are as follows *except*:
   a. Pubococcygeus b. Iliococcygeus
   c. Ischiococcygeus d. External anal sphincter

ANSWERS

1. c **2.** d **3.** d **4.** a **5.** d

35

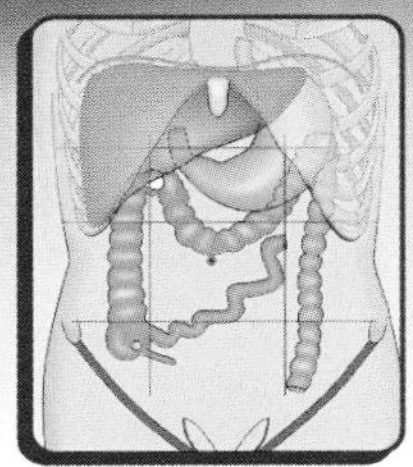

Surface Marking of Abdomen and Pelvis

It is easy to hate but it is healthy to love
—S Radhakrishanan

PLANES AND REGIONS OF THE ABDOMEN

Two horizontal (transpyloric and transtubercular) and two vertical (right and left lateral) planes divide the abdomen into nine regions (Fig. 35.1). These are described in Chapter 18.

SURFACE MARKING

Viscera

Spleen

1 It is marked on the left side of the back, with its long axis corresponding with that of the 10th rib.
2 The upper border corresponds to the upper border of the 9th rib, and the lower border to the lower border of the 11th rib (Fig. 35.2).
3 The medial end lies 4 to 5 cm from the posterior midline; and the lateral end on the left midaxillary line.

Stomach

1 *Cardiac orifice:* It is marked by two short parallel lines 2 cm apart, directed downwards and to the left on 7th costal cartilage, 2.5 cm to the left of median plane (Fig. 35.3).

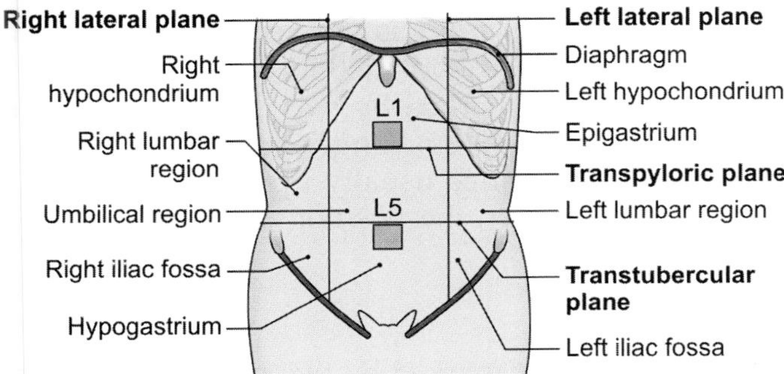

Fig. 35.1: Surface marking of regions of the abdomen

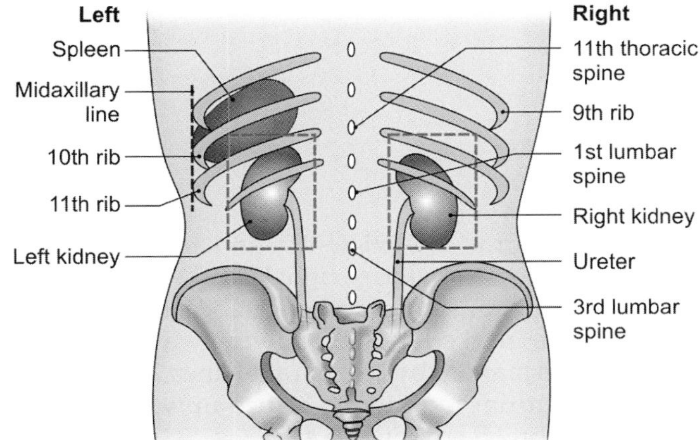

Fig. 35.2: Position of spleen, kidney and ureter from the posterior aspect

2 *Pyloric orifice:* It is marked by two short parallel lines 2 cm apart, directed upwards and to the right, on transpyloric plane, 1.2 cm to the right of the median plane.
3 *Lesser curvature:* It is marked by joining the right margin of the cardiac orifice with upper margin of the pyloric orifice by a J-shaped curved line. The lowest point of this line reaches a little below the transpyloric plane.
4 *Fundus:* This is marked by a line convex upwards drawn from the left margin of the cardiac orifice to highest point in the left 5th intercostal space just below the nipple.
5 *Greater curvature:* This is marked by a curved line convex to the left and downwards, drawn from the fundus to the lower margin of the pyloric orifice. It cuts the left costal margin between the tips of the 9th and 10th costal cartilages and extends down to the subcostal plane, i.e. level of lumbar 3 vertebra.

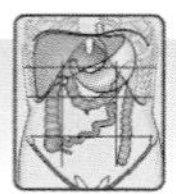

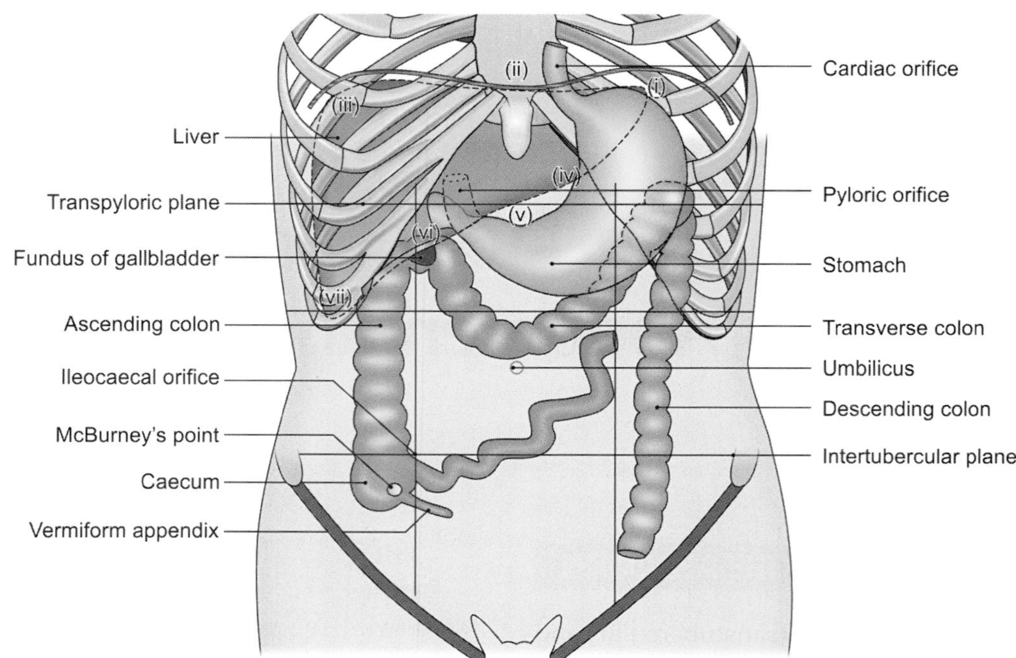

Fig. 35.3: Surface marking of some abdominal organs

Duodenum

The duodenum is 2.5 cm wide, and lies above the umbilicus. Mark the pylorus, right lateral vertical plane, median plane, transpyloric plane, subcostal plane. Its four parts are marked in the following way.

1. *First part* is marked by two parallel lines 2.5 cm apart extending from the pyloric orifice upwards and to the right for 2.5 cm (Fig. 35.4).
2. *Second part* is marked by similar lines on the right lateral vertical plane extending from the end of the first part downwards for 7.5 cm.
3. *Third part* is marked by two transverse parallel lines 2.5 cm apart on the subcostal plane, extending from the lower end of the second part towards the left for 10 cm. It crosses the median plane above the umbilicus.
4. *Fourth part* is marked by two lines extending from the left end of the third part to the duodenojejunal flexure which lies 1 cm below the transpyloric plane, and 3 cm to the left of the median plane. This part is 2.5 cm long.

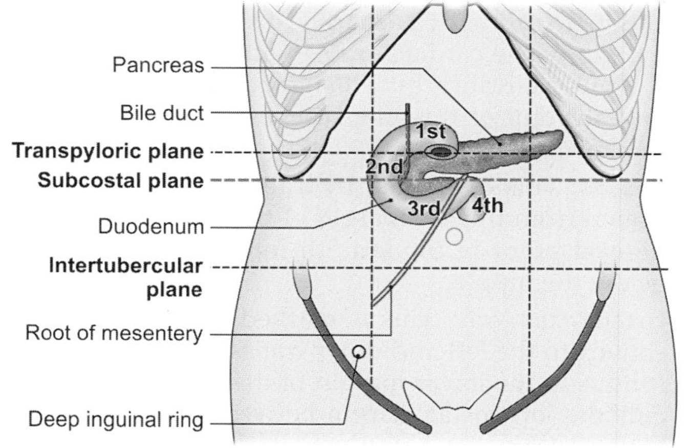

Fig. 35.4: Position of duodenum, pancreas, root of mesentery

Caecum

The caecum is marked in the right iliac fossa between inguinal ligament, right lateral plane and intertubercular plane. It is about 6 cm long and 7.5 cm broad. Its axis is directed downwards and slightly medially (Fig. 35.3).

Ileocaecal Orifice or Valve

Ileocaecal orifice is marked on the point of intersection of the right lateral and transtubercular planes (Fig. 35.3).

Appendix

1. The *appendicular orifice* is marked at a point 2 cm below the ileocaecal orifice (Fig. 35.3).
2. The *appendix* is marked by two parallel lines 1 cm apart and 7 to 10 cm long, extending from the appendicular orifice usually upwards behind the caecum. However, the position of the appendix is highly variable.

Ascending Colon

Ascending colon is marked by two parallel lines 5 cm apart, immediately to the right of the right lateral

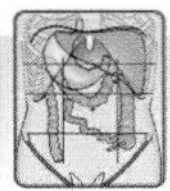

vertical plane, from the level of the intertubercular plane (upper end of caecum) to the upper part of the 9th costal cartilage (right colic flexure) (Fig. 35.3).

Transverse Colon

Transverse colon is marked by two parallel lines 5 cm apart. It begins at the upper part of the 9th costal cartilage (right colic flexure), runs downwards and medially to the umbilicus, and then upwards and laterally, crossing the transpyloric plane and also the left lateral vertical plane, to end at the 8th costal cartilage (left colic flexure) (Fig. 35.3).

Descending Colon

Descending colon is marked by two parallel lines 2.5 cm apart. It begins at the 8th costal cartilage (left colic flexure), runs downward immediately lateral to the left lateral vertical plane, and ends at the fold of the groin (inguinal ligament) (Fig. 35.3).

Rectum and Anal Canal

Rectum and anal canal are marked on the back by drawing two lines joining the posterior superior iliac spines to the anus. The lower parts of these lines (from 1 cm below the second sacral spine) represent the rectum and anal canal.

Liver

In surface projection from anterior aspect the liver is triangular in shape when seen from the front.

Planes to be drawn:

- Right midclavicular line
- Left midclavicular line
- Median line
- Transpyloric plane
- Subcostal plane

a. The *upper border* (Fig. 35.3) is marked by joining the following points:
   - First point (i) in the left 5th intercostal space below and medial to left nipple.
   - Second point (ii) at the xiphisternal joint.
   - Third point (iii) at the upper border of the right 5th costal cartilage in the right lateral vertical plane.

b. The *lower border* (Fig. 35.3) is marked by a curved line joining the following points.
   - First point (i) in the left 5th intercostal space below and medial to left nipple.
   - Fourth point (iv) at the tip of the 8th costal cartilage on the left costal margin.
   - Fifth point (v) at the transpyloric plane in the midline.
   - Sixth point (vi) at the tip of the 9th costal cartilage on the right costal margin.
   - Seventh point (vii) 1 cm below the right costal margin at the tip of 10th costal cartilage.

c. The *right border* is marked on the front by a curved line convex laterally, drawn from a point little below the right nipple to a point 1 cm below the right costal margin at the tip of the 10th costal cartilage (points number (iii) and (vii).

Gallbladder

The fundus of the gallbladder (Fig. 35.3) is marked by a small convex area at the tip of right 9th costal cartilage.

Bile Duct

Bile duct is marked by a line 7.5 cm long. The line is vertical in its upper half and inclines to the right in its lower half. The line extends from a point 5 cm above the transpyloric plane and 2 cm to the right of the median plane, to the middle of the medial border of the second part of the duodenum (Fig. 35.4).

Pancreas

First draw duodenum.

1 The *head* is marked within the concavity of the duodenum (Fig. 35.4).
2 The *neck* passes upwards and to the left behind the pylorus in the transpyloric plane.
3 The *body* is marked by two parallel lines 3 cm apart, drawn upwards and to the left for 10 cm from the neck, occupying the upper two-thirds of the space between the transpyloric and subcostal planes.

Kidney

The kidney measures 11 × 5 cm. It can be marked both on the back as well on the front.

On the back, it is marked within *Morrison's parallelogram* which is drawn in the following way. Two horizontal lines are drawn, one at the level of the 11th thoracic spine and the other at the level of the 3rd lumbar spine (Fig. 35.2).

On the front, the bean-shaped kidney is marked with following specifications.

a. On the right side the *centre of the hilum* lies 5 cm from the median plane a little below the transpyloric plane; and on the left side it lies 5 cm from the median plane a little above the transpyloric plane, just medial to the tip of the 9th costal cartilage.
b. The *upper pole* lies 4 to 5 cm from the midline, half way between the xiphisternum and the transpyloric plane (right one, a little lower).
c. The *lower pole* lies 6 to 7 cm from the midline on the right side at the umbilical plane and on the left side at subcostal plane (Fig. 35.5).

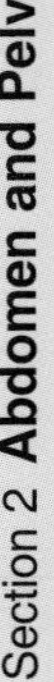

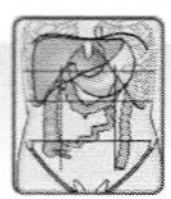

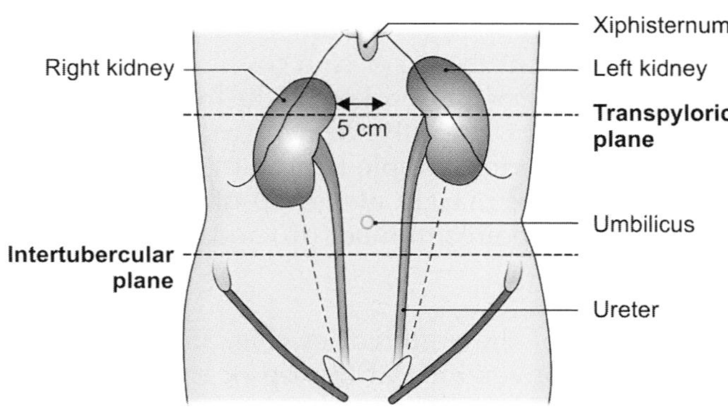

Fig. 35.5: Surface marking of kidneys from anterior aspect

Ureter

The ureter can also be marked both on the front as well as on the back.

1 *On the front,* it is marked by a line running downwards and slightly medially from the tip of the 9th costal cartilage to the pubic tubercle. The upper 5 cm of this line represents the renal pelvis (Fig. 35.5).
2 *On the back,* it is marked by a line running vertically upwards from the posterior superior iliac spine to the level of the second lumbar spine. The lower end of the renal hilum lies at this level (Fig. 35.2).

Vessels

Abdominal Aorta

Abdominal aorta is marked by two parallel lines 2 cm apart, extending from a point 2.5 cm above the transpyloric plane in the median plane to a point 1.2 cm below and to the left of the umbilicus (level of vertebra L4).

Common Iliac Artery

Common iliac artery is represented by the upper one-third of a broad line drawn from the lower end of the abdominal aorta to the midinguinal point (midpoint between ASIS and pubic symphysis).

External Iliac Artery

External iliac artery is represented by the lower two-thirds of a line drawn from the lower end of the abdominal aorta to the midinguinal point.

Coeliac Trunk and its Branches

The coeliac trunk is marked as a point 1 cm below the beginning of the abdominal aorta (Fig. 35.6).

The *left gastric artery* is marked by a line passing from the coeliac artery upwards and to the left towards the cardiac end of the stomach.

The *splenic artery* is marked by a broad line passing from the coeliac artery towards the left and slightly upwards for about 10 cm.

The *common hepatic artery* is marked by a line passing from the coeliac artery towards the right and slightly downwards for 2.5 cm, and then vertically upwards for 3 cm as proper hepatic artery.

Superior Mesenteric Artery

Superior mesenteric artery is marked by a curved line convex to the left, extending from the abdominal aorta just above the transpyloric plane to the point of intersection of the transtubercular and right lateral planes.

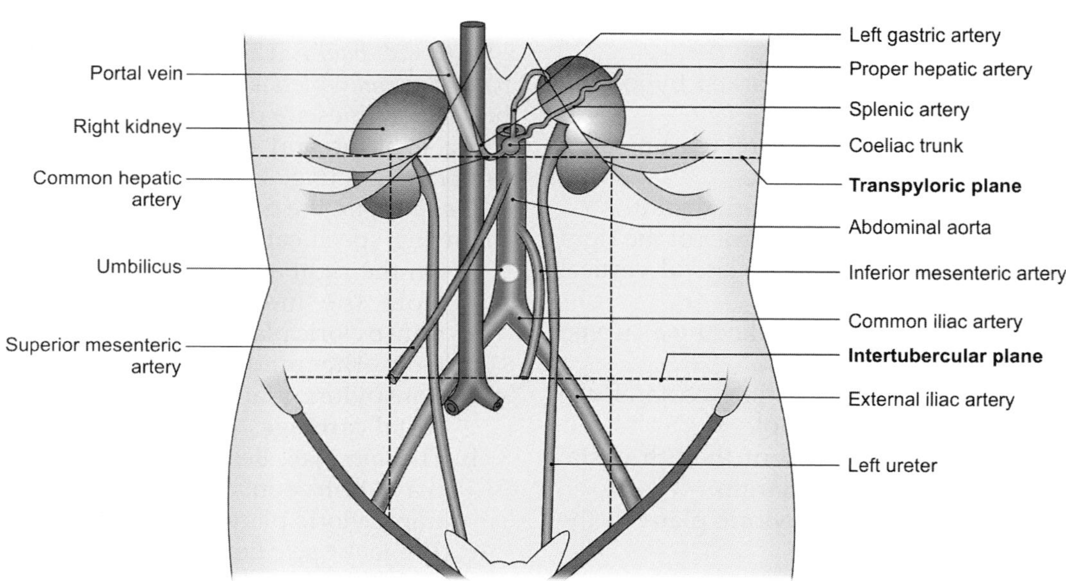

Fig. 35.6: Surface marking of various blood vessels and kidneys

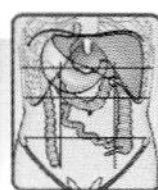

Inferior Mesenteric Artery

Inferior mesenteric artery is marked by a curved line slightly convex to the left, extending from the abdominal aorta 4 cm below the transpyloric plane to a point 4 cm below the umbilicus, and about the same distance to the left of median plane (Fig. 35.6).

Inferior Vena Cava

Inferior vena cava is marked by two vertical parallel lines 2.5 cm apart, a little to the right of the median plane. It extends from a point just below the trans-tubercular plane to the sternal end of the right 6th costal cartilage.

Portal Vein

Portal vein is marked by a broad line extending from a point on the transpyloric plane 1.2 cm to the right of the median plane upwards and to the right for about 8 cm (Fig. 35.6).

Miscellaneous

Inguinal Canal

Inguinal canal is marked by two parallel lines 1 cm apart and about 3.7 cm long, above the medial half of the inguinal ligament, extending from the deep to the superficial inguinal rings.

The *deep inguinal ring* is marked 1 cm above the midinguinal point, as a vertical oval ring (Fig. 35.7).

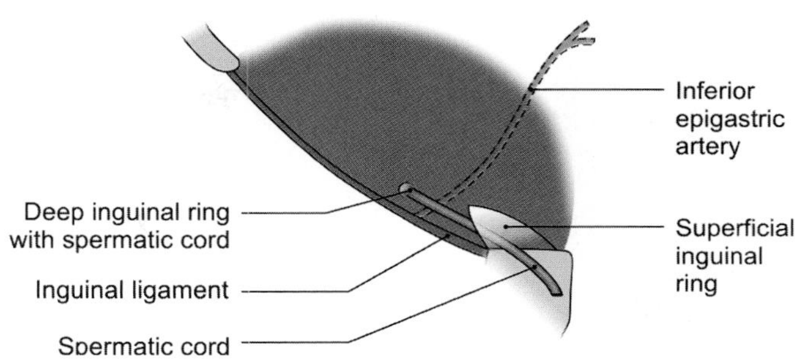

Fig. 35.7: Superficial and deep inguinal rings

Superficial inguinal ring lies above and lateral to the pubic crest. Pubic crest forms the base of the triangle; the margins are called the crura. Each crus meets laterally to form an obtuse apex, which lies above and lateral to pubic tubercle. Lateral crus is thicker and curved while medial crus is thinner and oblique.

Root of Mesentery

Root of mesentery is marked by two parallel lines close together, extending from the duodenojejunal flexure to the junction to the right lateral and transtubercular planes. The duodenojejunal flexure lies 1 cm below the transpyloric plane and 3 cm to the left of the median plane (Fig. 35.4).

36

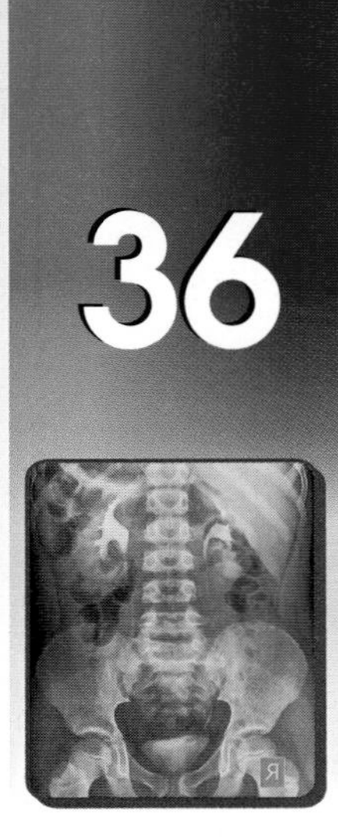

Radiological and Imaging Procedures

Never forget that it is not a pneumonia, but a pneumonic man who is your patient
—WW Gull

The common radiological methods used for the study or investigation of abdomen include the following.
1 Plain radiography.
2 Barium studies for the gastrointestinal tract.
3 Ultrasonography for the gallbladder, cystic duct, bile duct, pancreas, kidneys, spleen, abdominal vessels, uterus, ovaries and prostate.
4 Hysterosalpingography for uterus and fallopian tubes.
5 Aortography and selective angiography for coeliac, superior and inferior mesenteric vessels, iliac vessels and renal vessels.

PLAIN SKIAGRAM OF ABDOMEN

Nomenclature

Anteroposterior plain skiagram of the abdomen has been variously named, as the straight film, survey film, scout and KUB film. When done in a case of acute abdomen, it is often called a straight film. A scout film is obtained before taking a contrast radiograph. A KUB film is taken primarily for examining the kidney, ureter, and urinary bladder, for which the acronym KUB stands.

Preparation

In cases of emergency, requiring urgent surgical intervention, a straight film is taken without any preparation. However, in chronic conditions it is better to prepare the patient to obtain a clear and good picture. The object of preparation is to make the gastrointestinal tract as empty as possible, free from food in the stomach and from gases and faecal matter in the intestines. This may be achieved by:
1 Using antiflatulents for 3 days antiflatulents, like enzyme preparations, charcoal tablets and laxatives.
2 Avoiding oral feeds for about 12 hours before the investigation. Constipated subjects may require an enema to empty their bowels.

In a picture taken without any preparation, the shadows of the gases and faecal matter may completely mask the significant findings.

Reading of Skiagram

The plain skiagram of the abdomen can be studied systematically in the following way.

Bony Shadows

The radiograph (Fig. 36.1) shows:
1 The lower ribs.
2 Lumbar vertebrae.
3 Upper parts of the hip bones.
4 Sacrum with the sacroiliac joints.

However, the whole of the pelvis may have been included in the exposure. The bony shadows are used as landmarks for the assessment of the position of viscera and of existing abnormalities. Any variation in the ribs and vertebrae, if present, may be noted.

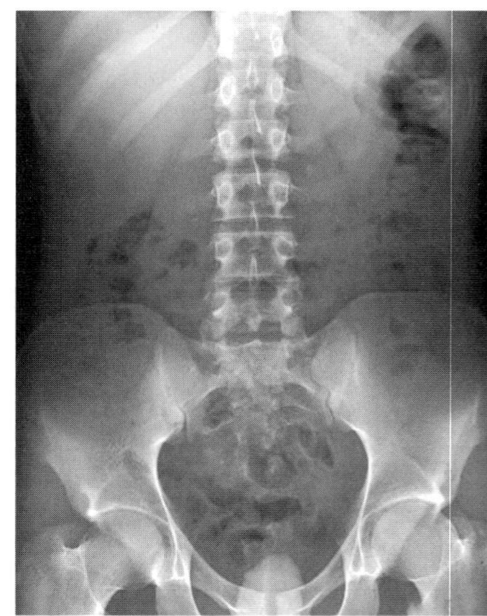

Fig. 36.1: Plain X-ray abdomen

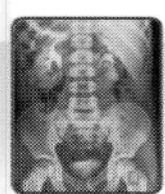

Soft Tissue Shadows

The faint shadows of the following structures may be seen.

1 Domes of the diaphragm.
2 Psoas major.
3 Kidney, made visible by the perirenal fat.
4 Liver, beneath the right dome of diaphragm.
5 The spleen.

Gas Shadows

Gas shadows are seen as black shadows because gases are radiolucent.

1 Gas in the fundus of stomach appears as a large bubble under the left dome of diaphragm.
2 The scattered intestinal gas shadows are often intermixed with the shadows of faecal matter.

Abnormal Shadows

Various abnormal shadows may be seen in different diseases.

ALIMENTARY CANAL: BARIUM STUDIES

Contrast Medium

The alimentary canal can be visualized and examined radiologically by using a suspension of barium sulphate in water. Barium is radio-opaque because of its high molecular weight. Barium sulphate is absolutely harmless to the body and is not absorbed from the gastrointestinal tract. Barium sulphate is not soluble in water, and can make only a suspension or emulsion in it.

Principle Involved

The passage of barium through the lumen outlines the mucosal patterns, which can be examined under a screen (fluoroscopy) or radiographed on a film.

Barium Swallow

50% suspension of barium sulphate is to be swallowed 2–3 times with patient standing behind fluoroscopic screen. Barium swallow shows the normal position of oesophagus as it lies posterior to aortic arch, left bronchus and the left atrium of heart (Fig. 36.2).

Enlargement of left atrium would show narrowed oesophagus.

Barium Meal Examination

Preparation

The subject is instructed not to eat or drink anything for 12 hours before the examination.

Administration of Contrast Medium

The patient is made to drink 300 to 400 cc (10 to 15 oz.) of a 5% barium sulphate suspension in water, and then

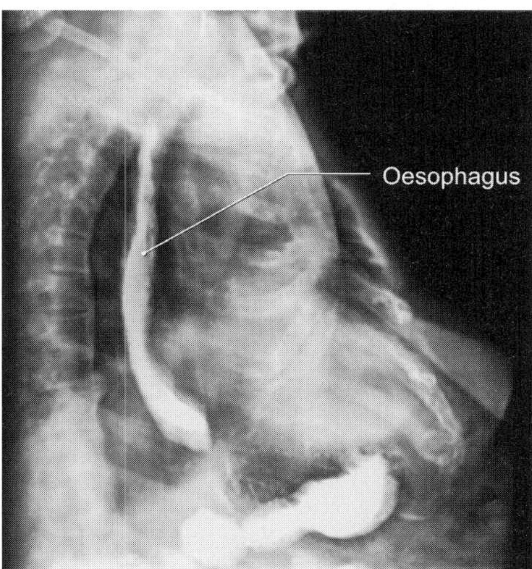

Fig. 36.2: Barium swallow

examined under fluoroscopy. Thus, the entire alimentary canal can be examined by following the barium and taking successive radiographs. The stomach and duodenum are visualized immediately after the barium drink (Fig. 36.3). The medium reaches the ileocaecal region in 3 to 4 hours, the hepatic flexure of the colon in about 6 hours, the splenic flexure of the colon in about 9 hours, the descending colon in 11 hours, and the sigmoid colon in about 16 hours. It is usually evacuated in 16 to 24 hours. However, some barium may persist in the large intestine for several days.

Stomach

As barium enters the stomach, it tends to form a triangular mass below the air in the fundus. It then descends in a narrow stream (canalization) to the

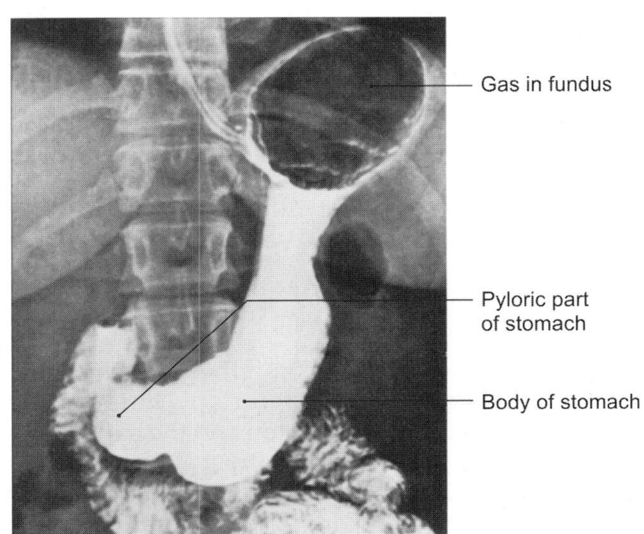

Fig. 36.3: Barium meal

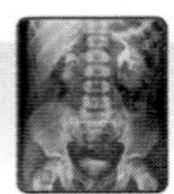

pyloric part of the stomach. In addition, the shape, curvatures, peristaltic waves, and the rate of emptying of the stomach can also be studied.

Duodenum

The beginning of the first part of duodenum shows a well-formed *duodenal cap* produced by poorly developed circular folds of mucous membrane and protruding pylorus into it. The rest of the duodenum has a characteristic feathery or floccular appearance due to the presence of well-developed circular folds.

Jejunum and Ileum

The greater part of the small intestine presents a feathery or floccular appearance due to the presence of transverse mucosal folds and their rapid movements. However, the terminal part of the ileum is comparatively narrow and shows a homogeneous shadow of barium.

Large Intestine

It is identified by its smooth outline marked by characteristic haustra or sacculations which are most prominent in the proximal part and may disappear in the distal part. Acute curvatures at the flexures cause superimposition of the shadows. Occasionally, the appendix may also be visible. Diseases of the large intestine are better examined by barium enema which gives a better filling.

Barium Enema

Preparation

1 A mild laxative is given on two nights before the examination.
2 A plain warm water enema on the morning of the examination.

Contrast Medium

About 2 litters of barium sulphate suspension are slowly introduced through the anus, from a can kept at a height of 2 to 4 feet. The enema is stopped when the barium starts flowing into the terminal ileum through the ileocaecal valve (as seen under the fluoroscopic screen).

Appearance

The rectum and sigmoid colon appear much dilated, and the colon shows characteristic haustrations (Fig. 36.4). The outline of the colon and the haustra may be accentuated by the double-contrast method in which the barium is evacuated and air is injected through the anus to distend the colon. In the background of air, the barium still lining the mucosa makes it clearly visible.

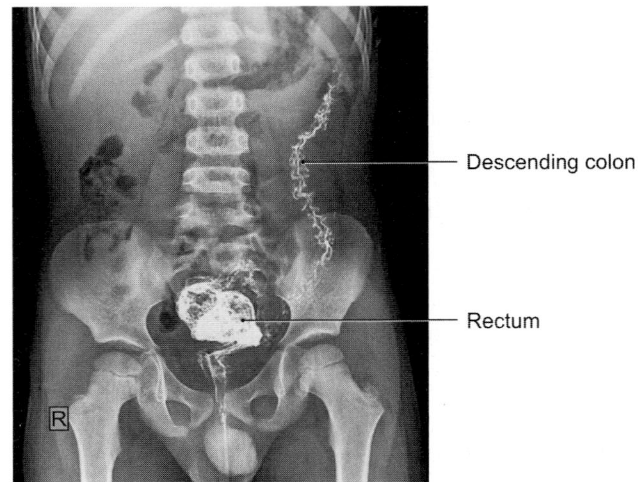

Fig. 36.4: Barium enema

PYELOGRAPHY

Pyelography (urography) is a radiological method by which the urinary tract is visualized. The radiograph thus obtained is called a *pyelogram*. It can be done in two ways depending on the route of administration of the radiopaque dye. When the dye is injected intravenously, it is called the *excretory* (*intravenous* or *descending*) *pyelography*. When the dye is injected directly into the ureter, through a ureteric catheter guided through a cystoscope, the technique is called *retrograde* (*instrumental* or *ascending*) *pyelography*.

Excretory (Intravenous or Descending) Pyelography

Preparation

In addition to routine abdomen preparation:

1 For 8 hours before pyelography, the patient is not given anything orally, all fluids are withheld, and diuretics are discontinued.
2 Patient is asked to empty his bladder just before the injection of the dye (Fig. 36.5).

Administration of the Dye

20–40 cc of a warm iodine compound (urograffin 60% or 76% Conray 420 or Conray 280) which is selectively excreted by the kidneys, is slowly injected intravenously. Care is taken not to push any dye outside the vein because it is an irritant and may cause sloughing.

Exposures

Serial skiagram (excretory pyelograms) are taken at 5, 15 and 30 minutes after the injection of the dye. Maximum concentration is reached in 15 to 20 minutes, and by 30 minutes the dye fills the urinary bladder.

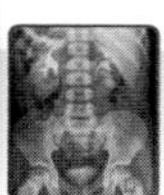

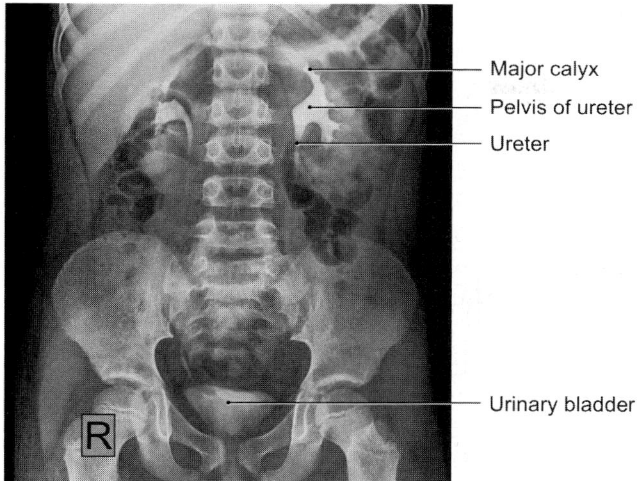

Fig. 36.5: Intravenous pyelogram

Reading

Intravenous pyelography is an anatomical as well as a physiological test because it permits not only visualisation of the urinary tract but also helps in assessment of the functional status of the kidney. Normally:

1. Minor calices are cup shaped due to the renal papillae projecting into them.
2. Renal pelvis is funnel-shaped.
3. Course of the ureter is clearly seen along the tips of the lumbar transverse processes, the sacroiliac joint and the ischial spine, up to the bladder.
4. Bladder appears oval or triangular in shape.

Retrograde (Instrumental or Ascending) Pyelography

Preparation

Preparation of the patient is similar to that for descending pyelography.

Injection of Dye

The technique is quite difficult and can be done only by urologists. A cystoscope is passed into the urinary bladder through the urethra. Then the ureteric catheter is guided into the ureteric opening and passed up to the renal pelvis. Through the catheter, 5 to 10 ml of a sterile solution of 6–8% sodium iodide (Conray 280) is injected. As the renal pelvis is filled to its capacity, the patient begins to complain of pain, when further injection must be stopped. General anaesthesia is therefore, contraindicated because of the risk of overdistension of the pelvis. If the renal pelvis admits more than 10 ml of the dye, hydronephrosis is suspected.

An ascending pyelogram can be distinguished from a descending pyelogram because:

a. Only one pelvis is outlined.
b. The catheter through which the dye is injected can be seen.

BILIARY APPARATUS

Investigation of Choice

The investigation of choice for gallbladder is *ultrasonography*. It can be undertaken on a fasting patient. Gallbladder is seen as a cystic oval shadow with a narrow neck in the right upper quadrant along with visualisation of the bile duct and portal vein. However, endoscopic retrograde cholangio-pancreaticography (ERCP) can be carried out to outline the intrahepatic radicals, bile duct, pancreatic duct and gallbladder through the oral route via an endoscope through which a catheter is inserted and the contrast is injected into the common bile duct.

Ultrasonography of abdomen shows pancreas and related structures (Figs 36.6a and b).

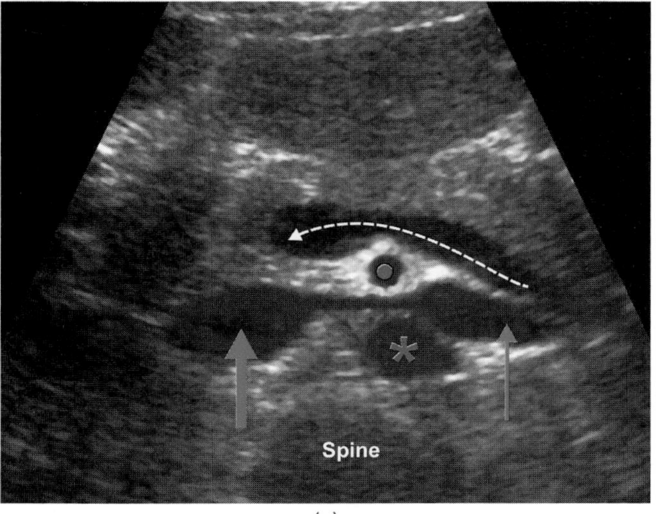

(a)

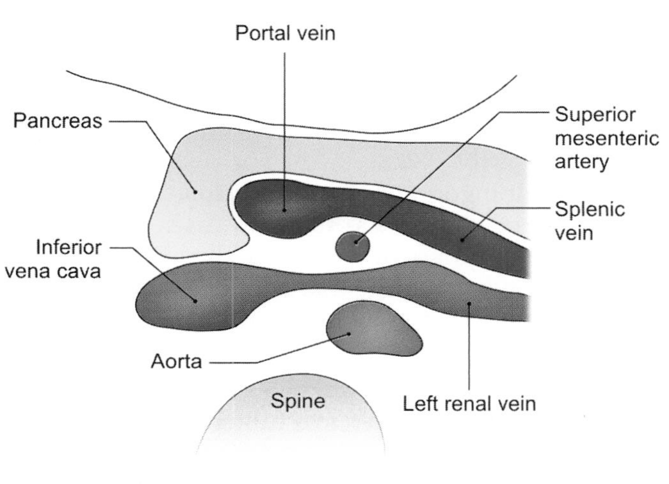

(b)

Figs 36.6a and b: Ultrasound image of pancreas and related structures

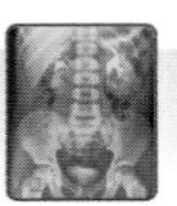

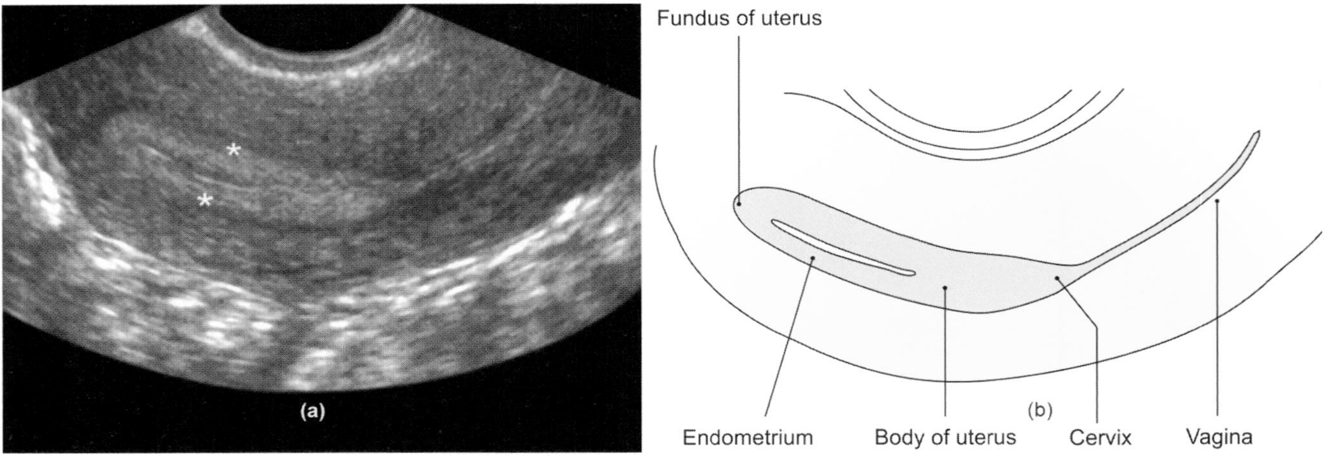

Figs 36.7a and b: Ultrasound image of uterus and cervix

Oral cholecystography is an outdated method for visualising the gallbladder by taking radiopaque dye which is exclusively excreted by the liver and concentrated by the gallbladder. The contrast is taken overnight and X-rays are taken 14–16 hours after the intake of the dye and gallbladder, cystic duct and bile duct can be seen. It is, however, dependent on the proper absorption from intestines.

Uterus of the female pelvis is seen by ultrasonography (Figs 36.7a and b).

HYSTEROSALPINGOGRAPHY

This is a radiological method by which the uterus and uterine tubes are visualized and their patency confirmed. The radiograph thus obtained is called a *hysterosalpingogram*.

The investigation is done preferably within the first 5 to 10 days of the menstrual cycle. A tight-fitting cannula is introduced into the internal os of the cervix. The cannula is connected to a syringe through which 5 to 10 ml of an iodized oil (lipiodol) are injected, and the skiagram taken.

The shape and size of the uterus and of the uterine tubes are studied. Spilling of the dye into the peritoneal cavity is noted (Fig. 36.8).

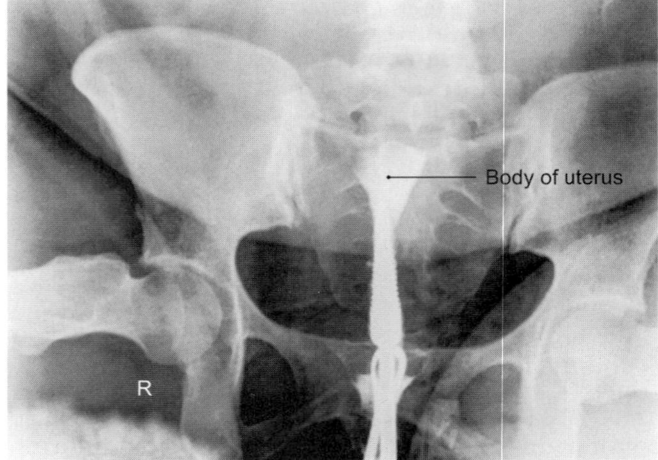

Fig. 36.8: Hysterosalpingogram

Hysterosalpingography is usually done to determine the patency of the uterine tubes in cases of sterility. However, it is also of value in the diagnosis of anomalies of the female genital tract. The female pelvic organs can also be seen by ultrasound.

FOETOGRAM

Plain X-ray of the abdomen in a fullterm pregnant lady showing the foetus with vertex presentation. The shaft of bones of upper and lower limbs and body of vertebrae can easily be identified and appreciated (Fig. 36.9).

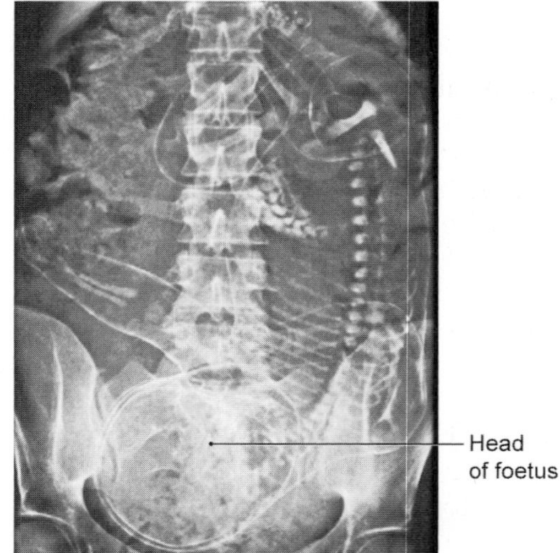

Fig. 36.9: Foetogram

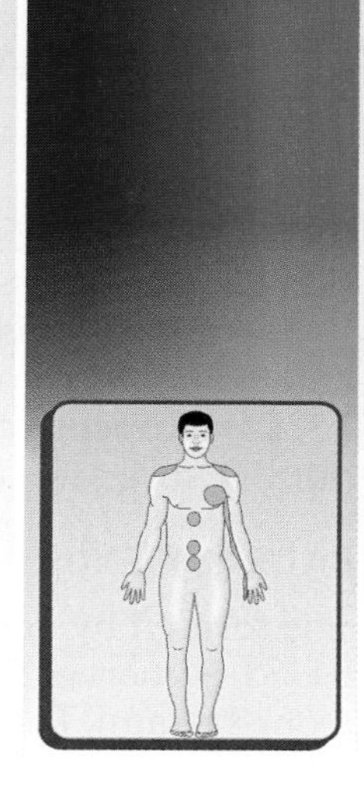

Appendix 2

And lo, the Hospital, grey, quiet, old where Life and Death like friendly chafferes meet
—Wilhan Errest Henley

NERVES OF ABDOMEN

LOWER INTERCOSTAL NERVES

Course

The ventral rami of T7–T11 pass forwards in the intercostal spaces below respective intercostal vessels. At the back of chest they lie between the pleura and posterior intercostal membrane but in most of their course they lie between internal intercostal and intercostalis intimi.

As they reach the anterior ends of their respective spaces, the 7th and 8th nerves curve upwards and medially across the deep surface of costal margin, passing between digitations of transverses abdominis then piercing the posterior layer of internal oblique, to enter the rectus sheath, and continue to run upwards and medially parallel to the costal margin. After supplying rectus abdominis, they pierce the anterior wall of the rectus sheath to reach the skin. 7th nerve supplies skin of the epigastrium and 8th below it.

At the anterior ends of 9th, 10th and 11th intercostal spaces, the 9th, 10th and 11th intercostal nerves pass between digitations of transversus abdominis to lie between it and the internal oblique and run in this plane. The 9th nerve runs horizontally, but 10th and 11th run downwards and medially.

When they reach the lateral margin of rectus abdominis, they pierce the posterior layer of rectus sheath, enter it, pierce the muscle and its anterior sheath to supply the skin. The 10th nerve supplies the band of skin which includes the umbilicus.

The ventral ramus of T12 is larger than the others. It accompanies the subcostal artery along the lower border of 12th rib and passes behind the lateral arcuate ligament. It lies behind the kidney, anterior to quadratus lumborum, pierces the aponeurosis of transversus abdominis and runs in the interval between transversus and internal oblique.

Branches

Muscular

The intercostal and subcostal nerves and their collateral branches supply intercostal muscles and muscles of anterolateral abdominal wall. T12 supplies pyramidalis also, if present.

Cutaneous

The terminal parts of T7–T12 nerves are called as the anterior cutaneous branches. These supply the skin close to the anterior median line. T10 supplying the skin around umbilicus; T7, the skin of epigastrium and T8, T9 the intervening skin between epigastrium and the umbilicus. T11, T12 and iliohypogastric (L1) supply the skin between umbilicus and pubic symphysis.

The lateral cutaneous branches of the T7–T11 intercostal nerves divide into anterior and posterior branches to supply the skin of lateral side of abdomen and back.

The lateral cutaneous branch of T12 supplies the skin of anterior part of the gluteal region.

UPPER LUMBAR NERVES

1 Iliohypogastric.
2 Ilioinguinal.
3 Genitofemoral.
4 Lateral cutaneous nerve of thigh.

All these nerves are described in Chapter 27.

LUMBAR PLEXUS

Formed by ventral rami of L1, L2, L3 and part of L4. These rami divide into dorsal and ventral divisions. From the ventral divisions of these rami arise

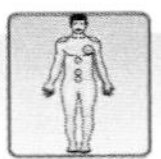

ilioinguinal (L1), genitofemoral (L1, L2), obturator (L2, L3, L4), accessory obturator (L3, L4) nerves.

The dorsal divisions of these rami give rise to lateral cutaneous nerve of thigh (L2, L3), femoral nerve (L2, L3, L4) (Appendix 1). Iliohypogastric contains fibres of both ventral and dorsal divisions (L1).

SACRAL PLEXUS

It is formed by ventral rami of part of L4, whole of L5, S1, S2, S3 nerves. Few muscular branches are given off from the rami. Then these divide into ventral and dorsal divisions.

Branches arising from ventral divisions are:

1. Nerve to quadratus femoris (L4, L5, S1): Supplies quadratus femoris, inferior gemellus and hip joint.
2. Nerve to obturator internus (L5, S1, S2): Supplies obturator internus and superior gemellus.
3. Pudendal nerve (S2, S3, S4) is described below.
4. Perforating cutaneous nerve (S3, S4): Supplies small area of skin of gluteal region.
5. Tibial part of sciatic nerve (L4, L5, S1, S2, S3): Supplies hamstrings, all muscles of the calf and of the sole.
6. Posterior cutaneous nerve of thigh (S1, S2): Supplies skin of back of thigh.

Branches from dorsal divisions are:

1. Superior gluteal nerve (L4, L5, S1): Supplies gluteus medius, gluteus minimus and tensor fascia latae.
2. Inferior gluteal nerve (L5, S1, S2): Supplies only gluteus maximus.
3. Common peroneal part of sciatic nerve (L4, L5, S1, S2): Supplies evertors and foot and dorsiflexors of ankle joint and extensor digitorum brevis.

Pudendal Nerve

Pudendal nerve supplies the skin, external genital organs and muscles of perineum. It is concerned with micturition, defaecation, erection, ejaculation and in females, with parturition. It is accompanied by internal pudendal vessels.

Root value: It arises from the sacral plexus in the pelvis. Its root value is ventral rami of S2, S3, S4 segments of spinal cord.

Course: It starts in the pelvis, enters the gluteal region through greater sciatic notch, lies on the sacrospinous ligament, leaves the gluteal region through lesser sciatic notch. It just peeps into the gluteal region to enter the pudendal canal in the lateral wall of the ischiorectal fossa.

Branches

1. *Inferior rectal nerve:* Skin around anus, external anal sphincter and lining of anal canal below the pectinate line.
2. *Perineal nerve:* Medial and lateral scrotal/labial branches. Muscular branches to deep transversus perinei, ischiocavernosus, bulbospongiosus, external anal sphincter, levator ani, corpus spongiosum, penis and urethra, lower 2.5 cm of vagina.
3. *Dorsal nerve of penis/clitoris:* Passes through deep perineal space, then runs on the dorsum of penis/clitoris and ends in the glans; supplying skin of body of penis/clitoris and of the glans.

Clinical Anatomy

Pudendal nerve block is given in some vaginal operations and may be given during delivery.

ABDOMINAL PART OF SYMPATHETIC TRUNK

Sympathetic trunk runs along the medial border of psoas major muscle. It is continuous with the pelvic part by passing behind the common iliac vessels. There are 4 ganglia in the lumbar or abdominal part. Only upper two ganglia receive white ramus communicans from the ventral primary rami of first and second lumbar nerves.

Branches

1. Grey rami communicans to the lumbar spinal nerves. These pass along the spinal nerves to be distributed to the sweat glands, cutaneous blood vessels and arrector pili muscles (sudomotor, vasomotor and pilomotor).
2. Postganglionic fibres pass medially to the aortic plexus.
3. Postganglionic fibres pass in front of common iliac vessels to form hypogastric plexus, which is also supplemented by branches of aortic plexus.

Aortic Plexus

This plexus is formed by preganglionic sympathetic, postganglionic sympathetic, preganglionic parasympathetic and visceral afferent fibres around the abdominal aorta. The plexus is concentrated around the origin of ventral and lateral branches of abdominal aorta. These are known as coeliac plexus, superior mesenteric plexus, inferior mesenteric plexus, and renal plexus.

PELVIC PART OF SYMPATHETIC TRUNK

It runs in front of sacrum, medial to ventral sacral foramina. Caudally the two trunks unite and fuse into a single *ganglion impar* in front of coccyx. There are 4 ganglia in this part of sympathetic trunk. Their branches are:

1. Grey rami communicans to the sacral and coccygeal nerves.
2. Branches to the pelvic plexuses.

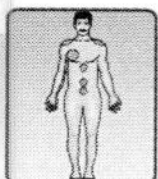

COLLATERAL OR PREVERTEBRAL GANGLIA AND PLEXUSES

Coeliac Plexus

It is the largest of the three autonomic plexuses, e.g. coeliac, superior mesenteric and inferior mesenteric plexuses. It is a dense network of nerve fibres which unite the two coeliac ganglia. The ganglia receive the greater splanchnic nerves, lesser splanchnic nerves of both sides including some filaments of vagi and phrenic nerves.

Coeliac ganglia are two irregularly shaped ganglia. Each ganglion receives greater splanchnic nerve. The lower part of the ganglion receives lesser splanchnic nerve and is also called as aorticorenal ganglion. The aorticorenal ganglion gives off the renal plexus which accompanies the renal vessels.

Secondary plexuses arising from coeliac and aorticorenal plexuses are distributed along the branches of the aorta, namely phrenic, splenic, left gastric, hepatic, intermesenteric, suprarenal, renal, gonadal, superior and inferior mesenteric plexuses, and abdominal aortic plexus.

Superior Hypogastric Plexus

This plexus lies between the two common iliac arteries and is formed by:

1 Aortic plexus.
2 Branches from third and fourth lumbar sympathetic ganglia.

It divides into right *and left inferior hypogastric plexus* (pelvic plexus); which runs on the medial side of internal iliac artery and is supplemented by pelvic splanchnic nerves (parasympathetic nerves). Thus inferior hypogastric plexus contains both sympathetic and parasympathetic nerves. These are for the supply of the pelvic viscera along the branches of the arteries. The plexuses supply gastrointestinal tract and genitourinary tract.

AUTONOMIC NERVE SUPPLY OF VARIOUS ORGANS

Gastrointestinal Tract

Oesophagus

It receives its nerve supply from vagus and sympathetic.

Cervical part of oesophagus receives branches from recurrent laryngeal nerve of vagus and middle cervical ganglion of sympathetic trunk.

Thoracic part gets branches from vagal trunks and oesophageal plexus as well as from sympathetic trunks and greater splanchnic nerves.

Abdominal part receives fibres from vagal trunk (i.e. anterior and posterior gastric nerves), thoracic part of sympathetic trunks, greater splanchnic nerves and plexus around left gastric artery. The nerves form a plexus called *myenteric* plexus between two layers of the muscularis externa and another one in the submucous layer.

Stomach

Sympathetic supply reaches from coeliac plexus along gastric and gastroepiploic arteries. A few branches also reach from thoracic and lumbar sympathetic trunks.

Parasympathetic supply is derived from vagus nerves. The left vagus forms anterior gastric, while right vagus comprises posterior gastric nerve. The anterior gastric nerve supplies cardiac orifice, anterior surface of body as well as fundus of stomach, pylorus and liver.

Posterior gastric nerve supplies posterior surface of body and fundus till pyloric antrum. It gives a number of coeliac branches, which form part of the coeliac plexus.

Vagus is secretomotor to stomach. Its stimulation causes secretion which is rich in pepsin. Sympathetic inhibits peristalsis and is motor to the pyloric sphincter. It also carries pain fibres from stomach. Spasm, ischaemia and distension causes pain.

Small Intestine

The nerves of this part of the gut are derived from coeliac ganglia formed by posterior gastric nerve (parasympathetic) and the plexus around superior mesenteric artery. These nerves form myenteric plexus and submucous plexus. Parasympathetic fibres relay in the ganglion cells present in these plexuses. Sympathetic inhibits the peristaltic movements of intestine but stimulates the sphincters.

Large Intestine

Large intestine except the lower half of anal canal is supplied by both components of autonomic nervous system. The derivatives of midgut, i.e. caecum, vermiform appendix, ascending colon and right two-thirds of transverse colon receive their sympathetic nerve supply from coeliac and superior mesenteric ganglia and parasympathetic from vagus nerve.

Left one-third of transverse colon, descending colon, sigmoid colon, rectum and upper half of anal canal (developed from hindgut and anorectal canal) receive their sympathetic nerve supply from lumbar part of sympathetic trunk and superior hypogastric plexus through the plexuses on the branches of inferior mesenteric artery. Its effect is chiefly vasomotor. Parasympathetic supply of colon is received from pelvic splanchnic nerves.

Pelvic splanchnic nerves give fibres to inferior hypogastric plexuses to supply rectum and upper half

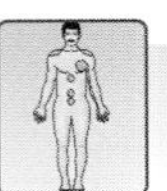

of anal canal. Some fibres of inferior hypogastric plexus pass up through superior hypogastric plexus and get distributed along the branches of inferior mesenteric artery to the left one-third of transverse colon, descending and sigmoid colon.

Rectum and Anal Canal

Sympathetic fibres pass along inferior mesenteric and superior rectal arteries also via superior and inferior hypogastric plexuses.

Parasympathetic supply is from pelvic splanchnic nerve, which joins inferior hypogastric plexus. This supply is motor to muscles of rectum and inhibitory to internal sphincter.

The external anal sphincter is supplied by inferior rectal branch of pudendal nerve. Afferent impulses of physiological distension of rectum and sigmoid colon are carried by parasympathetic, whereas pain impulses are conveyed both by sympathetic and parasympathetic nerves.

Pancreas

Branches of coeliac plexus pass along the arteries. Sympathetic is vasomotor. The nerve fibres make synaptic contact with acinar cells before innervating the islets. The parasympathetic ganglia lies in sparse connective tissue of the gland and in the islet cells.

Liver

Nerves of the liver are derived from hepatic plexus which contain both sympathetic and parasympathetic fibres. These accompany the blood vessels and bile ducts. Both types of nerve fibres also reach the liver through various peritoneal folds.

Gallbladder

Parasympathetic and sympathetic nerves of gallbladder are derived from coeliac plexus, along the hepatic artery (hepatic plexus) and its branches. Fibres from the right phrenic nerve (C4) through the communication of coeliac and phrenic plexus also reach gallbladder in the hepatic plexus. The reason of pain in the right shoulder (from where impulses are carried by lateral supraclavicular nerve C4) in cholecystitis is the stimulation of phrenic nerve fibres (C4) due to the communication of phrenic plexus and hepatic plexus via coeliac plexus.

Genitourinary Tract

Kidneys

The kidneys are supplied by renal plexus formed from coeliac ganglion, coeliac plexus, lowest thoracic splanchnic nerve, and first lumbar splanchnic nerve. The plexus runs along the branches of renal artery to supply the vessels, renal glomeruli and tubules. These are chiefly vasomotor in function.

Ureter is supplied in its upper part from renal and aortic plexus, middle part from superior hypogastric plexus and lower part from hypogastric nerve and inferior hypogastric plexus.

Vesical Plexus

Sympathetic fibres arise from T11 and T12 segments and L1 and L2 segments of spinal cord. Parasympathetic fibres arise from sacral S2, S3, S4 segments of spinal cord, which relay in the neurons present in and near the wall of urinary bladder. Parasympathetic is motor to the muscular coat and inhibitory to the sphincter; sympathetic is chiefly vasomotor. Emptying and filling of bladder is normally controlled by parasympathetic only.

Male Reproductive Organs

Testicular plexus accompanies the testicular artery to reach the testis. It is formed by renal and aortic plexus, and also from superior and inferior hypogastric plexuses. This plexus supplies the epididymis and ductus deferens.

Prostatic plexus is formed from inferior hypogastric plexus and branches are distributed to prostate, seminal vesicle, prostatic urethra, ejaculatory ducts, erectile tissue of penis, penile part of urethra and bulbourethral glands. Sympathetic nerves cause vasoconstriction, parasympathetic nerves cause vasodilatation.

Female Reproductive Organs

Ovary and uterine tube receive their nerve supply from plexus around the ovarian vessels. This plexus is derived from renal, aortic plexuses and also superior and inferior hypogastric plexuses. Sympathetic fibres derived from T10 and T11 segments of spinal cord are vasomotor in nature whereas parasympathetic fibres are probably vasodilator in function.

Uterus

It is supplied by uterovaginal plexus, formed from the inferior hypogastric plexus. The sympathetic fibres are derived from T12 and L1 segments of spinal cord. Parasympathetic fibres arise from S2, S3, S4 segments of spinal cord. Sympathetic causes uterine contraction and vasoconstriction, while parasympathetic nerves produce vasodilatation and uterine inhibition. Vagina is supplied by nerves arising from inferior hypogastric plexus and uterovaginal plexus. These supply wall of vagina including vestibular glands and clitoris. Parasympathetic fibres contain vasodilator effect on the erectile tissue.

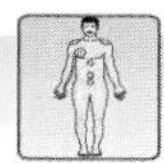

Pouch of Douglas: The rectouterine pouch in females is the deepest or most dependent part of peritoneal cavity in sitting position. It lies at a depth of 5.5 cm from the skin of perineum (*see* Fig. 18.30).

Gastric ulcers: The gastric ulcers are common along the lesser curvatures as the fluids (hot/cold), alcoholic beverages pass along lesser curvature. The blood supply is also relatively less along the lesser curvature so the ulcers are common here. Gastric pain is felt in the epigastrium because the stomach is supplied from segments T6–T9 of the spinal cord, which also supply the upper part of the abdominal wall.

Referred pain in early appendicitis: The visceral peritoneum over vermiform appendix is supplied by lesser splanchnic nerve which arises from thoracic 10 sympathetic ganglion. T10 spinal segment also receives the sensation of pain from umbilical area. Since somatic pain is better appreciated than visceral pain, pain of early appendicitis is referred to umbilical region. Later on there is pain in right fossa due to inflammation of local parietal peritoneum.

Intestinal obstruction: Intestinal obstruction is caused by tubercular ulcers not typhoid ulcers. In tubercular ulcers, the lymph vessels are affected, these pass circularly around the gut wall. During healing, these cause constriction of the gut wall and subsequent obstruction. Typhoid ulcers lie longitudinally along the antimesenteric border of the gut. These do not cause obstruction during healing.

Intussusception: Rarely a segment of intestine enters into the lumen of proximal segment of intestine, causing obstruction, and strangulation. It may be ileoileal or ileocolic.

Meckel's diverticulum: The apex of midgut loop is connected to secondary yolk sac by vitellointestinal duct. The proximal part of vitellointestinal duct may persist as Meckel's diverticulum. It is 2 inches long present at the antimesenteric border of ileum, 2 feet away from ileocaecal junction. Meckel's diverticulum may be connected to umbilicus by a fibrous band around which intestine may rotate and get obstructed (*see* Fig. 20.16b).

Internal haemorrhoids: The superior rectal artery divides into right and left branches. Only the right branch divides further into anterior and posterior branches. The veins follow the arteries. The venous radicles are in 3, 7, 11 o'clock positions. The internal piles are accordingly in 3, 7, 11 o'clock positions (*see* Fig. 33.14).

Cholecystitis: Inflammation of the gallbladder is called cholecystitis. There is pain over right hypochondrium, radiating to the inferior angle of right scapula or to the right shoulder (*see* Fig. 22.11).

Cholelithiasis: Stone formation in the gallbladder is called cholelithiasis (*see* Fig. 22.12).

Splenomegaly: Enlargement of spleen is called splenomegaly. It occurs mostly in malaria and blood disorders (*see* Fig. 23.9).

Splenectomy: Removal of spleen is called splenectomy. One must be careful of the tail of pancreas during splenectomy.

Diabetes mellitus: Deficiency of insulin causes diabetes mellitus.

Carcinoma of head of pancreas: Carcinoma of head of pancreas causes pressure over the underlying bile duct which leads to persistent obstructive jaundice.

Hepatitis: Inflammation of liver is referred to as hepatitis. It may be *infective* or *amoebic* hepatitis.

Cirrhosis: Due to malnutrition or alcohol abuse, the liver tissue undergoes fibrosis and shrinks. This is called cirrhosis of the liver.

Common diseases of kidney: The common diseases of kidney are nephritis, pyelonephritis, tuberculosis of kidney, renal stones and tumours. Common manifestations of a kidney disease are renal oedema and hypertension. Renal transplantation can be tried in selected cases. Lithotripsy is being used for removal of stones.

Ureteric colic: The ureteric colic is referred to T11–T12 segments. The pain radiates from loin to the groin (*see* Fig. 24.33).

Hysterectomy: The procedure of removing uterus for various reasons is called hysterectomy. One has to carefully ligate the uterine artery, which crosses the ureter lying below the base of broad ligament. The integrity of ureter has to be maintained.

Tubectomy: This is a simple operative procedure done in females for family welfare. The peritoneal cavity has to be opened in females. The fallopian tube or uterine tube is ligated at two places and intervening segment is removed. The procedure is done on both sides (*see* Figs 31.7 and 31.8).

Rupture of male urethra: The membranous part of urethra is likely to be ruptured. The urine fills superficial perineal space, scrotum, penis and lower part of anterior abdominal wall. It cannot go into the thighs because of firm attachment of membranous layer of superficial fascia to their boundaries (*see* Fig. 28.15).

Tubal pregnancy: Sometimes the fertilized ovum instead of reaching the uterus adheres to the walls of the uterine tube and starts developing there. This is known as *tubal pregnancy.* The enlarging embryo mostly leads to rupture of the fallopian tube.

Prolapse of the uterus: Sometimes the uterus passes downwards into the vagina, invaginating it.

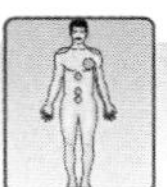

It is called the prolapse of the uterus, and is caused by weakened supports of the uterus.

Intrauterine contraceptive device: Insertion of a foreign body into the uterus can prevent implantation of the fertilized ovum. This is the basic principle underlying the use of various intrauterine contraceptive devices for preventing pregnancy (*see* Fig. 31.19).

Enucleation of the prostatic adenoma: The prostate has a false capsule and a true capsule. The prostatic venous plexus lies between the true and false capsules.

In benign hypertrophy of prostate the adenoma only is enucleated, leaving both the capsules and the venous plexus and normal peripheral part of gland.

Vasectomy: It is a simple surgical procedure done for family welfare. A segment of vas deferens is exposed from a small incision on the upper part of scrotum. The two ends are tied and a small piece of vas deferens is removed. The procedure is done on both sides. Since hormones continue to be produced and circulated through blood, person remains potent. But, since the sperms cannot pass in the distal part of vas and into ejaculatory duct, the person becomes sterile after 3–4 months (*see* Fig. 32.4).

Hydrocoele: The testis invaginates the processus vaginalis so that there is a visceral layer and a parietal layer of peritoneum. Collection of excess of fluid in between the two layers is called *hydrocoele*.

Cryptorchidism: If testis do not come down to the scrotum at birth or soon after, these are hidden anywhere along its path or these may have gone astray (*see* Fig. 17.12).

The testis may be undescended and be in lumbar region, iliac fossa, inguinal canal, superficial inguinal ring or at the upper end of scrotum. The testes may have gone astray (ectopic testis) to be in the region of inguinal canal and may be seen at superficial inguinal ring, root of penis, in perineum or in thigh (*see* Fig. 17.13).

Varicocoele: The dilatation and tortuosity of the pampiniform plexus in the spermatic cord is called *varicocoele*. It occurs more commonly on the left side. The factors are:

a. Left testis hangs a little lower than right (*see* Fig. 17.14).
b. Left testicular vein drains into left renal vein at right angle.
c. Loaded pelvic colon may press upon the left testicular vein and prevent its proper drainage.

Varicocoele may lead to infertility.

Ischioanal abscess: It is common as ischioanal fossae are situated on the two sides of the anal canal, deep to the skin of perineum. It is less painful compared to the perianal abscess. The perianal space is situated between ischial tuberosity and subcutaneous part of sphincter ani externus. The septa in this space are small and fat is tightly disposed, so infections are very painful.

Pudendal nerve block: This is an anaesthetic procedure used during vaginal deliveries or forceps delivery. The pudendal nerve is the nerve of perineum and after anaesthesia, the vaginal delivery becomes almost painless. The nerve is blocked by the anaesthetic drug as it lies on the ischial spine. The blockage can be done through vagina or from the perineum (*see* Fig. 28.26).

MULTIPLE CHOICE QUESTIONS

A. Match the following on the left side with their appropriate answers on the right side.

1. Plane — Vertebral level

a. Subcostal plane	i. L1
b. Transtubercular plane	ii. L3
c. Transpyloric plane	iii. L4
d. Highest point of iliac crest	iv. L5

2. Arterial branches and their origin

a. Splenic artery	i. Aorta
b. Testicular artery	ii. Superior mesenteric artery
c. Ileocolic artery	iii. Coeliac trunk
d. Inferior rectal artery	iv. Internal pudendal artery

3. Lymphatic drainage

a. Greater curvature of stomach	i. Pancreaticosplenic nodes
b. Testis	ii. Internal iliac nodes
c. Prostate gland	iii. Superior mesenteric nodes
d. Head of pancreas	iv. Para-aortic nodes

4. Venous drainage

a. Left gastric vein	i. Splenic vein
b. Inferior mesenteric vein	ii. Left renal vein
c. Left testicular vein	iii. Inferior vena cava
d. Right testicular vein	iv. Portal vein

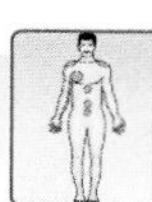

B. For each of the statements or questions below, one or more answers given is/are correct.

A. If only a, b, c are correct
B. If only a, c are correct
C. If only b, d are correct
D. If a, b, c, d are correct
E. If only d is correct
F. If all are correct

1. Contents of spermatic cord is/are:
  a. Ductus deferens
  b. Testicular artery
  c. Pampiniform plexus of veins
  d. Ilioinguinal nerve

2. Epiploic foramen is bounded:
  a. Superiorly by the left lobe of the liver
  b. Posteriorly by the inferior vena cava
  c. Inferiorly by pylorus of stomach
  d. Anteriorly by lesser omentum containing hepatic artery, portal vein and bile duct

3. Parasympathetic nerves innervating stomach:
  a. Increase the mobility of the stomach
  b. Are inhibitory to pyloric sphincter
  c. Increase the secretion of pepsin and HCl
  d. Are the chief pathway for pain sensation

4. The following statements are true regarding appendix:
  a. Appendicular orifice is situated on the posterolateral aspect of caecum.
  b. Sympathetic innervation is derived from T10 spinal segment.
  c. Pelvic position is the most common position of appendix.
  d. Referred pain caused by appendicitis is first felt in the region of umbilicus.

5. Lymphatics of the uterus drain into the following lymph nodes:
  a. External iliac
  b. Internal iliac
  c. Superficial inguinal
  d. Deep inguinal.

ANSWERS

A. 1. a – ii, b – iv, c – i, d – iii, 2. a – iii, b – i, c – ii, d – iv,
3. a – i, b – iv, c – ii, d – iii, 4. a – iv, b – i, c – ii, d – iii

B. 1. D 2. C 3. A 4. C 5. A

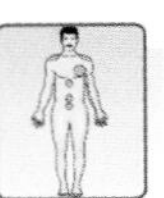

FURTHER READING

- Brodel M. The intrinsic blood vessels of the kidney and their significance in nephrotomy. John Hopkins Hosp *Bull* 1911; 12:10–13.
- Buccione R, Schroeder AC, Eppig JJ. Interactions between somatic cells and germ cells throughout mammalian oogenesis *Biol Reprod* 1990; 43:543–7.
- Burkhill GJC, Healy JC. Anatomy of the retroperitoneum. *Imaging* 2000; 12:10–20.
- Buschard K, Kjaeldgaard A. Investigations and analysis of the positions, fixation, length and embryology of the vermiform appendix, *Acta Chir Scand* 1973; 139:293–8.
- Chanecellor MB, Yoshimura N. *Physiology and pharmacology of the bladder and urethra.* In: Walsh PC et al (Eds) Campbell's Urology study Guide, 2nd edn. Philadelphia; Saunders; Chapter 23; 2002.
- D, Panjabi MM. Normal motion of the lumbar spine related to age and gender. *Eur Spine J* 1995; 4:18–23.
- Delancey JO. Anatomy. In: Stanton SL, Monga A (Eds) *Clinical Urogynaecology*, 2nd edition. London: Churchill Livingstone 2000.
- Didio L J, Anderson MC. The 'Sphinctres' of the Digestive System. Baltimore: Williams and Wilkins 1968.
- Dunaif A, Thomas A. Current concepts in the polycystic ovarian syndrome. *Annu Rev Med* 2001; 52:401–19.
- Ellis H (eds) Applied Radiological Anatomy. Cambridge, UK: Cambridge University Press.
- Jackson JE. Vascular anatomy of the gastrointestinal tract. In: Butler P, Mitchell AWM 1999.
- Kerr JB. Ultrastructure of the seminiferous epithelium and intertubular tissue of the human testis. *J electron Microsc Tech* 1991; 19:215– 40.
- Klutke CG, Siegel CL. Functional female pelvic anatomy. *Urol Clin North Am* 1995; 22 (3): 487–98.
- Kruyt RH, Delemarre JB, Doornbos J, Vogel HJ. Normal anorectum, dynamic MR imaging anatomy. *Radiology* 1991; 179 (1):159–63.
- Lunnis PJ, Phillips RK. Anatomy and function of anal longitudinal muscle. *Br J Surg* 1992; 79 : 882–4.
- Lytle WJ. Inguinal anatomy. *J Anatomy* 1979; 128:581–94.
- Meyers M. Dynamic Radiology of the Abdomen. Normal and pathologic Anatomy. New York: Springer 1994.
- Mitchell AWM, Dick R. Liver, gallbladder, pancreas and spleen. In: Butler P, Mitchell AWM, Ellis H (Eds) Applied Radiological Anatomy. Cambridge: Cambridge University Press; 1999; 239–58.
- Mundy AR, Fitzpatrick J, Neal D, George N (Eds). Male sexual function. In: The Scientific Basis of Urology, Chapter 12. Isis Medical Media: 1999; 243–53.
- Mundy AR, Fitzpatrick J, Neal D, George N (Eds). The prostate and benign prostatic hyperplasia. In : The Scientific Basis of Urology, Chapter 13. Oxford; *Isis Medical Media*: 1999; 257–76.
- Novick AC. Anatomic approaches in nephron-sparing surgery for renal cell carcinoma. *Atlas Urol Clin North Am* 1998; 6:39.
- Paquet KJ. Causes and pathomechanics of oesophageal varices development. *Med Sci Monit* 6: 2000; 915–28.55.Dvorak J, Vajda EG, Grob
- Pearcy M, Protek I, Shepherd J. a. Three-dimensional X-ray analysis of normal movement in lumbar spine. Spine 1984; 9:582–7.
- Reilly FD. Innervation and vascular pharmaco-dynamics of the mammalian spleen. *Experientia* 1985; 41:187–92.
- Rizk NN. A new description of the anterior abdominal wall in man and mammals *J Anat* 1980; 131:373–85.
- Shah PM, Scarton HA, Tsapogas MJ. Geometric anatomy of the aortocommon iliac bifurcation. *J Anat* 1978; 126: 451–8.
- Smith PH, Porte D Jr. Neuropharmacology of the pancreatic islets. *Annu Rev Pharmacol Toxicol* 1976; 16:269–85.
- Spornitz UM. The functional morphology of the human endometrium and decidua. *Adv Anat Embryol Cell Biol* 1992; 124:1–99.
- Suzuki M, Akasihi S, Rikiyama T, Naitoh T, Rahman MM, Mastsuno S. Laparoscopic cholecystectomy, Calot's triangle and variations in cystic arterial supply. *Surgical Endoscopy* 2000; 14:141–4.
- Taylar JR, Twomey LT. Sexual dimorphism in human vertebral shape. *J Anat* 1984; 138:281–6.
- Vinecnt JM, Morrison ID, Armstrong P, Reznek RH. The size of normal adrenal glands on computed tomography. *Clin Radiol* 1994; 49:453–55.
- Wendell Smith CP, Wilson PM. The vulva, vagina and urethra and the musculature of the pelvic floor. In: Philipp E, Setchell M, Ginsburg J (eds) *Scientific Foundations of Obstetrics and Gynecology*. Oxford: Butterworth–Heinemann; 1991; 84–100.
- Yamaguchi S, Kuroyanagi H, Milson JW, Sim R, Shimada H. Venous anatomy of the right colon, Precise structure of the major veins and gastrocolic trunk in 58 cadavers. *Dis Colon Rectum* 2002; 45:1337–40.

SPOTS ON LOWER LIMB

1 a. Indentify the highlighted structure.
b. Write its nerve supply.

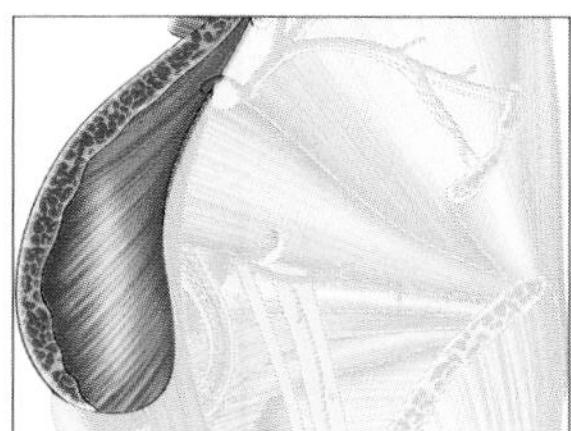

2 a. Identify the highlighted structure.
b. Write its action.

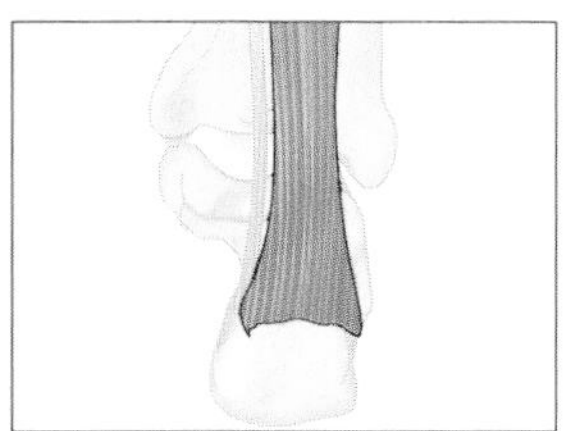

3 a. Name the highlighted structure.
b. Write its nerve supply.

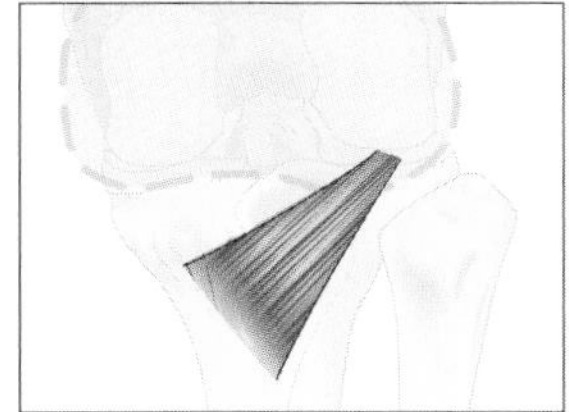

4 a Identify the area marked.
b. Name the structure attached to it.

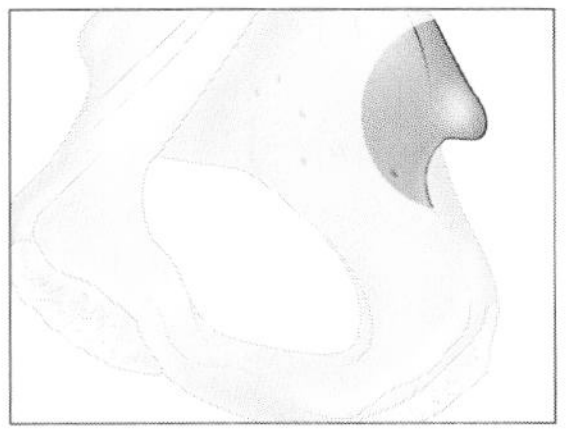

5 a. Identify the highlighted structure.
b. What is its nerve supply?

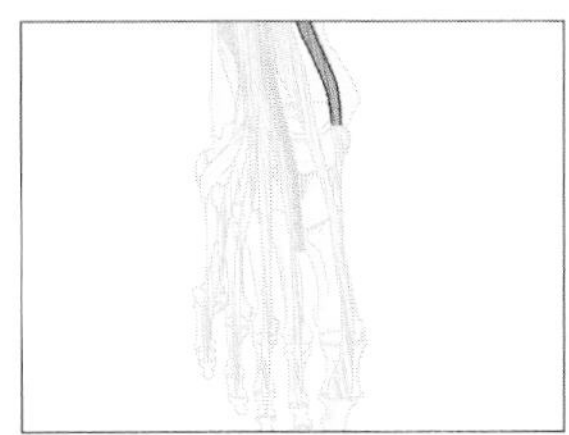

6 a. Identify the area marked.
b. Name the structure attached to it.

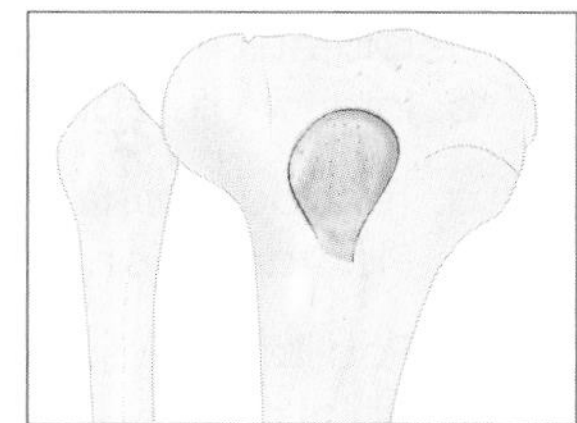

7 a. Identify the highlighted structure.
b. Name its terminal branches.

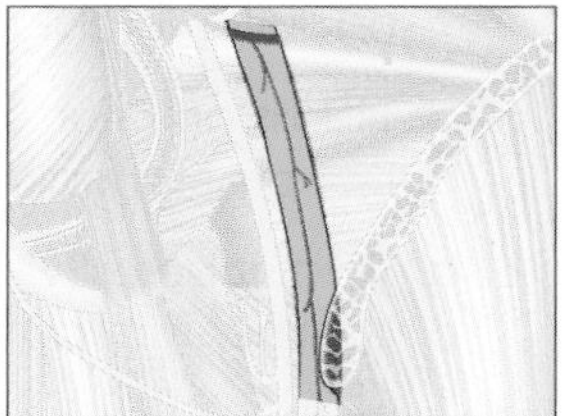

8 a. Identify the highlighted part.
b. Name the structure attached to this part.

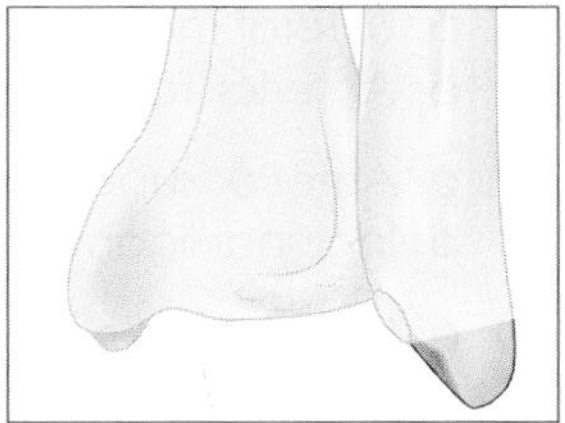

9 a. Identify the highlighted part.
b. Name the structures attached to it.

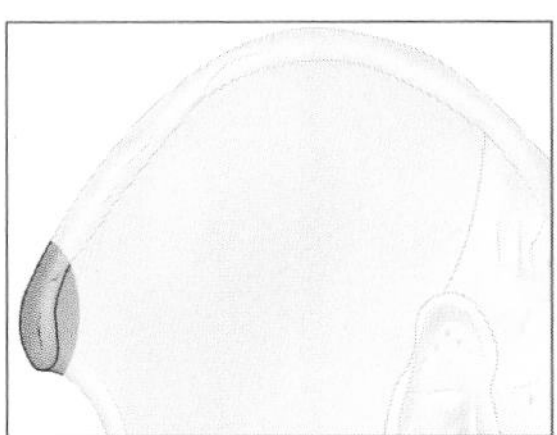

10 a. Identify the area marked.
b. Name the ligament attached. Name its other attachments.

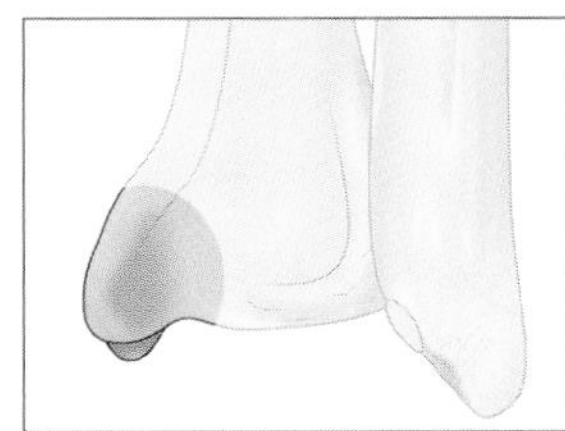

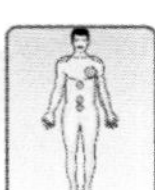

ANSWERS ON LOWER LIMB

1. a. Gluteus maximus
   b. Inferior gluteal nerve
2. a. Tendocalcaneus
   b. Plantar flexion of foot at the ankle joint
3. a. Popliteus muscle
   b. Tibial nerve
4. a. Anterior inferior iliac spine
   b. (1) Straight head of rectus femoris
   (2) Iliofemoral ligament
5. a. Tibialis anterior
   b. Deep peroneal nerve
6. a. Tibial tuberosity
   b. Ligamentum patellae
7. a. Sciatic nerve
   b. 1. Tibial nerve
   2. Common peroneal nerve
8. a. Lateral malleolus
   b. Anterior talofibular ligaments
9. a. Anterior superior iliac spine
   b. Inguinal ligament and sartorius muscle
10. a. Medial malleolus of tibia.
    b. Deltoid ligament. Other attachments:
    - Medial surface of talus, sustentaculum tali, medial tubercle of posterior process of talus
    - Spring ligament including tuberosity of navicular

SPOTS ON ABDOMEN AND PELVIS

1 a. Identify the highlighted structure.
b. What is its nerve supply?

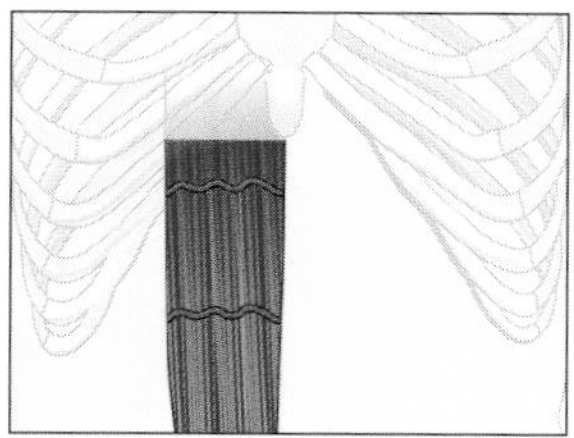

6 a. Identify the marked organ.
b. What are its muscular and ligamentous supports?

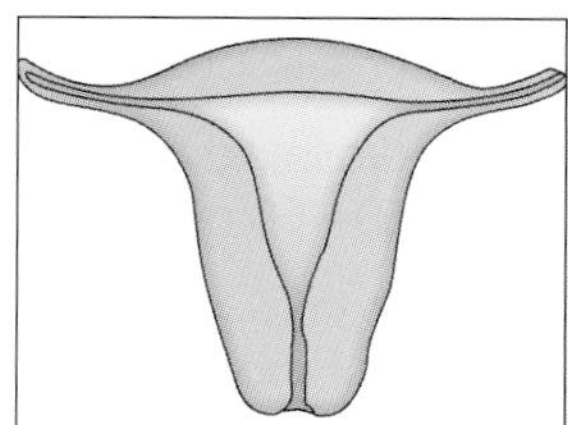

2 a. Identify the highlighted organ.
b. What its capacity?

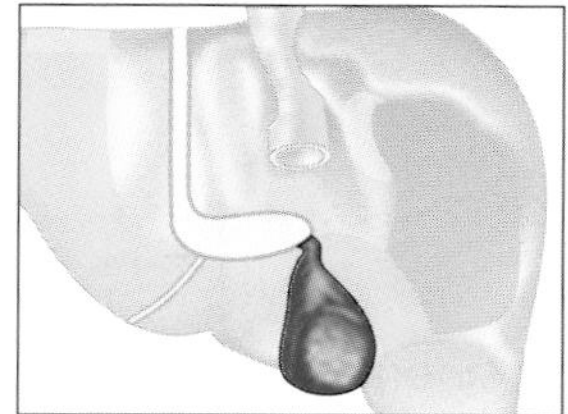

7 a. Identify the marked structure.
b. Name its ventral, branches.

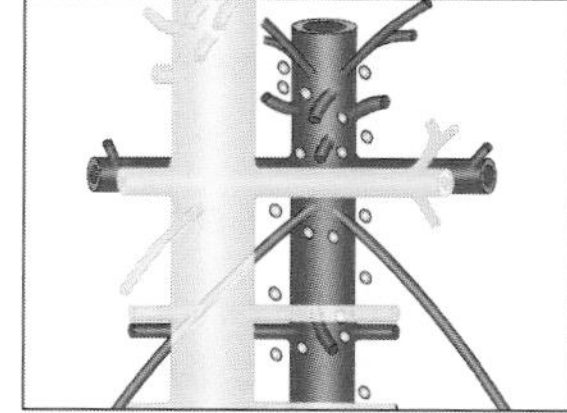

3 a. Identify the organ.
b. Write the arterial supply of its fundus.

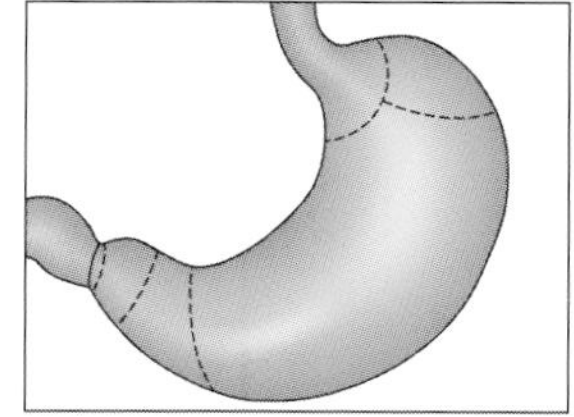

8 a. Identify the organ.
b. Name the main veins related to it.

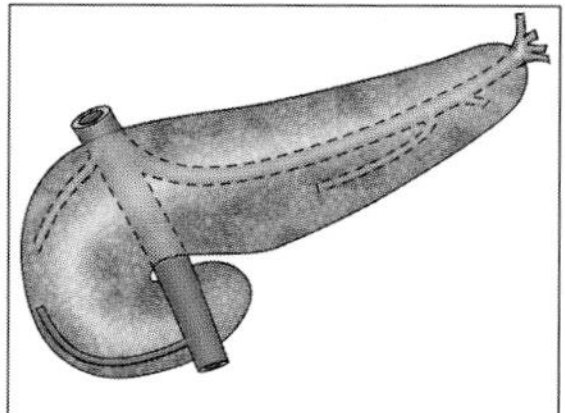

4 a. Identify the highlighted area.
b. Write its boundaries.

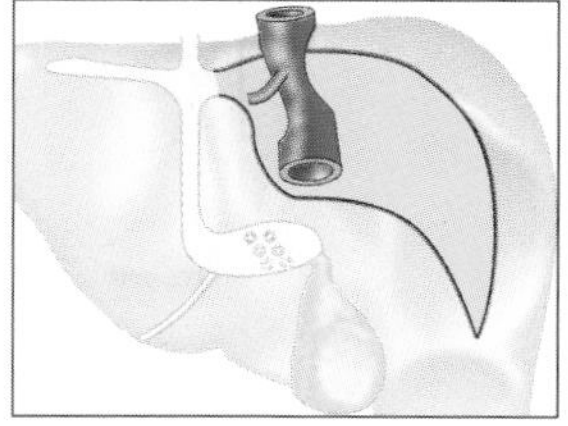

9 a. Identify the organ.
b. Name the viscera related to it.

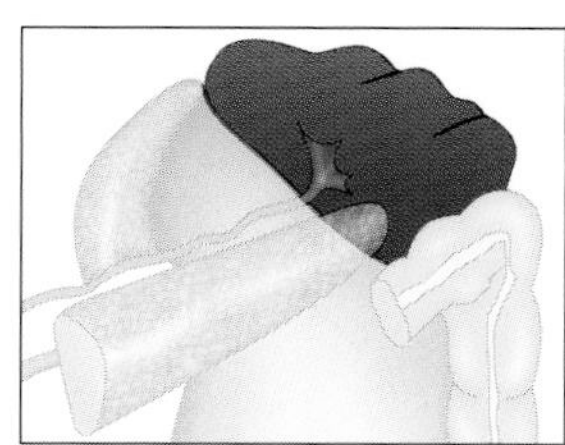

5 a. Identify the highlighted organ.
b. Name its commonest position.

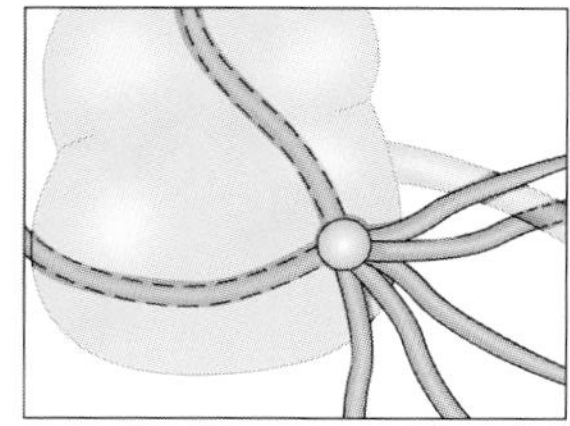

10 a. Identify the organ and its side.
b. Name viscera related to its anterior surface.

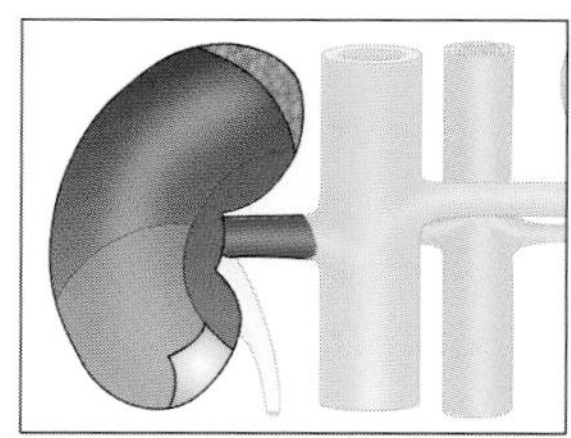

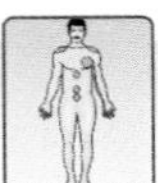

ANSWERS ON ABDOMEN AND PELVIS

1. a. Rectus obdominis
   b. Lower intercostal nerves
2. a. Gallbladder
   b. 50–100 ml
3. a. Stomach
   b. 5-7 short gastric arteries, branches of splenic artery
4. a The bare area of liver
   b. Superior and inferior layer of coronary ligaments, inferior vena cava and right triangular ligament
5. a. Vermiform appendix
   b. Retrocaecal/retrocolic
6. a. Uterus
   b. Levator ani and lateral cervical ligament
7. a. Abdominal aorta
   b. Coeliac axis, superior mesenteric and inferior mesenteric arteries
8. a. Pancreas
   b. Splenic, superior mesenteric and portal veins
9. a. Spleen
   b. Pancreas, stomach, left kidney and splenic flexure
10. a. Right kidney
    b. Right suprarenal, liver, coils of intestine, duodenum and ascending colon

Left Inguinal canal

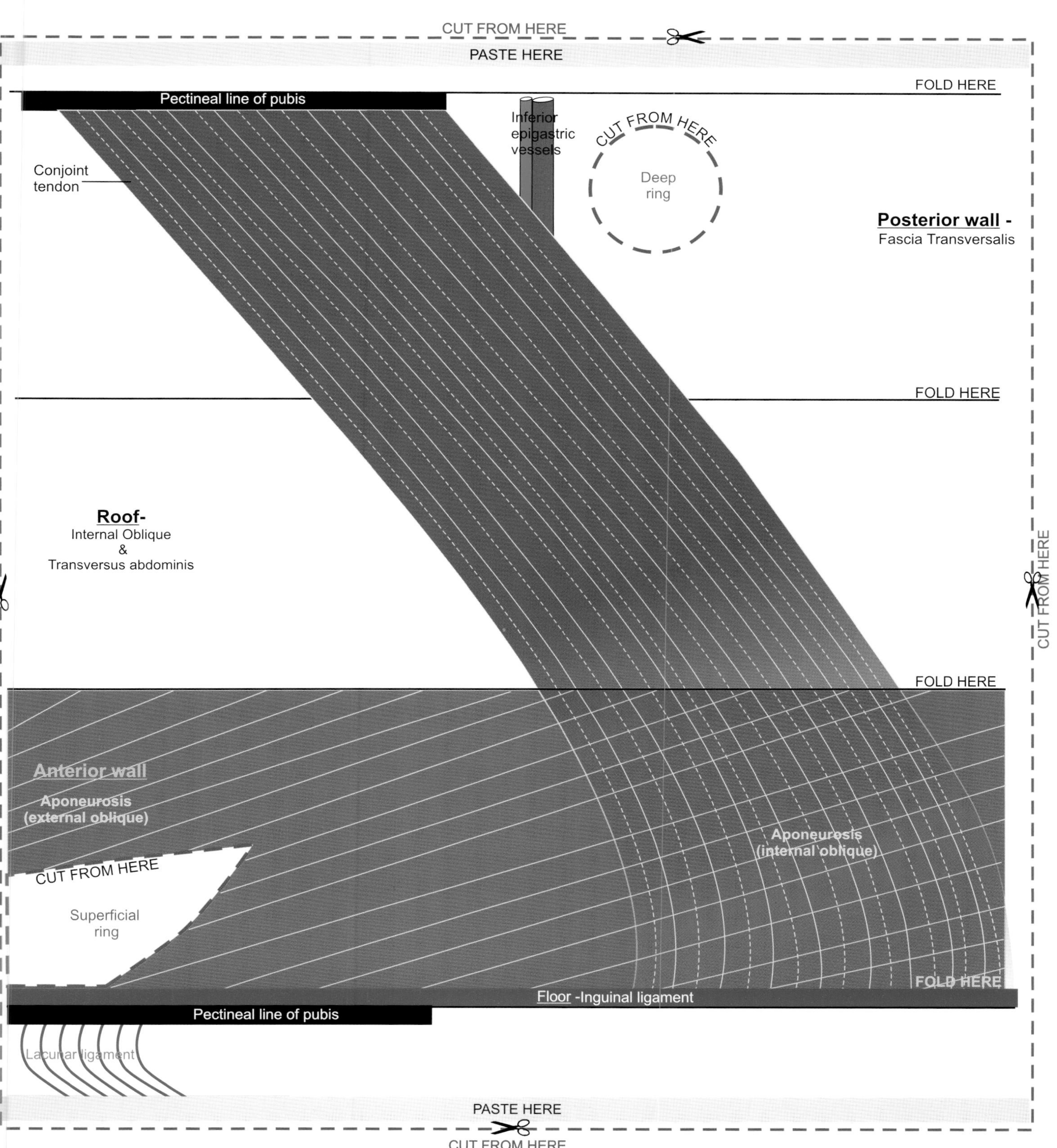

Index

A

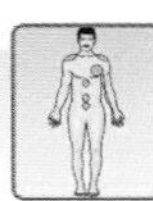

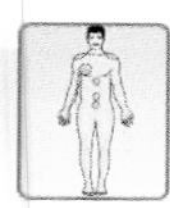

D

E

F